# Handbook of Experimental Pharmacology

Continuation of Handbuch der experimentellen Pharmakologie

## Vol. 68/I

# Antimalarial Drugs I

## Biological Background, Experimental Methods, and Drug Resistance

Contributors

A. L. Ager, Jr. · V. Boonpucknavig · S.-C. Chou · K. A. Conklin
D. W. Davidson, Jr. · R. E. Desjardins · M. Fernex · P. C. C. Garnham
H. M. Gilles · M. H. Heiffer · D. W. Korte, Jr. · M. R. Levy
G. H. Mitchell · W. Peters · S. Punyagupta · W. H. G. Richards
K. H. Rieckmann · R. N. Rossan · I. W. Sherman · T. Srichaikul
G. A. T. Targett · D. C. Warhurst

Editors

W. Peters and W. H. G. Richards

Springer-Verlag
Berlin Heidelberg GmbH 1984

WALLACE PETERS, M.D., DSc, FRCP, DTM & H
Professor of Medical Protozoology,
London School of Hygiene and Tropical Medicine,
Keppel Street,
London WC1E 7HT,
Great Britain

WILLIAM H. G. RICHARDS, BSc, Ph.D.
Manager, Scientific Advisory Services,
Wellcome Research Laboratories,
Ravens Lane,
Berkhamsted, Herts. HP4 2DY,
Great Britain

With 93 Figures

**ISBN 978-3-662-34991-5 ISBN 978-3-662-35326-4 (eBook)**
**DOI 10.1007/978-3-662-35326-4**

Library of Congress Cataloging in Publication Data. Main entry under title: Antimalarial drugs. (Handbook of experimental pharmacology; v. 68, 1–2) Includes bibliographies and index. Contents: 1. Biological background, experimental methods, and drug resistance – 2. Current antimalarials and new drug developments. 1. Antimalarials. 2. Malaria–Chemotherapy. I. Peters, W. (Wallace), 1924–. II. Richards, W.H.G. (William H.G.), 1928–. III. Series. [DNLM: 1. Antimalarials–Pharmacodynamics. 2. Antimalarials–Therapeutic use. W1 HA51L v. 68 pt. 1–2/QV 256 A631] QP905.H3 vol. 68, 1–2 615'.1s [616.9'362061] 83-16977 [RC159.A5]


Originally published by Springer-Verlag Berlin Heidelberg New York in 1984
Softcover reprint of the hardcover 1st edition 1984



Product liability: The publisher can give no guarantee for information about drug dosage and application thereof contained in this book. In every individual case the respective user must check its accuracy by consulting other pharmaceutical literature.

Typesetting,
2122/3130-543210

# List of Contributors

A. L. Ager, Jr., Director, Rane Research Laboratory, Department of Microbiology, University of Miami, School of Medicine, 5750 NW 32nd Avenue, Miami, FL 33142, USA

V. Boonpucknavig, Professor and Chairman, Department of Pathology, Faculty of Medicine, Ramathibodi Hospital, Rama VI Road, Bangkok 4, Thailand

S.-C. Chou, Professor of Pharmacology, Department of Pharmacology, School of Medicine, University of Hawaii, Honolulu, HI 96822, USA

K. A. Conklin, Department of Anesthesiology, UCLA School of Medicine, Center for the Health Sciences, Los Angeles, CA 90024, USA

D. W. Davidson, Jr., Chief, Department of Parasitology, Division of Experimental Therapeutics, Walter Reed Army Institute of Research, Walter Reed Army Medical Center, Washington, DC 20012, USA

R. E. Desjardins, Head, Anti-Infectives Section, Department of Clinical Investigation, Burroughs Wellcome Co., 3030 Cornwallis Road, Research Triangle Park, NC 27709, USA

M. Fernex, Professor of Tropical Medicine, Medical Faculty, University of Basel, 4002 Basel, Switzerland

P. C. C. Garnham, Southernwood, Farnham Common, Bucks. SL2 3PA, Great Britain

H. M. Gilles, Department of Tropical Medicine, Liverpool School of Tropical Medicine, Pembroke Place, Liverpool L3 5QA, Great Britain

M. H. Heiffer, Chief, Department of Pharmacology, Division of Experimental Therapeutics, Walter Reed Army Institute of Research, Walter Reed Army Medical Center, Washington, DC 20012, USA

D. W. Korte, Jr., Department of Pharmacology, Division of Experimental Therapeutics, Walter Reed Army Institute of Research, Walter Reed Army Medical Center, Washington, DC 20012, USA

M. R. Levy, Department of Biological Sciences, Southern Illinois University, Edwardsville, IL 62026, USA

G. H. Mitchell, Department of Chemical Pathology, Guy's Hospital Medical School, St. Thomas Street, London SE 1, Great Britain

W. PETERS, Professor of Medical Protozoology, London School of Hygiene and Tropical Medicine, Keppel Street, London, WC1E 7HT, Great Britain

S. PUNYAGUPTA, Medical Director, Vichaiyut Hospital, 114/4 Setsiri Road, Payathai, Bangkok, Thailand, and Consultant Physician, Infectious Diseases Hospital, Ministry of Public Health and Phra Mongkutklao Army Hospital, Bangkok, Thailand

W. H. G. RICHARDS, Wellcome Research Laboratories, Ravens Lane, Berkhamsted, HP4 2DY Herts., Great Britain

K. H. RIECKMANN, 35/64 Buxton Street, North Adelaide, S.A. 5006, Australia

R. N. ROSSAN, Gorgas Memorial Laboratory, APO Miami, FL 34002, USA

I. W. SHERMAN, Professor of Zoology, Department of Biology, University of California, Riverside, CA 92521, USA

T. SRICHAIKUL, Consultant Professor, Haematology Unit, Faculty of Medicine, Ramathibodi Hospital, and Director of Haematology Division, Department of Medicine, Phra-Mongkutklao Army Hospital, Bangkok, Thailand

G. A. T. TARGETT, Professor of Immunology of Protozoal Diseases, London School of Hygiene and Tropical Medicine, Keppel Street, London WC 1E 7HT, Great Britain

D. C. WARHURST, Department of Medical Protozoology, London School of Hygiene and Tropical Medicine, Keppel Street, London, WC1E 7HT, Great Britain

# Preface

Of all the parasitic diseases that beset man in the warmer parts of the world, malaria is still the major cause of morbidity and mortality. In spite of intensive efforts to interrrupt its transmission malaria still threatens over 800 million people, more than one-fifth of the world's population. Malignant tertian malaria caused by *Plasmodium falciparum* probably kills a million every year. Vivax malaria temporarily incapacitates millions more. The search for antimalarial drugs, both natural and synthetic, has been and continues to be one of the most challenging and, at times, rewarding exercises ever undertaken by chemists and biologists. The magnitude of the effort is reflected by the fact that, in the last 15 years, well over 250000 compounds have been screened for antimalarial activity in just one programme, that carried out under the auspices of the Walter Reed Army Institute of Research, not to mention sporadic studies undertaken by other research workers and organisations.

While most people engaged in the search for new drugs agree that a rational approach based on knowledge of the intimate biochemical pathways of the target cells would be ideal as well as intellectually satisfying, most are reluctantly obliged to concede that, up to the present time, the chances of success following a more or less empirical search have been far greater. Spectacular advances in molecular biology and biochemistry in recent years, however, are rapidly changing this situation. New techniques for the study of the biology of malaria parasites and the host-parasite interface, and for the cultivation of both intraerythrocytic and tissue stages of *Plasmodium* have opened up new avenues, not only for such fundamental studies, but also for drug screening *in vitro* and the investigation of the modes of action of antimalarial drugs. We can anticipate, therefore, that future research on antimalarial chemotherapy will hinge more on an intimate knowledge of the basic biology of the target organism and less on 'random' screening.

It is remarkable that, over 100 years after the first discovery of the malaria parasites of man, yet one more stage of the cycle has been revealed, namely the tissue-dwelling 'hypnozoite' that we now believe is responsible for relapses of benign tertian vivax and ovale malaria. Much has been learned of the metabolic pathways used by the blood-dwelling stages of these and other species, but almost nothing of the metabolism of the tissue stages. New culture techniques, apart from their value for metabolic studies, are now being widely used for screening and these and other *in vitro* models, as well as animal models, are described in some detail. Drugs are, in a sense, simply an aid to Nature. Without an active immune response on the part of the host, it is unlikely that any antimalarial used today will cure a patient of his malaria. For this reason detailed reviews are given of the response of the host to malarial infection, and the interaction between immunity and chemotherapy.

The course of antimalarial (as indeed any other) drug development spans the field from primary screening to advanced clinical trials in man. The different stages in this process are reviewed in order to provide guidelines for future investigators who would otherwise have to search widely scattered literature covering these activities.

The main stimulus for antimalarial drug development today (although by no means the only one) is the rapid rate of emergence of *P. falciparum* strains resistant to existing compounds. It is therefore essential to provide substantial background data on this problem and the last three chapters of Part 1 reflect this need.

Even while this volume was being conceived and prepared for publication an increasing flow of reports was being received by the World Health Organization and appearing in the medical press of patients with malignant tertian malaria who failed to respond to treatment with the best available drugs. The rapid geographical spread of such strains and the widening range of drugs to which the parasites are becoming resistant are such that the need for radically new types of antimalarial chemotherapy is becoming one of the most urgent requirements in what is, after all, becoming an ever shrinking world. Recognising this urgency, the Editorial Board of this series and Springer-Verlag have generously agreed to publish this volume *in toto*, in two parts, rather than trying to compress the material into their standard format.

In Part 2 of this volume, our contributions review in detail the range of drugs that are in current use, describe some novel approaches to their deployment and give an account of developments in different chemical series over the past decade.

We are deeply grateful to all our contributors and the staff of Springer-Verlag for their generous collaboration in this work.

WALLACE PETERS
WILLIAM H. G. RICHARDS

# Contents

## The Malaria Parasites

CHAPTER 1

**Life Cycles.** P. C. C. GARNHAM. With 4 Figures



CHAPTER 2

**Metabolism.** I. W. SHERMAN. With 6 Figures

CHAPTER 7

**Use of Avian Malarias (In Vivo).** W. H. G. Richards. With 1 Figure



CHAPTER 8

**Rodent Malaria Models.** A. L. Ager, Jr.



CHAPTER 9

**Malaria Models in Simian Hosts.** R. N. Rossan. With 1 Figure

## Preclinical and Clinical Trial Techniques

CHAPTER 12

**Preclinical Testing.** M. H. HEIFFER, D. E. DAVIDSON, JR., and D. W. KORTE, JR. With 1 Figure



CHAPTER 13

**Clinical Trials – Phases I and II.** M. FERNEX. With 2 Figures

CHAPTER 14

**Clinical Trials – Phases III and IV and Field Trials**
M. FERNEX. With 1 Figure



CHAPTER 15

**Pharmacogenetic Factors in Antimalarial Drug Testing.** H. M. GILLES
With 4 Figures



## Antimalarial Drug Resistance

CHAPTER 16

**History and Current Status of Drug Resistance.** W. PETERS
With 5 Figures

# Contents of Companion Volume 68, Part II

# The Malaria Parasites

CHAPTER 1

# Life Cycles

P. C. C. GARNHAM

## A. Introduction

There are at least one hundred species of malaria parasites, of which four occur in man. The others are important for the following reasons: (a) certain species affect domestic animals and epizootics may be a problem in veterinary medicine; (b) some species are widely used in malaria research in studies of the human disease, including experimental pharmacology; and (c) various species have proved to be invaluable for the solution of fundamental problems of the life cycle. The investigation of the group as a whole is of great interest to zoologists and parasitologists.

Malaria parasites include the true species belonging to the genus *Plasmodium*, but it is convenient to consider briefly other members of the suborder which, from time to time, have also borne the name of malaria parasites. In fact, some species are still placed in this category, to which they clearly do not belong. The following classification (necessary for the understanding of the cycle) includes the subphylum Apicomplexa on the basis of ultrastructural characteristics which are shared by the motile stages of the Coccidia as a whole. The two suborders which interest us (from the similarity of the respective life cycles and response to drugs) are the Eimeriina and the Haemosporina. The former contains two important families – the Eimeriidae (with one host) and the Toxoplasmidae (with two obligatory vertebrate hosts in the life cycle). The latter includes the Plasmodiidae, Haemoproteidae, and Leucocytozoidae.

The family Plasmodiidae comprises the true malaria parasites, belonging to a single genus, *Plasmodium*, and is defined as parasites exhibiting two types of schizogony (exoerythrocytic without pigment and erythrocytic with pigment) in the vertebrate host, and a sexual stage terminating in sporogony in the mosquito host. For convenience, the genus is split into a number of subgenera, three in mammals (*Plasmodium*, *Laverania* and *Vinckeia*), four in birds (*Haemamoeba*, *Giovannolaia*, *Novyella* and *Huffia*), and two in reptiles (*Carinamoeba* and *Sauramoeba*).

The Haemoproteidae differ from the Plasmodiidae by possessing only a single type of schizogony (in the tissues), pigmented gametocytes being the blood forms, while sporogony occurs in a variety of biting Diptera. This family does not occur in man or in the higher apes, but commonly parasitises monkeys and is useful for the study of infection confined to gametocytes, either for genetic or chemotherapeutic purposes. There are three genera in mammals (*Hepatocystis*, *Nycteria*, and *Polychromophilus*) and two genera in reptiles (*Haemocystidium* in lizards and *Simondia* in turtles). This family has little or no pathogenicity, but its (very numer-

**Table 1.** Minimum duration of stages in life cycle of human malaria parasites (in days). Modified from GARNHAM (1980)

| Species | Exoerythrocytic schizogony | Erythrocytic schizogony | Sporogony in mosquito |
|---|---|---|---|
| *P. vivax* | 8 | 2 | 8 |
| *P. ovale* | 9 | 2 | 12 |
| *P. falciparum* | 5½ | 2 | 9 |
| *P. malariae* | 15 | 3 | 16 |

ous) species were at one time placed among the true malaria parasites, with which it is sometimes, even today, confused.

The Leucocytozoidae differ from the two other families in producing no pigment (haematin) at any stage of the life cycle, and in having no schizogony in the blood where non-pigmented gametocytes alone occur. Two genera are recognised, both in birds, *Leucocytozoon* and *Akiba*. Some of the species are highly pathogenic to the avian host and chemotherapy has only been applied on a small scale.

## B. General Characters of *Plasmodium* s.l.

Apart from the characters which are embodied in the formal classification,there are additional features common to the genus *Plasmodium*. An important character is chronobiology which is applicable at subspecific level or even lower. The phenomena of periodicity during different stages of the life cycle are highly significant and provide criteria for the preliminary diagnosis into quotidian, tertian or quartan groups as regards the blood cycles, and for more sophisticated classification into closely related groups of parasites. Table 1 shows the minimum duration of stages in the four human species, though it must be appreciated that Nature rarely follows a precise timetable and that, exceptionally, the intervals may be a few hours shorter or longer than those shown. Moreover, the length of schizogony in the blood is the only easily available measurement, and even that may be confusing if two or more broods of parasites are present, or if, as in certain avian and rodent and in all saurian species, there is lack of synchronicity of the blood cycle. The duration of the sporogonic cycle is temperature dependent and should always be recorded. The termination of the exoerythrocytic cycle in mammalian malaria is best determined by subinoculation of blood at appropriate intervals after sporozoite infection but, under experimental conditions when excessive numbers have been inoculated, a careful watch for the first appearance of tiny rings in the peripheral blood will prove satisfactory.

The other features common to all or most malaria parasites include the following: destruction of erythrocytes, enlargement of spleen, deposition of pigment in many organs, acquisition of immunity, and pyrexia (except in rodent malaria). Many of the details of events in the life cycle are similar in all species, but the three main groups, primate, rodent and avian, have patterns of their own as shown in Table 2. The life cycle is still incompletely known in a considerable number of par-

**Table 2.** Differential features of life cycle of primate, rodent and avian malaria parasites. Modified from GARNHAM (1980)

| Feature | Primate species | Rodent species | Avian species |
|---|---|---|---|
| Invertebrate host | *Anopheles* spp. | *Anopheles* spp. | Usually culicine mosquito |
| Number of generations of pre-erythrocytic schizogony | One | One | Two |
| Length of pre-erythrocytic schizogony | Five days or more | Three days or less | Three days |
| Site of pre-erythrocytic schizogony | Liver parenchyma | Liver parenchyma | Mesoderm |
| Number of pre-erythrocytic merozoites per schizont | 2,000 or more | 2,000 or more | 200 or less |
| Origin of exoerythrocytic schizonts | Invariably sporozoites | Invariably sporozoites | Sporozoites and merozoites |

**Table 3.** Differential characters of the subgenera of mammalian species of *Plasmodium*. Modified from GARNHAM (1966)

| Subgenus | Vertebrate host | Shape of gametocytes | Pigment in gametocytes | Stippling of erythrocytes | Duration of EE schizogony |
|---|---|---|---|---|---|
| *Plasmodium* | Primates | Spherical | Widespread | Present | More than 5 days |
| *Laverania* | Primates | Crescentic | Perinuclear | Present | More than 5 days |
| *Vinckeia* | Lemurs and lower mammals | Spherical | Widespread | Absent | Less than 5 days |

asites, especially in lizard malaria, in which sporogonic stages are only now beginning to be recognised.

Each species, however, represents a separate entity. It is important to refrain from assuming that species of *Plasmodium* in animals are necessarily good models in every respect for the human species. The best model for the human species is man himself or, failing that, susceptible primates, among which chimpanzees presumably represent the nearest example. The ethics of using primates, particularly the rarer species, have to be carefully considered and, now that good culture methods are available for some stages of certain species, these should be substituted whenever possible. Rodent malaria parasites have been much used in research, since their original discovery by VINCKE and LIPS (1948), but they belong to a different subgenus and in some ways are nearer to the avian than to the primate species. COATNEY et al. (1971) suggested that *Plasmodium coatneyi* of Malayan macaques might prove to be a good model for *P. (Laverania) falciparum* of man, but a similar

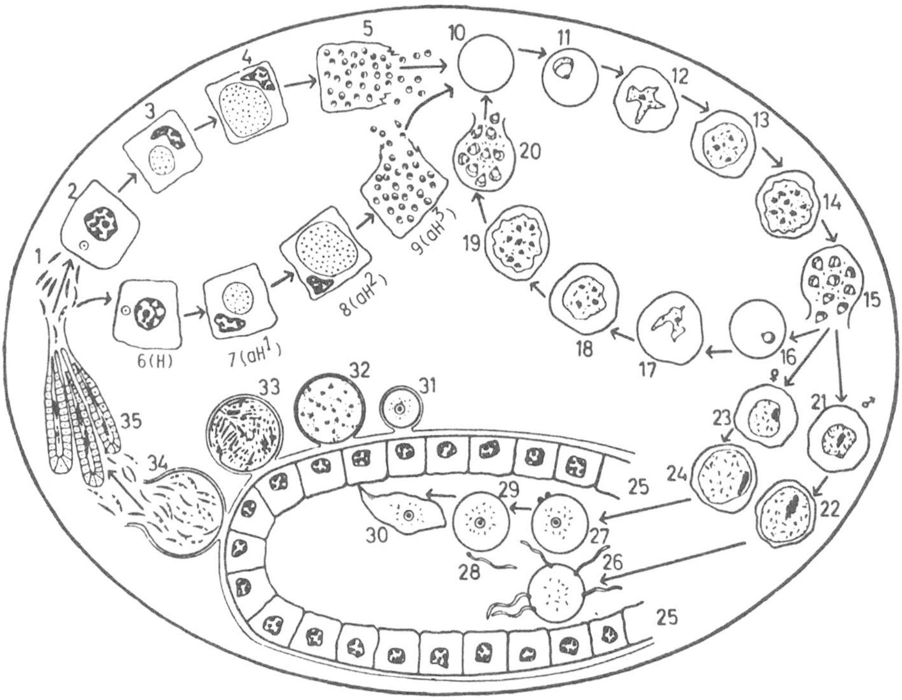


**Fig. 1.** Life cycle of *Plasmodium vivax*. L., sporozoites of two types penetrating hepatocytes (*1*); one type initiates immediate exoerythrocytic schizogony (*2–4*) and the other type becomes hypnozoites and eventually relapse forms (H and aH's); *2–4*, growing exoerythrocytic schizonts; *5*, mature and rupturing exoerythrocytic schizont; merozoites enter red blood cells (RBCs) (*10*); *6*, (H) hypnozoite in hepatocyte; *7–9*, aH's, $aH^2$, $aH^3$ activated hypnozoites; *10*, $aH^3$ mature activated form; merozoites enter RBCs (*10*); *11*, *12*, trophozoites in RBC; *13*, *14*, immature schizonts in RBCs; *15*, mature erythrocytic schizont discharging merozoites; *16–20*, merozoite re-establishes blood cycle; *21*, *22*, developing microgametocytes in blood; *23*, *24*, developing macrogametocytes in blood; *25*, entry of gametocytes into midgut of *Anopheles; 26*, exflagellation of microgametocyte with production of microgametes (only six of the eight are shown); *27*, macrogamete released from RBC (note polar bodies); *28*, free microgamete; *29*, macrogamete about to be fertilised by *28; 30*, zygote elongating into ookinete; *31–33*, oocysts on surface of midgut; *34*, rupture of mature oocyst and discharge of sporozoites into haemocoele; *35*, invasion of salivary glands by sporozoites

criticism applies in that, again, the model belongs to a different subgenus (see Table 3).

Certain avian models have proved useful in the past but have fundamental differences, while reptilian malaria is so unrelated to the human species that it has scarcely been used in chemotherapeutic studies.

The general structure of the life cycle is shown diagrammatically in Fig. 1 and relates specifically to *P. vivax* and other species in which true relapses occur. In the majority of species, the stages of hypnozoites are lacking and revival of infection takes place by repeated recrudescences in the blood stream (10–20), sometimes for many years.

This diagram serves as a representation of all malaria parasites *sensu lato*, if the following modifications are made:
1. As it stands – *P. vivax* and other species with true relapses.
2. Without *6–9–11* other species of mammalian malaria parasites.
3. Substitution of *1–5* and *6–10* by cryptozoic (an exoerythrocytic) generations in mesoderm, etc. – avian and reptilian malaria parasites.
4. Omission of *10–20* retention of *21–24* – Haemoproteidae and Leucocytozoidae. (The exoerythrocytic stages may be either in hepatocytes as shown or in other fixed tissue cells.)

## C. Life Cycle of *Plasmodium* Species

The development of species of *Plasmodium* will now be described and compared in the three broad groups, mammalian, avian, and reptilian, with particular emphasis on the first.

### I. Life Cycle in Mammalian Malaria

Except in the subgenus *Vinckeia*, the details of the three stages of the infection are known in most parasites of the other subgenera. These stages occur in the liver and blood of the vertebrate host and in the midgut and salivary glands of the invertebrate.

#### 1. Liver Stages

The infection is initiated by the entry of the sporozoite into the mammal, usually by the bite of an anopheline mosquito. The parasite is either immediately inoculated into a capillary by the proboscis or a blood vessel is torn, a pool of blood collects and the sporozoites are deposited therein (O'Rourke 1956). In both cases, the sporozoites quickly reach the general circulation, where they remain for 30–60 min. Many are undoubtedly phagocytosed, but a varying proportion reach the liver, where they undergo exoerythrocytic schizogony. While the exact course of early development in this organ is still unsettled, recent experimental work is discussed under *P. cynomolgi* (p. 21) and *P. berghei* (p. 24). However, within 10–48 h of their entry, the parasites start to develop inside the hepatocyte, the nuclei divide, the schizont grows and, after a genetically determined interval, the parasite becomes mature (Fig. 2) and the merozoites escape into the neighbouring sinusoid. The duration of this stage varies according to the species of *Plasmodium* but lies within strict limits (at least on the lower side). The invasion of the blood by the merozoites determines the characteristic prepatent period (i.e. when parasitaemia is initiated) of each species. Frequently, however, laggards occur, so that merozoites may continue to be discharged into the blood for several days or even a week or more after the original invasion.

The length of exoerythrocytic schizogony bears a certain relationship to the length of the other two stages of the life cycle. This is best seen in the quartan par-

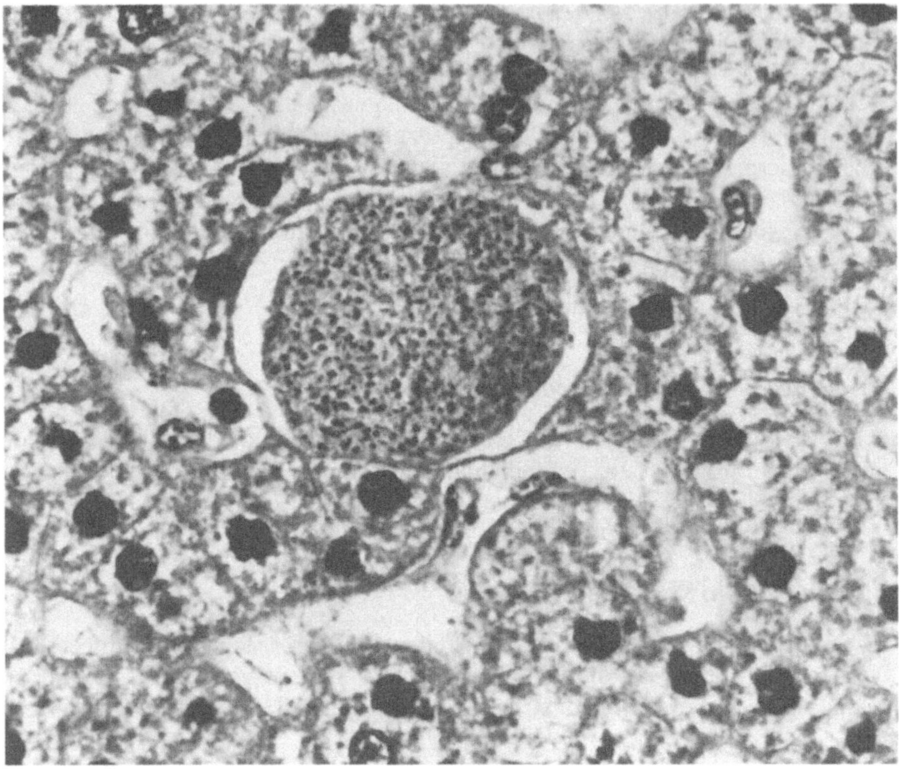

**Fig. 2.** Pre-erythrocytic schizont of *Plasmodium cynomolgi bastianellii* in section of liver of a rhesus monkey on the 7th day after sporozoite infection. Giemsa-colophonium stain, ×830

asites of primates in which the liver stage lasts from 12–15 days (according to species), the blood stage for 3 days and sporogony for 16 days. The shortest length is under 2 days for the liver stage of *P. yoelii*, possibly 1 day for erythrocytic schizogony and less than 12 days for sporogony. Rapidity of growth is also exhibited by *P. knowlesi*, which takes 5 days in the liver, 1 day in the blood and 9 days in the mosquito. The tertian parasites of *Plasmodium* (*Plasmodium*) in primates vary between 6 and 9 days in duration of exoerythrocytic schizogony. Among the 23 or more species of the subgenus *Vinckeia*, details of exoerythrocytic schizonts were said to be known in only three (KILLICK-KENDRICK 1978). These were all rodent parasites with very short tissue cycles, but recently LANDAU and BOULARD (1978) have shown that this stage in *P. atheruri* (of another West African small mammal) lasts as long as 6 days.

The liver stages of all mammalian malaria parasites are initiated only by the injection of sporozoites in which a single generation of exoerythrocytic schizogony follows, contrary to the theory of SHORTT and GARNHAM (1948), in which repeated cycles of species in the *vivax* group were said to occur. This subject and the related phenomenon of latency and relapses are discussed in Sect. C.I.

## 2. Blood Stages

The onset of parasitaemia is best determined in experimental work by the subinoculation of blood into clean animals, for if the dosage of sporozoites is low, it may take several generations of schizogony before enough parasites are produced to be detected by visual examination, or for symptoms to occur. The duration then is referred to as the incubation period.

The exoerythrocytic merozoites are first visible in the erythrocytes as tiny rings, i.e. a portion of cytoplasm alongside a deeply staining nucleus. A vacuole forms within the cytoplasm, which begins to grow (Fig. 3a) and, in some species, exhibits marked amoeboidicity (Fig. 3b). The parasite feeds on the haemoglobin of the host cell but the metabolism is incomplete and grains of pigment (haematin) remain scattered in the cytoplasm. The parasite at this stage is uninucleate and is termed a trophozoite. Within a day, or less or more according to the species, the nucleus divides by accelerated mitosis into two, and subsequently into 4, 8, 16 or 32. The pigment collects into a few pieces and the cytoplasm condenses around the final nuclei (Fig. 3c) to produce merozoites, each with a typical apicomplexan structure. Rupture of the much disorganised erythrocyte follows and the merozoites escape into the plasma (Fig. 3d). Their extracellular life is short, only a few seconds, and they then invade new erythrocytes by attachment to and invagination of the surface membrane.

The details of these developmental processes are best observed by electron microscopy (see AIKAWA and SEED 1980).

The asexual cycles in the blood continue and result in infections of two types (SERGENT 1963), either without restraint, the host succumbing to an overwhelming multiplication of the parasite, or the immunity mechanism is sufficient to dampen the infection, which becomes extinguished or progresses to latency. The quartan parasites, with their low rate of multiplication and production of few merozoites, allow immunity to intervene. *P. knowlesi* on the other hand produces many parasites every 24 h and soon kills its host. There are all types of response between these extremes, in which the natural as well as acquired immunity of the host plays an essential role. At the time of crisis, the infection is of course much disturbed, synchronicity is lost, the morphology of the parasites becomes more ragged and the number of merozoites is reduced.

The exact mechanism which causes the parasites to line up at a precise time to undergo schizogony and rupture has never been satisfactorily explained. The process could be regarded as of genetic origin and part of the characteristic chronobiology, but how can one reconcile the inevitable fluctuations in the composition of the different stages of the parasite in the blood with the maintenance of an orderly sequence? The only precise way of changing the rhythm is by artificial reversal of night and day, when eventually the time at which schizogony occurs can be altered by as much as 12 h. The effect of changes in the body temperature of the host has received little attention, though the few experiments in which it has been lowered artificially showed that some prolongation of schizogony occurred (NYE 1961).

The second major event in the life cycle in the blood is the production of gametocytes. Usually several generations of erythrocytic schizogony elapse before

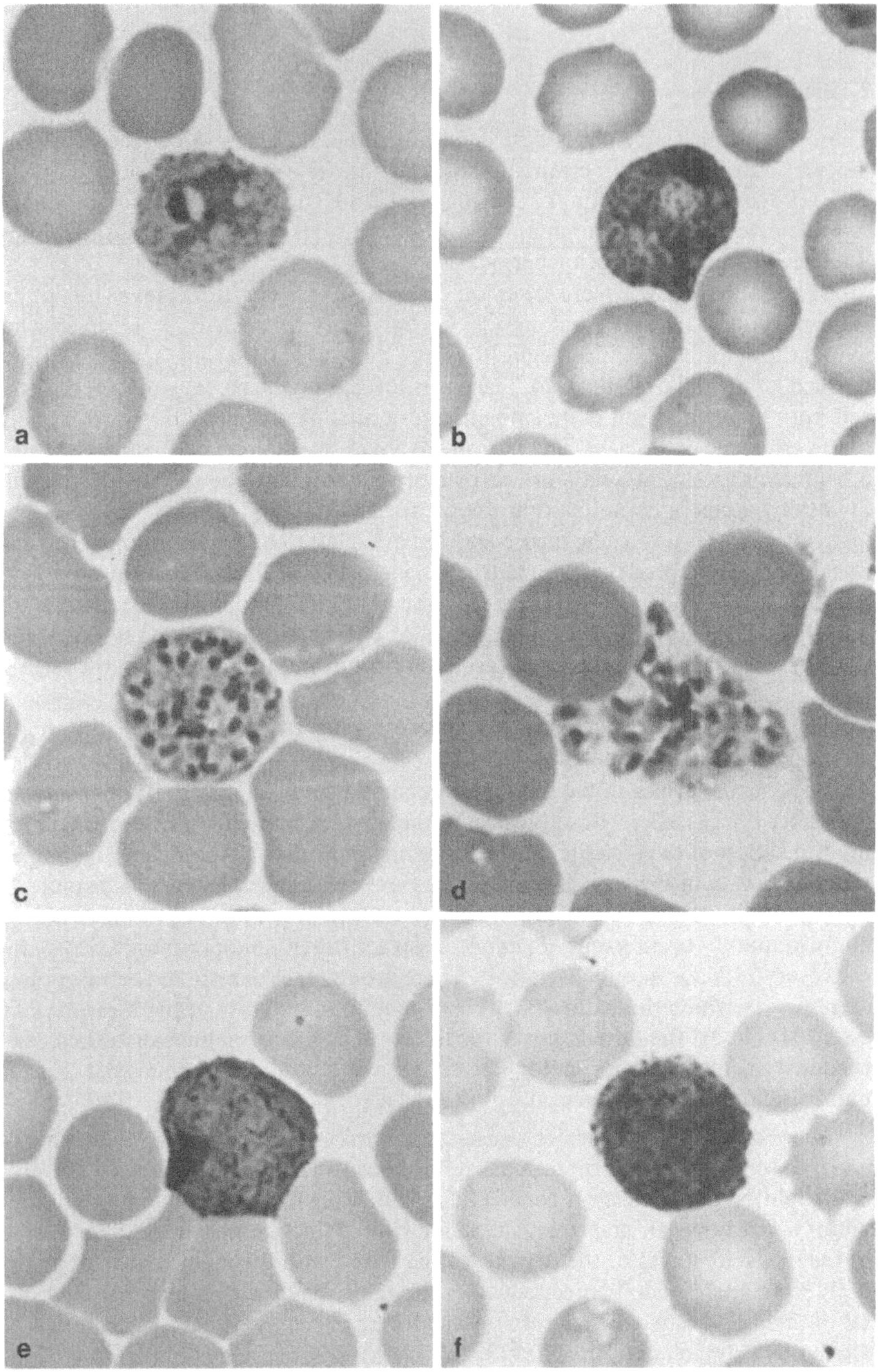


**Fig. 3a–f.** Asexual and sexual erythrocytic stages of *Plasmodium vivax* in blood of man. **a, b** Young, amoeboid trophozoites. **c** Nearly mature schizont with about 32 merozoites. **d** Merozoites erupted from schizont (note "ghost" red-cell envelope in background. **e** Macrogametocyte. **f** Microgametocyte (note the compact, clearly defined nucleus of the female, compared with the diffuse, pale staining nucleus of the male). Giemsa stain, × 1 900

their products become sexual. In spite of a few reports to the contrary it is doubtful if gametocytes of *Plasmodium* spp. can arise directly from exoerythrocytic schizonts in primate malaria, though KILLICK-KENDRICK and WARREN (1968) showed that they could in rodent malaria. Gametogony is subject to various influences, of which the most important are the following: the nature of the host (gametocytes fail to develop in some unnatural hosts), the presence of active immunity in the host (gametocytes are damaged in many species directly antibodies are produced), and repeated transmission of laboratory strains by blood instead of sporozoite transfer sooner or later may result in the disappearance of viable gametocytes. A rather extraordinary contradiction to this generalisation is provided by the observations of CARTER and MILLER (1979) on continuous culture of *P. falciparum* for 1 1/2 years, during which the cultures maintained their ability to produce plentiful crescents and exflagellation occurred.

Young gametocytes are usually unvacuolated, solid bodies which grow at half the speed of asexual forms. Amoeboidicity is slight or absent and the pigment remains scattered in the cytoplasm in most species, instead of becoming condensed into masses as in asexual parasites, or assuming a perinuclear distribution as in *P. (L) falciparum* crescents. Sexual dimorphism quickly becomes apparent, the cytoplasm of the macrogametocyte (Fig. 3e) staining a fairly dense blue with Giemsa stain and the nucleus remaining condensed and heavily stained, while the cytoplasm of the microgametocyte (Fig. 3f) is much paler and the nucleus spreads over a large area, perhaps more than half of the cytoplasm. The two sexes do not, as a rule, enter the blood simultaneously, the microgametocytes often appearing a day or two later, and often in smaller numbers.

The later life of the gametocyte in the vertebrate host has been investigated in recent years by HAWKING et al. (1966), who showed how quickly gametocytes degenerate in the blood and how their period of infectivity to mosquitoes is confined to the hours of darkness. These ideas conflict with the personal experience of malariologists from the time of ROSS and GRASSI until today, as it has repeatedly been shown that good mosquito-induced infections may be obtained by feeding the insects predominantly in the daytime. Nevertheless, HAWKING'S work has been confirmed by himself and a few other investigators and this theory fits in well with the fact that the main time that mosquitoes feed is at night, i.e. when the gametocytes are supposed to be most infective. In the words of GILLETT (1971), "the circadian rhythm of the parasite is brought into phase with that of the vector." HAWKING emphasises that the phenomenon can only be elicited in infections which are highly synchronous. In other cases the results are likely to be obscure and impossible to interpret.

### 3. Sporogonic Stages

While sporogony starts with the formation of gametocytes in the vertebrate host, the main sexual events take place in the anopheline mosquito. Only certain species can act as vectors, either because they have the suitable feeding preference or because they have the correct host-parasite relationship. The latter is more fundamental and, in most mammalian malarias, and especially the human forms, a wide range of species of *Anopheles* can act as vectors. However, in nature the range is more limited and, as MATTINGLY (1969) has pointed out, only certain species in the four common subgenera of *Anopheles* are natural vectors of *Plasmodium* spp. Now that subspecies or lower divisions are recognised, the specificity of the various combinations are seen to be quite strict. For example, the closely allied forms known originally as *Anopheles maculipennis* have markedly different vectorial capacities; *A. gambiae* is an ideal vector of African *P. falciparum* but is incapable of transmitting the European variety of the parasite, whereas *A. atroparvus* is an excellent host for European *P. falciparum*, but is a very poor host of the African variety.

These features of the host-parasite relationships deeply concern the life history and it is of primary importance to consider them in all experimental work involving mosquito transmission.

The mosquito bites an animal with gametocytes in its blood. The insect's mouthparts include two narrow tubes, one of which conveys saliva to the site while the other sucks back blood which eventually fills the midgut of the insect, either as the result of a single bite or often of two or more. The epithelial cells of the midgut secrete a mucus substance, probably containing chitin, which envelops the blood and localises it within a so-called peritrophic membrane (FREYVOGEL and STÄUBLI 1966). The exact sequence of events varies according to the species of *Anopheles*, both in regard to the composition of this membrane and to the clotting or digestion of the blood. Immediately on leaving the vertebrate host and on exposure to air, the gametocytes become active. The macrogametocyte becomes free of the erythrocyte and the nucleus undergoes changes preparatory to the formation of the macrogamete. The exact process has not been followed in *Plasmodium*, but it probably resembles the events which occur in the allied genus, *Haemoproteus*. GALUCCI (1974) described nuclear division, in which an intranuclear spindle is formed with the final discarding of one half of the material. This is thought to be the origin of the so-called polar bodies ascribed by the early workers to „*Kernreduktion.*“

The changes in the microgametocyte unlike the inconspicuous maturation of the female, are dramatic and well known. They are best observed at the ultrastructural level and are summarised by SINDEN (1981) in a brief communication based on many observations. He points out that essential cytological changes take place in the microgametocyte while it is still in the vertebrate host. These include the organisation of a microtubule centre, preparatory to the formation of axonemes of the gametes, while at the same time, but inside the nucleus, the octaploid genome is differentiated and this essential element of the gamete becomes linked to the microtubule organisation. These events are followed by "exflagellation" as described first by LAVERAN (1881). Eight microgametes emerge from the surface of the microgametocyte, this number being characteristic of all species of the Haemosporina. However, in practice, the number may appear to vary according to the perfection of the phenomenon. The extreme violence of the process frequently results in the gametes becoming entangled with one another or with remaining portions of the erythrocyte envelope, and the number is difficult to ascertain. Exflagellation begins in mammalian species of *Plasmodium* about 10 min after the mosquito has fed. It may be 1 min less and some parasites may not start exflagellating for 15 min or even later. While it was difficult to understand how the nucleus was able to divide in such a short time, SINDEN'S (1981) showed that DNA replication takes place "at leisure" while the gametocyte is still in the vertebrate host.

The microgametes become free in the content of the midgut of the mosquito and move actively in search of a macrogamete. Probably their energy is exhausted in 1/2 h or less, but usually fertilisation is rapidly achieved. The plasmalemma of the two gametes fuse and eventually, possibly some hours later, the two nuclei fuse. The zygote assumes various forms, often in the shape of a retort which straightens out into an elongate, travelling vermicule or ookinete.

The locomotion of the ookinete has been studied by various observers, with conflicting results. FREYVOGEL and STÄUBLI (1966) studied the problem in different species by direct observations and by time-lapse ciné films (16 mm). The maximum speed of an ookinete was 30 μm/min and the average speed 1 μm/min; the movement was often interrupted for short intervals. The motion is spiral-like and gives rise to a gliding movement as seen in gregarines. The parasite has to travel quite a distance from the blood in the centre of the midgut through the thin peritrophic membrane and the microvilli of the epithelial cell, and finally across the latter cell to emerge at its outer border beneath the thin basal lamina. This process is lengthy as compared with the rapidity of the earlier stages leading to fertilisation. The growth of the ookinete is slow. It does not attain its full length of about 15 μm (in *P. cynomolgi*) until about 24 h after the mosquito has fed (GARNHAM et al. 1962), while another 16 h is required for its passage across the gut wall. The ultrastructure of the ookinete has some striking features (GARNHAM et al. 1969), which include the pellicular folds at the anterior end (probably connected with the spiral movements), the crystalloids in the cytoplasm, which persist in the early oocyst, and the transition of the mitochondria from an acristate to a cristate state.

The timing of these events varies according to the ability of the ookinete to reach its destination, which may be as short as 15 h, or as long as 72 h. It now rounds up into a small, spherical object about 10 μm in diameter, the pellicle thickens and it is then termed an oocyst. The oocyst grows in size and projects into the haemocoelomic cavity. The rate of growth is strictly dependent upon the temperature at which the mosquito is maintained, and upon the species of *Plasmodium*. The chronobiology is as important at this stage as at any other stage of the life cycle, but it is particularly necessary here to note the *minimum* intervals and the *optimum* time for sporogony (see below under special features of rodent parasites).

The cytological changes within the oocyst are not described in detail here (see also AIKAWA 1971; SINDEN 1978). The nucleus remains single for about 36–48 h, but it increases greatly in size and becomes lobulate. Nuclear division starts on the 2nd or 3rd day and the cytoplasm becomes transformed into a deeply furrowed mass. The nuclei line the margins of each fold and, opposite each nucleus, a little finger-like process of cytoplasm is formed into which the nucleus, apical complex and other organelles are drawn. This process is the origin of the sporozoite, and is the usual interpretation of the development. In many species, however, the cytoplasmic mass appears to become cleft to give rise to separate nucleated islands or sporoblastoids. In some species (e.g. *P. gonderi:* GARNHAM et al. 1958) the little spheres are originally uninucleate and grow into multinucleate cytomeres, there being, apparently, no cytoplasmic bridges between them. Nevertheless, it is probably wrong to regard these bodies as true sporoblasts (as in other coccidians), as no cyst wall is developed later and no actual sporocysts are formed.

**Table 4.** Longevity of untreated human malaria parasites. Modified from GARNHAM (1970)

| Species | Average duration (years) | Probable maximum duration (years) |
| --- | --- | --- |
| *P. falciparum* | 1 | ? 4 (so-called longevity of over 2 years' duration) |
| *P. vivax* | 2 | 5 (or longer) |
| *P. ovale* | 1 | 5 |
| *P. malariae* | 4 | 53 |

The dimensions of the oocysts, their rate of growth and the sporozoite content vary greatly according to the species (COLLINS and AIKAWA 1977 – their Table IV). When mature, the weakened oocyst wall collapses and large rents are produced, or small holes or pores form through which the sporozoites escape. These phenomena are well seen in scanning electron microscope studies (SINDEN 1975). The rupture of oocysts is spread over several days but, after 3 or 4 days from the first burst, feew or no oocysts will be seen, nor even the empty "shells."

The sporozoites vary in length from 9 μm in some species to over 20 μm in others (e.g. *P. yoelii nigeriensis:* KILLICK-KENDRICK 1973). They drift in the haemocoelomic fluid to all parts of the body of the mosquito, but congregate in the salivary glands, particularly in the middle gland of each pair. The stimulus of probing by the host induces a flow of saliva and the sporozoites escape in this fluid in the acinal duct, and are deposited at the site of the bite. Varying numbers of from 1 000 to 10 000 sporozoites are quoted as being produced by each oocyst; the sporozoite content of the salivary glands is often as high as 50 000. In a recent experiment (KROTOSKI et al. 1982) 3 000 mosquitoes (*Anopheles dirus*) were found to contain approximately $207 \times 10^6$ sporozoites, i.e. nearly 70 000 in each mosquito.

It has frequently been stated, on not very precise evidence, that sporozoites need a little time to become infective, and that infectivity of sporozoites from the rupturing oocyst or even from the haemocoelomic fluid was much less than those from the salivary gland. VANDERBERG (1975) estimated that there was a 10 000-fold increase in infectivity of *P. berghei* sporozoites after they had reached the glands. On the other hand DAHER and KRETTLI (1980) have shown that *P. gallinaceum* sporozoites (in doses of 5 000–50 000) taken from oocysts (8 or 9 days old) were highly infective on inoculation to chicks. Mosquitoes are thought to lose their infectivity with time. SHUTE (1945), in a series of experiments with *P. falciparum* and *Anopheles atroparvus*, showed that the numbers of sporozoites in the salivary glands declined little until after 50 days, although the mosquitoes were allowed to feed on rabbits every 3 rd day.

## 4. Longevity

Estimations of the total length of life of malaria parasites have been made and Table 4 shows the approximate duration and maximum figures of the human species. These figures are merely an indication and not even the quoted durations of *P. malariae*, [32 years (SHUTE 1944), 36 years (SPITLER 1948), and 53 years (GUAZZI and GRAZI 1963)] are entirely reliable. There are at least two difficulties. First, patients undergoing malaria therapy are likely to be discharged or to die before a "maximum" duration is reached and, second, many reports of late relapses of malaria are not confirmed by positive blood films. On the other hand, experimental infections of monkey or chimpanzee malaria (*P. malariae, P. inui,* and *P. brasilianum*) have been watched for 9 years and confirm the long life of these quartan parasites.

## II. Life Cycle in Avian Malaria

Table 2, which compares the life cycles of mammalian and avian malaria, demonstrates the profound differences which exist in the two groups. It will be seen that these principally affect the nature of exoerythrocytic schizogony. The type of invertebrate host is probably of considerable phylogenetic significance, though sporogony in *Anopheles* and culicine mosquitoes runs much the same course in both, as it does in the other families of the suborder (see below, Sect. II.3).

### 1. Tissue Stages

An infected mosquito bites the bird between the insertions of the feathers, around the eyes or on the wing skin. The sporozoites are deposited at the site of the bite and their further development was followed in great detail in the researches of HUFF and COULSTON (1944) and HUFF (1947). The complete cycle was demonstrated in *Plasmodium (Haemamoeba) relictum, P. (H) cathemerium, P. (H) gallinaceum, P. (Giovannolaia) lophurae,* and *P. (G) fallax.* Other workers described certain stages of the pre-erythrocytic cycle of *P. (Huffia) elongatum,* notably RAFFAELE (1936), in so-called reticuloendothelial cells of greenfinches and goldfinches after sporozoite infection. The later, exoerythrocytic stages of many species of avian parasites have also been reported, but they form part of a different type of cycle which may persist in birds for months. Their products are termed "phanerozoites" and are described below.

The American investigator (HUFF 1969) followed the course of development of the sporozoite from inoculation or bite of infected mosquitoes, in the wing skin and internal organs of suitable birds. The steps are as follows:

a) Sporozoites are present in phagocytes from 1/2 h–6 h. They die rapidly in polymorphonuclear leucocytes but start to develop as cryptozoites in lymphoid-macrophage cells by the end of this period.

b) The cryptozoite assumes an oval or spherial shape and grows rapidly. The nucleus divides and, by 36 h, increases in number to 100. Schizogony is completed during the next 12 h, when elongate merozoites collect in parallel rows on the periphery.

c) The schizont then ruptures, the cryptozoic merozoites quickly invade adjacent macrophages and the second or metacryptozoic generation begins. The multiplication which takes place in the cryptozoic stages entails a greater concentration of parasites in the area and, by 72 h, mature metacryptozoic schizonts are formed.

d) Metacryptozoites invade further tissue cells in the vicinity, or enter erythrocytes in the blood stream. The prepatent period is thus seen to be about 75 h.

e) Some cryptozoites and metacryptozoites escape into the blood and are carried to various organs such as the spleen, heart, kidney, brain, and liver, where they develop in lymphoid-macrophage or endothelial cells.

f) These cycles of exoerythrocytic schizogony in avian malaria gradually lose their synchronicity and, after a few days, the schizonts often contain as many as 500–1 000 similar merozoites.

g) Sporozoites may enter the blood directly if introduced either naturally or artificially into a blood vessel and, in such instances, the tissue stage may start in any of the internal organs. In the same way, the cryptozoic merozoites rupturing in the skin may enter the blood and initiate secondary cycles elsewhere.

The foregoing account, which relates directly to *P.* (*H.*) *gallinaceum*, except in small details applies also to *P.* (*G.*) *lophurae*, and probably *P.* (*G.*) *fallax*. Pre-erythrocytic schizogony of *P.* (*H.*) *relictum* differs from that of *P.* (*H.*) *gallinaceum* in that the schizonts tend to be smaller and to contain fewer cryptozoites, but strains of the former vary considerably in these details. *P.* (*H.*) *cathemerium* resembles *P. relictum* except that nuclear division of the cryptozoite does not start until after 16 h instead of after 9 h, merozoites are fewer (35), and the prepatent period is possibly shorter.

The phanerozoite cycles of the above parasites are better known, as they are easier to elicit; they also occupy exoerythrocytic sites. They are responsible for the fundamental difference in the biological behaviour of the avian and mammalian parasites, the former being initiated by the inoculation of both sporozoites and blood forms, and the latter solely by sporozoites. They were most brilliantly demonstrated by James and Tate (1937) in brains of chickens inoculated with *P. gallinaceum*, in which profuse exoerythrocytic schizogony was produced in the cerebral capillaries. Actually phanerozoites may appear in many organs, and their production can continue for weeks. Phanerozoites of some species (e.g. *P. relictum*) are more easily produced by sporozoite than blood inoculation, while continuous blood transmission may entirely abolish the ability of the strain to give rise to a tissue phase.

The nature of the tissue stages of the above parasites is thus fairly uniform. The one exception is the subgenus *Huffia*, which contains one important and cosmopolitan species, *P.* (*Hu.*) *elongatum*. The life cycle is still incompletely known although it was the first parasite in which exoerythrocytic schizogony was recognised, by Raffaele in 1934. However, his compatriot, Corradetti (Corradetti et al. 1968), finally isolated a strain of *P. elongatum* from an owl in Udine, which proved to be easily transmissible by *Culex pipiens*, and which gave rise to clear-cut pre-erythrocytic cycles in canaries. Cryptozoites were first seen 60 h after sporozoite infection and subsequently at various intervals up to 120 h. They were present in macrophages and Kupffer cells of the liver and in the spleen, while they were scantier in the lungs, bone marrow, kidney, and heart. The mature schizonts contained 60–120 cryptozoic (or metacryptozoic) merozoites. At 120 h, the blood and bone marrow became invaded while, after this time, development in the lymphoid-macrophage system ceased entirely. Exoerythrocytic schizogony persisted, however, in the cells of the haemopoietic system particularly in the bone marrow and, because of this invasion, the canaries invariably died of anaemia following the fulminating infection.

Experimental pharmacologists might well find *P. elongatum* a useful model for comparing the action of drugs in the fixed macrophages of the prepatent stage and in the haemopoietic system in the developed infection with the very different life cycles of the other avian malaria parasites.

## 2. Blood Stages

The main features of the asexual cycle in the blood and the initiation of gametogony are similar in avian and mammalian malaria parasites. There are, however, a few rather striking differences which may have pharmacological significance.

### a) Mitochondrion

This organelle is fully developed in avian species and shows the typical protozoan morphology (AIKAWA 1971) with a double membrane, the inner being folded into microtubular cristae. In most mammalian species, the mitochondrion is replaced by a simple, double, membrane-bound structure, sometimes described as "multilaminate" or "whorled," and devoid of contents. The same composition of the mitochondrion is seen in the gametocytes of the two groups, though the matrix is denser in the sexual forms of the avian group.

### b) Blockage of Capillaries

Cerebral malaria occurs in both avian and mammalian malaria as a result of the interruption of the circulation of blood in the brain. In both instances the condition is limited to certain species of *Plasmodium*, but the pathogenesis is entirely different. In *P. (L.) falciparum* infections, schizogony is practically confined to the internal organs including the brain, where the erythrocytic schizonts grow and occlude the vessels. In avian malaria (e.g. *P. gallinaceum*) occlusion often occurs, but now as the result of the tremendous *exoerythrocytic* schizogony in the endothelial cells lining the cerebral capillaries. Both types lead to a fatal termination.

### c) Effect of Immunity on the Life Cycle

Mammalian malaria is often followed by the complete disappearance of parasites from the blood and a sterile immunity is the result. Avian malaria is characterised by the persistence of parasites in the blood. They are not entirely destroyed at the crisis, but may survive the immune processes and remain in a state of balance ("premunition") with the host's defences. In neither instance is this the inevitable outcome, for some mammalian species (e.g. *P. malariae*) may linger in low numbers in the blood of the host for life, while some avian species (e.g. *P. gallinaceum*) may kill the bird if it is young, or a new importation into an enzootic area. GABALDON and ULLOA (1980), describing the high mortality of nestlings (of pigeons and ducks) in heronries in Venezuela as the result of heavy infections of several species of *Plasmodium*, concluded that malaria was a powerful factor in controlling the size of the population of these birds in localised areas.

## 3. Sporogonic Stages

The avian malaria parasites develop naturally in at least six genera of mosquitoes, *Aedes*, *Aedomyia*, *Culex*, *Culiseta*, *Psorophora*, and *Mansonia* (GABALDON et al.

1977). The list is longer (nine genera) if laboratory vectors are included. *Anopheles* can become infected under such conditions and natural avian infections in species of this genus have been mistakely suspected of being part of the life cycle of human species of *Plasmodium*. The American genus *Wyeomyia* has been shown to be a good vector, in the laboratory and probably in the forest, of the turkey malaria parasite (*P. hermani*) by NAYAR et al. (1980). There is some relationship between the subgenera of *Plasmodium* and the genus of mosquito host. *Culex* seems to be the most preferred host of avian malaria parasites in general, and of *Haemamoeba* and *Huffia* of passerine birds in particular. *Aedes* carries *P.* (*H.*) *gallinaceum* of gallinaceous birds and also various species of *Giovannolaia* (*fallax* and *lophurae*) experimentally. *Aedomyia* is a natural vector of *P.* (*G.*) *circumflexum* in Africa but, in Sri Lanka, the vector is *Mansonia*. *Culiseta* also harbours *P.* (*G.*) *polare*. The mosquito hosts of species of *Novyella* are poorly known [though the type host of *P.* (*N.*) *rouxi* is the invertebrate *Culex pipiens* in which it was first identified]. The widespread *P.* (*N.*) *juxtanucleare* of chickens is carried by *Culex sitiens*, in which unique, pedunculated, oocysts are formed (BENNETT et al. 1963).

The cytological features of the sporogonic stages of avian malaria parasites have only an indirect bearing on the life cycle. The ultrastructural details have been described by numerous observers and the latest work by MELHORN et al. (1980) again confirms the *intra*-rather than *inter*cellular passage of the ookinete through the epithelium of the midgut. Their observations challenge the long-held belief that the first division of the nucleus of the zygote (i.e. ookinete) is meiotic. They describe the simultaneous formation of *several* nuclei, which they suggest cannot be "typical meiosis."

## III. Life Cycle in Reptilian Malaria

Reptilian malaria parasites are very common in lizards in subtropical and tropical regions of the world. *Plasmodium* is confined to one named species, *Plasmodium wenyoni* GARNHAM, 1965 (syn. *tomadoni* PESSOA, 1973) in snakes, and is absent in chelonians and the crocodilia. These parasites are clearly of very ancient origin and perhaps date back to the dinosaur age, as they betray very primitive characteristics. Unfortunately the life history of none of them is completely known, and it was not until 1970 that the sporogonic cycle in sandflies was discovered (AYALA 1970b).

In view of the paucity of data relating to malaria in lizards, it has only been possible to provide a tentative and arbitrary division of the parasites into two subgeneric groups, based on size, *Sauramoeba* for the larger and *Carinamoeba* for the smaller (GARNHAM 1966). A third subgenus was created for the sole malaria parasite of snakes, *Plasmodium* (*Ophidiella*) *wenyoni*.

Up to 1966, 23 species of malaria parasites in lizards were recognised. Since that the date, a few workers have devoted much time investigating the subject, PELAEZ and PEREZ-REYES (1952) in Mexico, AYALA (1970a, b) in California and South America, and particularly TELFORD (1977) in both the Old World and New World tropics, and LAINSON and co-workers in Brazil (LAINSON et al. 1975). The last group have raised the question of the correct taxonomy of their species, chiefly in relation to the presence or absence of pigment in the blood stages. As some of the Amazonian parasites fail entirely to produce pigment, even though schizogony occurs in the erythrocytes, they have relegated these species to a new family, Garniidae. Similar unpigmented parasites in the former haemoproteid group have been transferred to the new genus *Fallisia*. TELFORD (1973) disagrees with these taxonomic changes and would prefer to keep them in *Plasmodium* and *Haemocystidium* (Haemoproteidae) respectively. It is unlikely that a good solution will be found until the full life cycles are known and the definitions accordingly amended or not.

In this section, the subject will not be treated under the formal divisions of the life cycle as so little is known. Moreover, reptilian malaria offers little to experimental pharmacology at present.

Multiplication in the blood stream may assume fulminating proportions and sometimes in a wide spectrum of hosts in which the morphology may alter from species to species. There is little synchronicity of schizogony and the duration of this process is difficult to estimate. Reptiles are poikilothermic animals and offer potentialities for studies of development at different temperatures, but so far little work has been done.

The pre-erythrocytic development is totally unknown but exoerythrocytic schizogony has been observed in a number of species. The most interesting form is seen in *P. mexicanum*, where tissue stages occur in two sites, the haemopoietic system (similar to the avian parasite, *P. elongatum*) and the fixed endothelium of the tissues and organs ("gallinaceum type"). It was thought at one time that this mixed developmental cycle (the so-called mexicanum type) was confined to *P. mexicanum*, but probably it occurs also in other species. The differentiation may be difficult, because "fixed" cells may become detached and circulate in the blood. All these forms, of course, contain no malaria pigment.

AYALA (1970 b) showed that the sandfly, *Lutzomyia vexator occidentis*, became infected up to the sporozoite stage after feeding on *Sceloporus occidentalis* with *P. mexicanum* gametocytes in its blood. Sporogony took 7–10 days. The oocysts grew normally on the surface of the midgut and, on rupture, the rather sturdy sporozoites invaded the salivary glands. The only previous worker to obtain a partial success was JORDAN (1964), who observed oocysts of *P. floridense* in three species of *Culex*. In fact, few people have ever been able to elicit exflagellaton of the microgametocyte in various species of saurian *Plasmodium*.

Attempts to confirm AYALA's (1970 b) work have met with only limited success. YOUNG (1977) in Gainesville, Florida, obtained oocysts fairly easily in *Lutzomyia vexator* which had fed on fence lizards infected with *P. floridense*. Later, KIRMSEY (personal communication) has apparently succeeded in infecting *Lutzomyia trinidadensis* by feeding it on *Anolis limifrons* parasitised with *P. tropiduri*. Oocysts with sporozoites were said to be present in the lumen of the midgut.

LAINSON's attempts to infect sandflies or other biting insects have met with no success, and he informs me (LAINSON, personal communication) that he is by no means certain that sandflies are the sole vector. This is confirmed by the discovery of sporogony of *P. agamae* in *Culicoides* (PETIT et al., 1984).

## D. Specific Examples

The life cycle of malaria parasites is liable to be affected by a number of external and internal factors, and the examples which follow have been chosen to illustrate

**Table 5.** Species of primate malaria parasites with and without relapses

| Species with relapses | | Species probably without relapses |
|---|---|---|
| Confirmed | Probable | |
| *P. vivax*[a] | *P. silvaticum* | *P. falciparum* |
| *P. cynomolgi*[a] – subspp[a] | *P. simium* | *P. malariae* |
| *P. ovale* | *P. schwetzi* | *P. inui* |
| *P. simiovale*[b] | | *P. brasilianum* |
| *P. fieldi*[b] | | *P. knowlesi* |
| | | *P. fragile* |
| | | *P. coatneyi* |

[a] Hypnozoites seen
[b] See COLLINS and CONTACOS (1974)

special conditions, particularly in the human species of *Plasmodium* and to a lesser extent in a few animal species. When the latter are directly related, or almost identical with the human species, they will be considered together.

## I. Human Species of *Plasmodium*

### 1. *Plasmodium vivax* and Closely Related Forms Present in Monkeys and Apes

The most important part of the life cycle relates today to the relapse phenomenon, which, as Table 5 shows, is confined to this group of tertian, "Schüffner's-dots-producing," malaria parasites. "Relapses" have to be distinguished from "recrudescences," using these terms in the following technical way (WHO 1963):

A "recrudescence" is a renewed manifestation (of malaria) due to the survival of the infection in the blood. It may follow either blood- or sporozoite-induced malaria, and is curable by appropriate schizontocidal drugs. Recrudescences occur in all species of *Plasmodium*.

A "relapse" is a renewed manifestation due to the persistence and reactivation of latent, exoerythrocytic forms in the liver. It only occurs in sporozoite-induced infections, and may not be cured by schizontocidal drugs. Relapses are confined to the special group under discussion.

A preliminary to research on relapses is to determine the fate of sporozoites after introduction into the body of the vertebrate host, i.e. man or a substitute animal. Attempts have been made to grow sporozoites in vitro and only in recent years have they been successful, first by STROME et al. (1979) using turkey tissue cells and other exotic strains, then by SMITH et al. (1981) and, with most success, by HOLLINGDALE et al. (1981). DANFORTH et al. (1980) showed that sporozoites of *P. knowlesi* became attached to peritoneal macrophages and even to Kupffer cells, invaded the cells and remained alive for 1 h. The actual demonstration (by immunofluorescence) of sporozoites in Kupffer cells in vivo has been claimed by VERHAVE et al. (1980), while these workers and others (SMITH et al. 1981) have demonstrated that macrophage blocking agents (e.g. silica particles) can greatly reduce the numbers of exoerythrocytic schizonts in the parenchyma cells of the liver. It is suggested that this result is best explained on the assumption that *intact* Kupffer cells are necessary for the transport of sporozoites into the parenchyma cells. Practically all the foregoing experiments involved the use of *P. berghei* and rodents and have not been repeated using the vivax group of parasites and monkeys. The extraordinary path of the sporozoite, first from the oocyst and salivary glands, through the circulation of the primate, and the final tortuous passage in the space of Disse amongst the processes of the Kupffer cells, the undifferentiated endothelium of the sinusoid and the microvilli of the parenchyma cells, must constitute an "obstacle race," which perhaps *does* need the help of a transporting agent to guide the sporozoite to its destination (see MEIS et al., 1983).

SHORTT and GARNHAM (1948) advanced the theory that repeated cycles of exoerythrocytic schizogony of the *P. vivax* type of parasites occur every 8 days or so, and that a small number of histiocytic merozoites are produced in each generation which re-enter liver cells. In the meantime, the cycle in the blood reaches a peak, after which parasitaemia declines with the establishment of immunity. Eventually immunity is lost and the merozoites of the occult cycle in the liver are able to invade erythrocytes and a relapse ensues. SHORTT still adheres to this theory, but most people including the writer have discarded it in favour of the persistence of a latent stage, arising from a special type of sporozoite.

The existence of two types of sporozoites in some strains (e.g. the North Korean) of *P. vivax* was demonstrated by SHUTE et al. (1976), although the nature of the second (latent) form remained unknown. MARKUS (1976) named this "x body" the "dormozoite," later changed to "hypnozoite" (as suggested to the author by HOARE).

The hypnozoite (Fig. 4) was finally demonstrated (first by immunofluorescence, later by Giemsa staining) by KROTOSKI et al. (1980) in monkeys infected with large numbers of sporozoites of *P. cynomolgi bastianellii*. Biopsies of the liver were taken at various intervals up to 105 days and the small, always uninucleate, spherical or oval hypnozoites were seen at 3 days, 5 days, 7 days (when they reach their largest size, about 5 µm) and then at frequent intervals until 105 days. The hypnozoites remain unchanged throughout, but a proportion apparently became reactivated at various times, accompanied by a decline in number of the hypnozoites. The hypnozoite cycle is shown diagrammatically in Fig. 1 (H, $aH^1$, $aH^2$, $aH^3$). The reactivated forms (= "relapse forms") resemble those described by SHORTT and GARNHAM (1948) and later by other workers. Their dimensions varied from 16–38 µm.

Hypnozoites have now been seen in *P. cynomolgi cynomolgi, P.c. bastianellii* (Fig. 4), and *P. vivax* by immunofluorescence techniques. So far they have not been demonstrated in the limited amount of material available of infections of the non-relapsing species. The presence of hypnozoites indicates that the species concerned is likely to present "true relapses" in its life cycle. The absence of hypnozoites is an indication that relapses would not occur. Table 5 compares the respective groups.

Prolonged incubation periods are characteristic of *P. vivax hibernans* NICOLAIEV, 1949 from Northern Russia and of similar strains in temperate regions of Europe and elsewhere (e.g. North Korea: GARNHAM et al. 1975). They probably have the same aetiology as relapses and, in *P. vivax*, the duration of prepatency is

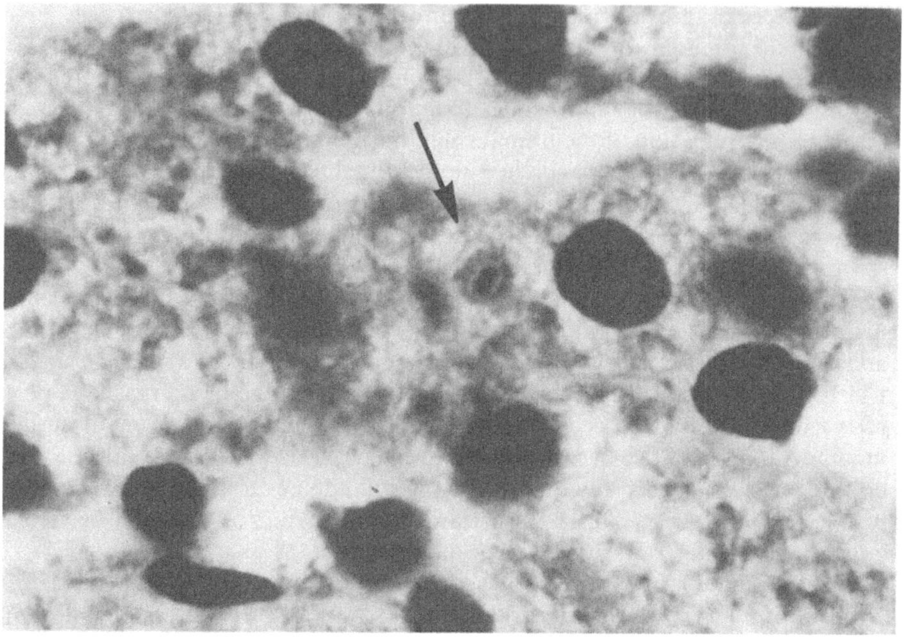

**Fig. 4.** Hypnozoite of *Plasmodium cynomolgi bastianellii* in section of liver of a rhesus monkey on the 7th day after sporozoite infection. This is the same biopsy as that containing the large, pre-erythrocytic schizont seen in Fig. 2. Note the minute, single-nucleated parasite *(arrowed)* in the cytoplasm of a hepatocyte. Giemsa-colophonium stain, ×2100

about 250 days (or as long as 628 days). Such prolonged periods apparently only occur in human infections and have never been reported in animals.

It might be mentioned here that "true relapses" are apparently absent in avian and saurian malaria. The situation must be quite different in the other families, Haemoproteidae, and Leucocytozoidae, in which no multiplication of the parasites occurs in the blood and the gametocytaemia must depend on a continuous supply of exoerythrocytic merozoites from the organs. The latter, presumably, is the result of repeated cycles, unless hypnozoites, derived from the original sporozoites, are the origin. DESSER et al. (1968) presented evidence that "spring relapses" of *Leucocytozoon simondi* in wild duck are due to cystic stages in the lungs and heart.

The *Plasmodium vivax* group shows another interesting feature in that the life cycle cannot apparently be established in the blood of the West African black. This race (unless mixed with Caucasian blood) is practically immune to *P. vivax*, *P. schwetzi*, and *P. cynomolgi*. On the other hand, it is fully susceptible to *P. ovale*. The explanation of the phenomenon was only discovered in 1976, when MILLER et al. (1976) showed that the absence of the Duffy factor on the surface of erythrocytes (a characteristic of this race) prevented the entry of the merozoites of *P. vivax*. Presumably the sporozoites of *P. vivax* are able to develop normally in the liver, but no invasion of the blood is possible. Unfortunately this phenomenon does not offer any lead to another, novel method of malaria control.

## 2. *Plasmodium ovale*

As mentioned above, this species exhibits certain differences from the *P. vivax* group and, in various ways, it has inexplicable characters, of which the following have some bearing on the life cycle:

1. The sporogonic and exoerythrocytic cycle are longer and the tissue stages larger.
2. Relapses are remarkable in that the number of merozoites in the erythrocytic schizont are doubled.
3. The rarity of infections seems almost incompatible with the scattered distribution – in Africa, New Guinea, and elsewhere. It is difficult to account for its survival, in spite of its possession of a true relapse mechanism.

## 3. *Plasmodium falciparum*

This example of the subgenus *Laverania* and its close relative, *P.* (*L.*) *reichenowi* in African apes, is unique in its possession of crescentic gametocytes with perinuclear pigment, which take a long time (about 10 days) to grow. It is nearly as fatal to man as *P. knowlesi* is to rhesus monkeys, *P. berghei* to mice, *P. elongatum* to canaries, and *P. floridense* to some species of lizards.

The erythrocytic cycle is peculiar in that half (or rather more) of it takes place in the peripheral blood and that half (or slightly less) is confined to the internal organs, where schizogony occurs. Thus the pigmented solid forms and schizonts are rarely seen in the peripheral blood. The same phenomenon is exhibited in the ape counterpart (*P. reichenowi*) but, in both man and ape, removal of the spleen causes a profound change. Schizogony now fulminates in the peripheral blood and may prove fatal, though this is not invariable even in man (see GARNHAM 1966).

Pernicious malaria in man is a dreaded effect of the infection due to the blockage of the internal capillaries by schizonts. Another sequela peculiar to *P. falciparum* is blackwater fever, in people sensitive to quinine after inadequate treatment (see also Chap. 5).

Various genetic conditions influence the life cycle of *P. falciparum*. Asexual multiplication of the parasite is partially inhibited by the presence of the haemoglobin S gene and to a lesser extent by a genetic deficiency of the enzyme glucose-6-phosphate dehydrogenase. A biological advantage operates for the heterozygotes of these traits in the human host. The Duffy blood group negative genotype is, however, not a factor in *P. falciparum* infection as was shown clearly in Central America, where SPENCER et al. (1978) showed that there was an equal distribution of *P. falciparum* between Duffy-negative and Duffy-positive individuals, whereas the only *P. vivax* infections (14) occurred in Duffy-positive cases (see also Chaps. 2, 4, 15).

## 4. *Plasmodium malariae* (*P. rodhaini syn.*) and *Plasmodium brasilianum*

These two quartan parasites of man (and chimpanzees) and New World monkeys respectively are considered together as they probably should all receive the same name, *P. malariae*. The synonymisation of *P. rodhaini* is now fully recognised and there is good evidence that *P. brasilianum*, the common malaria parasite of Latin American monkeys, is an example of a zoonosis in reverse (GARNHAM 1967), the human *P. malariae* having spread in the monkey population after the arrival of conquistadores or slaves in the early seventeenth century. Isoenzyme analysis of the respective strains could establish this theory.

The life cycle of *P. malariae* continues to cause controversy. Most British and American workers consider that no "true relapses" occur in this and other quartan strains. Instead, the very long course of infections is the result of recrudescences. The main evidence for this statement is as follows:

1. The parasites can be eradicated by blood schizontocides alone.
2. After the primary exoerythrocytic cycle in the liver no secondary tissue forms have been found.
3. Parasites persist in the blood for many years, even after blood inoculation (as in transfusion malaria), and there are no negative periods.
4. The above characters have all been demonstrated in *P. malariae*, *P. brasilianum*, and *P inui*.

It follows that if this evidence is acceptable, there is no need to administer a drug such as primaquine in addition to a full course of chloroquine or similar medicament, in order to produce a "radical cure."

## II. Rodent Malaria Parasites

The striking differences between these species of malaria parasites and those occurring in primates have been mentioned above (Sect. C.I). Three features deserve separate consideration in relation to the life cycle:

a) Effect of Temperature on Sporogony

Attempts at transmission of *P. berghei* were unsuccessful until YOELI (1965) investigated the natural conditions in the gallery forests of the High Katanga in Zaïre. He noticed at once that the ambient temperature was low and, on his return to New York, he dropped the temperature of his insectary from 25°–27 °C to 18 °C or 20 °C and achieved success. Above this latter temperature the sporozoites did not form or lost their viability. *P. vinckei* behaves in the same way, but most of the other species and subspecies undergo optimum sporogony at about 24 °C.

b) Relapses

Exoerythrocytic schizonts (of abnormal morphology) of *P. yoelii* have been found (LANDAU and BOULARD 1978) in the liver of *Thamnomys* up to 8 months after capture and maintenance in the laboratory in Paris. Moreover, relapses of parasitaemia occurred for 9 months after sporozoite inoculation with fluctuating negative intervals. LANDAU was also able to induce slow growth of the tissue forms after certain drugs, starvation or lowering of body temperature. The significance of this work and its relation to primate malaria is doubtful.

c) Absence of micropore at sporozoite stage

This organelle is a constant feature of all members of the Apicomplexa. It is present in the blood stages of the rodent species, but uniquely absent in the sporozoite stages (SINDEN and GARNHAM 1973). It is suggested that such sporozoites in the salivary glands may be at an incomplete stage of development and that residence in the Kupffer cells is necessary for the organelle to become differentiated and to allow exoerythrocytic schizogony to proceed in the parenchyma.

### III. *Hepatocystis kochi* (Syn. *Plasmodium kochi*)

The inclusion in this chapter of a haemoproteid parasite of African monkeys is justified for this reason: firstly, only gametocytes are produced in the blood and studies on gametocytocidal drugs could be facilitated by the use of such animals. Secondly, exoerythrocytic schizogony in the liver is macroscopic in the mature stages (merocysts measuring 2 mm) and could be observed easily in life.

The early liver stages resemble exoerythrocytic schizogony in mammalian malaria, as they develop in hepatocytes. The sporozoites initiate the infection through the bite of the vectors, various species of *Culicoides* (GARNHAM 1966).

The subject of other haemoproteids and members of the Leucocytozoidae is beyond the scope of this book, but various species have been used as models for human malaria in the past and studies of their life cycles may still provide clues to puzzles yet unsolved.

## E. Abnormal Modes of Transmission

The descriptions of sporogony in the foregoing sections suffice to indicate the part played by mosquito vectors in the life cycle of malaria parasites. These provide the normal routes, but occasionally in both human and animal malaria special instances occur and these include I, via the blood; II, involving an animal reservoir (zoonoses); and III, in abnormal hosts. They are briefly described below.

### I. Infection from a Blood Source

These include the following, not infrequent, examples, and they are all characterised by certain common features. As the sporozoite is not involved, relapses will be absent and cure should be easy with blood schizontocides (with one exception – see below). For the same reason, the attack will be preceded by no (biological) prepatent period and will merely depend upon the number of parasites introduced. In a heavily infected inoculum, the incubation could be practically non-existent or, if parasites are very scanty as after some blood transfusions, symptoms may not appear for weeks. In any such events, the infection may well arise in a non-endemic region, the eventual disease may not be recognised at once and the patient may die untreated.

#### a) Congenital Malaria

Congenital malaria arises in the infant from an infected mother, either transplacentally or during parturition. The former may be distinguished because parasites are visible in the baby's blood at birth and gametocytes may be present. In the latter, parasitaemia is not seen for 2 weeks or so and gametocytes will probably be absent. Attempts to induce congenital malaria in experimental animals have usually failed, although it occurs in all four species in man. In view of the excessive multiplication of *P. falciparum* in the human placenta (GARNHAM 1938; BRAY and SINDEN 1979) it is surprising that congenital malaria is so uncommon.

#### b) Transfusion Malaria

Transfusion malaria represents a danger both for the victim and for the community, because the infection may spread in a country from which it had been eradicated. This is especially so in countries like Rumania or S. Russia where quartan malaria probably still exists.

c) Malaria in Drug Addicts

This usually local condition was especially prevalent in the United States, when MOST (1940) vividly described how the infection is transmitted. The administration of heroin formed part of a social gathering in which the drug in a syringe was passed round without changing the needle so that, if one of the addicts was circulating parasites, they inevitably infected the subsequent members by its intravenous passage. In the twilight lives of these people fever passed unnoticed, and many of them died before receiving medical attention. Outbreaks of this sort are not uncommon when soldiers return from war campaigns with malaria and drug addiction.

d) Cannibalism

An unusual form of transmission occurs to an unknown extent in animals from *cannibalism*, when the parasites become transmitted by the mouth.

## II. Transmission from an Animal Reservoir

The susceptibility of man to a number of simian or ape parasites renders him a possible victim of "monkey malaria" in nature, and it is surprising how few cases have been reported. There appear to have been only four, three from Malaya (*P. knowlesi*) and one from Brazil (*P. simium*). Eight species have been shown to infect man experimentally (in volunteers) and laboratory infections of *P. cynomolgi* are known. Since deliberate surveys in enzootic areas have been completely negative, it is apparent that malaria as a zoonosis for man is rare.

On the contrary, the "veterinary zoonosis" is well known. *P. gallinaceum* of the jungle fowl gives rise to serious epizootics in domestic chickens, *P. juxtanucleare* is equally fatal to chickens from a feral source and *P. durae* kills turkeys in Kenya, the reservoir being the francolin.

A notable feature of monkey malaria in man is low parasitaemia and the mildness of the symptoms. If, however, the infection (*P. knowlesi*) is used in repeated blood passage in malaria therapy, it may become very severe.

## III. Life Cycle in Abnormal Hosts

Usually malaria parasites are fairly host specific and the only way to establish, for instance, a human species in an ape, is to splenectomise the animal, when the infection fulminates. However, in recent years monkeys of various species have been used with increasing success. CADIGAN et al. (1969) showed that the gibbon is highly susceptible to *P. falciparum*, while YOUNG et al. (1966) showed that *Aotus trivirgatus* takes *P. vivax* easily. Later the subspecies *griseimembra* of this monkey was shown also to be susceptible to *P. falciparum* and *P. malariae*. Other Latin American monkeys made less efficient hosts. The *Aotus* or owl monkey seems to be the most suitable animal, for it is able to produce viable gametocytes and the complete life cycle of several parasites can occur (though the exoerythrocytic stages in the liver are abnormal). SCHMIDT (1978) described in great detail the course of untreated *P. falciparum* and *P. vivax* in the blood of this animal, while COLLINS et al. (1981) have recently summarised a most extensive series of researches on human and monkey malaria parasites in splenectomised *Aotus trivirgatus* (*P. falciparum*, *P. vivax*, *P. fragile*, *P. knowlesi*, and *P. cynomolgi*) (see also Chap. 9).

Possibly the most surprising results in this field come from China, where JING-BO-JIANG et al. (1978) succeeded, by a novel device, in establishing the blood cycle of *P. falciparum* in rhesus monkeys after transfusing these animals with large quantities of human blood. Repeated passage of the parasite in monkeys, similarly transfused, resulted in heavy and sometimes fatal infections, with 46% parasitaemia.

## References


Aikawa M (1971) *Plasmodium:* The fine structure of malarial parasites. Exp Parasitol 30:284–320

Aikawa M, Seed TM (1980) Morphology of Plasmodia. In: Kreier JP (ed) Malaria vol 1. Academic, New York, pp 285–344

Ayala SC (1970a) Lizard malaria in California; description of a strain of *Plasmodium mexicanum*, and biogeography of lizard malaria in western North America. J Parasitol 56:417–425

Ayala SC (1970b) *Plasmodium mexicanum* in California: natural history and development in Phlebotomine sandflies (Diptera: Psychodidae). J Parasitol 56:13

Bennett GF, Eyles DE, Warren M, Cheong WH (1963) *Plasmodium juxtanucleare.* A newly discovered parasite of domestic fowl in Malaya. Singapore Med J 4:172–173

Bray RS, Sinden RE (1979) The sequestration of *Plasmodium falciparum* infected erythrocytes in the placenta. Trans R Soc Trop Med Hyg 73:716–719

Cadigan F, Ward RA, Chaicumpa V (1969) Further studies on malarial parasites in gibbons from Thailand. Milit Med 134:757–766

Carter R, Miller LH (1979) Evidence for environmental modulation of gametocytogenesis in *Plasmodium falciparum* in continuous culture. Bull WHO 57:37–52

Coatney JR, Collins WE, Warren M, Contacos PG (1971) The primate malarias. US Department Health, Education and Welfare, Bethesda

Collins WE, Aikawa M (1977) Plasmodia of non-human primates. In: Kreier JP (ed) Parasitic protozoa, vol 3. Academic, New York, pp 467–492

Collins WE, Contacos PG (1974) Observations on the relapse activity of *Plasmodium simiovale* in the rhesus monkey. J Parasitol 60:343

Collins WE, Contacos PG, Skinner JC, Stanfill PG, Richardson BB (1981) Susceptibility of Peruvian *Aotus* monkeys to infection with different species of *Plasmodium.* Am J Trop Med Hyg 30:26–30

Corradetti A, Neri I, Scanga M, Cavallini C (1968) I cicli pre-eritrocitico e sporogonico di *Plasmodium (Huffia) elongatum.* Parassitologia 10:133–143

Daher VR, Krettli AV (1980) Infectivity of *Plasmodium gallinaceum* sporozoites from oocysts. J Protozool 27:440–442

Danforth HD, Aikawa M, Cochrane AH, Nussenzweig RS (1980) Sporozoites of mammalian malaria: attachment to, interiorization, and fate within macrophages. J Protozool 27:193–202

Desser S, Fallis M, Garnham PCC (1968) Observations on relapse in ducks infected with *Leucocytozoon simondi* and *Parahaemoproteus nettionis.* Can J Zool 42:281–285

Freyvogel TA, Stäubli W (1966) Shape, movement *in situ*, and locomotion of *Plasmodium* ookinetes. Acta Trop (Basel) 23:201–222

Gabaldon A, Ulloa G (1980) Holoendemicity of malaria; an avian model. Trans R Soc Trop Med Hyg 74:501–507

Gabaldon A, Ulloa G, Godoz N, Marquez E, Pulido J (1977) *Aedomyia squamipennis* vector natural de malaria aviaria en Venezuela. Bol Dir Malariol San Amb 17:9–13

Galucci BB (1974) Fine structure of *Haemoproteus columbae* Kruse during macrogametogenesis and fertilisation. J Protozool 21:254–263

Garnham PCC (1938) The placenta in malaria with special reference to reticulo-endothelial immunity. Trans R Soc Trop Med Hyg 32:13–48

Garnham PCC (1966) Malaria parasites and other haemosporidia. Blackwell, London

Garnham PCC (1967) Malaria in mammals excluding man. Adv Parasitol 5:139–204

Garnham PCC (1970) Longevity of malaria parasites in man and its epidemiological significance. In: Ministry of Health, Georgian SSR (ed) Festschrift for Murashvili. Tbilisi, Georgia SSR, pp 71–78

Garnham PCC (1980) Malaria in its various vertebrate hosts. In: Kreier JP (ed) vol 1. Malaria Academic, New York, pp 95–144

Garnham PCC, Lainson R, Cooper W (1958) The complete life cycle of a new strain of *Plasmodium gonderi* from the drill (*Mandrillus leucophaeus*) including its sporogony in *Anopheles aztecus* and its pre-erythrocytic schizogony in the rhesus monkey. Trans R Soc Trop Med Hyg 52:509–517

Garnham PCC, Bird RG, Baker JR (1962) Electron microscope studies of motile stages of malaria parasites III: the ookinetes of *Haemamoeba* and *Plasmodium*. Trans R Soc Trop Med Hyg 56:116–120

Garnham PCC, Bird RG, Baker JR, Desser SS, El-Nahal HMS (1969) Electron microscope studies of motile stages of malaria parasites VI: the ookinete of *Plasmodium berghei yoelii* and its transformation into the early oocyst. Trans R Soc Trop Med Hyg 63:187–194

Garnham PCC, Bray RS, Bruce-Chwatt LJ, Draper CC, Killick-Kendrick R, Sergiev PG, Tiburskaya NA, Shute PG, Maryon M (1975) A strain of *Plasmodium vivax* characterised by long incubation. Bull WHO 52:21–30

Gillett JD (1971) Mosquitoes. Weidenfeld and Nicolson, London

Guazzi M, Grazi S (1963) Considerazionne su un caso de malaria quartana recidivante dopo 53 anni di latenza. Riv Malariol 42:55–59

Hawking F, Worms MJ, Gammage K (1966) The biological purpose of the blood cycles of the malaria parasite *Plasmodium cynomolgi*. Lancet 2:422–424

Hollingdale MR, Leef JL, McCullough M, Beaudoin RL (1981) *In vitro* cultivation of *Plasmodium berghei* and from sporozoites. Science 213:1021–1022

Huff CG (1947) Life cycle of malarial parasites. Ann Rev Microbiol 1:43–58

Huff CG (1969) Exoerythrocytic stages of avian and reptilian malarial parasites. Exp Parasitol 24:383–421

Huff CG, Coulston F (1944) The development of *Plasmodium gallinaceum* from sporozoite to erythrocytic trophozoite. J Infect Dis 75:231–249

James SP, Tate P (1937) New knowledge of the life cycle of malaria parasites. Nature 193:545

Jingbo-Jiang, Long Z, Zou J (1978) The successive passage and heavy infections of *Plasmodium falciparum* in the two species of macaques, the blood of which has been partly replaced by human blood (in Chinese with English summary). Acta Sci Nat Sunyatsen University, 52:5–15

Jordan H (1964) Lizard malaria in Georgia. J Protozool 11:52–56

Killick-Kendrick R (1973) Parasitic protozoa in the blood of rodents 1: the life-cycle and zoogeography of *Plasmodium berghei nigeriensis* sub. sp. nov. Ann Trop Med Parasitol 67:261–277

Killick-Kendrick R (1978) Taxonomy, zoogeography, and evolution. In: Killick-Kendrick R, Peters W (eds) Rodent malaria. Academic, London, pp 1–52

Killick-Kendrick R, Warren M (1968) Primary exoerythrocytic schizonts of a mammalian *Plasmodium* as a source of gametocytes. Nature 220:191–192

Krotoski WA, Krotoski DM, Garnham PCC, Bray RS, Killick-Kendrick R, Draper CC, Targett GAT, Guy MW (1980) Relapses in primate malaria: discovery of two populations of exoerythrocytic stages. Preliminary note. Br Med J 1:153–154

Krotoski WA, Bray RS, Garnham PCC, Gwadz RW, Killick-Kendrick R, Draper CC, Targett GAT, Krotoski DM, Guy MW, Koontz LC, Cogswell FB (1982) Observations on early and late post-sporozoite tissue stages in primate malaria. II. The hypnozoite of *Plasmodium cynomolgi bastianellii* from 3 to 105 days after infection, and detection of 36- to 30-hour pre-erythrocytic forms. Am J Trop Med Hyg 31:211–225

Lainson R, Shaw JJ, Landau I (1975) Some blood parasites of the Brazilian lizards *Plica-umbra* and *Uranoscodon superciliosa* (Iguanidae). Parasitology 70:119–141

Landau I, Boulard Y (1978) Life cycles and morphology. In: Killick-Kendrick R, Peters W (eds) Rodent malaria. Academic, London, pp 53–84

Laveran A (1881) Description d'un nouveau parasite découvert dans le sang des malades atteints de fièvre palustre. C R Séances Acad Sci 93:627–630

Markus MB (1976) Possible support for the sporozoite hypothesis of relapse and latency in malaria. Trans R Soc Trop Med Hyg 70:535

Mattingly PF (1969) The biology of mosquito-borne disease. Allen and Unwin, London

Mehlhorn H, Peters W, Haberkorn A (1980) The formation of kinetes and oocyst in *Plasmodium gallinaceum* (Haemosporidia), and considerations on phylogenetic relationships between Haemosporidia, Piroplasmida, and other Coccidia. Protistologica 16:135–154

Meis JFG, Verhave JP, Jap PHK, Meuwissen JHT (1983) An ultrastructural study of the role of Kupffer cells in the process of infection by *Plasmodium berghei* in rats. Parasitology 86:231–242

Miller LH, Mason SJ, Clyde DF, McGinniss MA (1976) The resistance factor to *Plasmodium vivax* in blacks. The Duffy blood group genotype FyFy. N Engl J Med 295:302–304

Most H (1940) Malignant malaria among drug addicts. Epidemiological, clinical, and laboratory studies. Trans R Soc Trop Med Hyg 34:139–172

Nayar JK, Joung MD, Forrester DJ (1980) *Wyeomyia vanduzeei* an experimental host for wild turkey malaria. J Parasitol 66:166–167

Nye A (1961) Temperature studies on chicks infected with *Plasmodium gallinaceum* (Brumpt, 1935) including some effects of cooling host and parasite. Expl Parasitol 11:77–89

O'Rourke FJ (1956) Observations on pool and capillary feeding in *Aedes aegypti* (L.). Nature 177:1087–1088

Pelaez D, Perez-Reyes R (1952) Estudios sobre hematozoarios. III. Las especies Americanos del genero *Plasmodium* en reptiles. Rev Palud Med Trop 4:137–160

Petit G, Landau I, Boulard Y, Gomes A, Touratier L (1984) Sporogonie de *Plasmodium agamae* chez *Culicoides nubeculosus* au laboratoire: 1. Expérimentation et déscription du cycle. Protistologica (in press)

Raffaele G (1934) Un ceppo italiano di *P. elongatum*. Riv Malariol 1:332–337

Raffaele G (1936) Il doppio ciclo schizogonico di *Plasmodium elongatum*. Riv Malariol 5:309–317

Schmidt LH (1978) *Plasmodium falciparum* and *Plasmodium vivax* infections in the owl monkey (*Aotus trivirgatus*). Am J Trop Med Hyg 27:671–702

Sergent E (1963) Latent infections and premunition. Some definitions of microbiology and immunology. In: Garnham PCC, Pierce AE, Roit A (eds) Immunity to protozoa. Blackwell, Oxford, pp 39–47

Shortt HE, Garnham PCC (1948) Demonstration of a persisting exoerythrocytic cycle in *Plasmodium cynomolgi* and its bearing on the production of relapses. Br Med J 1:1225–1228

Shute PG (1944) Relapse of quartan malaria after 12 and 21 years. Lancet 2:146

Shute PG (1945) An investigation into the number of sporozoites found in the salivary glands of *Anopheles* mosquitoes. Trans R Soc Trop Med Hyg 38:493–498

Shute PG, Lupascu G, Branzei P, Maryon M, Constantinescu P, Bruce-Chwatt LJ, Draper CC, Killick-Kendrick R, Garnham PCC (1946) A strain of *Plasmodium vivax* characterised by predominantly prolonged incubation: the effect of numbers of sporozoites on the length of the prepatent period. Trans R Soc Trop Med Hyg 70:474–481

Sinden RE (1975) The sporogonic cycle of *Plasmodium yoelii nigeriensis*. A scanning electron microscope study. Protistologica 11:31–39

Sinden RE (1978) Cell biology. In: Killick-Kendrick R, Peters W (eds) Rodent malaria. Academic, London, pp 85–168
Sinden RE (1981) Sexual development of malarial parasites in their mosquito vectors. Trans R Soc Trop Med Hyg 75:171–172
Sinden RE, Garnham PCC (1973) A comparative study on the ultrastructure of *Plasmodium* sporozoites within the oocyst and salivary glands, with particular reference to the incidence of the micropore. Trans R Soc Trop Med Hyg 67:631–637
Smith JE, Sinden RE, Beadle J, Hartley R (1981) The effect of silica treatment on the uptake and infectivity of *Plasmodium yoelii* sporozoites *in vivo* and *in vivo*. Trans R Soc Trop Med Hyg 75
Spencer AC, Miller LH, Collins WE, Hansen CK, McGinnis MH, Shiroishi T, Lobos RA, Feldman RA (1978) The Duffy blood group and resistance to *Plasmodium vivax* in Honduras. Am J Trop Med Hyg 27:664–670
Spitler DL (1948) Malaria relapse. Report of a case 36 years after original infection. N Engl Med J 2:38–39
Strome CPA, De Santis PL, Beaudoin RL (1979) The cultivation of the exoerythrocytic stages of *Plasmodium berghei* from sporozoites. In Vitro 15:531–536
Telford SR Jr (1973) Saurian malarial parasites from Guyana: their effect upon the validity of the family Garniidae and the genus *Garnia*, with descriptions of two new species. Int J Parasitol 3:829–842
Telford SR Jr (1977) The distribution, incidence, and general ecology of saurian malaria in Middle America. Int J Parasitol 7:299–314
Vanderberg JP (1975) Development of infectivity by the *Plasmodium berghei* sporozoite. J Parasitol 61:43–50
Verhave JP, Meuwissen T, Golensen J (1980) The dual role of macrophages in the sporozoite-induced malaria infection. A hypothesis. Int J Nucl Med Biol 7:149–156
Vincke IH, Lips M (1948) Un nouveau *Plasmodium* d'un rongeur sauvage du Congo, *Plasmodium berghei* n. sp. Ann Soc Belg Méd Trop 28:97–104
WHO (1963) Terminology of malaria and of malaria eradication. WHO, Geneva
Yoeli M (1965) Studies on *Plasmodium berghei* in nature and under experimental conditions. Trans R Soc Trop Med Hyg 59:255–276
Young DG (1977) PhD Thesis, University of Florida 1977
Young MD, Porter JA, Johnson MA (1966) *Plasmodium vivax* transmitted from man to monkey to man. Science 153:1006–1007

CHAPTER 2

# Metabolism

I. W. SHERMAN

## A. Introduction

The metabolism of *Plasmodium* has been under study for 4 decades, and periodically the accumulated literature has been reviewed (FULTON 1951; MCKEE 1951; FULTON and SPOONER 1955; MOULDER 1962; HONIGBERG 1967; PETERS 1969; FLETCHER and MAEGRAITH 1972; TRAGER 1970; OELSHLEGEL and BREWER 1975; HOMEWOOD 1978; SHERMAN 1979). The present chapter is designed to provide an introduction to the metabolic capabilities of malarial parasites; where possible, biochemical features that could provide insights into the mechanisms of drug action are emphasised.

## B. Biochemical Determinants of Parasite Specificity for the Host Cell

The invasion of a red cell by a malarial merozoite follows a definite sequence: the merozoite attaches, there is widespread deformation of the erythrocyte, a junction forms between the merozoite and red cell, the erythrocyte membrane invaginates to internalise the merozoite and then reseals after parasite entry has been completed. In the 1950 s MCGHEE (1953) showed that the merozoites of *P. lophurae* not only recognised different kinds of red blood cells, but that they preferentially invaded a particular erythrocyte. However, it was not clear from his experiments by what means the parasite was able to select a particular kind of red cell.

To clarify the nature of the red cell receptor MILLER and his colleagues treated human erythrocytes with a variety of enzymes and then subjected these to invasion by *P. knowlesi* merozoites (reviewed in MILLER 1977). Chymotrypsin and pronase blocked invasion, whereas trypsin and neuraminidase were without effect. The results suggested that the receptor on the human red cell for the *knowlesi* merozoite was a glycoprotein. Later, they (MASON et al. 1977) showed that Duffy blood group negative human erythrocytes were refractory to invasion by *P. knowlesi* merozoites. If Duffy-positive erythrocytes were treated with chymotrypsin the cells resisted invasion. MILLER (1977) suggested that there may be two *knowlesi* receptors on the human red cell. One receptor (chymotrypsin sensitive) is unrelated to the Duffy determinants $Fy^a/Fy^b$, whereas another receptor appears to play a role in junction formation. Indeed, although *knowlesi* merozoites treated with cytochalasin B did attach to Duffy-positive cells, invasion did not take place (MILLER et al. 1979). Moreover, cytochalasin B-treated merozoites did attach to Duffy-negative cells but no junction formed; consequently, parasite entry did not occur.

Thus, the Duffy-associated determinants seem to play a role in junction formation, but apparently are not involved in the initial attachment of the merozoite.

The prevalence of the Duffy-negative phenotype is extremely high in West Africa, where resistance to vivax malaria is also high. Based on this and other considerations MILLER postulated that Duffy factor might be involved in the susceptibility of human erythrocytes to *P. vivax* (MILLER et al. 1978). To test this postulate, 11 American blacks who had previously been exposed to *P. vivax*-infected mosquitoes were typed. The five Duffy negatives were resistant, whereas the six Duffy positives became infected. Thus, the available evidence tends to support the hypothesis that the Duffy-negative phenotype acts as a basis for resistance to vivax malaria. The chemical nature of the Duffy blood group receptor and how it specifically interacts with the merozoites of *P. vivax* and *P. knowlesi* is unknown. However, based on susceptibility studies of various erythrocytes, it appears that the red cell receptors for the two species of malaria are similar, but not identical. Since West Africans who are refractory to vivax malaria are susceptible to other human malarias, MILLER suggested that these other malaria species might have different erythrocyte receptors. Indeed, human red cells lacking Duffy and other blood group determinants were invaded by *P. falciparum* merozoites. Trypsin treatment of human red cells reduced their susceptibility for *P. falciparum*, but not *P. knowlesi* merozoites; conversely, chymotrypsin blocked *P. knowlesi* invasion but did not influence susceptibility to *P. falciparum* (MILLER 1977). Thus, the *P. knowlesi* (and probably the *P. vivax*) and *P. falciparum* receptors on the human red-cell surface differ from one another.

MILLER (1977) speculated that successful invasion of the red-cell involves two steps. First, the merozoite must react with a specific peptide or carbohydrate moiety on the red-cell surface; this provides for merozoite attachment. Second, reaction with another peptide must then occur; this triggers red-cell endocytosis with internalisation of the parasite. The widespread deformation of the erythrocyte, radiating from the point at which the merozoite makes contact, suggests that the merozoite releases material(s) which act(s) on the host cell membrane. This may be released from organelles at the merozoite's apical end and could induce red cell endocytosis, thus permitting merozoite entry into the host cell.

The end result of merozoite invasion is that the parasite is enclosed by a parasitophorous vacuolar membrane (PVM). The PVM is retained throughout the entire intraerythrocytic developmental cycle (LANGRETH and TRAGER 1973). The nature of the PVM has received considerable attention. Although its origins are erythrocytic it appears to come under the control of the growing parasite. This is not unexpected. The PVM increases in size as the parasite's volume expands; consequently, it must either stretch or be added to. Although small parasites showed a localisation of ATPase in the PVM that was typical of an invaginated red-cell membrane, as the parasite grew there was a reorientation of ATPase in the membrane. Similarly, NADH oxidase, an enzyme localised on the outer surface of the red cell, was not found on the inner surface of the PVM (as it would if it were simply an invaginated red cell membrane), but on the PVM's outer surface (LANGRETH 1977). STERLING (unpublished) has suggested that spectrin is absent from the PVM, which again suggests erythrocyte membrane modification. Furthermore, studies with cationised ferritin (TAKAHASHI and SHERMAN 1978), ferritin-conjugated lectins

(TAKAHASHI and SHERMAN 1980) and freeze-fracture (MCLAREN et al. 1977, 1979) techniques show that the PVM is dynamically altered by the parasite. How such alterations are induced, and by what mechanisms, remain unknown.

## C. Membrane Proteins of the Infected Erythrocyte

Some species such as *P. falciparum* and *P. malariae* induce electron-dense elevations or excrescences on the surface of the cells they infect (AIKAWA 1977). These knobs, as they are commonly referred to, appear to be underneath the erythrocyte membrane. The erythrocytic knobs tend to increase in number as the parasite grows. Some *P. falciparum* strains are better knob inducers than are others, and the knobs may be lost during prolonged in vitro culture (LANGRETH et al. 1979). As the intraerythrocytic parasite grows the knobs obscure the red-cell membrane, bizarre extensions may form and some of these appear to be sloughed from the surface of the erythrocyte. The knobs on the surface of erythrocytes infected with falciparum-type malarias, it has been claimed, contain a parasite-synthesised glycoprotein with a molecular weight of 80000 and homologous with the histidine-rich protein isolated from *P. lophurae* (KILEJIAN 1979, 1980). How such parasite materials become incorporated into the knobs has still not been determined.

Erythrocytes infected with ovale- and vivax-type malarias when examined with the electron microscope show many small invaginations (=caveolae) which are surrounded by small vesicles. The number of caveolae is correlated with the size of the parasite, cells with larger parasites usually having more. The caveolae are equivalent to Schüffner's dots (AIKAWA 1977). The caveolae-vesicle complex may be involved in micropinocytosis and could contribute to the enlargement of the ovale-vivax-infected cell.

In the rodent malarias *P. berghei* and *P. chabaudi* WEIDEKAMM et al. (1973) and KÖNIGK and MIRTSCH (1977) demonstrated a decrease in the staining of spectrin (bands 1 and 2), band 4 and PAS-1. Concomitantly with such reductions, bands 7, 8, and PAS-2 increased, and some new bands appeared (2a and $PAS_i$). The unique band, $PAS_i$ with a molecular weight of ~165000, was reported to be present in red cells infected with *P. berghei*, *P. yoelii* YM, *P. vinckei*, and *P. chabaudi* (YUTHAVONG et al. 1979). However, in some strains of *P. yoelii* (17x and 33x) such a distinct band did not appear, and instead there were several weak bands in the molecular weight range of 120000–200000. WEIDEKAMM et al. (1973) suggested that the decreased amounts of spectrin could be due to degradation by proteolysis and this would contribute to band 2a and the increased intensities of bands 7 and 8. Additionally, breakdown of band 4 could also intensify band 7 and 8. YUTHAVONG et al. (1979) tested this hypothesis by incubating normal mouse red-cell membranes with lyophilised preparations of *P. berghei*, and although there was degradation of spectrin no new bands of ~150000 molecular weight were evident. CHAIMANEE and YUTHAVONG (1979) showed the presence of a phosphorylated membrane protein with a molecular weight of 42000 to be present only in *P. berghei*-infected cells. The significance of this finding is obscure.

EISEN (1977) could not find a decrease in the total amount of spectrin in *P. chabaudi*-infected erythrocytes, and did not detect glycophorin in such cells. This is correlated with the report of TRIGG et al. (1977), where a decrease in the labelling (by galactose oxidase/tritiated borohydride after pretreatment of cells with neuraminidase) of band 3 in *P. knowlesi*-infected monkey erythrocytes was described. WALLACH and CONLEY (1977) found a decrease in PAS-1 and the iodinatable component of band 5 (50000 mol. wt.) in *P. knowlesi*-infected cells, new Coomassie blue staining bands (120000–200000 mol. wt.), and a parasite-specific glycoprotein (PAS-1p, 125000 mol. wt.). Band 2 decreased while band 4 increased. SHAKESPEARE et al. (1979a) confirmed the presence of three iodinatable membrane proteins in normal and infected monkey erythrocytes, but found no evidence for new radioactive peaks, and described a reduced iodinatability of *P. knowlesi*-infected cells. Additionally, these workers found that the *P. knowlesi*-infected red cell had about one-half the number of binding sites for concanavalin A as did the uninfected cell. Recently, SCHMIDT-ULLRICH and co-workers (1979, 1980) reported that at least three proteins (55000–90000 daltons) occurred in the membranes of erythrocytes bearing *P. knowlesi*, but these proteins were not found in parasites or normal red cells. By contrast, DEANS et al. (1978) found relatively few *P. knowlesi* antigens in infected red-cell membranes, and all of these were present in the intracellular parasite.

Modifications in the membranes of the duck red blood cell during infection with *P. lophurae* have been studied (SHERMAN and JONES 1979). Membrane vesicles prepared from normal duckling erythrocytes contained 79 nmol sialic acid/mg membrane protein, whereas those derived from infected cells had approximately half this amount. Furthermore, the iodinatability of infected red-cell membranes was reduced. When the Coomassie blue stained gel patterns of infected red-cell membranes from duckling erythrocytes bearing trophozoites or schizonts were compared with normal membranes, a reduction in bands 1, 2, and 3 and an intensification of bands 4–7 were observed. No new bands were found.

How do these changes in the host cell membranes come about? Modifications in band intensity, reduction in iodinatability and diminished sialic acid content could be due to the action of plasmodial enzymes, as well as changes in the lipid milieu of the membrane. Thus it is conceivable that the intracellular release of plasmodial proteases degrades some inner surface proteins such as spectrin and actin as well as proteins that span the entire red-cell membrane. As a consequence, the cytoskeletal framework of the erythrocyte is altered. Such alterations could also serve to modify the accessibility of outer surface proteins to reagents commonly employed for tagging the external surface of cells. Here it is of some interest to note that FITCH et al. (1978) found that treatment of normal mouse red cells with *Streptomyces griseus* protease induced a pattern of chloroquine accumulation resembling that found in chloroquine-sensitive malaria. Presumably, protease treatment exposed cryptic chloroquine-binding sites.

In malarias such as *P. knowlesi* and *P. falciparum* and in several species of rodent malaria plasmodial proteins appear to be introduced into the surface of the red cell. These so-called "neoproteins" could modify the antigenicity of the infected red cell, and may affect its function. The manner by which such proteins move to the red-cell surface, and how they are intercalated, remains unresolved.

# D. Plasmodial Membrane Proteins

Studies of plasmodial membranes are restricted to *P. lophurae*, *P. berghei*, and *P. knowlesi*.

*P. lophurae* can be removed from the red cell by treating infected red cells with a haemolytic antiserum prepared in rabbits followed by trypsin and DNase (TRAGER et al. 1972). Free *P. lophurae* were not agglutinated by lectins, nor was there evidence for the binding of ferritin-conjugated lectins to the surface of the parasitophorous vacuolar membrane (PVM) or parasite plasma membrane (PPM). An exception to this was the occasional binding of concanavalin A (con A) (TAKAHASHI and SHERMAN 1980). Similarly, SEED and KREIER (1976) reported a stage-independent binding of con A-ferritin to erythrocyte-free *P. berghei*, and BANNISTER et al. (1977) could not agglutinate *P. knowlesi* merozoites with phytohaemagglutinin, wheat germ agglutinin, ricin, and con A, but occasionally some con A-ferritin binding was observed. Such results show that the PVM, although derived from the red cell by endocytosis, is changed. This is corroborated by cytochemical (LANGRETH 1977) and freeze-fracture observations (MCLAREN et al. 1977, 1979).

Membrane vesicles of *P. lophurae* were deficient in their ability to incorporate radioactive iodine using the lactoperoxidase/glucose oxidase method (SHERMAN and JONES 1979) and contained only ~8 nmol sialic acid/mg protein, about one-tenth the amount found for red-cell membrane vesicles. [Reduced amounts of sialic acid were also reported for *P. berghei* (SEED et al. 1973)]. Plasmodial membranes analysed by sodium dodecyl sulphate (SDS)-polyacrylamide gel electrophoresis were distinctly different from those of the host cell. They could not be stained with PAS and no spectrin bands were present (SHERMAN and JONES 1979). WALLACH and CONLEY (1977) reported similar findings for erythrocyte-free *P. knowlesi*.

# E. Lipids of Malaria-Infected Erythrocytes

In general, the total lipid content as well as the amounts of lipid in the various fractions of malaria-infected erythrocytes is higher than that found in normal erythrocytes. In *P. knowlesi*-infected red cells the total lipid content is three to five times greater than that of the uninfected red cell. Similar increases, but of smaller magnitude, were reported for *P. berghei*-infected rat red cells and *P. lophurae*-infected duckling cells (reviewed in HOLZ 1977) (Table 1). Most of the increases in the infected cell lipid can be attributed to the plasmodial membrane phospholipids. Although the total cholesterol content of an infected erythrocyte tends to increase, the ratio of cholesterol to phospholipid falls because the parasite lipids contain proportionally more phospholipid (Table 1), and the infected red-cell membrane tends to lose cholesterol. How this occurs is not understood.

The major phospholipids of the uninfected red cell are phosphatidylethanolamine and phosphatidylcholine, with lesser amounts of sphingomyelin and phosphatidylinositol. The parasite has increased amounts of phosphatidylethanolamine and phosphatidylinositol, and decreased quantities of sphingomyelin (Table 2). The most common fatty acids of the normal erythrocyte are palmitic (16:0), stearic

**Table 1.** Lipid contents of normal and infected erythrocytes and *Plasmodium*. Modified from HOLZ (1977) and SHERMAN (1979)

| | Total lipid | Phospholipid (P) | Cholesterol (C) | Ratio P/C |
|---|---|---|---|---|
| Monkey RBC | 3.5 | 2.1 | 1.1 | 2.0 |
| *P. knowlesi*-infected RBC | 17.0 | 13.2 | 2.4 | 5.5 |
| *P. knowlesi* | 4.5 | 2.5 | 0.7 | 3.5 |
| Duck RBC | 6.5 | 4.8 | 1.3 | 3.6 |
| *P. lophurae*-infected RBC | 13.2 | 10.8 | 1.58 | 6.0 |
| Rat RBC | 5.3 | 4.0 | 1.26 | 3 |
| *P. berghei*-infected RBC | 8–10 | 6.5 | 2.11 | 3 |
| *P. berghei* | 8–28 | – | – | – |

Values expressed as milligrams per $10^{10}$ cells

**Table 2.** Per cent distribution of total lipids in various phospholipid classes. Modified from HOLZ (1977)

| | PE | PS | PI | PC | SM | Lysolipids |
|---|---|---|---|---|---|---|
| Duck RBC | 20 | < 1 | 1 | 40 | 11 | 1 |
| *P. lophurae* | 36 | < 1 | 4 | 40 | 2 | < 1 |
| Monkey RBC | 19 | 7 | 2 | 22 | 9 | 2 |
| *P. knowlesi* | 27 | 1 | 5 | 29 | 2 | 1 |
| Rat RBC | 10 | 7 | 1 | 35 | 13 | 7 |
| *P. berghei* | 18 | 9 | 3 | 29 | 7 | 6 |

PE, phosphatidylethanolamine; PS, phosphatidylserine; PI, phosphatidylinositol; PC, phosphatidylcholine; SM, sphingomyelin

**Table 3.** Fatty acid composition (in %) of normal erythrocytes and *Plasmodium*. HOLZ (1977)

| Fatty acid | Duck erythrocytes | *Plasmodium lophurae* | Monkey erythrocytes | *Plasmodium knowlesi* | Rat erythrocytes | *Plasmodium berghei* |
|---|---|---|---|---|---|---|
| 14:0 | 1 | < 1 | 1 | < 1 | – | 2 |
| 16:0 | 24 | 26 | 22 | 34 | 24 | 42 |
| 16:1 | 1 | 2 | – | – | < 1 | 4 |
| 18:0 | 10 | 16 | 15 | 9 | 17 | 15 |
| 18:1 | 18 | 33 | 18 | 36 | 8 | 21 |
| 18:2 | 21 | 12 | 15 | 15 | 11 | 7 |
| 18:3 | 1 | 1 | 1 | 1 | – | 2 |
| 20:2 | 1 | < 1 | < 1 | 1 | – | – |
| 20:3 | 1 | 1 | 2 | < 1 | – | – |
| 20:4 | 10 | 3 | 17 | 2 | 31 | 5 |
| 20:5 | 1 | 1 | 2 | < 1 | – | – |
| 22:5 | 2 | 1 | 2 | < 1 | 2 | – |
| 22:6 | 7 | 3 | 2 | < 1 | – | – |

(18:0), oleic (18:1), linoleic (18:2), and arachidonic (20:4). Upon infection striking increases are observed in the saturated fatty acids palmitic acid and oleic acid, and this is correlated with the fatty acid composition of the parasite (Table 3). Linoleic acid and arachidonic acid decline in both the avian and mammalian malarias. Stearic acid declined in *P. knowlesi* and *P. berghei*, but increased in *P. lophurae*-infected cells (HOLZ 1977). The enhanced amount of 18:1 in the *P. lophurae*-infected erythrocyte is probably associated with the red-cell membrane itself. (This is derived from the fact that the alkoxy form of phosphatidylethanolamine is not present in the lipids of *P. lophurae* but does occur in substantial amounts in the red cell where the content of 18:1 fatty acids was increased.)

The increased amounts of 18:1 in the erythrocytes of infected animals could influence the properties of the infected red-cell membrane by altering the fluidity of the inner and outer leaflets of the phospholipid bilayer. A consequence of this could be conformational changes in membrane proteins with an effect on transport and other membrane functions. Cholesterol, by imposing restraints on the movement of the phospholipid hydrocarbon chains, tends to stabilise membrane fluidity. Therefore, a loss of cholesterol and an increase in the erythrocyte's membrane phospholipid/cholesterol ratio (Table 1) could be reflected in reduced active transport, increased osmotic fragility, and enhanced passive permeability, characteristics of malaria-infected red cells.

## F. Plasmodial Membrane Lipids

Studies of the lipids of malaria parasites are prone to error because of the presence of undetermined amounts of contaminating erythrocytic membranes. Indeed, even in those reports describing the lipid composition of truly "free" parasites the isolated parasites remain enclosed within the PVM, itself a derivative of the red-cell membrane. However, the composition of the PVM may not substantially confound the analytic results since there is now evidence to show that, shortly after formation, the PVM assumes plasmodial characteristics.

These limitations aside, the membranes of malaria parasites have been found to be richer in unesterified fatty acids, triacylglycerols, polyglycerol phosphatides, 1,2-diacylglycerols, diacylphosphatidylethanolamine, and phosphatidylinositol, and to contain less cholesterol, phosphatidylserine, and sphingomyelin than the membranes of the red blood cell (reviewed in HOLZ 1977). The unique qualities of plasmodial membranes can be determined from several bits of evidence. Phosphatidylinositol, a significant phospholipid of *P. lophurae* and *P. knowlesi* membranes (4%–8%), was not present to a significant degree in erythrocytic membranes. Phosphatidylserine, a component of mammalian membranes, was virtually absent from plasmodial membranes. In *P. lophurae* less of the phosphatidylethanolamine was in the alkyl-1-enyl and alky-acyl forms than in the red cell (4% and 3% versus 35% and 9% respectively), whereas for phosphatidylinositol the reverse was true (10% and 15% versus 7% and 4% respectively).

Although the principal fatty acids of the red cell and *Plasmodium* phospholipids were similar, the proportion of 18:1 (oleic, *cis*-vaccenic) and saturated fatty acids (principally 16:0, palmitic acid, and 19:0, stearic acid) was increased in the plasmodial membrane, whereas the polyunsaturates (18:2, linoleic, 20:4, arachidonic, and

22:6, docosahexanoic) decreased (Table 3). This bias for 18:1 and the relative paucity of polyunsaturates in the malarial parasite phospholipids suggests that the plasmodia are deficient in desaturases and chain elongation enzyme systems. The parasites do differ from their host cells in the proportions of neutral and polar lipids, in the content of 1,2-diacylglycerols in the neutral lipids and the diphosphatidylglycerol and alkoxy lipids in the phospholipids, as well as the amounts of fatty acids in all lipids. It is thus apparent that, despite the parasites' inability to biosynthesise lipids from acetate (see p. 59), they can regulate their use of host-cell lipids and lipid precursors.

How does membrane biosynthesis by the intracellular plasmodium take place, and how is the asymmetry of the PVM changed? It seems plausible to assume that during intraerythrocytic feeding by the parasite much of the PVM is recycled, and such a mechanism could provide an opportunity for intercalation of new parasite-derived membrane materials into the PVM. The result is a topographic organisation of the PVM lipid bilayer similar to that of the red-cell and plasmodial plasma membranes. In addition to the lipids of the endocytosed cytoplasm and membranes of the host cell, the uptake of plasma phospholipids, cholesterol, fatty acids, phosphate, inositol, choline, glycerol, and ethanolamine could be utilised for parasite membrane synthesis. Incapable of de novo fatty acid biosynthesis, the parasite acts as a metabolic sink for host fatty acids, particularly oleic acid. As a consequence there is a net movement of this fatty acid from the blood plasma into the infected red cell, and membrane lipid enrichment in octadecenoic fatty acids results. There are no data on the transmembrane distribution of phospholipids in the membranes surrounding the parasite. Such information could be critical to an understanding of parasite membrane function.

## G. Metabolic Pathways

### I. Carbohydrate Transport and Metabolism

#### 1. Glucose Uptake

The earliest metabolic studies with malaria-infected erythrocytes showed that glucose disappeared rapidly when added to suspensions of such cells. However, uninfected erythrocytes used very little sugar (Table 4). It is not possible to state with certainty that the amount of glucose utilised by malaria-infected cells is a reflection of the metabolism of the parasite or the host-parasite complex, since in many instances no assessment of the contribution of contaminating white cells, platelets and reticulocytes was made (see HOMEWOOD 1978; SHERMAN 1979). Thus, the reported values should be regarded more as trends rather than as absolutes. Moreover, in each instance the magnitude of sugar utilisation is influenced by the species, the parasitaemia, the kind of red cell (mature versus reticulocyte), the stage of the parasite, the synchronicity of the infection, the presence of contaminants, the amount of substrate available, the pH and the ionic composition of the medium. Nevertheless, despite the influence of such complex variables the conclusion seems inescapable that a malaria-infected red cell utilises substantially more glucose than an uninfected erythrocyte. The plasma glucose is the chief energy source for *Plasmodium*, but it has been reported that other sugars and glycerol may be

**Table 4.** Glucose utilisation, oxygen consumption and products of glucose metabolism by intraerythrocytic stages of malaria (IRBC), their host cells (RBC) and free parasites

| | Glucose used µg $10^9$ $cells^{-1}$ $h^{-1}$ | $O_2$ used µlitre $10^9$ $cells^{-1}$ $h^{-1}$ | Lactate | Products (%) | |
|---|---|---|---|---|---|
| | | | | $CO_2$ | Other |
| Human RBC | 14–28 | | | | |
| *P. falciparum* IRBC | 360–457 [a] | | | | |
| *P. vivax* IRBC | 1,002–2,315 [a] | | | | |
| Monkey RBC | 25–50 [a, r] | 2–3 [a, r] | | | |
| *P. knowlesi* IRBC | 180–486 [a, r] | 79–224 [a, d] | 54–82 [r] | 17 [r] 11%–29% | Unaccounted |
| *P. cynomolgi* IRBC | 180–209 [a] | 52–171 [a] | | | |
| Mouse RBC | 156 [b] | 2–4 [b] | 70–80 [b, s] | | |
| Mature rat RBC | 50–91 [c] | 6 [c] | – | | |
| Rat/mouse reticulocyte | 410 [c] | 40 [d] | 74 [b, c] | | |
| *P. berghei* IRBC | 900–2,000 [b, e] | 88 [f] | 70–84 [b, o, s] | | |
| *P. chabaudi* IRBC | – | – | 80 [t] | – | |
| *P. yoelii* IRBC | 2,120 [f] | – | 66 [e] | | |
| Canary RBC | – | 2–12 [g, j] | – | – | |
| Chicken RBC | 6–43 [h, i, j, m] | 8–22 [h] | 50–70 [h] | 30–50 [h] | |
| Duckling RBC | 25–128 [k, l] | 48 [u] | 70 [u] | | |
| *P. lophurae* IRBC | 200 [q] | 14–418 [u] | 20 [u] | 20 | 10% citrate, succinate, 40% amino acids |
| *P. relictum* IRBC | 520 [k] | – | – | – | – |
| *P. gallinaceum* IRBC | 300–400 [i] | 60–320 [h, m] | 50–70 [h] | > 18 [m] | – |
| *P. hexamerium* IRBC | 354 [l] | – | – | – | |
| *P. cathemerium* IRBC | – | 99–253 [g] | – | – | |
| Free *P. berghei* | 350–920 [b, o] | 0.5 [b] | 73–85 [b, o, s] | < 2 | |
| Free *P. knowlesi* | 2,200 [d] | 60 [d] | 15–30 [p] | < 2 | 30%–50% acid volatile |
| Free *P. lophurae* | – | 100–300 [v] | 20 [u] | 56 | Pyruvate; 8% amino acids |
| Free *P. gallinaceum* | 1,800 [n] | 55 [n] | | 43 | Pyruvate; 34% acetate |

[a] McKee (1951); [b] Bowman et al. (1960, 1961); [c] Rickard (1969); [d] Fulton (1939); [e] Homewood (1978), [f] Fulton and Spooner (1956); [g] Velick (1942); [h] Silverman et al. (1944); [i] Manwell and Feigelson (1949); [j] Moulder (1948); [k] Warren and Manwell (1954); [l] Khabir and Manwell (1955); [m] Marshall (1948); [n] Speck et al. (1946); [o] Cenedella and Jarrell (1970); [p] Scheibel and Miller (1969); [q] Sherman et al. (1969); [r] Ball et al. (1948); [s] Bryant et al. (1964); [t] Coombs and Gutteridge (1975); [u] Bovarnick et al. (1946 a); [v] Christophers and Fulton (1939)

utilised in vitro (Table 5). The inferences drawn from some of these reports on substrate utilisation should be treated with a degree of scepticism since, in most cases, there was no measure of substrate depletion but, rather, an increase in oxygen uptake over a period of minutes to hours was taken as indicative of utilisation. The correlation may be inappropriate. Thus, glycerol which stimulated oxygen consumption for a short time in vitro could not support the in vitro growth of *P. knowlesi* for 24–48 h (Anfinsen et al. 1946).

**Table 5.** Relative utilisation of substrates by malarial parasites

| Substrate | *P. knowlesi*[a] | *P. knowlesi*[b] | *P. lophurae* *P. gallinaceum*[c] | *P. vivax*[d] | *P. falciparum*[e] | *P. berghei*[f] |
|---|---|---|---|---|---|---|
| Glucose | 100 | 100 | 100 | | 100 | + |
| Mannose | 46 | 125 | | | | |
| Fructose | 85 | 100 | | | | |
| Galactose | 0 | 0 | | | | |
| Maltose | 12 | 24 | | | 100 | |
| Glycerol | | 100 | + | | | |
| Lactate | 16 | 100 | 100 | | | |
| Pyruvate | | 0 | 100 | | | + |
| Succinate | | 0 | 30 | | | + |
| Malate | | 0 | + | | | |
| Fumarate | | | 30 | | | |
| Citrate | | 0 | | | | |

[a] FULTON (1939); [b] MCKEE (1951); MAIER and COGGESHALL (1941); [c] BOVARNICK et al. (1946a); MARSHALL (1948); [d] JOHNS (1930); [e] BASS and JOHNS (1912); [f] NAGARAJAN (1968a)

The dramatic increase in glucose consumption by red cells infected with malarial parasites (Table 4) presumably can be sustained only by an alteration in the permeability of the red-cell membrane since uninfected bird (chicken and duckling) and rodent (mouse) erythrocytes demonstrate a low sugar uptake. This suggestion, first proposed by HERMAN et al. (1966), was confirmed by SHERMAN and TANIGOSHI (1974b) using the nonmetabolisable sugar, 3-0-methylglucose (3-OMG). The permeability of the *P. lophurae*-infected red cell was found to be markedly enhanced for 3-OMG due to an increase in the simple diffusion component as well as a modification in the carrier-mediated portion of the entry process. Furthermore, the leakiness towards 3-OMG was greatest for erythrocytes bearing larger parasites. Although normal mouse red cells were shown to be impermeable to L-glucose (also non-metabolisable), *P. berghei*-infected cells readily took it up (HOMEWOOD and NEAME 1974; NEAME and HOMEWOOD 1975). It is significant that in an infected animal L-glucose entered red cells containing *P. berghei*, but not uninfected cells. Thus the malaria-infected red cell not only consumes more glucose than the normal red cell, but the presence of the parasite accelerates the entry of sugar by changing the permeability characteristics of the host cell. How the parasite alters host-cell permeability requires further clarification.

## 2. End Products of Glucose Metabolism

The end products of glucose metabolism vary with the species of *Plasmodium* (Table 4). In vitro, mammalian red cells infected with *P. knowlesi*, *P. berghei* or *P. chabaudi* convert 70%–85% of the added glucose to lactate (MCKEE et al. 1946; BALL et al. 1948; BOWMAN et al. 1961; CENEDELLA and JARRELL 1970; COOMBS and GUTTERIDGE 1975), whereas avian erythrocytes bearing *P. lophurae* or *P. gallinaceum* metabolise glucose more completely so that, in addition to lactate, $CO_2$, amino acids and organic acids are produced (SILVERMAN et al. 1944; SHERMAN et al. 1969, 1970). Careful balance sheets for the amount of glucose utilised and the quantity of products formed are not available for most species, and in several experiments 10%–30% of the end products were unaccounted for.

The pattern of glucose metabolism by infected erythrocytes is mirrored by that of free parasites (Table 4). Thus free *P. berghei* metabolised most of the added glucose to lactate (BOWMAN et al. 1960), but *P. lophurae* and *P. gallinaceum* metabolised a considerable portion of the added glucose to $CO_2$ (reviewed by SHERMAN 1979). SCHEIBEL and PFLAUM (1970) found that virtually all of the radioactive glucose added to suspensions of free *P. knowlesi* ended up as lactate or volatile compounds, particularly acetate, and formate. Aerobically the parasites utilised pyruvate and produced acetate, not $CO_2$. Free *P. gallinaceum* oxidised pyruvate at one-third the rate of the infected red cell, and large amounts of acetate as well as $CO_2$ were formed. MOULDER (1962) speculated that this metabolism by free parasites could be due to the plasmodia lacking coenzyme A and, as a consequence, pyruvate oxidation via the citric acid cycle was reduced. As noted by SPECK et al. (1946) however, it seems unlikely that acetate formation is an important metabolic pathway under physiological conditions, i.e. intraerythrocytically. Malaria parasites appear to be facultative aerobes, and under in vitro conditions the enzymes of the citric acid cycle may no longer function as a cycle. Thus instead of a typical cycle, some free parasites exhibit signs of having a branched pathway from oxaloacetate. One branch, the oxidative one, functions as in the original cycle forming α-ketoglutarate, whereas the other, the reductive branch, reverses the usual pathway and leads to succinate (Fig. 1). It is also possible that the observed

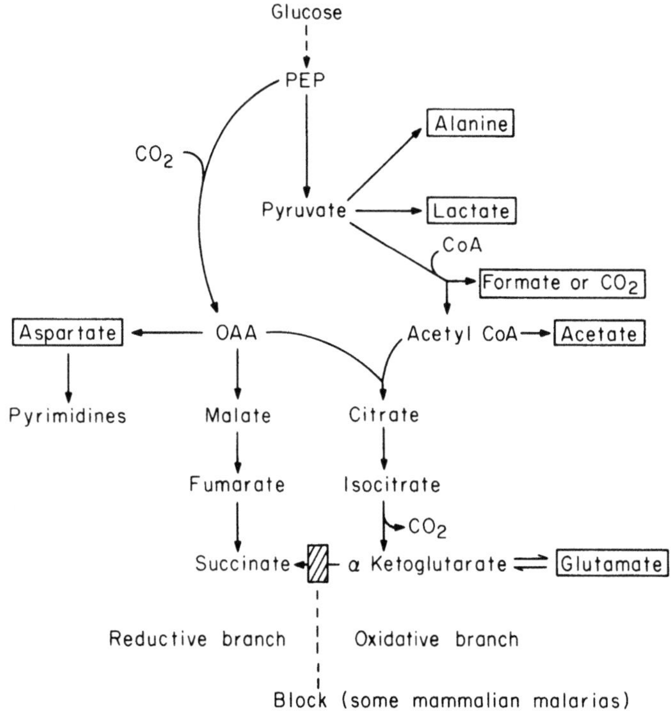


**Fig. 1.** An abbreviated pathway of glucose metabolism

metabolism of free parasites is due to damage incurred by the isolation procedure, or that the free parasites lack the necessary cofactors for complete oxidation of pyruvate. (However, the available evidence suggests that in "free" *P. lophurae* a conventional tricarboxylic acid cycle probably does exist.)

## 3. Enzymes of Carbohydrate Metabolism

### a) Glycolytic Enzymes

All species of malaria parasites appear to possess the glycolytic enzymes of the Embden-Meyerhoff pathway. However, for any one malaria species not a single complete sequence of glycolytic enzymes is known (Table 6). Assuming that the presence of an enzyme in one kind of malaria can be extrapolated to other species then evidence can be adduced for the existence of hexokinase, glucose phosphate isomerase (GPI), phosphofructokinase (PK), aldolase, glyceraldehyde-3-phosphate dehydrogenase, phosphoglyceric kinase, enolase, phosphoglycerate mutase, pyruvic kinase, and lactic dehydrogenase (LDH). Using this information the possible pathway for glucose metabolism by *Plasmodium* would be as shown in Fig. 2.

In some of the published reports it cannot be unequivocally decided whether the enzyme activity in a crude extract of parasites is entirely due to the plasmodium or reflects contaminants. However, for hexokinase, GPI, PK, and LDH where par-

**Table 6.** Enzymes of carbohydrate metabolism in *Plasmodium* species. Adapted from SHERMAN (1979)

| | *knowlesi* | *berghei* | *chabaudi* | *yoelii cinckei* | *falciparum* | *gallinaceum* | *lophurae* | *cathemerium* |
|---|---|---|---|---|---|---|---|---|
| Hexokinase | | + | | + | | + | | |
| Glucose phosphate isomerase | | + | | + | + | + | | |
| Phosphofructokinase | | + | | | | + | | |
| Aldolase | | + | | | | + | | |
| Triose phosphate isomerase | | | | | | + | | |
| Glyceraldehyde-3-$PO_4$ DH | | | | | | + | | |
| Phosphoglyceric kinase | | | | | | | + | |
| Phosphoglyceric mutase | | + | | | | | | |
| Enolase | | + | | | | + | | |
| Pyruvic kinase | + | + | | | | | + | |
| Lactic dehydrogenase | + | + | + | | + | + | + | |
| Isocitric dehydrogenase | | − | | | | | + | |
| Malic dehydrogenase | | ± | | + | | | + | |
| Succinic dehydrogenase | | − | | | | + | + | |
| Cytochrome oxidase | + | + | | | + | + | + | + |
| Phosphoenolpyruvate carboxylase | | + | | | | | | |
| Phosphoenolpyruvate carboxylkinase | | + | | | | | | |
| Glutamic dehydrogenase | | + | + | | | | + | |
| Glucose-6-$PO_4$ DH | − | ± | | − | − | − | − | |
| 6-phosphogluconate DH | + | + | | + | + | + | | |

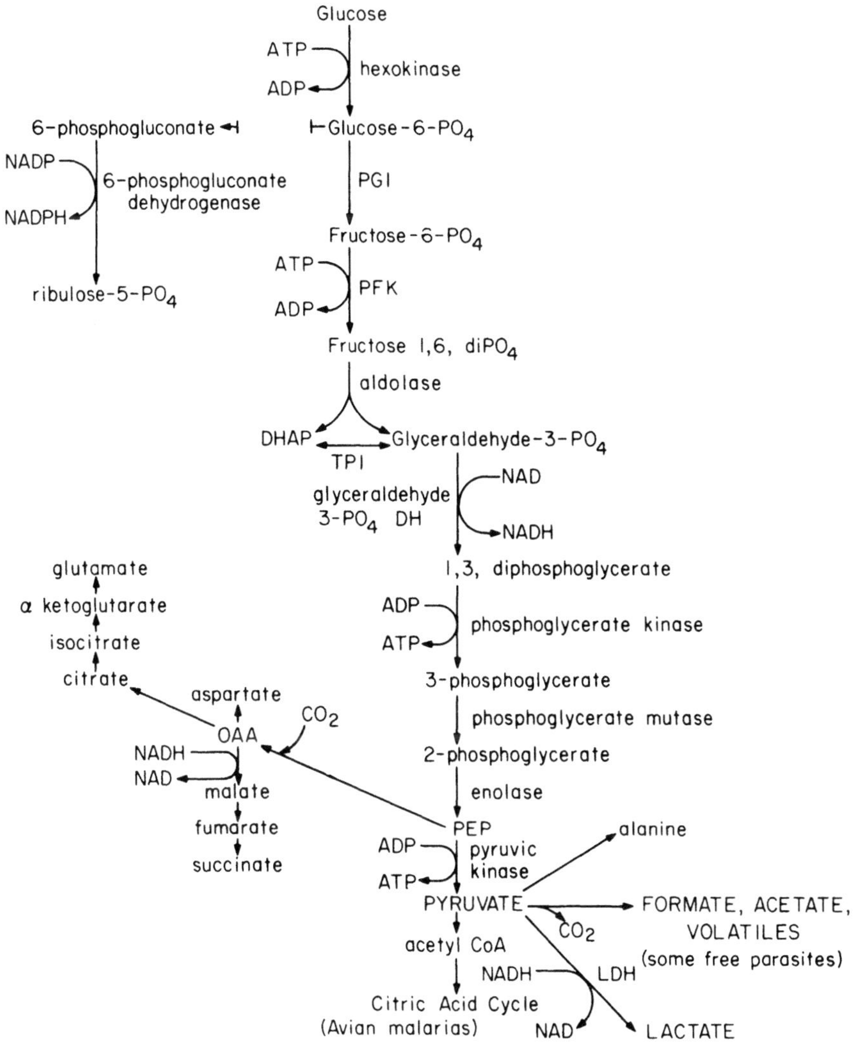


**Fig. 2.** Possible metabolic conversions of glucose by *Plasmodium*

asite-specific isoenzymes were identified (OELSHLEGEL et al. 1975; CARTER and WALLIKER 1977; SHERMAN 1961; MOMEN 1979a, b; PHISPHUMVIDHI and LANGER 1969; TSUKAMOTO 1974), it seems reasonable to ascribe such activities to the parasite itself and not to some other source. Hexokinase activity was inhibited by chloroquine and mepacrine[1] (FRASER and KERMACK 1957); quinine affected the formation of acetyl coenzyme A (MOULDER 1948, 1949); dapsone (DDS) inhibited glucose transport into the red cell (CENEDELLA and JARRELL 1970); and mepacrine also inhibited 6-phosphofructokinase (BOWMAN et al. 1961). In most of these stud-

1 Mepacrine is also known as atabrin, atebrin, quinacrine, and various other synonyms

ies, however, drug concentrations were exceedingly high (~1 m*M*), so that the specificity of inhibition remains questionable.

b) Citric Acid Cycle Enzymes

The only enzyme of the citric acid cycle identified with some degree of certainty in both rodent and avian malarias is malic dehydrogenase (SHERMAN 1966a; MOMEN 1979a; TSUKAMOTO 1974). The avian malaria (*P. lophurae*) malic dehydrogenase (MDH) appears to be extramitochondrial (i.e. soluble). It may play a role in the reoxidation of nicotinamide-adenine dinucleotide, reduced (NADH) for glycolysis (SHERMAN 1966a), and in this way could serve in a capacity similar to that of LDH. Isocitrate dehydrogenase specific for the bird malaria *P. lophurae* has been identified (SHERMAN, unpublished), but no evidence for its presence in the rodent malaria *P. berghei* was obtained (HOWELLS and MAXWELL 1973). There is, however, no cellular localisation of isocitrate dehydrogenase in *P. lophurae*. While it has been claimed that *P. lophurae* and *P. gallinaceum* have succinate dehydrogenase activity (SEAMAN 1953; SPECK et al. 1946), this enzyme could not be identified in *P. berghei* (HOWELLS 1970; NAGARAJAN 1968a–c), and yet, paradoxically, oxygen utilisation was stimulated by succinate. Thus there is suggestive evidence for citric acid cycle enzymes in the bird malarias *P. gallinaceum* and *P. lophurae*, but most enzymes of this pathway appear to be absent from the rodent malarias and *P. knowlesi*.

c) Carbon Dioxide-Fixing Enzymes

Several species of malaria parasites appear to be capable of fixing $CO_2$. That is, when cell suspensions of *P. knowlesi*, *P. berghei*- and *P. lophurae*-infected cells were incubated with radioactive $NaHCO_3$ (reviewed in SHERMAN 1977a, b, 1979) $^{14}C$ was incorporated into keto and other organic acids as well as amino acids. Aspartate formed in this way could serve for pyrimidine biosynthesis, and the glutamate formed could be used for the regeneration of nicotinamide-adenine dinucleotide phosphate, reduced (NADPH) or for energy via the citric acid cycle in avian malarias. Free *P. lophurae* were capable of fixing $CO_2$ (TING and SHERMAN 1966). However, only in the case of *P. berghei* have the enzymes of $CO_2$ fixation, phosphoenolpyruvate carboxylase, and phosphoenolpyruvate carboxykinase (Table 6) been definitively identified (SIU 1967). The phosphoenolpyruvate carboxylase seems to be unique to *P. berghei* since this enzyme has not been found in other animal tissues. Quinine and chloroquine ($10^{-4}$ *M*) were reported to inhibit the *P. berghei* phosphoenolpyruvate carboxykinase (MCDANIEL and SIU 1972).

d) Pentose Phosphate Pathway

The activity of the overall pentose pathway in the malaria-infected red cell appears to be low. Thus, only 2% of 1-[$^{14}C$]glucose was metabolised to $^{14}CO_2$ by free *P. berghei* and less than 20% of 1-[$^{14}C$]glucose was recovered as $^{14}CO_2$ in *P. knowlesi*-infected cells (BOWMAN et al. 1961; SHAKESPEARE and TRIGG 1973; SHAKESPEARE et al. 1979b). With "free" *P. knowlesi* 1-[$^{14}C$]glucose was incorporated into $CO_2$ to such a small degree that the existence of a pentose pathway was considered to be non-existent(SCHEIBEL and PFLAUM 1970). Little or no 6-phosphogluconate was formed by *P. berghei* from radioactive glucose (BRYANT et al. 1964). Similarly, HERMAN et al. (1966) and SHERMAN et al. (1970), using specifically radiolabelled glucose, came to the conclusion that the pentose pathway played a minor role in *P. gallinaceum* and *P. lophurae* glucose catabolism.

Although the glucose-6-phosphate dehydrogenase (G6PDH) activity of *P. knowlesi*-infected monkey erythrocytes increased with increasing parasitaemia, there was no evidence for the presence of G6PDH in the parasite itself (reviewed in SHERMAN 1979). What is paradoxical, moreover, about the pentose phosphate shunt and malaria parasites is that the second enzyme of the pathway, 6-phosphogluconate dehydrogenase (6PGDH), has been consistently identified in plasmodial extracts, and is electrophoretically distinct from the host-cell enzyme (CARTER and WALLIKER 1977); yet no known mechanism exists for the formation of the substrate for this enzyme since G6PDH, which catalyses the formation of 6-phosphogluconate from glucose-6-phosphate, has not been found in any of the malarias studied (Table 6).

Therefore it appears that for *Plasmodium* the pentose pathway is absent, or a novel, as yet undiscovered, pathway exists. The parasite could utilise some of the pentose pathway intermediates directly from the host cell, but to date no compelling evidence for this exists. The absence of a plasmodial G6PDH leaves the parasite without a mechanism for the regeneration of reduced NADP, a cofactor critical to several biosynthetic schemes. It has been suggested, however, that a plasmodial specific glutamic dehydrogenase could assume this role (SHERMAN et al. 1971; WALTER et al. 1974). If the pentose phosphate pathway of the parasite is incomplete, where do the pentoses required for plasmodial nucleic acid synthesis come from? Possibly pentoses arise from the action of erythrocytic and/or plasmodial nucleoside phosphorylases on host-cell ATP catabolites which, in turn, release a free base and ribose-1-phosphate.

## 4. Oxygen Utilisation and Electron Transport

Malaria-infected red cells show enhanced oxygen uptake with certain substrates when compared with uninfected red cells (Table 4). This increased oxygen consumption is demonstrable even under those circumstances where platelets, white cells and reticulocytes have been accounted for or removed. Interestingly, increased oxygen consumption by *P. gallinaceum*-infected red cells took place after exposure to 30000 R, a dose that destroyed parasite infectivity (CEITHAML and EVANS 1946). Undoubtedly some of the increased respiratory activity of the malaria-infected red cell is due to stimulation of the metabolism of the host cell, but the favouring effects of lower oxygen levels ($<5\%$) on the in vitro intraerythrocytic development of *P. lophurae*, *P. knowlesi*, and *P. falciparum* strongly suggest that the parasites are microaerophilic (SCHEIBEL et al. 1979b).

BOVARNICK et al. (1946a, b) found that "free" *P. lophurae* had an $O_2$ consumption rate with pyruvate and lactate equal to that with glucose, but with succinate and fumarate the rate was only one-third of this. Erythrocyte-free *P. lophurae* and *P. gallinaceum* had a lower $O_2$ consumption than did the intact infected red cell (SPECK et al. 1946), and in some cases the $O_2$ consumed was only one-sixth of that expected for complete oxidation of glucose. This implies that either free parasites were impermeable to the added substrates, were damaged during the isolation procedure, or that they lacked the cofactors necessary for further oxidation of pyruvate. The respiratory activity of such "free" parasite preparations was shown to be inhibited by cyanide (CN), suggesting that metalloenzyme catalysis was involved with oxygen uptake. Also *P. knowlesi*-infected cells seemed to contain a heavy metal catalyst since oxygen uptake was inhibited by CN and CO. However, in the latter case, the CO inhibition could not always be reversed by strong light (MCKEE et al. 1946).

Quinine and mepacrine, at concentrations of 1 m$M$, inhibited oxygen uptake by *P. knowlesi*- and *P. gallinaceum*-infected red cells by 50% (BOVARNICK et al. 1946 a, b; FULTON and CHRISTOPHERS 1938), but $3\times10^{-5}$ $M$ quinine sulphate or $5\times10^{-4}$ $M$ mepacrine had no effect on $^{14}CO_2$ liberation from radioactive glucose by *P. lophurae*-infected erythrocytes (SHERMAN et al. 1970). The significance of these findings remains unclear. Oxygen uptake may be difficult to correlate with the physiology of *Plasmodium* since many subtle factors interact with one another. For example, temperature, time, serum concentration, tonicity of the medium, pH, $pO_2$, and the reduced amounts of haemoglobin in infected cells may affect the buffering and oxygen-carrying capacity of the blood, and these in turn may influence $O_2$ uptake measurements. Since the malaria parasite utilises both haemoglobin and oxygen such factors assume special significance. Indeed, although the parasites live in an $O_2$-rich environment and can assimilate $O_2$, utilisation may not be substantial, e.g. *P. falciparum* grows optimally in vitro at 3% $O_2$ and survives at 0.5% and, in vivo, schizonts develop in the more anaerobic deep tissues (SCHEIBEL et al. 1979 b).

Save for the presence of cytochrome oxidase, cytochromes have not been isolated from plasmodia (Table 6). SCHEIBEL and MILLER (1969) identified cytochrome oxidase activity in platelet-free preparations of *P. knowlesi*, *P. berghei*, *P. cynomolgi*, and *P. falciparum*. Using electron microscope cytochemistry this activity was localised in the acristate mitochondria of *P. berghei* (THEAKSTON et al. 1969). Avian malarias possess cristate mitochondria, and cytochrome oxidase activity was found to be associated with this organelle (THEAKSTON et al. 1969; PLATZER 1977). *P. falciparum* as well as *P. brasilianum*, and *P. malariae* also have cristate mitochondria, but where cytochrome oxidase activity is localised in these species is uncertain.

The presence of cytochrome oxidase, of itself, is not indicative of a functional cytochrome-mediated electron transport system. In the absence of a complete citric acid cycle, as appears to be the case for most mammalian malarias, what can be the functional significance of cytochrome oxidase? It is conceivable that malaria parasites contain a unique, undiscovered electron transport chain, or that cytochrome oxidase serves not as a component of an aerobic energy-generating system, but functions in some other capacity. GUTTERIDGE et al. (1979) proposed that oxygen utilisation by plasmodia may be coupled to the de novo biosynthesis of pyrimidines. Dihydroorotate dehydrogenase catalyses the formation of dihydroorotate to orotate. This enzyme is mitochondrial, irreversible, and closely linked to the cytochrome chain to which electrons are passed directly via the ubiquinones, and for which oxygen is the terminal acceptor (Fig. 3). Dihydroorotate dehydrogenase was present in extracts from *P. gallinaceum*, *P. berghei*, and *P. knowlesi* and its activity was inhibited by CN and antimycin (GUTTERIDGE et al. 1979). Should such findings be confirmed and extended (i.e. are superoxides

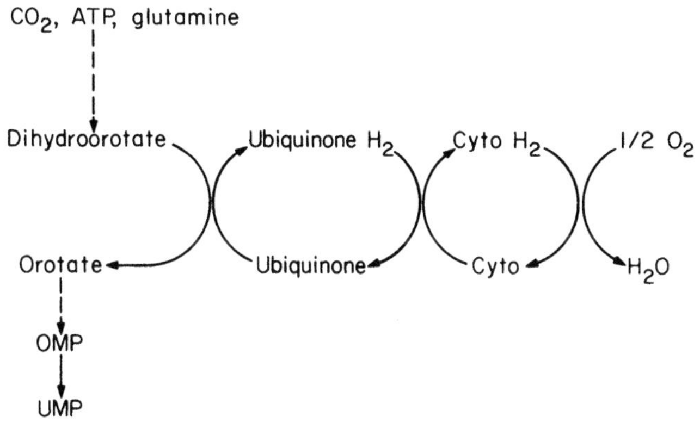


**Fig. 3.** Proposed conversion of dihydroorotate to orotate

formed or do the electrons pass directly to $O_2$ with the formation of water?), it would strongly support the notion that oxygen is used by *Plasmodium* for biosynthetic purposes, especially fabrication of nucleic acids. This idea is particularly intriguing in the light of the work of VELICK (1942), which showed a marked increase in $O_2$ consumption in *P. cathemerium*-infected cells at the time of schizogony.

SCHEIBEL et al. (1979a) reported that disulfiram (Antabuse) and its reduction product inhibit lactate production as well as the in vitro growth of *P. falciparum*. These findings prompted the suggestion that oxygen may be utilised via metalloprotein oxygenases other than cytochromes. Such oxygenases have not, as yet, been identified. It has been postulated, based on the indirect technique of measuring the effects of inhibitors on chloroquine-induced clumping of malarial pigment, that a branched electron transport system may exist in plasmodia (HOMEWOOD et al. 1972b). One branch in this proposed scheme would be CN sensitive, involve cytochromes, and would have oxygen as the terminal acceptor, whereas the other branch would be CN insensitive and would involve an unidentified electron acceptor. However, we do not know the mechanisms involved in clumping and rather high concentrations of inhibitors were needed to prevent the process of clumping. Therefore suggestions concerning an electron transport system based on pigment clumping in the presence of certain inhibitors is without strong foundation.

## II. Protein Synthesis

### 1. Biosynthesis of Amino Acids

Malaria parasites and malaria-infected erythrocytes fix $CO_2$, and by this mechanism a limited number of amino acids (alanine, aspartic, and glutamic acids) can be synthesised (see SHERMAN 1977a, b, 1979 for review). It is noteworthy that the free amino acid pool of the infected red cell is substantially increased in these same amino acids (SHERMAN and MUDD 1966). However, since very little of the amino acids formed via $CO_2$ fixation is incorporated into plasmodial proteins it appears that this is an anaplerotic pathway, i.e. glutamic acid oxidation coupled to the enzymes of the citric acid cycle could provide an ancillary source of energy (avian malarias). Indeed, free *P. lophurae* metabolised >60% of the added [$^{14}$C]glutamic acid to $^{14}CO_2$ (SHERMAN and TANIGOSHI 1971 b). In the rodent malarias (LANGER et al. 1970; WALTER et al. 1974) the conversion of glutamate to α-ketoglutarate could serve to regenerate NADPH needed for reductive syntheses.

## 2. Uptake of Free Amino Acids

Characteristically, malaria-infected red cells take up and incorporate exogenously supplied amino acids at an accelerated rate when compared with uninfected red cells, e.g. *P. knowlesi*- and *P. lophurae*-infected red cells accumulate isoleucine, methionine, leucine, cystine, and histidine. This feature has been useful (especially with isoleucine, which is readily incorporated) in a variety of malarias (i.e. *P. falciparum*, *P. berghei*, and *P. lophurae*) for monitoring plasmodial growth under different culture conditions, for measuring drug efficacy and for assessing viability after cryopreservation (reviewed in SHERMAN 1977 a, b).

Unfortunately, no detailed studies exist on the mechanism of transport of isoleucine (or any other amino acid for that matter) into erythrocytes infected with mammalian malarias. However, studies of amino acid uptake with the avian parasite *P. lophurae* may provide some clues as to the nature of the transport processes in these other malarias. It has been reported that duckling erythrocytes infected with *P. lophurae* tend to show diffusion entry of several amino acids (alanine, leucine, histidine, methionine, cysteine) which are ordinarily transported by carrier-mediated processes in the normal cell, and even with those amino acids that continue to be moved across the infected red-cell surface by carrier-mediated processes (glycine, serine, threonine, lysine, and arginine) there was an altered (increased) transport constant (SHERMAN and TANIGOSHI 1974 a). It was suggested that this leakiness of the infected cell was due to a depletion of host-cell ATP and plasmodium-induced (enzymic?) alterations in the erythrocyte membrane. However, an attempt to establish the transport characteristics of alanine, observed in malaria-infected cells by treating normal duckling red cells with parasite extracts and reducing the red-cell ATP content, was only partially successful.

SHERMAN and co-workers (reviewed in SHERMAN 1977 a, b) have studied amino acid uptake by *P. lophurae* "removed" from the host cell by saponin lysis. [It has been shown that such saponin-prepared parasites are not entirely removed and many parasites remain enclosed by red-cell membranes (see TRAGER et al. 1972).] Of all the amino acids tested only arginine, lysine, glutamic acid, aspartic acid, and cysteine entered the parasite by what appeared to be a carrier-mediated process; all others entered by simple diffusion. These studies with "free" parasites appear to support the contention (first formulated by MOULDER in 1962) that the parasites have a permeability defect. However, it remains uncertain whether the free parasites commonly used for these studies are highly permeable in situ (intracellularly) or whether this leaky condition is provoked by the techniques used to remove the parasites from the host cell. Until this dilemma can be satisfactorily resolved it will be difficult to ask critical questions regarding the transport properties of "free" parasites.

### 3. Proteolysis of Haemoglobin and the Formation of Malaria Pigment

Since de novo biosynthesis of amino acids is restricted in kind (see $CO_2$ fixation above), and because the free amino acid pool of the red cell is presumed not to be of sufficient quantity to serve for the synthesis of plasmodial proteins, erythrocyte haemoglobin is probably the principal source of amino acids for the malaria parasite. Early malariologists recognised that the golden brown-black pigment (= haemozoin) accumulated during the intraerythrocytic development of the parasites was related to haemoglobin destruction by the plasmodium. Therefore, characterisation of haemozoin should provide, in theory at least, clues to the parasite's ability to utilise haemoglobin. Early investigators believed that the pigment was melanin (reviewed in McKEE 1951) but later it was shown that haemozoin was ferriprotoporphyrin coupled to a denatured polypeptide. The nature of the polypeptide moiety has been the subject of controversy, one group believing it to be a partially degraded haemoglobin (SHERMAN et al. 1968), whereas others contended that the protein was synthesised by the plasmodium (HOMEWOOD et al. 1972a). Recent findings suggest that the malaria pigment of *P. lophurae* consists of insoluble monomers and dimers of haematin, plus ferriprotoporphyrin coupled to a plasmodial protein, and insoluble methaemoglobin (YAMADA and SHERMAN 1979). It is difficult to state with certainty that the extracted pigment is truly identical to the haemozoin formed in situ within parasite food vacuoles since haematin is known to bind avidly to many proteins, and during extraction some cytoplasmic constituents may be rereleased and bound adventitiously to the pigment. It is also not clear whether all malarias have haemozoins of similar composition. Several investigators have suggested that haemozoin formation is related to chloroquine resistance, and recent experiments by CHOU et al. (1980) provide presumptive evidence that the chloroquine receptor in the malaria parasite may be ferriprotoporphyrin IX. In what way this binding is related to chloroquine resistance has not been fully clarified (see also Chaps. 10 and 19).

The functional significance of haemozoin is not completely understood. It may be that plasmodial formation of insoluble ferriprotoporphyrin polymers enables the parasite to sequester in a benign form the excess haem derived from its digestion of haemoglobin, and by processing haemoglobin in this way the untoward effects of oxygen for the plasmodium may be reduced, or the ferriprotoporphyrin could be involved in red-cell haemolysis and release of merozoites.

The average intraerythrocytic plasmodium destroys between 25% and 75% of the host-cell haemoglobin (GROMAN 1951). During this process amino nitrogen is released and insoluble malaria pigment is deposited. When radiolabelled red cells were transfused into *P. lophurae-*, *P. knowlesi-*, and *P. berghei*-infected hosts and parasites were permitted to invade and grow in these tagged erythrocytes, the radioactive amino acids of haemoglobin became incorporated into plasmodial proteins (FULTON and GRANT 1956; SHERMAN and TANIGOSHI 1970; THEAKSTON et al. 1970). Studies with the electron microscope show that the destruction of erythrocytic haemoglobin occurs within the food vacuoles which are pinched off from the base of the parasite's special ingestive organelle, the cytostome (AIKAWA 1977). Involved in the degradation of haemoglobin are parasite proteases which are probably secreted into these food vacuoles. MOULDER and EVANS (1946) identified a proteolytic enzyme in extracts of *P. gallinaceum* with a pH optimum of 6.5, and COOK et al. (1961) and COOK et al. (1969) reported that extracts of *P. berghei* and *P. knowlesi* readily hydrolysed denatured haemoglobin. A major alkaline (pH 7-8) and a minor acid (pH 4-5) protease were detected in both of these species. Subsequently, LEVY and co-workers (LEVY and CHOU 1973, 1974) identified a cathepsin D-like proteinase from *P. berghei-*, *P. knowlesi-* and *P. falciparum*-infected red cells. The enzyme was believed to be membrane bound or enclosed in membranous vesicles since enzyme activity was enhanced by the presence of Triton X-100. These proteases were not inhibited by chloroquine. On the other hand, protease inhibitors did diminish macromolecular synthesis by *P. knowlesi* in vitro (LEVY and CHOU 1975). CHARET and co-workers (1980) described aminopeptidase activity in *P. yoelii nigeriensis* and *P. chabaudi*, and showed $10^{-3}$ *M* chloroquine, mepacrine, and primaquine to be potent inhibitors in vitro.

## 4. Mechanisms of Protein Synthesis

The available evidence indicates that for *P. knowlesi* (SHERMAN et al. 1975; SHERMAN 1976), *P. berghei* (MILLER and ILAN 1978), and *P. lophurae* (SHERMAN and JONES 1976, 1977) the molecular mechanisms involved in plasmodial protein synthesis are typically eukaryotic. Protein synthesis is sensitive to cycloheximide and puromycin, but not to chloramphenicol; the optimum $Mg^{2+}$ was 5–7 m*M* for an endogenous cell-free protein synthesising system; the parasite ribosomes had a sedimentation constant of 80S, and could be dissociated into 60S and 40S subparticles. The plasmodial ribosomal RNA was found to be typically protozoan in its base composition (see p. 52), and the ribosomal RNAs were distinct from other eukaryotes in both their sedimentation constant and electrophoretic mobility. Therefore all species of malaria appear to synthesise their proteins by utilising their own metabolic machinery and do not depend upon host-cell ribosomes.

## 5. Histidine Rich Protein

The only well-characterised protein from a malaria parasite is the histidine-rich protein (HRP) isolated from membrane-bound cytoplasmic granules of *P. lophurae* (KILEJIAN 1974). This acid-soluble protein with a molecular weight of 35 000–40 000 is particularly rich (~73%) in histidine residues (KILEJIAN et al. 1975) and is synthesised in large amounts by *P. lophurae*. It has been suggested that the HRP may be a component of the polar organelles (KILEJIAN 1976). KILEJIAN (1978) found that ducklings immunised with HRP were protected against ordinarily fatal infections with *P. lophurae*, but this work could not be verified (MCDONALD et al. 1981).

Evidence of an indirect nature was presented for the presence of an acid-soluble HRP in *P. falciparum* (KILEJIAN and JENSEN 1977). The *P. falciparum* HRP had a higher molecular weight (55 000) on SDS-polyacrylamide gel than did the protein obtained from *P. lophurae*. There has been no localisation of the falciparum HRP or a description of its possible function.

## III. Nucleic Acids

### 1. DNA: Characteristics and Synthesis

In the early 1940 s, using the Feulgen staining technique, it was shown that malaria parasites contained DNA. Later, WHITFELD (1952, 1953) and CLARKE (1952a, b) found that $^{32}P$ from $Na_2H^{32}PO_4$ was incorporated into nucleic acids by *P. berghei*-infected red cells, and *P. gallinaceum* growing either intracellularly or extracellularly. SCHELLENBERG and COATNEY (1961) used this same method, i.e. $^{32}P$ incorporation, to evaluate the intracellular growth of *P. berghei* and *P. gallinaceum* in the presence or absence of antimalarials. Quinine, chloroquine, mepacrine, pyrimethamine, and proguanil [2] all inhibited incorporation of $^{32}P$ into parasite DNA.

It has been suggested (SINDEN 1978) that the merozoite stage is haploid with a chromosome number of ten and contains $\sim 1 \times 10^{-13}$ g DNA, this amount increasing 10- to 20-fold during schizogony (Table 7). When during development is this chromosomal DNA made? In vitro studies using synchronous infections of intraerythrocytic *P. lophurae* showed a lag of $^{32}P$ incorporation into DNA for 2–4 h, maximum synthesis for the following 20 h, and then a levelling off of incorporation for the last 8–10 h of development (WALSH and SHERMAN 1968a). *P. lophurae* has a 36-h schizogonic cycle, and during the first 2–4 h in culture the predominant stages were early rings. The greatest incorporation took place when the red cells contained trophozoites and early schizonts whereas, during the last 8–10 h, schizogony was essentially complete. Similar in vitro results were obtained with *P. knowlesi*, a species with a 24-h asexual cycle. This showed, a lag of incorporation of radioactive orotic acid for 5–10 h, maximum synthesis for 10–15 h, and then an abrupt cessation of incorporation when schizogony began (GUTTERIDGE and TRIGG 1970; POLET and BARR 1968a). Increased amounts of incorporation took place during the late trophozoite and early schizont stages. In all of these studies, despite the variation in the duration of the asexual cycle, the synthesis of DNA appeared to occur continuously, and there was no evidence for a periodicity. Later, however, it was claimed that nucleic acid synthesis was discontinuous. GUTTERIDGE and TRIGG (1972a, b), using incorporation of tritiated adenosine into nucleic acids, found that the S phase of the *P. knowlesi* cell cycle occurred during the ring and trophozoite stages, with little or no synthesis taking place during schizogony. There was a very short ($\sim$1 h) $G_1$ phase and little indication of a $G_2$ phase. They were of the opinion that adenosine incorporation was a more valid measure of DNA synthesis than orotic acid incorporation because: (a) since the membranes of the red cell and parasite are relatively impermeable to pyrimidines, entry of orotic acid into the red cell could be limited during the early growth of the parasite, and (b) because orotic acid has to be added in high specific activity to see any incorporation, its incorporation represents a minimal amount of DNA synthesis. This contention was questioned by CONKLIN et al. (1973), who found DNA synthesis to occur primarily in late trophozoites and early schizonts using either orotic acid or adenosine as tracers. There has been no completely satisfactory resolution to these contradictory findings.

---

2 Proguanil is also known as chlorguanide in the United States

**Table 7.** DNA and RNA content and base ratios of *Plasmodium* and their hosts

| Cell type | DNA | | RNA | | Ref. |
|---|---|---|---|---|---|
| | Content g × $10^{-13}$ cells | Composition % G+C | Content g × $10^{-13}$ cells | Composition % G+C | |
| *P. lophurae* merozoite | 0.50 | 20, 19 | – | – | a, f |
| schizont | 10.00 | – | 65.0 | 35 | a |
| *P. gallinaceum* 8B | – | 18 | – | – | b |
| *P. knowlesi* ring | 0.76 | – | – | – | b |
| trophozoite | 11.2 | 37, 19 | 60.0 | 37 | b |
| schizont | 17.5 | – | – | – | b |
| *P. falciparum* | – | 18 | – | – | k |
| *P. berghei* NK65 | – | 24 | – | – | b |
| *P. berghei* N30 | – | 24 | – | – | b |
| *P. berghei* WLTM | – | 24 | – | – | b |
| *P. berghei* Whitfeld | 0.54 | 40 [j] | 1.09 | – | c |
| *P. berghei* RC | – | 23.5 | – | – | d |
| *P. berghei* NSL3 | – | 23.5 | – | – | d |
| *P. berghei* NS | – | 23.5 | – | – | d |
| *P. berghei yoelii* 17X | – | 23.5 | – | 37–43 | d |
| *P. berghei* N67 | – | 25.5, 17.3 | – | – | d |
| *P. vinckei* LPL5 | – | 23.5 | – | – | d |
| *P. vinckei* 52 | – | 24 | – | – | d |
| *P. chabaudi* LPL5 | – | 26.5, 17.3 | – | – | d |
| Rat liver cell | 20 | 40 | 58 | – | |
| Monkey reticulocyte | – | – | – | 67 | h |
| Mouse liver | 28 | 40 | 90 | 58–51 | c, i |
| Chicken red cell | 23–25 | 37 | 2 | – | e, a |
| Duck red cell | | 39 | – | 64 | f, g |

[a] BAHR (1966); [b] GUTTERIDGE et al. (1969, 1971); GUTTERIDGE and TRIGG (1972a); [c] WHITFELD (1952); [d] CHANCE et al. (1978); [e] SCHELLENBERG and COATNEY (1961); [f] WALSH and SHERMAN (1968a); [g] SHERMAN and JONES (1977); [h] SHERMAN et al. (1975); [i] MILLER and ILAN (1978); [j] GUTTERIDGE et al. found this value to be 24%; the 40% value of WHITFELD may be due to contamination with white blood cells. [k] POLLAK et al. (1982)

According to nuclear DNA base composition malaria parasites can be separated into three discrete categories, simian malarias having 37%, rodent malarias having 24%, and avian malarias and *P. falciparum* having 18%–20% G+C ratios (Table 7), In *P. lophurae* a mitochondrial DNA with a buoyant density of 1.679, identical in density to that of nuclear DNA, was shown to have circular contours of 10 μm (KILEJIAN 1975). The minor satellite bands observed in DNA preparations from *P. knowlesi. P. berghei,* and *P. chabaudi* (Table 7) could also represent mitochondrial DNA but, to date, DNA has not been isolated from mitochondria or mitochondrion-like bodies from these species.

The mode of antimalarial action of chloroquine remains unclear. CIAK and HAHN (1966) showed that chloroquine bound to the DNA of *Bacillus megaterium*, and that by such binding nucleic acid synthesis was inhibited. However, the binding constant of chloroquine to *P. knowlesi* DNA was similar to that of mammalian DNA (GUTTERIDGE et al. 1972). It was believed by these latter authors that chloroquine exerted its effects by depressing RNA, DNA, and protein synthesis, as well as lactate formation. THEAKSTON et al. (1972), using EM autoradiography, found evidence that chloroquine affects the transport properties of the infected red cell. We are thus left in a quandary as to the biochemical mode of action of chloroquine on chloroquine-sensitive strains of malaria.

## 2. RNA: Characteristics and Synthesis

The RNA content of the malarial parasite is about five times greater than the content of DNA (Table 7). Most of this RNA is localised in abundant cytoplasmic ribosomes which are present in the intraerythrocytic parasite. The ribosomal RNA (rRNA) of *P. lophurae* is typically protozoan in its sedimentation values of 25S and 17S [in contrast to the 28S and 18S of other eukaryotes (SHERMAN and JONES 1977)]. Similarly, *P. knowlesi* rRNA had sedimentation values of 24.2S and 17.4S (TRIGG et al. 1975) and that of *P. berghei* had values of 25S and 14.9S (TOKUYASU et al. 1969). The nucleotide base composition of the rRNAs of these three species was distinct from other eukaryotes, but akin to that of other protozoans, in having a low G+C ratio of ~35%. (Typically, the rRNA of the host was found to be ~64% G+C.) Apparently, chloroquine treatment of the host induces a breakdown of ribosomal RNA in *P. knowlesi* (WARHURST and WILLIAMSON 1970).

Although it was initially believed that the large rRNA of *P. berghei* ribosomes was provided by the host-cell (reticulocyte) ribosomes, this work could not be confirmed with *P. knowlesi* or *P. lophurae* (SHERMAN et al. 1975; SHERMAN and JONES 1977; TRIGG et al. 1975). Thus free *P. lophurae*, after being pulse-labelled in vitro with [$^3$H]adenosine, were shown to have radioactivity in both the large (60S) and small (40S) ribosomal subparticle, and *P. knowlesi*-infected cells incubated in the presence of radioactive adenosine had major peaks of radioactivity which corresponded to rRNAs of 24.2S and 16.6S. In a new study of the characteristics of *P. berghei* rRNA (MILLER and ILAN 1978) it was shown that the long delay in the labelling of the 25S component of the plasmodium after cells were incubated with $NaH_2{}^{32}PO_4$ or $^{14}$C-orotic acid (and which was taken to be evidence for an absence of plasmodial biosynthesis of the large ribosomal subparticle) was probably the result of uncontrolled ribonuclease activity by the parasite, which contributed to the degradation of the 25S rRNA. Although the large rRNA of *P. knowlesi* and *P. lophurae* was invariably recovered intact, in *P. berghei* it was always isolated in a partially degraded form. It has been suggested that this could be due to a "nicking" of the RNA, the in situ action of nucleases on an exposed portion of the RNA, or it might represent a natural occurrence during the maturation of this rRNA. Although ribonuclease was demonstrated in *P. gallinaceum* decades ago (MILLER and KOZLOFF 1947), the ribonuclease of *P. berghei* remains of considerable interest in that its activity appears not to be diminished by conventional RNA inhibitors, and its action is restricted to the large ribosomal RNA.

The pattern of rRNA synthesis is not completely understood for *Plasmodium*. The occurrence of 45S, 37.2S, and 23.7S RNA species in *P. knowlesi* suggests that the processing of rRNA may be typically eukaryotic (TRIGG et al. 1975), i.e. processing takes place in the nucleolus. Although avian malarias have a compact nucleolus, a compact nucleolus is absent from simian and rodent malarias.

The synthesis of RNA during the intraerythrocytic development of *P. knowlesi* has been studied in several laboratories. For example, POLET and BARR (1968a) followed the incorporation of [$^{14}$C]orotic acid into total RNA and observed a slight lag for the first 5 h, followed by a linear rate of incorporation. GUTTERIDGE and TRIGG (1970) found a similar in vitro pattern with [$^{3}$H]adenine and [$^{3}$H]orotic acid as the tracers, with a lag for 4–8 h, linear incorporation for ~10 h and then abrupt cessation as the parasites entered schizogony. However, with [$^{3}$H]adenosine no lag in incorporation was evident and maximum incorporation occurred at the late trophozoite stage before nuclear division took place. TRIGG and GUTTERIDGE (1972) found that when *P. knowlesi* were grown in vitro in cell suspension cultures there was a striking deficiency in the synthesis of RNA during the second growth cycle, and they proposed that this could in part account for the inability of the parasites to multiply in culture.

Although most workers have been unable to demonstrate incorporation of uracil or uridine into plasmodial RNA, one group (CONKLIN et al. 1973) claimed evidence for this. The discrepancy could be due to purity of the isotopes, presence of leucocytes, very high specific activity of the tracer and/or varied culture conditions. It is likely that uridine or uracil may be incorporated by malaria parasites only under highly artificial circumstances, i.e. when supplied in exceedingly high concentrations.

Despite there being limitations to the use of orotic acid for studying the timing of DNA synthesis, its incorporation or lack thereof has provided valuable information on the action of antimalarials. Thus POLET and BARR (1968b) showed that $10^{-7}$ *M* chloroquine inhibited the incorporation of orotic-5-[$^{3}$H] acid into both DNA and RNA of *P. knowlesi* after 17 h in vitro cultivation, and POLET and CONRAD (1969a, b) assessed the effects of isoleucine antagonists on in vitro growth using this method. Similarly, McCORMICK et al. (1974) studied the in vitro incorporation of orotic acid and adenosine into *P. knowlesi* DNA and RNA in order to evaluate prospective antimalarial compounds and to determine chemical structure-activity relationships. TRAGER et al. (1978, 1980) have reported that *S*-isobutyl adenosine and analogues of adenosylhomocysteine [3-deaza adenosine, 5′-deoxy-5′-(isobutylthio)-3-deazadenosine and sinefungin] inhibit the in vitro growth of *P. falciparum*. The exact mode of action of these drugs (synthesis of RNA?) is as yet undetermined. ILAN et al. (1970, 1977) reported that D-arabinosyladenine inhibited the growth of *P. berghei* in mice, as well as inhibiting protein synthesis.

### 3. Pyrimidine Biosynthesis

In 1967 and 1968 BÜNGENER and NIELSEN showed that *P. berghei*- and *P. vinckei*-infected erythrocytes incorporated tritiated hypoxanthine and adenosine, but not thymidine. The basis for these findings became clear when it was discovered that plasmodia could not synthesise the purine ring de novo, that is, labelled formate and glycine were not incorporated into plasmodial purines derived from nucleic acids (WALSH and SHERMAN 1968b). Therefore the purines necessary for the synthesis of nucleic acids and other metabolic functions had to be obtained by so-called salvage pathway mechanisms. By contrast, it was found that the plasmodia were able to incorporate [$^{14}$C]bicarbonate into pyrimidines (WALSH and SHERMAN 1968b). In keeping with the evidence for the de novo synthesis of pyrimidines has

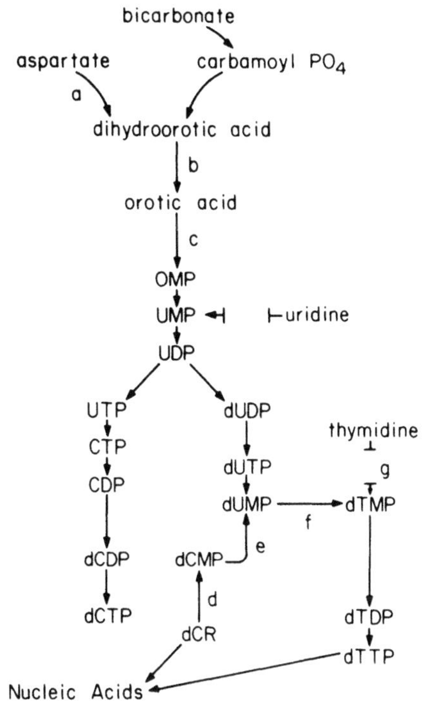


**Fig. 4.** Pyrimidine pathway *Plasmodium*. *a*, aspartate transcarbamylase (VAN DYKE et al. 1969, 1970); *b*, dihydroorotic dehydrogenase (GUTTERIDGE et al. 1979; KROOTH et al. 1969); *c*, orotidine monophosphate pyrophosphorylase (WALSH and SHERMAN 1968 b; O'SULLIVAN and KETLEY 1980); *d*, deoxycytidine kinase (KÖNIGK 1977); *e*, deoxycytidylate aminohydrolase (KÖNIGK 1977); *f*, thymidylate synthetase (WALSH and SHERMAN 1968 b; REID and FRIEDKIN 1973 b); *g*, thymidine kinase not present

been the identification of about a half-dozen enzymes associated with this pathway (Fig. 4). Thymidine kinase has not been found in plasmodia, but thymidylate synthetase has. In *P. berghei* thymidylate synthetase is distinct from that of the host cell in its higher molecular weight (REID and FRIEDKIN 1973 b).

It should be emphasised that in those cases where it has been studied, only the folate enzyme associated with pyrimidine biosynthesis (i.e. serine hydroxymethyltransferase) has been identified in plasmodial extracts, whereas the folate enzymes involved with purine metabolism are conspicuous by their absence (see below).

## 4. Purine Transport and Salvage Pathway Mechanisms

A clue to the requirement for exogenous sources of nucleic acid precursors by malaria parasites was evident from some of the earliest in vitro growth studies with *P. knowlesi* (reviewed in MCKEE 1951); namely, omission of the "purine + pyrimidine" component from the medium adversely affected the intraerythrocytic growth of the parasites. Later it was shown that, when mice and rats infected with *P. berghei* or *P. vinckei* were injected with the tritiated pyrimidines, uridine, and thymidine, there was no evidence of incorporation and in vitro incubation of *P.*

*vinckei*-infected mouse blood gave similar results. However, when exposed to radioactive adenosine, *P. berghei*-infected cells became heavily labelled (BÜNGENER and NIELSEN 1967, 1968). Autoradiographic studies using tritiated hypoxanthine showed similar patterns with *P. berghei*- and *P. vinckei*-infected erythrocytes, and when mouse erythrocytes labelled with [$^3$H]adenosine were transfused into mice infected with *P. vinckei*, radioactivity was incorporated into the malaria parasite (BÜNGENER and NIELSEN 1969).

The data on purine uptake by rodent malarias have been completely confirmed by studies with primate avian and human malarias. Thus intraerythrocytic *P. knowlesi* utilised adenine, adenosine, deoxyadenosine, guanosine, and hypoxanthine; thymine, thymidine, uracil, uridine, cytidine, and deoxycytidine were not incorporated. Only one pyrimidine, orotic acid, was incorporated into DNA and RNA (GUTTERIDGE and TRIGG 1970; POLET and BARR 1968 a). *P. lophurae*-infected red cells had a high uptake of adenosine, inosine, and hypoxanthine, with the degree of accumulation being directly related to size of the parasite (TRACY and SHERMAN 1972). In the case of adenine, the reverse was true as infected cells with multinucleate parasites took up less than red cells containing uninucleate forms. AMP, ATP, and IMP were taken up to a very limited degree. Adenosine uptake by infected cells was inhibited by the presence of hypoxanthine and inosine, but such mutual inhibition was not seen in normal cells and adenine, guanine, and ATP did not act as uptake inhibitors. TRACY and SHERMAN (1972) suggested that adenosine was deaminated to inosine shortly before or during uptake by the parasitised cell. Thus they concluded that adenosine, inosine, and hypoxanthine had a common 6-oxypurine transport site on the infected red-cell membrane.

Most workers have found that only purines are transported into the malaria-infected erythrocyte, whereas pyrimidines (except for orotic acid) seem to be excluded. NEAME et al. (1974) have disputed this. They incubated *P. berghei*-infected cells with purines (adenosine and guanosine) and pyrimidines (cytidine and thymidine) and showed that for all substrates tested there was equilibrium across the red-cell membrane, although only purines were incorporated. Thus according to these workers, the poor utilisation of pyrimidines was due not to their inability to permeate the red cell but, rather, to a deficiency of the enzymes necessary to effect phosphorylation or incorporation. It should be noted that in the in vitro studies of NEAME et al. incubation time was prolonged (1 h) and substrate concentrations were exceedingly high (1 mmol/litre). Probably pyrimidines (except for orotic acid) are not utilised in vivo by malaria-infected cells for several reasons: first, they are transported very slowly into the erythrocyte; second, the appropriate host cell and plasmodial enzymes to convert these into nucleotides are lacking; and third, the parasites synthesise pyrimidines de novo.

WALSH and SHERMAN (1968 b) speculated: "The parasite is capable of the de novo synthesis of pyrimidines including thymidylate and presumably utilises these compounds for the synthesis of DNA and RNA. *P. lophurae* synthesises purines de novo only to a limited extent and therefore must rely on exogenous sources of these compounds. The most obvious source is the host erythrocyte which contains a relatively high concentration of purines. ..."

What are the purine sources in the erythrocyte that the growing plasmodium requires? Approximately 80% of the red cell's purines are in the form of ATP, and potentially this could be utilised by the parasite. Indeed, TRAGER (1950) found that the extracellular survival of *P. lophurae* (freed from the host cell by haemolytic antiserum) was favoured by the addition of ATP to a red-cell extract (RCE) medium. Although ATP promoted extracellular development of the parasite, addition of AMP, and ATP both interfered with the uptake of radiolabelled adenine (TRAGER 1971). This suggests that the added AMP and ATP were altered after being added to the RCE, and the resultant nucleosides and nucleobases acted as competitors for the plasmodial adenine transport locus. In TRAGER's view, the role of exogenous ATP is for the active transport of materials across the two closely apposed membranes that separate the cytoplasms of red cell and parasite and, in support of this, TRAGER (1973) showed that bongkrekic acid, an inhibitor of mitochondrial ATPase and cation transport, inhibited the extracellular growth of *P. lophurae* and the intracellular development of *P. falciparum*. Addition of ATP (2–12 mmol/litre) reversed the bongkrekic acid (1.4–35 μg) effects. Atractyloside, a related inhibitor, was without effect, however. Despite such findings, there is still no direct evidence to show what role ATP exerts on parasite growth.

What purine is utilised in vivo by the intracellular parasite? Using saponin-"free" *P. lophurae*, a high uptake of hypoxanthine, adenosine, inosine, and guanine was demonstrated, whereas uptake of guanosine, xanthine, adenine, AMP, ATP, and IMP was low (TRACY and SHERMAN 1972). The magnitude of the uptake, the high distribution ratios ($>90\%$ of the available radioactivity, at low substrate concentrations, was inside the cell), the saturation kinetics at high purine levels and the phenomenon of mutual inhibition suggested that the "free" parasites transported adenosine, inosine, and hypoxanthine by a common carrier. Unfortunately, the transport studies were compromised by long (5-min) incubation periods and the fact that some substrate metabolism took place. TRACY and SHERMAN (1972) speculated that hypoxanthine might be the purine species available to *P. lophurae* in vivo and that the exogenously added adenosine was probably deaminated to inosine during uptake by "free" parasites in vitro. It is of interest to note that in vitro intraerythrocytic growth of *P. lophurae* took place in Weymouth's medium, which contains $2.5 \times 10^{-4}$ mol/litre hypoxanthine as the sole purine (WALSH and SHERMAN 1968) and that TRIGG and GUTTERIDGE (1971) found good *P. knowlesi* growth could be obtained in vitro with adenosine (40 $\mu M$) as the only added purine.

Purine uptake by mammalian erythrocytes infected with *P. knowlesi* and *P. berghei* has been used as a tool for studying drug effects. Thus, VAN DYKE and his associates (1969) found that mepacrine, DDS, daunomycin and actinomycin all inhibited the incorporation of adenosine-8-[$^3$H] into cells parasitised by *P. berghei*. TRIGG et al. (1971) reported that $10^{-6}$ $M$ cordycepin inhibited the incorporation of radioactive adenosine and hypoxanthine into *P. knowlesi* DNA and RNA, and MCCORMICK et al. (1974) used in vitro adenosine uptake by *P. knowlesi* to screen potential antimalarial compounds.

Despite there being many investigations with intracellular parasites, studies of purine uptake by erythrocyte-free mammalian plasmodia are limited to one species, *P. berghei* (reviewed in SHERMAN 1977a). Early studies with "saponin-freed" parasites in Krebs' buffer indicated that radioactivity from adenosine or ATP was incorporated into parasite nucleic acids and it was believed that ATP did not cross the parasite membrane directly, but first was degraded to adenosine by ATPase from contaminating red-cell stroma. Cytidine and uridine were not incorporated. When saponin-freed parasites were suspended in plasma, the pattern of tritium incorporation was AMP > ADP > ATP > adenosine, but no incorporation of label was obtained with ATP-$\gamma$-$^{32}$P or ATP-$\beta$,$\gamma$-$^{32}$P, suggesting that the $^{32}$P label was cleaved from the [$^{32}$P]ATP before the nucleoside, adenosine, penetrated the plasmodium. The higher efficiency of AMP-8-[$^{3}$H] when compared with adenosine-8-[$^{3}$H] was believed to be due to the former being a protected form of the nucleoside. AMP was not as easily deaminated as the utilisable adenosine and the slow dephosphorylation of AMP gradually released adenosine. Using this method LANTZ et al. (1971) and CARTER and VAN DYKE (1972) found that radioactive AMP incorporation by "free" parasites was inhibited by acridines, phenanthridine, ethidium, and mepacrine.

The use of plasma as a suspending medium coupled with the presence of red-cell stroma in the aforementioned experiments makes it uncertain as to which purine species was actually utilised. Although initially VAN DYKE and co-workers were of the opinion that adenosine was phosphorylated to AMP by the parasite, more recently they suggested the following scheme: adenosine → inosine → hypoxanthine in the extracellular medium, with phosphorylated compounds (IMP → AMP → ADP → ATP) being present in the parasite. Patterson's compound 555 (an inhibitor of adenosine transport) had no effect on adenosine incorporation, whereas $10^{-6}$–$10^{-4}$ $M$ purine-6-sulphonic acid-3*N*-oxide effectively blocked uptake and phosphorylation of tritiated hypoxanthine by both *P. berghei*-parasitised red cells and "free" parasites. Accordingly, the conclusion drawn was that hypoxanthine is the initial entry compound for free parasites (MANANDHAR and VAN DYKE 1975). However, no control preparations of red-cell ghosts [which routinely contaminate saponin-"freed" parasites (TRAGER et al. 1972)] were tested, total removal of leucocytes and platelets was not attempted and parasites entirely free of red-cell contaminants (e.g. plasmodia freed by haemolytic antiserum) were not employed in these studies. Since saponin-liberated parasites are leaky to macromolecules (YAMADA and SHERMAN, to be published), it is uncertain whether the added label or a resultant intermediate produced by plasmodial enzymes present in the incubation medium was being utilised.

Recently, YAMADA and SHERMAN (1981a) studied the purine sources and requirements of *P. lophurae*. They found that during the malarial infection there was a dramatic decline in the erythrocytic ATP level, and estimated that the purine pool, mainly in the form of ATP, could supply 25% of the purine requirements for the development of a uninucleate trophozoite to the schizont stage. Purine interconversion enzymes were identified in both the red cell and parasite and, based on enzyme activities, they proposed that adenylate nucleotide catabolism in the malarial infected red cell was directed towards the formation of hypoxanthine (YAMADA and SHERMAN 1981b). (This was based on the presence of 5′-adenylate deaminase, 5′IMP nucleotidase and purine nucleoside phosphorylase, which would catalyse: AMP → IMP → inosine → hypoxanthine.) On the other hand, no evidence for the production of adenosine or adenine was found, nor was there 5′AMP nucleotidase activity which would have been involved in adenosine formation. They contended that the hypoxanthine, present in the cytosol of the infected cell, was taken up and

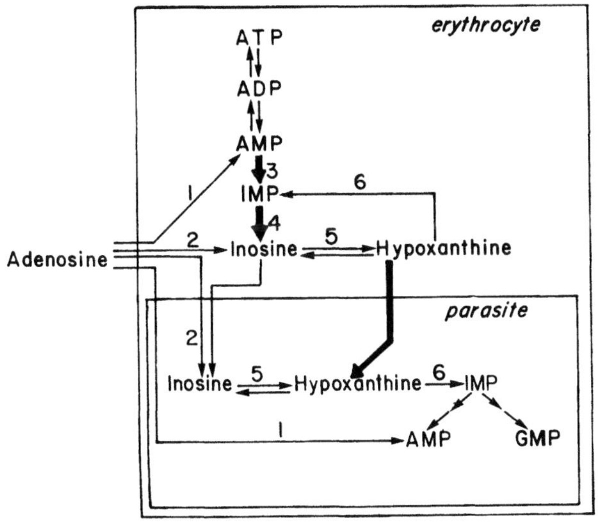


**Fig. 5.** Purine salvage pathway in the erythrocyte and *Plasmodium*. *1*, adenosine kinase; *2*, adenosine deaminase; *3*, 5′AMP deaminase; *4*, 5′IMP nucleotidase; *5*, inosine nucleoside phosphorylase; *6*, hypoxanthine phosphoribosyl transferase

utilised by the plasmodium. (The purine salvage pathway for *Plasmodium* and its host cell is summarised in Fig. 5).

It is of interest to note that BÜNGENER (1974) found that the addition of allopurinol to the drinking water of rats and mice enhanced the severity of *P. berghei*, *P. vinckei*, or *P. chabaudi* infections. Since allopurinol acts as an inhibitor of xanthine oxidase it may be that allopurinol treatment of the host increased blood levels of hypoxanthine. If we assume that purines may be a limiting factor in the multiplication of the parasites then the additional supplies of hypoxanthine in allopurinol-treated animals could contribute to parasite reproduction, although allopurinol could also have other effects.

## IV. Lipid Biosynthesis

Lipids constitute a significant fraction of the total solids of the malaria parasite and the plasmodia tend to be richer in phospholipid than their host. Approximately 80% or more of the fatty acids of the parasite total lipids are unsaturated (reviewed in HOLZ 1977). To date, direct evidence for the synthesis of long chain fatty acids from acetate by *Plasmodium* has not been obtained. Therefore what little is known about lipid biosynthesis by malaria parasites is derived from rather indirect, and often seriously compromised, observations.

Although *P. fallax* growing in turkey erythrocytes incorporated [$^{14}$C]acetate and $^{14}$C-labelled fatty acids (oleic, palmitic, and stearic) into phospholipids (primarily phosphatidylethanolamine), there was no critical examination as to whether this incorporation represented de novo biosynthesis (GUTIERREZ 1966). Indeed, CENEDELLA (1968) found that, despite the rapid incorporation of carbon from radioactive glucose into the phospholipid fraction of *P. berghei*-infected cells, less than 5% of the label was in the fatty acid portion, and the vast majority was recovered in the glycerol moiety. ROCK (1971a, b) performed similar experiments with *P. knowlesi*. He found that [$^{14}$C]palmitic, oleic, and stearic acids were readily incorporated during a 2-h in vitro incubation by infected cells and "free" parasites, whereas uninfected monkey red cells incorporated $<2\%$ of the extracellular label into lipids. Eighty to ninety per cent of the incorporated fatty acids were in the phospholipid fraction, primarily in phosphatidylethanolamine, phosphatidylcholine, and phosphatidylinositol; this was in marked contrast to the low rates of incorporation of labelled acetate, glucose or glycerol in the acyl portion of the lipid. Additionally, [$^{32}$P]orthophosphate incorporation into *P. knowlesi* was 80–100 times higher than in red-cell membranes. Incorporation was primarily into phospholipids in the parasite, whereas in the host cell it was into phosphatidic acid. The high rates of fatty acid incorporation and the low $^{32}$P-labelling pattern suggested that a rapid turnover of phosphorus rather than a net synthesis of parasite phospholipids occurred (ROCK et al. 1971). When parasites were exposed to [$^{14}$C]choline, incorporation was into phosphatidylcholine, whereas with [$^{14}$C]ethanolamine the label was recovered in phosphatidylethanolamine. Over 95% of the $^{14}$C from glucose was recovered in the glycerol moiety of the parasite phospholipids. If normal and *P. knowlesi*-infected red cells were incubated in vitro with labelled acetate, mevalonate, and cholesterol, only labelled cholesterol was recovered from the parasite membranes (TRIGG 1968). Confirmation of these metabolic studies comes from work (SIDDIQUI et al. 1967) in which it was shown that stearic acid and cholesterol enhanced the in vitro growth of *P. knowlesi*.

Thus malaria parasites appear to be incapable of fabricating fatty acids de novo. However, through the incorporation of acetate into existing fatty acids and by means of limited chain-lengthening reactions, the parasite is able to maintain a lipid fatty acid composition distinct from its host (Table 3). Since the parasite is unable to synthesise cholesterol or fatty acids, and its capabilities for desaturation are restricted, the parasite must satisfy a portion of its requirements for phospholipids, lysophospholipids, cholesterol, fatty acids, and phospholipid precursors (i.e. as glycerol, inositol, choline, and phosphorus) by participating in dynamic exchanges with components of the blood plasma during the turnover of erythrocyte lipids. Additionally, by endocytotic feeding of the parasite, both the membrane lipids of the parasite as well as those of the host cell become available for plasmodial lipid biosynthesis.

## V. Vitamins and Cofactors

### 1. Vitamin A

A dietary deficiency of vitamin A was reported to depress infections of *P. lophurae* in chicks (ROSS et al. 1946) and *P. berghei* in rats (FABIANI and GRELLET 1951). However, in another study, vitamin A deficiency produced a more acute *P. berghei* infection (BOUISSET and RUFFIE 1958). It is not clear from the available evidence whether the vitamin deficiency directly affected parasite growth or interfered with nutrition of the host.

### 2. Vitamin $B_1$ (Thiamine)

Thiamine deficiency was reported to depress *P. berghei* infections (RAMA RAO and SIRSI 1956a) and SINGER (1961) showed that the *P. berghei*-infected red cell contained more thiamine than normal cells.

### 3. Vitamin $B_2$ (Riboflavin)

A host deficiency of riboflavin decreased the severity of the course of infection of chickens with *P. lophurae* (SEELER and OTT 1944) and *P. gallinaceum* (RAMA RAO and SIRSI 1956b). This vitamin, the precursor for the coenzymes FAD and FMN, was reported to be present in *P. knowlesi* (BALL et al. 1948).

### 4. Biotin

In birds made severely deficient in biotin, infections of *P. lophurae* were of high intensity, suggesting that the vitamin deficiency impaired the immune response of the host. However, in ducklings made moderately deficient in biotin, *P. cathemerium* infections progressed slowly at first, but later the parasitaemia was considerably higher than in birds maintained on a diet having adequate amounts of biotin. It has been concluded that these results show that biotin is required by the parasite for growth, as well as by the host for developing resistance to the parasite (TRAGER 1977). There are, however, conflicting reports on the in vitro effects of biotin. SIDDIQUI et al. (1969) claimed that addition of biotin favoured the growth of *P. knowlesi* in monkey red cells, but with *P. lophurae* there was no effect, and blood from biotin-deficient monkeys did not adversely affect the in vitro growth of *P. knowlesi* (MCKEE 1951).

### 5. Nicotinic Acid (Niacin), Nicotinamide, and Pyridine Nucleotides

A deficiency of nicotinic acid in the diet of chicks produced a depression of parasitaemia with *P. lophurae* (ROSS et al. 1946), and in vitro *P. lophurae* required a high level of nicotinamide for good extracellular growth (TRAGER 1977).

The presence of NAD in *P. gallinaceum* (SPECK and EVANS 1945) and the pyridine content of *P. berghei*- and *P. lophurae*-infected red cells have been reported (SHERMAN 1966b; NAGARAJAN 1964). In both *P. lophurae* and *P. berghei* striking increases in the total pyridine nucleotides of infected cells were observed. In *P. berghei* the reduced forms increased nine fold whereas the oxidised forms increased only about twofold. Since NAD and NADP were not individually measured, and because *P. berghei* invades reticulocytes which have the capacity for pyridine nucleotide synthesis, it is possible that such increases reflect host-cell stimulation as well as the synthetic capabilities of the parasite itself. However, in *P. lophurae*, a parasite of mature erythrocytes, the NAD, NADH, and NADP levels were increased only twofold in the infected red cell and, during infection, the NADPH content remained unchanged. The NADH, NADPH, and NADP content of free *P. lophurae* was equivalent in amount to that found in the duckling red cell, whereas the NAD content of the parasite was 1.5 times greater. It was assumed that the parasites fabricated their own pyridine nucleotides since the total content of the *P. lophurae*-infected cell could be arrived at by simply summing the content of the free parasite with that of the uninfected erythrocyte. Direct utilisation of host-cell NADPH has been suggested for *P. berghei* (ECKMAN and EATON 1979).

### 6. Ascorbic Acid

A dietary deficiency of vitamin C (ascorbic acid) in rhesus monkeys greatly inhibited the multiplication of *P. knowlesi*, and administration of this vitamin reversed the effect (McKEE 1951). However, since absence of ascorbic acid in the in vitro culture medium had no effect on parasite growth, it was assumed that this vitamin acted indirectly via the host. No evidence for a change in the ascorbic acid content in the adrenal glands of chicks infected with *P. gallinaceum* was detected in spite of adrenal hypertrophy (McKEE 1951).

### 7. Vitamin E

The effect of vitamin E on the course of a malarial infection was tested indirectly. The addition of vitamin E was found to reverse the depressive effect of a cod-liver oil diet on *P. berghei* in mice (GODFREY 1957) and *P. gallinaceum* in chicks (TAYLOR 1958). In a more direct test vitamin E-deficient mice were found to be more resistant to *P. berghei* (EATON et al. 1976).

### 8. Vitamin $B_6$ Group

SEELER (1945) found that massive doses of pyridoxine reversed the antimalarial activity of quinine and mepacrine against *P. lophurae* and RAMAKRISHNAN (1954) noted that if rats were placed on a pyridoxine-deficient diet *P. berghei* infections were low. TRAGER (1977) suggested that the lower activity of pyridoxine kinase in the red cells of Africans might exert a selective advantage in such individuals if the parasite lacked this enzyme. However, PLATZER and KASSIS (1978) found pyridoxine kinase in *P. lophurae*, suggesting that plasmodial metabolism of vitamin $B_6$ was independent of the host cell. The *lophurae* enzyme had a lower affinity for pyridoxine than the host-cell enzyme. Thus if the host were limited in the availability of pyridoxine, the parasite would be deprived of this essential cofactor since the pyridoxine must first cross the host-cell cytoplasm before it can enter the plasmodium. Deoxypyridoxine competitively inhibited both the host-cell and parasite enzymes.

### 9. Pantothenate

Pantothenate when added in vitro to *P. lophurae*-infected erythrocytes maintained parasite infectivity and the viability of male gametocytes. In vivo studies with blood-induced *P. gallinaceum* infections in chickens showed that parasitaemias were lower in pantothenate-deficient birds (summarised in TRAGER 1977). Later, the role of pantothenate in the growth of the parasite became clearer. TRAGER found that pantothenate, a precursor of coenzyme A (CoA), when added to extracellular *P. lophurae* had no beneficial effects and that only CoA would lengthen the extracellular survival of the parasites (TRAGER 1952). CoA could not be replaced by phosphopantothenoyl cysteine, although some restoration of extracellular growth took place with phosphopantetheine and complete growth was achieved when the red-cell extract-containing medium was supplemented with dephospho CoA (TRAGER and BROHN 1975).

TRAGER hypothesised that the parasite required CoA, but was unable to synthesise it from pantothenate. Because the parasite was entirely dependent on the host to supply the intact coenzyme, TRAGER suggested that the plasmodia were obligately parasitic. This hypothesis was supported by the finding that, although all of the enzymes in the biosynthetic pathway from pantothenate to CoA were present in the red cell, none could be found in the free parasites (BENNETT and TRAGER 1967; BROHN and TRAGER 1975). The beneficial effects of phosphopantetheine and dephospho CoA on the extracellular growth of *P. lophurae* can be ascribed to the conversion of these by erythrocyte enzymes present in the red-cell extract of the culture medium and not by plasmodial activity. Indeed, because the CoA activity of the host cell declined as parasite growth increased, it tends to support the argument that the parasites destroy rather than contribute to the host-cell constituents. Moreover, since the CoA content of the liver of the host declines during the infection (SINGER 1956), it may be that the CoA required by the malaria parasite is synthesised in other organs and transported to the red cell.

CoA is required for the oxidation of glucose via the citric acid cycle and for the synthesis of cellular constituents by acetylation reactions. Therefore a deficiency in its availability could impair parasite growth. The antimetabolitic effects of pantothenate analogues on the in vitro intracellular growth of *P. falciparum* and *P. coatneyi* (TRAGER 1977) are undoubtedly related to this.

## 10. Vitamin K and Ubiquinones

Coenzymes Q (CoQ) are components of the electron transport system of mitochondria. Despite there being limited information concerning mitochondrial function in plasmodia, it has been speculated that the antimalarial activity of certain naphthoquinones could be related to their structural similarity to vitamin K and/or ubiquinone (WAN et al. 1974). An extensive search for vitamin K and its synthesis from shikimic acid proved to be fruitless. However, ubiquinones-8 and -9 (CoQ) were identified in *P. lophurae*-infected duck blood, but only $CoQ_{10}$ was found in *P. knowlesi*, *P. cynomolgi*, and *P. berghei* (RIETZ et al. 1967; SCHNELL et al. 1971; SKELTON et al. 1969, 1970). Although $Q_{10}$ and $Q_9$ as well as $Q_8$ occur in the blood of normal rhesus monkeys, and $Q_9$ and $Q_8$ are found in mouse blood, the predominance of $Q_8$ in the samples of infected blood suggests that this coenzyme is characteristic of the parasite.

Of the CoQ analogues tested for antimalarial activity only a few alkylmercaptoquinones were found to be effective (WAN et al. 1974). While these compounds do resemble $CoQ_8$ the biochemical basis for their antimalarial action is far from established, although it is suspected that their activity is not solely confined to the inhibition of $CoQ_8$ activity or its biosynthesis.

## 11. Folates

### a) Biosynthesis of Dihydrofolate and Tetrahydrofolate

Nutritional studies have amply confirmed the plasmodial requirement for para-aminobenzoic acid (PABA). The in vitro growth of *P. knowlesi* was improved by adding PABA to the medium, parasitaemias in *P. berghei*-infected rats and *P. cynomolgi*-infected monkeys were suppressed when the hosts were maintained on a milk diet low in PABA, *Aotus* monkeys kept on a milk diet did not support good growth of *P. falciparum*, and the severity of a *P. berghei* infection in mice was directly related to the PABA level of the diet (reviewed in FERONE 1977). The investigations on milk diet and PABA strongly suggested that malaria parasites synthesised their folate cofactors de novo and did not utilise exogenously supplied, intact folate molecules as did their hosts. Thus, sulphanilamide, sulphaquinoxaline, sulphadimethoxine, and dapsone, analogues of PABA, all probably act as antimalarials by preventing the synthesis of dihydropteroate, an intermediate in the formation of tetrahydrofolate.

Further confirmation of the folate biosynthetic pathway in malaria parasites has come from the identification of the enzymes involved in the formation of dihydrofolate and tetrahydrofolate. Extracts of *P. chabaudi*, *P. berghei*, *P. knowlesi*, *P. lophurae* and *P. gallinaceum* contained dihydropteroate synthetase, and extracts of *P. chabaudi* and *P. berghei* contained 2-amino-4-hydroxy-6-hydroxymethyl-dihydropteridine pyrophosphokinase (summarised by FERONE 1977). Dihydrofolate reductase has been found in *P. lophurae*, *P. berghei*, *P. chabaudi*, and *P. knowlesi* (FERONE et al. 1969; PLATZER 1974; GUTTERIDGE and TRIGG 1971). The activity of dihydrofolate (DHF) reductase markedly increased during the growth of *P. chabaudi* (WALTER and KÖNIGK 1971), with maximal activity occurring during schizogony. In both pyrimethamine-sensitive and abnormal strains of various plasmodial species the enzyme had a molecular weight of 100000–200000, which is five to ten times greater than the dihydrofolate reductase of birds, mammals, helminths, and bacteria, but of similar size to that reported for other protozoans. The DHF reductase of the parasite is exquisitely more sensitive to pyrimethamine than is the host-cell enzyme.

### b) Tetrahydrofolate Metabolism

Erythrocyte-free *P. berghei*, unlike the host cell, cannot reduce exogenously supplied folate to dihydrofolate, indicating that the parasites lack folate reductase (FERONE and HITCHINGS 1966). However, if *P. berghei* are supplied with dihydrofolate they are capable of forming tetrahydrofolates since they produce substances that promote the growth of *Pediococcus cerevesiae* (REID and FRIEDKIN 1973a). PLATZER (1972) reported that, although serine hydroxymethyltransferase (SHMT) was increased in *P. lophurae*-infected cells, the activities of formyltetrahydrofolate synthetase (FTHFS) and methylene tetrahydrofolate dehydrogenase (MTHFDH) were decreased in infected red cells. Indeed, neither of the latter two enzymes was demonstrable in extracts of free *P. lophurae*. The SHMT of *P. lophurae* was found to be cytosolic (PLATZER 1977) and distinctly different from the host-cell enzyme in molecular weight, pH optimum, and thermostability. Based on these findings, as well as the presence of DHF and thymidylate synthetase in extracts of *P. lophurae* (WALSH and SHERMAN 1968b), *P. chabaudi* (WALTER and KÖNIGK 1971), and *P. berghei* (REID and FRIEDKIN 1973b), PLATZER (1972) proposed the existence of a "thymidylate synthesis cycle" in plasmodia: dihydrofolate → tetrahydrofolate → $N^5$, $N^{10}$ methylene tetrahydrofolate → dihydrofolate. Such a cycle (Fig. 6) conveniently accounts for the de novo biosynthesis of pyrimidines by the parasite, and supports the contention that malaria parasites rely on salvage pathway enzymes for their purines, but are incapable of synthesising purines de novo.

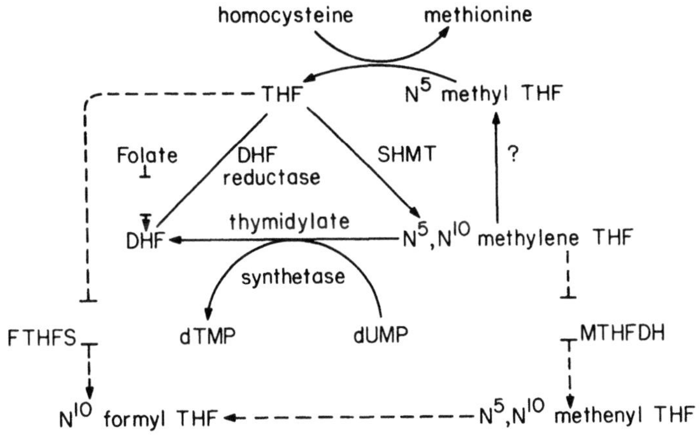


**Fig. 6.** Thymidylate synthesis cycle

Recently, reactions involving the synthesis of methionine and participation of $N^5$ methyl THF have been demonstrated in malaria-infected cells (SMITH et al. 1976). Thus it is possible that, in addition to the thymidylate synthesis cycle, another folate pathway exists. However, the enzymes involved in the formation of $N^5$ methyl THF have not been identified, and the conversion rate of homocysteine to methionine was low. If malaria parasites synthesise THF de novo, and require only PABA for the formation of DHF, then how can one explain the beneficial effects of added folic and folinic acid ($N^5$ formyl THF) on plasmodia growing intracellularly and extracellularly (SIDDIQUI and TRAGER 1966), and the finding that these materials and PABA reversed the inhibition of DNA synthesis by sulphalene but not pyrimethamine? The simplest explanation is that pteridines or para-aminoglutamic acid (pABG) were contaminants in the samples of folic or folinic acid, and/or media contained host enzymes which were able to break down the added folates into pABG, and then this was converted by the parasite to utilisable THF (FERONE 1977).

It appears then that malarial parasites do not use exogenous folates supplied from the host cell for two reasons: they are impermeable to these molecules, and they lack the appropriate enzymes for conversion to utilisable THF cofactors.

## H. Biochemical Characteristics of the Erythrocyte and Host-Parasite Relationships

### I. Sickle Cell Haemoglobin

It is now an accepted fact that carriers of sickle cell haemoglobin are resistant to *P. falciparum*. The molecular basis for such protection has been elucidated by using in vitro cultures of malaria parasites in erythrocytes bearing this abnormal haemoglobin. Although minimal retardation in invasion and growth of *P. falciparum* was in evidence in heterozygous (AS) and homozygous (SS) cells maintained aerobically (~18% $O_2$), when these infected cells were exposed to low oxygen tensions (1%–5%) parasite growth was severely limited (FRIEDMAN 1978; FRIEDMAN et al.

1979a; PASVOL et al. 1978). In vitro, after about 6 h exposure to low $O_2$, the parasites in SS red cells were found to be mechanically disrupted by needle-like aggregates of deoxygenated sickle cell haemoglobin, and this ultimately ruptured the parasite membranes (FRIEDMAN 1979a). In AS red cells physical disruption at low $O_2$ tensions did not take place, but instead the parasites showed extensive vacuolisation and a leaching of the cytoplasm. This occurred, according to FRIEDMAN et al. (1979a), because of a parasite-induced drop in the red-cell intracellular pH as well as a leakage of red-cell potassium.

Since parasitised AS red cells sickle more readily than unparasitised erythrocytes when deoxygenated in vitro (ROTH et al. 1978), and *falciparum*-infected red cells are sequestered in the deep tissues where oxygen tensions are low, it has been suggested that intracellular death of the parasite may occur during the sickling process itself. However, it is also possible that parasite death may occur with the removal of infected sickled erythrocytes by the phagocytic elements of the spleen.

## II. Other Haemoglobins and Thalassaemia

### 1. Haemoglobin F

At birth red cells contain mainly fetal haemoglobin (HbF), and during the 1st year of life this is replaced by adult haemoglobin (HbA). Young red cells containing HbA were shown to be preferentially invaded by *P. falciparum* in vitro when compared with HbA cells from the adult, and the rate of development in both kinds of cells was not the same. When HbA and HbF cells of the same age were compared it was found that the invasion rate was similar, but the growth of *P. falciparum* was retarded in HbF-containing cells (PASVOL et al. 1977; WILSON et al. 1977). This result was not due to an age effect of the red cells since adult cells having the genetic abnormality (hereditary persistence of fetal haemoglobin) were used. Thus it would seem that younger red cells, whether they contain HbF or HbA, are preferentially invaded by *P. falciparum* (PASVOL et al. 1980); in HbF cells parasite growth is retarded, but invasion is unaffected. The degree of plasmodial growth inhibition was directly correlated with the amount of erythrocyte HbF. The mechanisms involved in growth retardation are as yet unknown.

### 2. Haemoglobin C

Haemoglobin C carries a $\beta$-chain mutation which in vivo increases intermolecular attraction and produces some haemoglobin aggregation, deoxygenation in vitro producing crystallisation of the haemoglobin. The in vitro growth rate of *P. falciparum* in HbA/HbC cells was similar to that in HbA/HbA cells, but multiplication was sharply limited in HbC/HbC erythrocytes. No effect of reduced oxygen on growth of *P. falciparum* in the HbA/HbC cells was observed. Although the multiplication of parasites in HbS/HbC cells was unaffected when fully oxygenated, the parasites were killed when the cells were placed in an atmosphere containing 3% $O_2$. Since red cells under these circumstances have an enhanced rate of sickling (because HbC interacts with HbS to promote crystallisation), crystals of haemoglobin were responsible for disrupting the parasite. The mechanism by which parasite growth is impaired in HbC/HbC cells is not known, but it could involve the enhanced tendency of HbC to crystallise in the infected red cell (FRIEDMAN et al. 1979 b).

### 3. Thalassaemias

PASVOL et al. (1977) did not find a significant reduction in the maturation rate of *P. falciparum* in in vitro cultures of thalassaemic red cells however. FRIEDMAN (1979b) was of the opinion that in thalassaemic red cells parasite development was impaired by oxidative stress. Riboflavin (2 μ*M*), menadione (2.5 μ*M*), and high $O_2$ (25%) were inhibitory to parasite growth in vitro. He suggested that the sensitivity of the thalassaemic cells to riboflavin was due to the sensitivity of these cells to free radicals, since vitamin E (α-tocopherol) reversed the effect. In addition, dithiothreitol protected thalassaemic red cells from menadione-induced production of $H_2O_2$. FRIEDMAN hypothesised that oxidant damage to the thalassaemic red cell causes an increase in cation permeability, and leakage of this sort leads to an impairment of parasite metabolism. Indeed, in a medium lacking reduced glutathione, parasites could be protected if the medium contained increased amounts of potassium (150 m*M*). Presumably, the high potassium medium acted to prevent the loss of red-cell potassium, and therefore, despite damage to the red-cell membrane, the parasite was spared.

## III. Glucose-6-phosphate Dehydrogenase Deficiency and Reduced Glutathione Content

The gene *Gd* for glucose-6-phosphate dehydrogenase (G6PDH) is sex-linked in humans. Because of random X-chromosome inactivation, females heterozygous for G6PDH deficiency (Gd+/Gd−) are genetic mosaics, whereas males are either Gd+ or Gd−. In the early 1960s it was suggested that an erythrocytic deficiency of G6PDH could afford some protection against *P. falciparum*. In a survey of females with acute febrile malaria, parasite rates were lower in heterozygotes and, within the blood of such individuals, the G6PDH (+) cells invariably had more parasites than did the G6PDH (−) erythrocytes. However, in vivo parasite development in Gd− males has been shown to be essentially normal. Thus in vivo resistance to malaria appears to be restricted to the heterozygous female, but why this is so remains unclear. In vitro studies with *P. falciparum* showed that parasite growth was impaired in G6PDH (−) red cells if they were subjected to high $O_2$ (30%), menadione (2.5 μ*M*) or riboflavin (2 μ*M*). These effects were only partly reversed by vitamin E, but dithiothreitol (DTT) was more effective. Based on these findings, FRIEDMAN (1979b) suggested that, in G6PDH (−) cells, the production of peroxide by the parasite tends to overload the reducing capacity of the red cell and, as a consequence, there is a depletion of reduced glutathione, and peroxide damage to the erythrocyte membrane ensues. The addition of DTT to the medium serves to reduce the intracellular oxidised glutathione, protects red-cell catalase, and the $H_2O_2$ level is lowered. Since addition of catalase (50 μg/ml) to the medium also protected parasites in G6PDH (−) cells, it was contended that the enhanced survival of carriers of this trait was related to the oxidant sensitivity of these cells (FRIEDMAN 1979b). However, as noted above, this does not explain why in vivo the growth of *P. falciparum* in the G6PDH (−) male is normal (see also LUZZATTO 1979).

The hexose monophosphate shunt of the red cell provides NADPH for the reduction of oxidised glutathione (GSSG → GSH). In G6PDH (−) cells, the formation of NADPH is low and, when subjected to oxidant stress, such cells lose GSH, haemoglobin is oxidised and ultimately these cells are removed by the phagocytic elements of the reticuloendothelial system. FLETCHER and MAEGRAITH (1970) found no change in the level of GSH in *P. berghei*-infected red cells, but with *P. knowlesi* they observed a decrease. SHERMAN (1965) claimed that there was no reduction in the amount of GSH in *P. lophurae*-infected cells. However, PICARD-MAUREAU et al. (1975) recorded both a ten fold increase in the level of GSH in *P. vinckei*-infected red cells, and a concomitant decline in the level of G6PDH. Recently, ECKMAN and EATON (1979) found that *P. berghei*-infected erythrocytes had more than twice the GSH content of uninfected red cells, and that most of this GSH was localised in the parasite. Additionally, infected cells had significantly higher levels of NADP-specific glutathione reductase, and this was related to the presence of a parasite enzyme. Since all of the malaria parasites examined to date lack G6PDH activity, these authors proposed that the NADPH for glutathione reduction came from the red cell, perhaps via a NADPH-linked reduction of parasite GSSG. If this were the case, they contended, then the presence of excess NADP in the infected cell would contribute to the observed increase in oxidant sensitivity, as well as the acceleration of pentose shunt activity of infected cells.

Malaria parasites do lack the capacity for NADP reduction via the hexose monophosphate shunt by virtue of the fact that G6PDH is absent from all species of *Plasmodium*, but they do have an NADP-specific glutamic dehydrogenase which could serve in this capacity. Further, although *P. knowlesi*-infected erythrocytes utilised significantly more glucose than uninfected erythrocytes, the mean percent of glucose metabolised via the shunt declined from 10% in normal red cells to 4% in infected blood samples (BARNES and POLET 1969). A similar pattern of glucose metabolism has been found in *P. falciparum* growing in vitro (ROTH, personal communication). Thus there is neither evidence for the direct utilisation of host-cell NADPH by the intraerythrocytic plasmodium, nor does there appear to be preferential stimulation of the shunt. It seems that the parasites synthesise and/or accumulate red-cell glutathione which can be reduced by a parasite-specific glutathione reductase.

## IV. Adenosine Triphosphate Deficiency

In 1950 TRAGER found that addition of ATP to in vitro cultures of extracellular *P. lophurae* enhanced survival, growth, and reproduction of the parasite. He concluded that the malaria parasite had an essential requirement of ATP. Indeed, in most experimental malarias, the ATP content of the erythrocyte declines dramatically during plasmodial growth, and the fall in blood ATP levels is correlated with the proportion of infected red cells. In a study of non-immune blacks infected with falciparum malaria, a significant positive correlation between the preinfection level of ATP in the red cell and the rise in parasitaemia early in the course of infection was found (BREWER and POWELL 1965). Based on this, it was proposed that the erythrocytic ATP level might affect the severity of malaria in the host. If the ATP levels in the erythrocyte were low enough it might slow the rate of increase in parasitaemia and permit immune mechanisms to come into play before high parasitaemia-related mortality occurred. Following this line of reasoning, EATON and BREWER (1969) found a strong positive correlation between peak parasitaemia and preinfection ATP levels in rhesus monkeys infected with *P. cynomolgi*, and BREWER and COAN (1969) reported that hyperoxia diminished, at least initially, the rise in parasitaemia in *P. vinckei-* and *P. berghei*-infected rodents. The exact mechanism for the hyperoxic effect was not determined, but it was suggested that ATP might be involved. Quite possibly an ATP-deficient cell has a reduced survival time after infection and therefore parasite schizogony cannot be completed, or an ATP-deficient cell cannot provide those substances (whatever they may be) essential for parasite growth and reproduction. However, there are no data to indicate which, if any, of these operate in vivo.

## J. Cation Alterations

OVERMAN et al. (1949) showed that a profound cationic imbalance existed in the plasma and erythrocytes of monkeys infected with *P. knowlesi*. Similar findings were reported for *P. gallinaceum* in chickens (OVERMAN et al. 1950), *P. lophurae* in ducklings (SHERMAN and TANIGOSHI 1971 a), *P. coatneyi* in monkeys, *P. falciparum* in chimpanzees, and *P. berghei* in hamsters (DUNN 1969 a, b). The most significant increases of potassium occur in the plasma, whereas in the erythrocyte the most striking change is an elevation in the level of sodium. DUNN (1969 a) studied sodium alterations in some detail and found that red blood cell sodium level was increased disproportionately to the parasitaemia. This increase persisted for several days after drug therapy had eradicated the infection and non-parasitised as well as parasitised erythrocytes were abnormal in their capacity for sodium extrusion. The ATP content of the red cells also increased two to three times and this paralleled the increases in parasitaemia and intracellular sodium.

DUNN postulated that the elevated sodium level was a consequence of a circulating toxin that diminished the efflux of sodium, while promoting its influx. However, cross-incubation experiments with malarious plasma did not produce sodium transport changes identical to those found in the infected animal. Since the disruption of the cation gradient was found to be both gradual and unrelated to immunological phenomena, it seems more plausible to ascribe these events not to a toxin, but to a modification of proteins involved in the sodium pump. Membrane protein changes could also contribute to the osmotic fragility of non-parasitised cells in the malarious host.

## K. Conclusion

Successful invasion of the erythrocyte by a merozoite involves specific binding of the parasite to a surface receptor and induction of endocytosis. Malaria parasites may alter the red-cell surface but the exact mechanisms whereby such parasite-provoked changes come about is uncertain. The malaria parasite is incapable of de novo synthesis of fatty acids and of cholesterol. Intraerythrocytically, bird, and mammalian malarias appear to derive energy by changing glucose into lactic acid via a conventional scheme of anaerobic glycolysis. Avian parasites oxidise a portion of the pyruvate to $CO_2$ and $H_2O$ by means of the citric acid cycle, whereas rodent and primate malarias, lacking a functional citric acid cycle, are unable to do so, and have lactate as their primary end product. There is no evidence for a pentose phosphate shunt in malaria parasites since the first enzyme in the pathway (G6PDH) is absent.

Evidence for an energy-yielding electron transport chain is at best circumstantial. In all the malarias studied, the only enzyme found to be associated with this system is cytochrome oxidase.

Malaria parasites are incapable of de novo purine biosynthesis, but pyrimidines are synthesised de novo. The mechanism of protein synthesis by the parasites is typically eukaryotic. The capacity of the parasite for de novo amino acid biosynthesis is limited, and it seems probable that the host-cell haemoglobin provides most of the amino acids. The only well-characterised plasmodial protein is the histidine-rich protein (HRP) of *P. lophurae*.

Information regarding the vitamin requirements of malaria parasites is scanty.

Characteristically, malaria-infected erythrocytes show an elevated sodium content due to an inability of the cell to extrude this cation. It has been postulated that this alteration is provoked by a circulating toxin, but it is also possible to ascribe such a change to modifications in membrane lipid-protein architecture.

*Acknowledgements.* The work reported here was supported by research grants from the National Institute of Allergy and Infectious Diseases. U.S. Public Health Service (AI-05226) and the National Science Foundation (PCM 782216). Portions of this review were modified from SHERMAN (1979).

## References

Aikawa M (1977) Variations in structure and function during the life cycle of malarial parasites. Bull WHO 55:139–156

Anfinsen CB, Geiman QM, McKee RW, Ormsbee RA, Ball EG (1946) Studies on malarial parasites. VIII. Factors affecting the growth of *Plasmodium knowlesi* in vitro. J Exp Med 84:607–621

Bahr GF (1966) Quantitative cytochemical study of erythrocytic stages of *Plasmodium lophurae* and *Plasmodium berghei*. Milit Med 131:1064–1070

Ball EG, McKee RW, Anfinsen CB, Cruz WO, Geiman QM (1948) Studies on malarial parasites. IX. Chemical and metabolic changes during growth and multiplication in vivo and in vitro. J Biol Chem 175:547–571

Bannister L, Butcher G, Mitchell G (1977) Recent advances in understanding the invasion of erythrocytes by merozoites of *Plasmodium knowlesi*. Bull WHO 55:163–170

Barnes MG, Polet H (1969) The influence of methylene blue on the pentose phosphate pathway in erythrocytes of monkeys infected with *Plasmodium knowlesi*. J Lab Clin Med 74:1–11

Bass CC, Johns FM (1912) The cultivation of malarial plasmodia (*Plasmodium vivax* and *Plasmodium falciparum*) in vitro. J Exp Med 16:567–579

Bennett TP, Trager W (1967) Pantothenic acid metabolism during avian malaria infection: pantothenate kinase activity in duck erythrocytes and in *Plasmodium lophurae*. J Protozool 14:214–216

Bouisset L, Ruffie J (1958) Course of *Plasmodium berghei* malaria in white rats deficient in vitamin A. Ann Parasitol Hum 33(3):209–217

Bovarnick MR, Lindsay A, Hellerman L (1946a) Metabolism of the malarial parasite, with reference particularly to the action of antimalarial agents. I. Preparation and properties of *Plasmodium lophurae* separated from the red cells of duck blood by means of saponin. J Biol Chem 163:523–533

Bovarnick MR, Lindsay A, Hellerman L (1946b) Metabolism of the malarial parasite, with reference particularly to the action of antimalarial agents. II. Atabrine (quinacrine) inhibition of glucose oxidation in parasites initially depleted of substrate. Reversal by adenylic acid. J Biol Chem 163:535–531

Bowman IBR, Grant PT, Kermack WO (1960) The metabolism of *Plasmodium berghei*, separated from the host cell. Exp Parasitol 9:131–136

Bowman IBR, Grant PT, Kermack WO, Ogston D (1961) The metabolism of *Plasmodium berghei*, the malaria parasite of rodents. 2. An effect of mepacrine on the metabolism of glucose by the parasite separated from its host cell. Biochem J 78:472–478

Brewer GJ, Coan CC (1969) Interaction of red cell ATP levels and malaria, and the treatment of malaria with hyperoxia. Milit Med 134:1056–1067

Brewer GJ, Powell RD (1965) A study of the relationship between the content of adenosine triphosphate in human red cells and the course of falciparum malaria: a new system that may confer protection against malaria. Proc Nat Acad Sci USA 54:741–745

Brohn FH, Trager W (1975) Coenzyme A requirement of malarial parasites: enzymes of coenzyme A biosynthesis in normal duck erythrocytes and erythrocytes infected with *Plasmodium lophurae*. Proc Nat Acad Sci USA 72:2456–2458

Bryant C, Voller A, Smith MJH (1964) The incorporation of radioactivity from [$^{14}$]glucose into the soluble metabolic intermediates of malaria parasites. Am J Trop Med Hyg 13:515–519

Büngener W (1974) Einfluß von Allopurinol auf Zyklusdauer und Vermehrungsrate von *Plasmodium vinckei* in der Ratte. Tropenmedizin Parasitol 25:464–468

Büngener W, Nielsen G (1967) Nukleinsäurenstoffwechsel bei experimenteller Malaria. 1. Untersuchungen über den Einbau von Thymidin, Uridin und Adenosin in Malariaparasiten (*Plasmodium berghei* and *Plasmodium vinckei*). Z Tropenmed Parasitol 18:456–462

Büngener W, Nielsen G (1968) Nukleinsäurenstoffwechsel bei experimenteller Malaria. 2. Einbau von Adenosin und Hypoxanthin in die Nukleinsäuren von Malariaparasiten (*Plasmodium berghei* and *Plasmodium vinckei*). Z Tropenmed Parasitol 19:185–197

Büngener W, Nielsen G (1969) Nukleinsäurenstoffwechsel bei experimenteller Malaria. 3. Einbau von Adenin aus dem Adeninnukleotidpool der Erythrozyten in die Nukleinsäuren von Malariaparasiten. Z Tropenmed Parasitol 20:66–73

Carter G, Van Dyke K (1972) Drug effects on the phosphorylation of adenosine and its incorporation into nucleic acids of chloroquine sensitive and resistant erythrocyte-free malarial parasites. Proc Helminth Soc Wash 39:244–249

Carter R, Walliker D (1977) Biochemical markers for strain differentiation in malarial parasites. Bull WHO 55:339–345

Ceithaml J, Evans EA Jr (1946) The biochemistry of the malaria parasite. IV. The in vitro effects of X-rays upon *Plasmodium gallinaceum*. J Infect Dis 78:190–197

Cenedella RJ (1968) Lipid synthesis from glucose carbon by *Plasmodium berghei* in vitro. Am J Trop Med Hyg 17:680–684

Cenedella RJ, Jarrell JJ (1970) Suggested new mechanisms of antimalarial action for DDS involving inhibition of glucose utilization by the intraerythrocytic parasite. Am J Trop Med Hyg 19:592–598

Chaimanee P, Yuthavong Y (1979) Phosphorylation of membrane proteins from *Plasmodium berghei*-infected red cells. Biochem Biophys Res Comm 87:953–959

Chance ML, Momen H, Warhurst DC, Peters W (1978) The chemotherapy of rodent malaria, XXIX. DNA relationships within the subgenus *Plasmodium* (*Vinckeia*). Ann Trop Med Parasitol 72:13–22

Charet P, Aissi E, Maurois P, Bouquelet S, Biguet J (1980) Aminopeptidase in rodent *Plasmodium*. Comp Biochem Physiol [B] 65:519–524

Chou AC, Chevli R, Fitch CD (1980) Ferriprotoporphyrin IX fulfills the criteria for identification as the chloroquine receptor of malaria parasites. Biochemistry 19:1543–1549
Christophers SR, Fulton JD (1939) Experiments with isolated malaria parasites (*Plasmodium knowlesi*) free from red cells. Ann Trop Med Parasitol 33:161–170
Ciak J, Hahn F (1966) Chloroquine: Mode of action. Science 151:347–349
Clarke DH (1952a) The use of phosphorus 32 in studies on *Plasmodium gallinaceum*. I. The development of a method for the quantitative determination of parasite growth and development in vitro. J Exp Med 96:439–450
Clarke DH (1952b) The use of phosphorus 32 in studies on *Plasmodium gallinaceum*. II. Studies on conditions affecting parasite growth in intact cells and in lysates. J Exp Med 96:451–463
Conklin KA, Chou SC, Siddiqui WA, Schnell JV (1973) DNA and RNA syntheses by intraerythrocytic stages of *Plasmodium knowlesi*. J Protozool 20:683–688
Cook L, Grant PT, Kermack WO (1961) Proteolytic enzymes of the erythrocytic forms of rodent and simian species of malarial plasmodia. Exp Parasitol 11:372–379
Cook RT, Aikawa M, Rock RC, Little W, Sprinz H (1969) The isolation and fractionation of *Plasmodium knowlesi*. Milit Med 134:866–883
Coombs GH, Gutteridge WE (1975) Growth *in vitro* and metabolism of *Plasmodium vinckei chabaudi*. J Protozool 22:555–560
Deans JA, Dennis ED, Cohen S (1978) Antigenic analysis of sequential erythrocytic stages of *Plasmodium knowlesi*. Parasitology 77:333–344
Dunn MJ (1969a) Alterations of red blood cell sodium transport during malarial infection. J Clin Invest 48:674–684
Dunn MJ (1969b) Alterations of red blood cell metabolism in simian malaria: evidence for abnormalities of nonparasitized cells. Milit Med 134:1100–1105
Eaton JW, Brewer GJ (1969) Red cell ATP and malaria infection. Nature 222:389–390
Eaton JW, Eckman JR, Berger E, Jacob HS (1976) Suppression of malaria infection by oxidant-sensitive host erythrocytes. Nature 264:758–760
Eckman JR, Eaton JW (1979) Dependence of plasmodial glutathione metabolism on the host cell. Nature 278:754–756
Eisen H (1977) Purification of intracellular forms of *Plasmodium chabaudi* and their interactions with the erythrocyte membrane and serum albumin. Bull WHO 55:333–338
Fabiani G, Grellet P (1951) Etude chez le rat blanc des rapports entre la carence en vitamine A et le paludisme expérimental à *Plasmodium berghei*. C R Soc Biol (Paris) 146:441–444
Ferone R (1977) Folate metabolism in malaria. Bull WHO 55:291–298
Ferone R, Hitchings GH (1966) Folate cofactor biosynthesis by *Plasmodium berghei*. Comparison of folate and dihydrofolate as substrates. J Protozool 13:504–506
Ferone R, Burchall JJ, Hitchings GH (1969) *Plasmodium berghei* dihydrofolate reductase. Isolation, properties, and inhibition by antifolates. Mol Pharmacol 5:49–59
Fitch CD, Ng R, Chevli R (1978) Erythrocyte surface: novel determinant of drug susceptibility in rodent malaria. Antimicrob Agents Chemother 14:185–193
Fletcher KA, Maegraith BG (1970) Erythrocyte reduced glutathione in malaria (*Plasmodium berghei* and *P. knowlesi*). Ann Trop Med Parasitol 64:481–486
Fletcher KA, Maegraith BG (1972) The metabolism of the malaria parasite and its host. Adv Parasitol 10:31–48
Fraser DM, Kermack WO (1957) The inhibitory action of some antimalarial drugs and related compounds on the hexokinase of yeasts and *Plasmodium berghei*. Br J Pharmacol Chemother 12:16–23
Friedman M (1978) Erythrocyte mechanism of sickle cell resistance to malaria. Proc Nat Acad Sci USA 75:1994–1997
Friedman M (1979a) Ultrastructural damage to the malaria parasite in the sickled cell. J Protozool 26:195–199
Friedman M (1979b) Oxidant damage mediates variant red cell resistance to malaria. Nature 280:245–247
Friedman M, Roth E, Nagel R, Trager W (1979a) *Plasmodium falciparum:* physiological interactions with the human sickle cell. Exp Parasitol 47:73–80

Friedman M, Roth E, Nagel R, Trager W (1979b) The role of hemoglobins C, S, and $N_{Balt}$ in the inhibition of malaria parasite development in vitro. Am J Trop Med Hyg 28:777–780

Fulton JD (1939) Experiments on the utilization of sugars by malarial parasites (*Plasmodium knowlesi*). Ann Trop Med Parasitol 33:217–227

Fulton JD (1951) The metabolism of malaria parasites. Brit Med Bull 8:22–27

Fulton JD, Christophers SR (1938) The inhibitive effect of drugs upon oxygen uptake by trypanosomes (*Trypanosoma rhodesiense*) and malaria (*Plasmodium knowlesi*). Ann Trop Med Parasitol 32:77–93

Fulton JD, Grant PT (1956) The sulphur requirements of the erythrocytic form of *Plasmodium knowlesi*. Biochem J 63:274–282

Fulton JD, Spooner DF (1955) The biochemistry and nutrition of *Plasmodium berghei*. Indian J Malariol 9:161–176

Fulton JD, Spooner DF (1956) The in vitro respiratory metabolism of erythrocytic forms of *Plasmodium berghei*. Exp Parasitol 5:59–78

Godfrey D (1957) Antiparasitic action of dietary cod liver oil upon *Plasmodium berghei* and its reversal by vitamin E. Exp Parasitol 6:555–565

Groman NB (1951) Dynamic aspects of the nitrogen metabolism of *Plasmodium gallinaceum* in vivo and in vitro. J Infect Dis 88:126–150

Gutierrez J (1966) Effect of the antimalarial chloroquine on the phospholipid metabolism of avian malaria and heart tissue. Am J Trop Med Hyg 15:818–822

Gutteridge WE, Trigg PI (1970) Incorporation of radioactive precursors into DNA and RNA of *Plasmodium knowlesi* in vitro. J Protozool 17:89–96

Gutteridge WE, Trigg PI (1971) Action of pyrimethamine and related drugs against *Plasmodium knowlesi* in vitro. Parasitology 62:431–444

Gutteridge W, Trigg W (1972a) Periodicity of nuclear DNA synthesis in the intraerythrocytic cycle of *Plasmodium knowlesi*. J Protozool 19:378–381

Gutteridge WE, Trigg PI (1972b) Some studies on the DNA of *Plasmodium knowlesi*. In: Van den Bossche H (ed) Comparative biochemistry of parasites. Academic, New York, pp 199–218

Gutteridge WE, Trigg PI, Williamson DH (1971) Properties of DNA from malarial parasites. Parasitology 62:209–219

Gutteridge WE, Trigg PI, Williamson DH (1969) Base compositions of DNA from some malarial parasites. Nature 224:1210–1211

Gutteridge WE, Trigg PI, Bayley PM (1972) Effects of chloroquine on *Plasmodium* in vitro. Parasitology 64:37–45

Gutteridge WE, Dave D, Richards WHG (1979) Conversion of dihydroorotate to orotate in parasitic protozoa. Biochim Biophys Acta 582:390–401

Herman YF, Ward RA, Herman RH (1966) Stimulation of the utilization of 1-$^{14}$-glucose in chicken red blood cells infected with *Plasmodium gallinaceum*. Am J Trop Med Hyg 15:276–280

Holz GG Jr (1977) Lipids and the malarial parasite. Bull WHO 55:237–248

Homewood CA (1978) Biochemistry. In: Killick-Kendrick R, Peters W (eds) Rodent malaria. Academic, New York, pp 170–211

Homewood CA, Neame KD (1974) Malaria and the permeability of the host erythrocyte. Nature 252:718–719

Homewood CA, Jewsbury JM, Chance ML (1972a) The pigment formed during haemoglobin digestion by malarial and schistosomal parasites. Comp Biochem Physiol 43B:517–523

Homewood CA, Warhurst DC, Peters W, Baggaley VC (1972b) Electron transport in intraerythrocytic *Plasmodium berghei*. Proc Helminth Soc Wash 39:382–386

Honigberg BM (1967) Chemistry of parasitism among some protozoa. In: Kidder GW (ed) Chemical zoology, vol I. Protozoa. Academic, New York, pp 695–814

Howells RE (1970) Mitochondrial changes during the life cycle of *Plasmodium berghei*. Ann Trop Med Parasitol 64:181–187

Howells RE, Maxwell L (1973) Further studies on the mitochondrial changes during the life cycle of *Plasmodium berghei:* electrophoretic studies on isocitrate dehydrogenases. Ann Trop Med Parasitol 67:279–283
Ilan J, Tokuyasu K, Ilan J (1970) Phosphorylation of D-arabinosyl adenine by *Plasmodium berghei.* and its partial protection of mice against malaria. Nature 228:1300–1301
Ilan J, Pierce DR, Miller FW (1977) Influence of 9-β-D-arabinofuranosyladenine on total protein synthesis and on differential gene expression of unique proteins in the rodent malarial parasite *Plasmodium berghei.* Proc Nat Acad Sci USA 74:3386–3390
Johns FM (1930) Influence of dextrose and of low temperature on preservation, transportation, and viability of malaria parasites. Proc Soc Exp Biol Med 28:743–745
Khabir PA, Manwell RD (1955) Glucose consumption of *Plasmodium hexamerium.* J Parasitol 41:595–603
Kilejian A (1974) A unique histidine-rich polypeptide from the malaria parasite, *Plasmodium lophurae.* J Biol Chem 249:4650–4655
Kilejian A (1975) Circular mitochondrial DNA from the avian malarial parasite *Plasmodium lophurae.* Biochim Biophys Acta 390:276–284
Kilejian A (1976) Does a histidine-rich protein from *Plasmodium lophurae* have a function in merozoite penetration? J Protozool 23:272–277
Kilejian A (1978) Histidine-rich protein as a model malaria vaccine. Science 201:922–924
Kilejian A (1979) Characterization of a protein correlated with the production of knob-like protrusions on membrane of erythrocytes infected with *Plasmodium falciparum.* Proc Nat Acad Sci USA 76:4650–4653
Kilejian A (1980) Homology between a histidine-rich protein from *Plasmodium lophurae* and a protein associated with the knob-like protrusions on membranes of erythrocytes infected with *Plasmodium falciparum.* J Exp Med 151:1534–1538
Kilejian A, Jensen JB (1977) A histidine-rich protein from *Plasmodium falciparum* and its interaction with membranes. Bull WHO 55:191–198
Kilejian A, Liao T-H, Trager W (1975) Studies on the primary structure and biosynthesis of a histidine-rich polypeptide from the malaria parasite, *Plasmodium lophurae.* Proc Nat Acad Sci USA 72:3057–3059
Königk E (1977) Salvage syntheses and their relationship to nucleic acid metabolism. Bull WHO 55:249–252
Königk E, Mirtsch S (1977) *Plasmodium chabaudi* infection of mice: specific activities of erythrocyte membrane-associated enzymes and patterns of proteins and glycoproteins of erythrocyte membrane preparations. Tropenmed Parasitol 28:17–22
Krooth RS, Wuu K-D, Ma R (1969) Dihydroorotic acid dehydrogenase: introduction into erythrocyte by the malaria parasite. Science 164:1073–1075
Langer BW Jr, Phisphumvidhi P, Jiampermpoon D (1970) Malarial parasite metabolism: the glutamic acid dehydrogenase of *Plasmodium berghei.* Exp Parasitol 28:298–303
Langreth S (1977) Electron microscope cytochemistry of host-parasite membrane interactions in malaria. Bull WHO 55:171–178
Langreth SG, Trager W (1973) Fine structure of the malaria parasite *Plasmodium lophurae* developing extracellularly in vivo. J Protozool 20:606–613
Langreth S, Reese R, Motyl M, Trager W (1979) *Plasmodium falciparum:* loss of knobs on the infected erythrocyte surface after long-term cultivation. Exp Parasitol 48:213–219
Lantz CH, Van Dyke K, Carter G (1971) *Plasmodium berghei:* in vitro incorporation of purine derivatives into nucleic acids. Exp Parasitol 29:402–416
Levy MR, Chou SC (1973) Activity and some properties of an acid proteinase from normal and *Plasmodium berghei*-infected red cells. J Parasitol 59:1064–1070
Levy MR, Chou SC (1974) Some properties and susceptibility to inhibitors of partially purified acid proteases from *Plasmodium berghei* and from ghosts of mouse red cells. Biochim Biophys Acta 334:423–430
Levy MR, Chou SC (1975) Inhibition of macromolecular synthesis in the malarial parasites by inhibitors of proteolytic enzymes. Experientia 31:52–54
Levy MR, Siddiqui WA, Chou SC (1974) Acid protease activity in *Plasmodium falciparum* and *P. knowlesi* and ghosts of their respective host red cells. Nature 247:546–549
Luzzatto L (1979) Genetics of red cells and susceptibility to malaria. Blood 54:961–976

Maier J, Coggeshall LT (1941) Respiration of malaria plasmodia. J Infect Dis 69:87–96
Manandhar MSP, Van Dyke K (1975) Detailed purine salvage metabolism in and outside the free malarial parasite. Exp Parasitol 37:138–146
Manwell RD, Feigelson P (1949) Glycolysis in *Plasmodium gallinaceum*. Proc Soc Exp Biol Med 70:578–582
Marshall PB (1948) The glucose metabolism of *Plasmodium gallinaceum*, and the action of antimalarial agents. Br J Pharmacol 3:1–7
Mason SJ, Miller LH, Shiroishi T, Dvorak JA, McGinnis MH (1977) The Duffy blood group determinants: their role in the susceptibility of human and animal erythrocytes to *Plasmodium knowlesi* malaria. Br J Haematol 36(3):327–336
McCormick GJ, Canfield CJ, Willet GP (1974) In vitro antimalarial activity of nucleic acid precursor analogs in the simian malaria *Plasmodium knowlesi*. Antimicrob Agents Chemo 6:16–21
McDaniel HG, Siu PML (1972) Purification and characterization of phosphoenolpyruvate carboxylase from *Plasmodium berghei*. J Bacteriol 109:385–390
McDonald V, Hannon M, Tanigoshi L, Sherman I (1981) *Plasmodium lophurae:* immunization of Pekin ducklings with different antigen preparations. Exp Parasitol 51:195–203
McGhee RB (1953) The infection by *Plasmodium lophurae* of duck erythrocytes in the chick embryo. J Exp Med 97:773–782
McKee RW (1951) Biochemistry of *Plasmodium* and the influence of antimalarials. In: Hutner SH, Lwoff A (eds) Biochemistry and physiology of protozoa, vol I. Academic, New York, pp 251–322
McKee RW, Ormsbee RA, Anfinsen CB, Geiman QM, Ball EG (1946) Studies on malarial parasites. VI. The chemistry and metabolism of normal and parasitized (*P. knowlesi*) monkey blood. J Exp Med 84:569–582
McLaren DJ, Bannister LH, Trigg PI, Butcher GA (1977) A freeze-fracture study on the parasite-erythrocyte interrelationship in *Plasmodium knowlesi* infections. Bull WHO 55:199–204
McLaren DJ, Bannister LH, Trigg PI, Butcher GA (1979) Freeze-fracture studies on the interaction between the malaria parasite and host erythrocyte in *Plasmodium knowlesi* infections. Parasitology 79:125–139
Miller FW, Ilan J (1978) The ribosomes of *Plasmodium berghei:* isolation and ribosomal ribonucleic acid analysis. Parasitology 77:345–365
Miller LH (1977) Hypothesis on the mechanism of invasion of erythrocytes by malaria merozoites. Bull WHO 55:157–162
Miller LH, Aikawa M, Johnson J, Shiroishi T (1979) Interaction between cytochalasin B-treated malarial parasites and erythrocytes. J Exp Med 149:172–184
Miller LH, McGinniss MH, Holland PV, Sigmon P (1978) The Duffy blood group phenotype in American blacks infected with *Plasmodium vivax* in Vietnam. Am J Trop Med Hyg 27:1069–1072
Miller ZB, Kozloff LM (1947) The ribonuclease activity of normal and parasitized chick erythrocytes. J Biol Chem 170:105–120
Momen H (1979a) Biochemistry of intraerythrocytic parasites: I. Identification of enzymes of parasite origin by starch-gel electrophoresis. Ann Trop Med Parasitol 73:109–115
Momen H (1979b) Biochemistry of intraerythrocytic parasites: II. Comparative studies in carbohydrate metabolism. Ann Trop Med Parasitol 73:117–121
Moulder J (1962) The biochemistry of intracellular parasitism. University of Chicago Press, Chicago, Illinois, pp 13–42
Moulder JW (1948) Effect of quinine treatment of the host upon the carbohydrate metabolism of the malarial parasite *Plasmodium gallinaceum*. J Infect Dis 83:262–270
Moulder JW (1949) Inhibition of pyruvate oxidation in the malarial parasite *Plasmodium gallinaceum* by quinine treatment of the host. J Infect Dis 85:195–204
Moulder JW, Evans EA Jr (1946) The biochemistry of the malaria parasite. VI. Studies on the nitrogen metabolism of the malaria parasite. J Biol Chem 164:145–147
Nagarajan K (1964) Pyruvate and lactate levels in relationship to the nicotinamide adenine dinucleotide levels in malarial parasites (*Plasmodium berghei*). Biochem Biophys Acta 93:176–179

Nagarajan K (1968a) Metabolism of *Plasmodium berghei*. I. Krebs cycle. Exp Parasitol 21:19–26
Nagarajan K (1968b) Metabolism of *Plasmodium berghei*. II. $^{32}P_i$ incorporation into high-energy phosphates. Exp Parasitol 22:27–32
Nagarajan K (1968c) Metabolism of *Plasmodium berghei*. III. Carbon dioxide fixation and role of pyruvate and dicarboxylic acids. Exp Parasitol 22:33–42
Neame KD, Homewood CA (1975) Alterations in the permeability of mouse erythrocytes infected with the malaria parasite, *Plasmodium berghei*. Int J Parasitol 5:537–540
Neame KD, Brownbill PA, Homewood CA (1974) The uptake and incorporation of nucleosides into normal erythrocytes and erythrocytes containing *Plasmodium berghei*. Parasitology 69:329–335
Oelshlegel FJ Jr, Brewer GJ (1975) Parasitism and the red blood cell. In: Mac D, Surgenor N (eds) The red blood cell, 2nd edn. vol 2. Academic, New York, pp 1263–1302
Oelshlegel FJ Jr, Sander BJ, Brewer GJ (1975) Pyruvate kinase in malaria host-parasite interaction. Nature 255:345–347
O'Sullivan WJ, Ketley K (1980) Biosynthesis of uridine monophosphate in *Plasmodium berghei*. Ann Trop Med Parasitol 74:109–114
Overman RR, Hill TS, Wong UT (1949) Physiological studies in the human malarial host. I. Bood, plasma, "extracellular" fluid volumes, and ionic balance in therapeutic *P. vivax* and *P. falciparum*. J Nat Malar Soc 8:14–31
Overman RR, Bass AC, Tomlinson TH Jr (1950) Ionic alterations in chickens infected with *Plasmodium gallinaceum*. Fed Proc Fed Am Soc Exp Biol 9:96–97
Pasvol G, Weatherall DJ, Wilson RJM (1977) Effects of fetal hemoglobin on susceptibility of red cells to *Plasmodium falciparum*. Nature 270:171–173
Pasvol G, Weatherall DJ, Wilson RJM (1978) Cellular mechanism for the protective effect of haemoglobin S against *P. falciparum* malaria. Nature 274:701–703
Pasvol G, Weatherall DJ, Wilson RJM (1980) The increased susceptibility of young red cells to invasion by the malarial parasite *Plasmodium falciparum*. Br J Haematol 45:285–295
Peters W (1969) Recent advances in the physiology and biochemistry of plasmodia. Trop Dis Bull 66:1–29
Phisphumvidhi P, Langer BW Jr (1969) Malarial parasite metabolism: the lactic acid dehydrogenase of *Plasmodium berghei*. Exp Parasitol 24:37–41
Picard-Maureau A, Hempelmann E, Krammer G, Jackisch R, Jung A (1975) Glutathionstatus in *Plasmodium vinckei* parasitierten Erythrozyten in Abhängigkeit vom intraerythrozytären Entwicklungsstadium des Parasiten. Tropenmed Parasitol 26:405–416
Platzer EG (1972) Metabolism of tetrahydrofolate in *Plasmodium lophurae* and duckling erythrocytes. Trans NY Acad Sci, Series II, 34:200–208
Platzer EG (1974) Dihydrofolate reductase in *Plasmodium lophurae* and duckling erythrocytes. J Protozool 21:400–405
Platzer EG (1977) Subcellular distribution of serine hydroxymethyltransferase in *Plasmodium lophurae*. Life Sci 20:1417–1424
Platzer EG, Kassis JA (1978) Pyridoxine kinase in *Plasmodium lophurae* and duckling erythrocytes. J Protozool 25:556–559
Pollack Y, Katzen AL, Spira DT, Golenser J (1982) The genome of *Plasmodium falciparum* I. DNA base composition. Nucleic Acid Res 10:539–546
Polet H, Barr CF (1968a) DNA, RNA, and protein synthesis in erythrocytic forms of *Plasmodium knowlesi*. Am J Trop Med Hyg 17:672–679
Polet H, Barr CF (1968b) Chloroquine and dihydroquinine. In vitro studies of their antimalarial effect upon *Plasmodium knowlesi*. J Pharmacol Exp Ther 164:380–386
Polet H, Conrad ME (1969a) In vitro studies on the amino acid metabolism of *Plasmodium knowlesi* and the antiplasmodial effect of the isoleucine antagonists. Milit Med 134:939–944
Polet H, Conrad ME (1969b) The influence of three analogs of isoleucine on in vitro growth and protein synthesis of erythrocytic forms of *Plasmodium knowlesi*. Proc Soc Exp Biol Med 130:581–586
Rama Rao R, Sirsi M (1956a) Avian malaria and B complex vitamins. I. Thiamine. J Indian Inst Sci 38:108–114

Rama Rao R, Sirsi M (1956b) Avian malaria and B complex vitamins. II. Riboflavin. J Indian Inst Sci 38:186–189
Ramakrishnan SP (1954) Studies on *Plasmodium berghei* Vincke and Lips 1948. XIX. The course of blood induced infections in pyridoxine or vitamin $B_6$ deficient rats. Indian J Malar 8:107–113
Reid VE, Friedkin M (1973a) *Plasmodium berghei:* folic acid levels in mouse erythrocytes. Exp Parasitol 33:424–428
Reid VE, Friedkin M (1973b) Thymidylate synthetase in mouse erythrocytes infected with *Plasmodium berghei.* Mol Pharmacol 9:74–80
Rickard MD (1969) Carbohydrate metabolism in *Babesia rodhaini:* differences in metabolism of normal and infected rat erythrocytes. Exp Parasitol 25:16–31
Rietz PJ, Skelton FS, Folkers K (1967) Occurrence of ubiquinones-8 and -9 in *Plasmodium lophurae.* Int J Vit Res 37:405–411
Rock RC (1971a) Incorporation of $^{14}C$-labelled non-lipid precursors into lipids of *Plasmodium knowlesi* in vitro. Comp Biochem Physiol 40B:657–669
Rock RC (1971b) Incorporation of $^{14}C$-labelled fatty acids into lipids of rhesus erythrocytes and *Plasmodium knowlesi* in vitro. Comp Biochem Physiol 40B:893–906
Rock RC, Standefer J, Little W (1971) Incorporation of $^{33}P$-orthophosphate into membrane phospholipids of *Plasmodium knowlesi* and host erythrocytes of *Macaca mulatta.* Comp Biochem Physiol 40B:543–561
Roos A, Hegsted D, Stare F (1946) Nutritional studies with the duck. IV. The effect of vitamin deficiencies on the course of *P. lophurae* infection in the duck and the chick. J Nutr 32:473–484
Roth E, Friedman M, Ueda Y, Tellez I, Trager W, Nagel R (1978) Sickling rates of human AS red cells infected in vitro with *Plasmodium falciparum* malaria. Science 202:650–652
Scheibel LW, Miller J (1969) Glycolytic and cytochrome oxidase activity in plasmodia. Milit Med 134:1074–1080
Scheibel LW, Pflaum WK (1970) Carbohydrate metabolism in *Plasmodium knowlesi.* Comp Biochem Physiol 37:543–553
Scheibel W, Adler A, Trager W (1979a) Tetraethylthiuram disulfide (Antabuse) inhibits the human malaria parasite *Plasmodium falciparum.* Proc Nat Acad Sci USA 76:5303–5307
Scheibel LW, Ashton SH, Trager W (1979b) *Plasmodium falciparum:* Microaerophilic requirements in human red blood cells. Exp Parasit 47:410–418
Schellenberg KA, Coatney GR (1961) The influence of anti-malarial drugs on the nucleic acid synthesis in *Plasmodium gallinaceum* and *Plasmodium berghei.* Biochem Pharmacol 6:143–152
Schmidt-Ullrich R, Wallach DFH, Lightholder J (1979) Two *Plasmodium knowlesi*-specific antigens on the surface of schizont-infected rhesus monkey erythrocytes induce antibody production in immune hosts. J Exp Med 150:86–99
Schmidt-Ullrich R, Wallach DFH, Lightholder J (1980) Metabolic labelling of *P. knowlesi*-specific glycoproteins in membranes of parasitized rhesus monkey erythrocytes. Cell Biol Int Rep 4:555–561
Schnell JW, Siddiqui WA, Geiman QM (1971) Biosynthesis of coenzymes Q by malarial parasites. 2. Coenzyme Q synthesis in blood cultures of monkeys infected with malarial parasites (*Plasmodium falciparum* and *P. knowlesi*). J Med Chem 14:1026–1029
Seaman GR (1953) Inhibition of the succinic dehydrogenase of parasitic protozoans by an arsono and a phosphano analog of succinic acid. Exp Parasitol 2:366–373
Seed TM, Kreiser JP (1976) Surface properties of extracellular malaria parasites: electrophoresis and lectin-binding characteristics. Infect Immun 14:1339–1347
Seed TM, Aikawa M, Sterling CR (1973) An electron microscope-cytochemical method for differentiating membranes of host red cells and malaria parasites. J. Protozool 20:603–605
Seeler AO (1945) The inhibitory effect of pyridoxine on the activity of quinine and atabrine against avian malaria. J Nat Malar Soc 4:13–19
Seeler AO, Ott W (1944) Effect of riboflavin deficiency on the course of *Plasmodium lophurae* infections in chicks. J Inf Dis 75:175–178

Shakespeare PG, Trigg PI (1973) Glucose catabolism by the simian malaria parasite *Plasmodium knowlesi.* Nature 241:538–540
Shakespeare P, Trigg P, Tappenden L (1979a) Some properties of membranes in the simian malaria parasite. Ann Trop Med Parasit 73:333–343
Shakespeare P, Trigg P, Kyd S, Tappenden L (1979b) Glucose metabolism in the simian malaria parasite *Plasmodium knowlesi:* activities of the glycolytic and pentose phosphate pathways during the intraerythrocytic cycle. Ann Trop Med Parasitol 73:407–415
Sherman IW (1961) Molecular heterogeneity of lactic dehydrogenase in avian malaria (*Plasmodium lophurae*). J Exp Med 114:1049–1062
Sherman IW (1965) Glucose-6-phosphate dehydrogenase and reduced glutathione in malaria-infected erythrocytes (*Plasmodium lophurae* and *P. berghei*). J Protozool 12:394–396
Sherman IW (1966a) Malic dehydrogenase heterogeneity in malaria (*Plasmodium lophurae* and *P. berghei*). J Protozool 13:344–349
Sherman IW (1966b) Levels of oxidized and reduced pyridine nucleotides in avian malaria (*Plasmodium lophurae*). Am J Trop Med Hyg 15:814–817
Sherman IW (1976) The ribosomes of the simian malaria *Plasmodium knowlesi.* II. A cell-free protein synthesizing system. Comp Biochem Physiol 53B:447–450
Sherman IW (1977a) Transport of amino acids and nucleic acid precursors in malarial parasites. Bull WHO 55:211–225
Sherman IW (1977b) Amino acid metabolism and protein synthesis in malarial parasites. Bull WHO 55:265–276
Sherman IW (1979) Biochemistry of *Plasmodium* (malarial parasites). Microbiol Rev 43:453–495
Sherman IW, Jones LA (1976) Protein synthesis by a cell-free preparation from the bird malaria, *Plasmodium lophurae.* J Protozool 23:277–281
Sherman IW, Jones LA (1977) The *Plasmodium lophurae* (avian malaria) ribosome. J Protozool 24:331–334
Sherman IW, Jones LA (1979) *Plasmodium lophurae:* Membrane proteins of erythrocyte-free plasmodia and malaria-infected red cells. J Protozool 26:489–501
Sherman IW, Mudd JB (1966) Malaria infection (*P. lophurae*): changes in free amino acids. Science 154:287–289
Sherman IW, Tanigoshi L (1970) Incorporation of $^{14}C$-amino-acids by malaria (*Plasmodium lophurae*). IV. In vivo utilization of host cell haemoglobin. Int J Biochem 1:635–637
Sherman IW, Tanigoshi L (1971a) Alterations in sodium and potassium in the red blood cells and plasma during the malaria infection (*Plasmodium lophurae*). Comp Biochem Physiol 40A:543–546
Sherman IW, Tanigoshi L (1971b) Incorporation of $^{14}C$-amino-acids by malaria (*Plasmodium lophurae*). III. Metabolic fate of selected amino-acids. Int J Biochem 2:41–48
Sherman IW, Tanigoshi L (1974a) Incorporation of $^{14}C$-amino acids by malarial plasmodia (*Plasmodium lophurae*). VI. Changes in the kinetic constants of amino acid transport during infection. Exp Parasitol 35:369–373
Sherman IW, Tanigoshi L (1974b) Glucose transport in the malarial (*Plasmodium lophurae*) infected erythrocyte. J Protozool 21:603–607
Sherman IW, Ting IP, Ruble JA (1968) Characterization of the malaria pigment (hemozoin) from the avian malaria parasite *Plasmodium lophurae.* J Protozool 15:158–164
Sherman IW, Ruble JA, Ting IP (1969) *Plasmodium lophurae:* [U-$^{14}C$]-glucose catabolism by free plasmodia and duckling host erythrocytes. Exp Parasitol 25:181–192
Sherman IW, Ting IP, Tanigoshi L (1970) *Plasmodium lophurae:* glucose-*1*-$^{14}C$ and glucose-6-$^{14}C$ catabolism by free plasmodia and duckling host erythrocytes. Comp Biochem Physiol 34:625–639
Sherman IW, Petersen I, Tanigoshi L, Ting IP (1971) The glutamate dehydrogenase of *Plasmodium lophurae* (avian malaria). Exp Parasitol 29:433–439
Sherman IW, Cox RA, Higginson B, McLaren DJ, Williamson J (1975) The ribosomes of the simian malaria, *Plasmodium knowlesi.* I. Isolation and characterization. J Protozool 22:568–572
Siddiqui WA, Trager W (1966) Folic and folinic acids in relation to the development of *Plasmodium lophurae.* J Parasitol 52:556–558

Siddiqui WA, Schnell JV, Geiman QM (1967) Stearic acid as plasma replacement for intracellular in vitro culture of *Plasmodium knowlesi*. Science 156:1623–1625
Siddiqui WA, Schnell JV, Geiman QM (1969) Nutritional requirements for in vitro cultivation of a simian malarial parasite, *Plasmodium knowlesi*. Milit Med 134:929–938
Silverman M, Ceithaml J, Taliaferro LG, Evans EA Jr (1944) The in vitro metabolism of *Plasmodium gallinaceum*. J Infect Dis 75:212–230
Sinden R (1978) Cell biology. In: Killick-Kendrick R, Peters W (eds) Rodent malaria. Academic, New York, pp 85–168
Singer I (1956) Coenzyme A changes in liver, spleen, and kidneys of rats with infections of *Plasmodium berghei*. Proc Soc Exp Biol Med 91:315–318
Singer I (1961) Tissue thiamine changes in rats with experimental trypanosomiasis or malaria. Exp Parasitol 11:391–401
Siu PML (1967) Carbon dioxide fixation in plasmodia and the effect of some antimalarial drugs on the enzyme. Comp Biochem Physiol 23:785–795
Skelton FS, Lunan KD, Folkers K, Schnell JV, Siddiqui WA, Geiman QM (1969) Biosynthesis of ubiquinones by malarial parasites. I. Isolation of [$^{14}$C]ubiquinones from cultures of rhesus monkey blood infected with *Plasmodium knowlesi*. Biochem 8:1284–1287
Skelton FS, Rietz PJ, Folkers K (1970) Coenzyme Q. CXXII. Identification of ubiquinone-8 biosynthesized by *Plasmodium knowlesi*, *P. cynomolgi*, and *P. berghei*. J Med Chem 13:602–606
Smith CC, McCormick GJ, Canfield CJ (1976) *Plasmodium knowlesi:* in vitro biosynthesis of methionine. Exp Parasitol 40:432–437
Speck JF, Evans EA Jr (1945) The biochemistry of the malarial parasite. II. Glycolysis in cell-free preparations of the malaria parasite. J Biol Chem 159:71–81
Speck JF, Moulder JW, Evans EA Jr (1946) The biochemistry of the malaria parasite. V. Mechanism of pyruvate oxidation in the malaria parasite. J. Biol Chem 164:119–144
Takahashi Y, Sherman IW (1978) *Plasmodium lophurae:* Cationized ferritin staining, an electron microscope cytochemical method for differentiating malarial parasite and host cell membranes. Exp Parasitol 44:15–154
Takahashi Y, Sherman IW (1980) *Plasmodium lophurae:* Lectin mediated agglutination of malaria-infected red cells and fine-structure cytochemical detection of lectin binding sites on plasmodial and host cell membranes. Exp Parasitol 49:233–247
Taylor AER (1958) Effects of cod liver oil and vitamin E on infections of *Plasmodium gallinaceum* and *Treponema duttoni*. Ann Trop Med Parasitol 52:139–144
Theakston RDG, Howells RE, Fletcher KA, Peters W, Fullard J, Moore GA (1969) The ultrastructural distribution of cytochrome oxidase activity in *Plasmodium berghei* and *P. gallinaceum*. Life Sci 8:521–529
Theakston RDG, Fletcher KA, Maegraith BG (1970) The use of electron microscope autoradiography for examining the uptake and degradation of haemoglobin by *Plasmodium berghei*. Ann Trop Med Parasitol 64:63–71
Theakston RDG, Ali SN, Moore GA (1972) Electron microscope autoradiographic studies on the effect of chloroquine on the uptake of tritiated nucleosides and methionine by *Plasmodium berghei*. Ann Trop Med Parasitol 66:295–302
Ting IP, Sherman IW (1966) Carbon dioxide fixation in malaria-I. Kinetic studies in *Plasmodium lophurae*. Comp Biochem Physiol 19:855–869
Tokuyasu K, Ilan J, Ilan J (1969) Biogenesis of ribosomes in *Plasmodium berghei*. Milit Med 134:1032–1038
Tracy SM, Sherman IW (1972) Purine uptake and utilization by the avian malaria parasite *Plasmodium lophurae*. J Protozool 19:541–549
Trager W (1950) Studies on the extracellular cultivation of an intracellular parasite (avian malaria). I. Development of the organisms in erythrocyte extracts, and the favoring effect of adenosine triphosphate. J Exp Med 92:349–366
Trager W (1952) Studies on the extracellular cultivation of an intracellular parasite (avian malaria). II. The effects of malate and of coenzyme A concentrates. J Exp Med 96:465–476
Trager W (1970) Recent progress in some aspects of the physiology of parasitic protozoa. J Parasitol 56:627–633

Trager W (1971) Malaria parasites (*Plasmodium lophurae*) developing extracellularly in vitro: incorporation of labeled precursors. J Protozool 18:392–399
Trager W (1973) Bongkrekic acid and the adenosinetriphosphate requirement of malaria parasites. Exp Parasitol 34:412–416
Trager W (1977) Cofactors and vitamins in the metabolism of malarial parasites. Bull WHO 55:285–289
Trager W, Brohn FH (1975) Coenzyme A requirement of malaria parasites: effects of coenzyme A precursors on extracellular development in vitro of *Plasmodium lophurae*. Proc Nat Acad Sci USA 72:1834–1837
Trager W, Langreth SC, Platzer EG (1972) Viability and fine structure of extracellular *Plasmodium lophurae* prepared by different methods. Proc Helminthol Soc Wash 39:220–230
Trager W, Robert-Gero M, Lederer E (1978) Antimalarial activity of *S*-isobutyl adenosine against *Plasmodium falciparum* in culture. FEBS Letters 85:264–266
Trager W, Tershakovec M, Chiang P, Cantoni G (1980) *Plasmodium falciparum:* antimalarial activity in culture of sinefungin and other methylation inhibitors. Exp Parasitol 50:83–90
Trigg PI (1968) Sterol metabolism of *Plasmodium knowlesi* in vitro. Ann Trop Med Parasitol 62:481–487
Trigg PI, Gutteridge WE (1971) A minimal medium for the growth of *Plasmodium knowlesi* in dilution cultures. Parasitology 62:113–123
Trigg PI, Gutteridge WE (1972) A rational approach to the serial culture of malaria parasites. Evidence for a deficiency in RNA synthesis during the first cycle in vitro. Parasitology 65:265–271
Trigg PI, Gutteridge WE, Williamson J (1971) The effects of cordycepin on malaria parasites. Trans Soc Trop Med Hyg 65:514–520
Trigg PI, Shakespeare PG, Burt SJ, Kyd SI (1975) Ribonucleic acid synthesis in *Plasmodium knowlesi* maintained both in vivo and in vitro. Parasitology 71:199–209
Trigg P, Hirst S, Shakespeare P, Tappenden L (1977) Labelling of membrane of glycoprotein in erythrocytes infected with *Plasmodium knowlesi*. Bull WHO 55:205–210
Tsukamoto M (1974) Differential detection of soluble enzymes specific to a rodent malaria parasite, *Plasmodium berghei*, by electrophoresis on polyacrylamide gels. Trop Med 16:55–69
Van Dyke K, Szustkiewicz C, Lantz CH, Saxe LH (1969) Studies concerning the mechanism of action of antimalarial drugs – inhibition of the incorporation of adenosine-8-$^3$H into nucleic acids of *Plasmodium berghei*. Biochem Pharmacol 18:1417–1425
Van Dyke K, Tremblay GC, Lantz CH, Szustkiewicz C (1970) The source of purines and pyrimidines in *Plasmodium berghei*. Am J Trop Med Hyg 19:202–208
Velick SF (1942) The respiratory metabolism of the malaria parasite, *P. cathemerium*, during its developmental cycle. Am J Hyg 35:152–161
Wallach DFH, Conley M (1977) Altered membrane proteins of monkey erythrocytes infected with simian malaria. J Molec Med 2:119–135
Walsh CJ, Sherman IW (1968 a) Isolation, characterization, and synthesis of DNA from a malaria parasite. J Protozool 15:503–508
Walsh CJ, Sherman IW (1968 b) Purine and pyrimidine synthesis by the avian malaria parasite, *Plasmodium lophurae*. J Protozool 15:763–770
Walter RD, Königk E (1971) Synthese der Desoxythymidylat-Synthetase und der Dihydrofolat-Reduktase bei synchroner Schizogonie von *Plasmodium chabaudi*. Z Tropenmed Parasitol 22:250–255
Walter RD, Nordmeyer J-P, Königk E (1974) NADP-specific glutamate dehydrogenase from *Plasmodium chabaudi*. Hoppe-Seyler's Z Physiol Chem 355:495–500
Wan Y-P, Porter TH, Folkers K (1974) Antimalarial quinones for prophylaxis based on rationale of inhibition of electron transfer in *Plasmodium*. Proc Nat Acad Sci USA 71:952–956
Warhurst DC, Williamson J (1970) Ribonucleic acid from *Plasmodium knowlesi* before and after chloroquine treatment. Chemico-Biol Inter 2:89–106
Warren L, Manwell RD (1954) Rate of glucose consumption by malarial blood. Exp Parasitol 3:16–24

Weidekamm E, Wallach DFH, Lin PS, Hendricks J (1973) Erythrocyte membrane alterations due to infection with *Plasmodium berghei*. Biochim Biophys Acta 323:539–546
Whitfeld PR (1952) Nucleic acids in erythrocytic stages of a malaria parasite. Nature 169:751–752
Whitfeld PR (1953) Studies on the nucleic acids of the malaria parasite, *Plasmodium berghei* (Vincke and Lips). Aust J Biol Sci 6:234–243
Wilson RJM, Pasvol G, Weatherall DJ (1977) Invasion and growth of *Plasmodium falciparum* in different types of erythrocytes. Bull WHO 55:179–186
Yamada KA, Sherman IW (1979) *Plasmodium lophurae:* Composition and properties of hemozoin, the malarial pigment. Exp Parasitol 48:61–74
Yamada K, Sherman I (1981 a) *Plasmodium lophurae:* Malaria induced nucleotide changes in duckling (*Anas domesticus*) erythrocytes. Mol Biochem Parasitol 1:187–198
Yamada K, Sherman I (1981 b) Purine metabolizing enzymes of the avian malaria *Plasmodium lophurae* and its host cell, the duckling (*Anas domesticus*) erythrocyte. Mol Biochem Parasitol 2:349–358
Yamada K, Sherman I (to be published) Regulation of purine uptake and metabolism by avian malarial parasite *Plasmodium lophurae*. Mol Biochem Parasitol
Yuthavong Y, Wilairat P, Panijpan B, Potiwan C, Beale G (1979) Alterations in membrane proteins of mouse erythrocytes infeced with different strains and species of malaria parasites. Comp Biochem Physiol 63B:83–85

CHAPTER 3

# In Vitro Culture Techniques

W. H. G. RICHARDS

## A. Introduction

The control of malaria by chemotherapy, the use of pesticides, and public health measures has been curtailed by the increasing spread of drug resistance of the parasite, especially *Plasmodium falciparum*, while increased tolerance of the mosquito vectors to the older insecticides has exacerbated the global malaria problem by facilitating the return of infection to areas recently freed from the disease. The search for new chemotherapeutic agents and investigations aimed at a better understanding of existing antimalarials is an expensive and time-consuming task, usually only undertaken in the more sophisticated laboratories. The successful in vitro cultivation of the blood, tissue and sporogonic stages of the malaria parasite could quickly and easily provide the means to examine compounds against the target species, or an acceptable experimental model. It should allow for a better understanding of the mechanism of parasite invasion, biochemistry, physiology, chemotherapy, drug resistance, and immunology.

The relative slowness with which techniques for continuous in vitro cultivation have been developed is mainly due to the inadequate knowledge of the biochemistry of the parasites, the host tissue cells and their constituents. The great diversity of plasmodia infecting a variety of vertebrate and invertebrate hosts has resulted in studies using avian, rodent, simian, and human parasites. While some notable successes have been achieved and individual cycles, e.g., the asexual, erythrocytic cycle of *P. falciparum*, established, there is still no complete malaria cycle in continuous cultivation. The recent work of TRAGER (1976) and TRAGER and JENSEN (1976), demonstrating the cultivation of *P. falciparum* using a continuous flow system (TRAGER 1971) and a simple dilution system in Petri dishes, gave increased hope and impetus to in vitro culture systems in laboratories around the world.

## B. Asexual Intraerythrocytic Stages

### I. Basic Problems of In Vitro Culture

#### 1. Erythrocytes

The dependence of the malaria asexual intraerythrocytic parasites and gametocytes on the host erythrocyte is demonstrated by their ability to invade and develop only inside the host cell. The maintenance of the integrity of the red cell in vitro is of primary importance for long-term cultivation. This has to be viewed in relation to the associated blood plasma and/or surrounding medium that has to support and maintain the erythrocytes, and to support the merozoites for the limited period when they are released following schizogony and prior to their entering a fresh host erythrocyte.

Few studies have been carried out on erythrocytes incubated at 37 °C for prolonged periods. The osmotic fragility of the red cells increases markedly when they are incubated in vitro (HAUT et al. 1962). GOMPERTS (1967) demonstrated that the erythrocytes degenerate metabolically after only 24 h at 37 °C. After 24 h there was a decrease in glucose consumption with a subsequent decrease in the rate of phosphorylation of adenosine 5′-(tetrahydrogen triphosphate) ATP; this is a phenomenon similar to that seen in aging red cells. The importance of the red cell was demonstrated by TRAGER (1950, 1952), who grew the asexual blood stages of the avian parasite *P. lophurae* extracellularly and showed that the parasite was dependent on the host red cell for ATP. TRIGG and SHAKESPEARE (1976a, b) have shown that normal rhesus monkey red blood cells incubated for periods up to 48 h in vitro are less susceptible to invasion by *P. knowlesi* than normal erythrocytes taken from a monkey, immediately before use.

Recent work, whilst emphasising the importance of the host erythrocyte, also demonstrates that the problem is not as difficult as was imagined in the past. SIDDIQUI and his co-workers (1970a), using homologous *Aotus* monkey blood, were able to achieve a limited twofold multiplication of *P. falciparum* during a single cycle in vitro. Increased multiplication occurred (TRAGER 1971) by mixing the donor parasitised blood from *Aotus* monkeys with human erythrocytes. Group B or AB cells will not agglutinate with *Aotus* cells whereas group A will. TRIGG (1975) showed that *P. falciparum* parasites appeared to invade preferentially human group 0 red cells rather than the original cells from an *Aotus* monkey. Later, in 1976, HAYNES et al., using *P. falciparum* from a chimpanzee, found that the parasites invaded erythrocytes from chimpanzees or humans equally well, but no conclusions were drawn from this observation because of the small number of experiments. Successful long-term cultivation, however, was achieved from both lines in human erythrocytes from all three A, B, and 0 groups.

Other factors have been examined and THEAKSTON and FLETCHER (1971), using $^{59}Fe$ for autoradiographic and scintillation counting techniques, demonstrated that the rodent malaria *P. berghei* had a predilection for young, immature erythrocytes compared with the more mature cells. PASVOL et al. (1976), who studied the susceptibility of human cells containing fetal haemoglobin, HbF, to invasion by *P. falciparum*, concluded that the susceptibility of erythrocytes to invasion is related to their age rather than to the presence of HbF. Parasite development, however, is retarded inside erythrocytes containing HbF.

It appears that, although erythrocytes from all the human A, B, and 0 groups are able to support the long-term growth of *P. falciparum* in vitro, there is variation amongst donors in the innate ability of their erythrocytes to support the parasites in vitro.

For many years those workers involved with the cultivation of intracellular parasites believed that the erythrocytes used in their systems should be from freshly collected blood. Lack of success may have been due to the inhibitory presence of leucocytes; certainly VERNES (1980) reported the engulfment of *P. falciparum* by monocytes in vivo in man and also the same phagocytic activity in vivo with *P. fal-*

*ciparum* in chimpanzee blood. BASS and JOHNS (1912) stressed the necessity for removing leucocytes from infected blood for the successful cultivation of *P. falciparum,* in the first recorded attempt at in vitro maintenance. RICHARDS and WILLIAMS (1973) recognised that many of the in vitro studies relied on the biochemical inertness of the host erythrocyte for quantitation of the parasite's metabolic activity by measuring the incorporation of radioactive precursors into plasmodial protein, RNA or DNA. Leucocytes which may be present in the cell population also synthesise these biopolymers and consequently interfere with the quantitation of parasite activity. They recognised that the accepted methods for removal of leucocytes were not completely effective. Using *P. berghei* as a model they developed a technique whereby infected blood diluted in culture medium was passed through a CF-11 cellulose column, removing all the leucocytes but allowing the parasites to pass through and remain viable. It is interesting that the first successful attempts at the continuous cultivation of *P. falciparum* concentrated on the removal of leucocytes either by aspiration (TRAGER and JENSEN 1976) or by passage through a CF-11 cellulose column (HAYNES et al. 1976). It is now accepted that, for the successful culture of *P. falciparum,* human blood collected in acid-citrate-dextrose (ACD) or citrate-phosphate-dextrose (CPD) can be used for up to 4 weeks when stored at 4 °C (TRAGER 1980). After 1 week's storage the leucocytes are no longer viable while the erythrocytes are still susceptible to invasion by *P. falciparum.* The immediate availability of time-expired blood bank cells therefore offers the opportunity for increased in vitro cultivation.

## 2. Culture Medium

In the original culture of *P. falciparum,* BASS and JOHNS (1912) used a very simple glucose medium. Since then the culture media have become more complex. The original work on the cultivation of *P. knowlesi* in vitro used the Harvard growth medium (BALL et al. 1945; ANFINSEN et al. 1946), which was based on a chemical analysis of monkey plasma. Modifications of the Harvard medium gave improved growth and multiplication of *P. knowlesi* (TRIGG 1968; COHEN and BUTCHER 1971). SIDDIQUI et al. (1970b) sought to replace the Harvard medium by a commercially available culture medium CMRL-1066, produced by the Grand Island Biological Company, and found it to be comparable. The authors indicated that the readily available medium would be suitable for drug testing against *P. falciparum* in vitro. Many workers including PHILLIPS et al. (1972) used a modified "199" culture medium with limited success. HAYNES et al. (1976) also used a modified 199 medium for the continuous cultivation of *P. falciparum* in vitro. They used cryopreserved chimpanzee blood infected with *P. falciparum* in a simple dilution system incubated at 38 °C. The medium was changed every 1–2 days and, when the parasites had matured to the schizont stage, they were resuspended and inoculated into new cultures containing fresh human erythrocytes. These cultures were maintained for 22 days.

The work of TRAGER has now shown that a commercially available medium is satisfactory for the continuous growth of *P. falciparum* in vitro. The events leading to this finding (TRAGER and JENSEN 1978) showed that a slow flow of medium over a settled layer of infected erythrocytes was favourable to *P. coatneyi* and *P. falciparum.* The medium RPMI 1640 with HEPES buffer, originally designed as a leucocyte culture medium, supported good growth of *P. coatneyi* in rocker flasks. A raised $CO_2$ and decreased $O_2$ gaseous phase also favoured parasite growth. No better culture medium than RPMI 1640 with 25 m*M* HEPES buffer has yet been found.

### 3. Maintenance of pH

The maintenance of a suitable pH in the culture medium is vital to the successful development of malaria parasites in vitro. The large amount of lactic acid produced by the parasites lowers the pH. GEIMAN and his co-workers (1966) stated that a pH of 7.3–7.5 is critical to parasite growth, and indicated that the zwitterionic buffer glycyl-glycine with a pKa 7.9 at 37 °C, when used at 5 m*M*, gave an improved growth of *P. knowlesi* in vitro. While zwitterionic buffers have the advantage that they maintain pH stability during the period when the cultures are held outside a $CO_2$-rich atmosphere, they would undoubtedly be of greater use with a pKa closer to a pH of 7.3–7.5. SIDDIQUI and SCHNELL (1973) and HAYNES et al. (1976) used TES in their culture systems with success. The work of TRAGER and JENSEN (1976), using a 25 m*M* HEPES buffer with a pKa 7.31 at 37 °C, appeared to show that this was the best buffer for the thin-cell layered cultures and the small-volume continuous flow cultures. The large volume cultivation of malaria parasites will obviously pose fresh problems, necessitating precise monitoring and adjustment during the growth of the cultures.

### 4. Gas Phase

Work in recent years has provided continuous cultures, of *P. falciparum,* but in a situation allowing for a thin layer of cells in medium with a large surface area to allow for adequate gas exchange. TRAGER and JENSEN (1978) showed that burning a candle in a dessicator containing cultures produced an atmosphere of 2%–3% $CO_2$ and an $O_2$ content of 15%–18%. This ratio of $CO_2/O_2$ appears to be beneficial to the cultures and can be supplied via commercial gas cylinders. A potential problem for the future could be with the bulk culture of malaria parasites. Care will need to be exercised to ensure that, whatever culture system is employed, the optimum level of dissolved oxygen in the medium is maintained.

## II. Techniques of Cultivation

Since the early work of BASS and JOHNS (1912), in which they observed the development of *P. falciparum* in a static layer of cells, relatively few techniques have been utilised for the cultivation in vitro of intraerythrocytic malaria parasites. The majority of these studies were made with the rocker-dilution technique first developed by GEIMAN et al. (1946) which involved the dilution of an infected blood suspension with nutrient medium, followed by gentle rocking in a continuous stream of 5% $CO_2$/95% air mixture. A variation on this theme was used by POLET (1966), who incubated culture tubes on a roller rotating at 20 rph. These dilution systems are simple but did not allow for anything other than very short-term cultivation. TRAGER (1971) and then TRAGER and JENSEN (1976) further developed the dilution technique to a continuous flow system capable of continuous cultivation of *P. falciparum*. The system allowed for the production of large numbers of parasites and

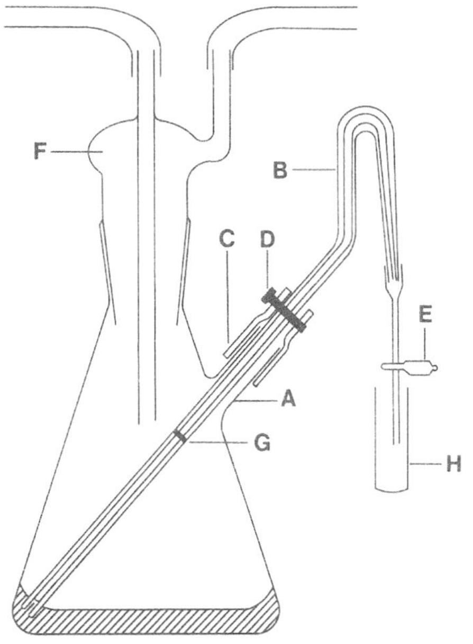


**Fig. 1.** A modified 100-ml Erlenmeyer flask for repeated aseptic sampling of culture material. *A*, side arm; *B*, swan-necked capillary sampling tube; *C*, rubber pressure tubing to give an air-tight seal; *D*, plastic clip; *E*, artery clip; *F*, dreschel bottle head; *G*, mark for predetermined volume required for examination; *H*, collecting vessel

could prove useful in biochemical and immunological studies. The Petri dish culture technique described by the same authors is ideal for chemotherapeutic studies, as is the microtitre plate technique reported by RIECKMANN et al. (1978). The shape and size of culture vessels used for cultivation of malarial parasites has varied greatly over the years. The majority of vessels have either been complicated and difficult to use, or simple and used for a single determination only. A flask developed by WILLIAMS and RICHARDS (1972) enables repeated samples to be removed easily, quickly, and aseptically (Fig. 1). The culture vessel is a modified 100-ml Erlenmeyer flask with a ground glass neck and a Dreschel bottle head to facilitate an appropriate gas mixture to be passed at positive pressure through the flask. A side arm is fitted onto the flask through which a swan-necked capillary tube is passed and an air-tight seal made using rubber pressure tubing. The lower end of the capillary rests in the culture medium and the capillary at the upper end is fitted with a piece of fine bore silicone rubber tubing which is closed with an artery clip. Samples may be collected by releasing the artery clip and allowing culture material to be forced up the capillary by positive pressure in the flask created by the gas flow. Many analytical procedures may be performed on small volumes obtained from a single culture using this technique. The design allows for each flask to be maintained in a 37 °C water bath and to be continually monitored with greater control throughout each experiment, thus alleviating the need to continually open and remove the flask from the incubator.

The primary criteria for parasite growth in vitro prior to the mid-1950s were generally limited to morphological observations. It soon became evident that both morphological and biochemical criteria were essential to interpret experimental results. The utilisation of glucose and conversion to lactate by *P. knowlesi* was determined by MCKEE et al. (1946) and TRIGG and GUTTERIDGE (1971) as a measure of carbohydrate metabolism. POLET and CONRAD (1969) and COHEN et al. (1969) correlated the morphological growth of the parasite with the incorporation of amino acids into parasite protein, and GUTTERIDGE and TRIGG (1970) correlated morphological growth with the incorporation of purines into parasite DNA and RNA. It must be remembered that the simple incorporation of a radioisotope into the parasite does not measure net synthesis of any macromolecule unless the pool sizes of the compound are taken into account. In assessing growth over a short period of time, biochemical measurements must always be used in conjunction with morphological findings and not in isolation. This was shown by the work of GUTTERIDGE and TRIGG (1971) in which pyrimethamine-treated cultures of *P. knowlesi* parasites showed similar patterns of incorporation of amino acids into protein to those of untreated control cultures, although the drug-treated parasites were morphologically abnormal. RICHARDS and WILLIAMS (1975) found that in vitro labelling with radio-tracers may sometimes give a better indication of the mode and speed of action of a drug, but do not necessarily establish the death of the parasite, which can only be done unambiguously by titration into clean cultures, or into fresh, susceptible hosts. *Aotus trivirgatus* monkeys with established infections of *P. falciparum* were treated orally with either chloroquine or a novel compound, 1-amidino-3-(3-chloro-4-cyanophenyl) urea. Blood samples were cultured in vitro 18 h after treatment, when no morphological abnormalities were apparent. The incorporation of radioactive leucine from the medium by the blood of treated monkeys was compared with that of the undosed control, and parasite maturation was also examined. Both chloroquine and the amidinourea were effective against the strain of *P. falciparum*, and the combined use of an in vivo and in vitro test demonstrated that biochemical disturbance of the parasite may be demonstrable before morphological effects are seen.

It should be emphasised that to facilitate meaningful comparison of work between different laboratories, the parasites should be characterised as far as possible, the method of storage standardised and the culture techniques be as standard as possible.

## III. Drug Testing

Recent advances in in vitro techniques allow for a much more meaningful approach to drug testing. Although without doubt the majority of the studies will be carried out using the human parasite *P. falciparum*, in exploring potential chemical leads rodent and simian models will also need to be used. Using the assessment of activity in vivo in conjunction with in vitro culture appears to offer considerable advantages, although the combined system has not yet been widely used, for example:

1. The infected cells can be exposed to a controlled concentration of drugs.

2. The concentration of drug attainable in vitro may be much higher than that possible for plasma levels in vivo. This may enable less active compounds to be assessed, which greatly improves the statistical correlations between physicochemical properties and biological activity.
3. Compounds found to be active in vivo and inactive in vitro indicate that an active metabolite is present.
4. Only microgram quantities of an active metabolite would be required to be isolated to demonstrate activity in vitro.
5. The mechanism of drug action can be investigated.
6. Metabolic pathways in plasmodia may be traced which may lead to the design of new antimalarials.
7. Considerable economies can be achieved when primates are used since several experiments in vitro can be run concomitantly with an experiment in vivo, all using the same animal.

## IV. New Developments

The developments of in vitro cultivation since 1976 have opened a new approach to malaria chemotherapy and the investigation of parasite metabolism. This was highlighted in a symposium reported by RICHARDS et al. (1980), e.g.:

1. HAYNES described a study of the purine metabolism of *P. falciparum* which utilises preformed purines provided by the host. Examining five purine salvage enzymes he found high levels of a parasite-specific adenosine deaminase which could be differentiated from that of the host. When the enzymes were inhibited by deoxycoformycin or low concentrations of adenosine or deoxyadenosine, at levels comparable to that in vivo, they inhibited the growth of the parasite. It was also found that the toxicity of cordycepin, an adenosine analogue with known antimalarial activity, was increased 1 000-fold by the inhibition of adenosine deaminase, thus demonstrating the ability of the enzyme to detoxify adenine nucleosides and analogues. The differences between host and parasite enzymes could be further exploited in the development of adenosine analogues as potential antimalarial agents.

2. SCHEIBEL in the same symposium suggested that the malaria parasite does not rely on oxygen for energy metabolism to the same degree as aerobic mammalian tissue, but acts to a greater degree through metalloprotein biosynthetic oxygenases rather than electron transport. He therefore studied as antimalarials the activity of known chelating agents, tetraethylthiuram disulphide (Antabuse), and diethyldithiocarbamate. Both agents in vitro exhibited an antimalarial effect at 0.1 µg/ml, which is 1/100 of the blood level found in vivo. Antabuse at 1 µg/ml also inhibited parasite glycolysis without affecting glycolysis in human red cells.

3. The activity of standard antimalarials against *P. falciparum* was also described by RICHARDS at the same symposium. Also demonstrated was the bioassay of human plasma after dosing with pyrimethamine. Serum samples taken at various time intervals after dosing were incubated in Petri dish cultures of *P. falciparum*. This study showed that a maximum concentration of pyrimethamine was reached in 2 h and a protective level maintained for 7 days. These findings were corroborated by gas-liquid chromatographic methods. These techniques will undoubtedly feature prominently in future clinical trials, where initially it will be possible to es-

tablish inhibitory drug concentrations without the need to challenge volunteers with the parasite.

### V. Conclusion

The earlier attempts at culture of the asexual stages of the malaria parasite remained ineffective and almost static for the first half of this century. The outbreak of World War II and the continuing conflict in Southeast Asia provided the stimulus for greater effort and, coupled with the skill and dedication of a relatively small group of workers, has seen, certainly in the 1970s, a dramatic success in the cultivation of plasmodia. *P. falciparum* is now isolated and kept in continuous cultivation with relative ease. This opens up the possibility of large-scale production and possible vaccine production, as well as greater chemotherapeutic potential with increased possibilities for monitoring clinical trials, drug testing and the study of drug resistance.

Workers in the field, however, are aware that there are still many areas that need to be improved and expanded. The other human malarias need to be isolated and maintained in continuous cultivation. The simian and rodent malarias, vitally important in chemotherapeutic and immunological studies, need to be brought into continuous cultivation. Changes in parasite status, especially that of drug sensitivity, also need to be studied during prolonged cultivation.

Although commercially available culture media are used successfully for the in vitro cultivation of plasmodia, it is important that this is improved, at least to the stage where the serum component can be replaced with a defined constituent.

Malaria has remained a major health problem until now even though active drugs and insecticides are available. Improved cultivation of malaria parasites could be a major factor in successfully controlling the disease.

## C. Tissue Stages

### I. Introduction

Attempts to culture the exoerythrocytic stages of the malaria parasite began almost a quarter of a century after the work of BASS and JOHNS (1912). All the early work was carried out using avian models, the first recorded attempt being that of HUFF and BLOOM (1935). Their objectives were simply to observe the exoerythrocytic stages of *P. elongatum* in canary bone marrow culture. The in vitro culture was not very successful but parasites were still viable after 48 h and able to infect clean canaries. The persistence and longevity of avian parasites was also demonstrated by GAVRILOV et al. (1938). They attempted to culture exoerythrocytic material from birds infected with *P. gallinaceum* but without any obvious success, although the material after in vitro culture for 7 and 10 days was able to infect fresh birds. HAWKING (1945), also using *P. gallinaceum*, maintained the culture for 89 days. The primary cultures using infected spleens were able to demonstrate the presence of parasites, but attempts at continuous cultivation were unsuccessful.

### II. Avian Studies

DE OLIVEIRA and MEYER (1955) were the first to record the successful subcultivation of exoerythrocytic malaria parasites. The initial culture from plasma clot was successfully transferred to roller tube culture and maintained by alternate subculture for 1 year and, in a subsequent report by MEYER and MUSACCHIO (1959), they described a 4-year continuous culture with the parasites still viable and able to infect susceptible birds.

Outstanding in the field were HUFF and his co-workers, who in 1966 (DAVIS et al. 1966) developed a system for the continuous cultivation of large numbers of malaria parasites. Using embryonic turkey brains infected with *P. fallax* the exoerythrocytic cycle was maintained in vitro. This was an important finding; it emphasised that culture of malaria-infected embryonic cells was more successful than mature cells and that, with large-scale production, it would be possible to study the morphology and biochemistry of the parasite as well as allowing for chemotherapy and immunological studies.

BEAUDOIN et al. (1969) were quick to realise this potential and modified the techniques to study the action of primaquine against the tissue phases. AIKAWA and BEAUDOIN (1970), using very sophisticated techniques, developed the findings further. Morphological changes following treatment with the 8-aminoquinoline, primaquine, suggested that the primary site of activity was at the parasite mitochondrion. Then using $^3$H-primaquine in autoradiographic studies, *P. fallax* was examined after drug treatment by the use of the electron microscope. Primaquine localised within the mitochondria as early as 2 h after treatment and the evidence suggested that there was a localisation of the drug which precedes the swelling of the organelle. Although it was generally believed that primaquine binds to DNA, these workers found no evidence of exposed silver grains overlying the parasite nucleus. Although further work with other tritiated 8-aminoquinolines was not carried out, the authors suggest that, together with primaquine, pentaquine, isopentaquine, and the pentaquine metabolite 8(5-isopropylaminopentyl amino)-5,6-quinolinediol trihydrobromide act in a similar manner, with the primary site of action being the mitochondrion in the exoerythrocytic stages of the avian malaria parasite.

A number of studies examined the immunogenicity of the exoerythrocytic parasites. HOLBROOK et al. (1974, 1976) showed that formalin-killed merozoites from exoerythrocytic cultures were able to form the basis for a successful homologous vaccine and challenge. When the same type of preparation was used to vaccinate mice there was good protection against challenge with *P. berghei* when the merozoites were from young cultures. Merozoites from cultures of more than 3 months' duration offered no protection against challenge. BEAUDOIN and PACHECO (1980), reporting on further work by HOLBROOK, suggest that avian merozoites from exoerythrocytic cultures do not provide protection in rodents against a challenge with rodent sporozoites.

## III. Rodent Models

Experimental work on mammalian exoerythrocytic cultures was many decades behind that of the avian work. The existence of a mammalian exoerythrocytic cycle was not demonstrated until 1948 in the liver of a rhesus monkey infected with *P. cynomolgi* and, later, in a man infected with *P. vivax*. Rodent malaria exoerythrocytic stages were not described until 1965 (YOELI and MOST). For many years progress was restricted by the belief that host-specific or, at least, mammalian hepatocytes were a prerequisite for successful culture. There has only been one report of the exoerythrocytic stages of *P. vivax* being cultured in vivo (DOBY and BARKER 1976) and this with very limited success.

Cultivation of the exoerythrocytic stages of rodent malaria parasites began with short-term culture of infected rat liver cells (FOLEY et al. 1978). Two groups of workers, BEAUDOIN and his colleagues in the United States and SINDEN in the United Kingdom, developed a technique using sporozoites of *P. berghei* to infect rat and turkey embryonic brain (STROME et al. 1979; SINDEN and SMITH 1980). This work demonstrated that a rigid requirement for host-cell specificity did not exist and that it was possible to obtain development from sporozoite to immature tissue schizonts in vitro. The sporozoite infectivity was only 0.01%–0.04%, 2 to 3 orders of magnitude lower than that found in vivo. An interesting finding by SINDEN was that, when mosquito salivary glands, either infected or uninfected, were added to the embryonic rat brain cells in vitro, they inhibited the normal multiplication rate of the cells.

STROME et al. (1979) reported that sporozoites of *P. berghei* entered and developed in embryonic rat liver and brain cells as well as embryonic turkey brain cells in vitro. In culture all host cells appeared fibroblastic in appearance and the parasites generally were found to be located close to the host-cell nucleus.

Cultivation of the complete exoerythrocytic cycle of rodent malaria has now been demonstrated in vitro (HOLLINGDALE et al. 1981). Both rat embryonic brain cells and human embryonic lung cells (line W138) were equally susceptible to both *P. berghei* and *P. yoelii*. The time to development was comparable to that found in vivo when schizont size was used as the criterion. The growth rate of both species in rat cells grown in NCTC 135 medium was good and resembled the expected in vivo development. The improved infectivity, 400-fold over previous reports, allowed the workers to use immunofluorescent staining of the developing exoerythrocytic parasites which could then be examined by phase contrast microscopy, the parasites being easily located under ultraviolet light and then observed by transmitted light.

The remarkable advances made in a few years with the exoerythrocytic forms of rodent malaria in culture hold out great hope for the future cultivation of human parasites.

## D. Gametocytogenesis In Vitro

One of the earliest reports on gametocytes in vitro was by ROW (1929). Using the culture technique of BASS and JOHN (1912) he found that the crescents of *P. falciparum*, in a medium poor in proteins, do not grow and usually degenerate and macerate whether they are inside or outside the pale vacuolated erythrocytes.

Following the successful continuous cultivation of *P. falciparum* by TRAGER and JENSEN (1976), CARTER and BEACH (1977) and COX (1977) reported that, by increasing the serum content of the medium from 10%–50%, morphologically mature gametocytes could be found in vitro after 8 days' cultivation. It was suggested that it should now be possible to complete the asexual and sexual cycles of *P. falciparum* without the need for a mammalian host. JENSEN (1979) observed that current culture methods could not provide a continuous supply of functionally mature gametocytes of *P. falciparum*. He found that, although the gametocytes were morphologically mature after 8–9 days, they would not exflagellate even after 14–18 days of development.

SMALLEY (1976), using fresh infected patient's blood cultured in vitro, found that 10 days are required for the progressive development of gametocytes, rather than an inductive process and a shorter period of development. His concern was that the development of functionally mature gametocytes was inhibited and limited by the ability of the erythrocytes to survive in vitro at 37 °C for prolonged periods. A very careful and detailed series of experiments were described by SINDEN and SMALLEY (1979), again using fresh blood from human patients with *P. falciparum* infections, as well as the same material after storage in liquid nitrogen. The gametocytes' development was observed over a 9-day growth period, and four distinct phases characterised the cell cycle.

1. A $G_1$ period, which lasts only a few hours.
2. The S phase, where DNA synthesis occurs, occupying the remainder of the first 2 days of development.
3. A $G_2$ stage, which is composed of two distinct sections: $G_{2A}$ in which significant RNA and protein synthesis continue to occur, and $G_{2B}$ where there is a progressive transcription control with a resulting depression of both RNA and protein synthesis. This stage sees the production of a functionally mature gametocyte.
4. The final M stage. This is characterised by the brief and dramatic gametogenesis during which time there is a period of de novo protein synthesis.

The same workers also reported on the activity of a number of chemical compounds. Test solutions were added on each day over a period of 9 days, the drug being left in contact with the parasites for 48 h. The cultures were made in commercially available microtitration plates and incubated using the TRAGER and JENSEN (1976) technique. The results reported were that mitomycin C, an inhibitor of DNA replication, stopped development of the gametocyte for the first 3 days of culture. With increasing age the gametocyte became more refractory to treatment and by day 9 was unaffected even at dose levels 725 times greater than that effective against the early stages. 8-Azaguanine, even when used at 200 μg/ml, was without effect. Rifampicin was effective at 8 μg/ml and higher and actinomycin D was lethal at $5 \times 10^{-8}$ *M*. Emetine, cycloheximide, and puromycin were the most potent of the antimetabolites tested at levels of $2.4 \times 10^{-6}$ *M*, $5.8 \times 10^{-6}$ *M*, and $1.2 \times 10^{-7}$ *M*, respectively. It was interesting that colchicine at levels that did not kill the sexual or asexual parasites maintained gametocyte numbers at or above the untreated control cultures.

CARTER and MILLER (1979) studied the effect of culture dilution with fresh erythrocytes on the conversion rate to gametocytes. Using the now conventional TRAGER and JENSEN (1976) system, when *P. falciparum* cultures were diluted to lower the parasitaemia using fresh erythrocytes, there was a correlated reduction in the conversion to and production of gametocytes. The levels rose after several days' growth in culture. The donor cultures continued to maintain a high conversion rate. Although the environmental factors involved in mediating the changes in conversion rate are not known, the authors suggested that the effect is not just associated with the aging of the erythrocytes but is probably associated with changes in the medium following a period of growth in culture. Following this work Kaushal et al. (1980) found that gametocyte production is rare in culture conditions conducive to rapid growth of the cultures but frequent when parasite densities were static. Using cultures of *P. falciparum* they demonstrated that almost 100% of the ring stages develop into gametocytes in response to 1 m*M* cyclic AMP in static cultures, whereas the same treatment in rapidly growing cultures had little or no effect.

Smalley and Brown (1981) also studied gametocytogenesis stimulation. They reported that the presence of lymphocytes with parasites in European serum had no effect on the conversion rate of *P. falciparum* gametocytes isolated in The Gambia. Lymphocytes from naturally infected indigenous children significantly increased the conversion rate and subsequent number of developing gametocytes. They admit that the mechanism is still unknown. Ifediba and Vanderberg (1981) postulate that, although RPMI-1640 is able to supply all the nutritional needs of the asexual parasites of *P. falciparum,* the gametocytes may require additional growth factors. They suggest that the depleted hypoxanthine reserves of the host erythrocyte need to be supplemented in vitro. Added hypoxanthine 50 μg/ml allowed for the production of mature gametocytes of *P. falciparum* on a regular basis. Mosquitoes allowed to feed on these cultures developed midgut infections with subsequent development to sporozoites in the salivary glands.

Two other groups of workers, Campbell et al. (1980) and Ponnudurai et al. (1980), have successfully cultured *P. falciparum* gametocytes and infected *Anopheles freeborni* and *Anopheles gambiae,* respectively.

## E. Sporogonic Stages

Very little work apart from that of Ball and Chao (1971) and their co-workers has been reported on the cultivation of sporogonic stages of malaria parasites. Much of the early work was done using *P. relictum* where different stages were maintained in the mosquito stomach. As yet it has not been possible to culture the complete cycle in any one culture in vitro. The techniques involved are intricate and complicated by the need to achieve and maintain sterility of material removed from mosquitoes. Schneider (1968a, b), using mature, 8- to 9-day-old oocysts of *P. gallinaceum,* was able to maintain them in Grace's *Antheraea eucalypti* cell line and demonstrate the production of sporozoites, thus showing that older and preferably unattached oocysts are able to grow better in vitro than the younger stages and that the mosquito stomach was not a strict prerequisite. Ball and Chao (1971) also showed improved growth in insect cell-line culture and almost doubled the time in culture of a single isolate of *P. relictum.*

In mammalian models, again little work has been done. Alger (1968) incubated blood at room temperature from *P. berghei*-infected mice, containing both male and female gametocytes, in capillary tubes, and was able to obtain ookinete formation. In the same year Yoeli and Upmanis (1968) were unable to repeat this finding until an aqueous extract of the midgut of *Anopheles stephensi* was added to the cultures. It was possible to obtain ookinete formation if the blood was collected from a mosquito whilst feeding on a mouse infected with *P. berghei.* Using epithelial cell lines from fat-head minnow and primary cultures of *Anopheles stephensi,* Rosales-

RONQUILLO and SILVERMAN (1974) were able to obtain ookinete formation from *P. berghei*-infected blood. In the same year together with NIENABER the same workers (ROSALES-RONQUILLO et al. 1974) grew *P. berghei* ookinetes intracellularly in fat-head minnow cells.

More recently CHEN (1981) reported on the in vitro cultivation of *P. yoelii yoelii*-infected blood containing gametocytes. The blood, collected from the tail vein or orbits of infected mice, was mixed with different media in various proportions and incubated at 19–25 °C. Mature ookinete formation occurred in four kinds of medium: (a) a mosquito extract with heparinised mouse blood, (b) BME synthetic medium with mouse blood, (c) Locke's solution with mouse blood, and (d) simply in mouse blood with heparin. The first two media gave better results than the latter two. A number of findings were recorded: the morphology of the ookinete was similar to that seen in the ookinete structures developing in the mosquito haemocoele; the optimum temperature range is 19–25 °C with temperatures higher than this being inhibitory to the formation of microgametes; the best time to take gametocyte containing blood is 3–5 days after the mice are infected and with no more than five generations away from cyclical transmission; the presence of leucocytes is inhibitory to growth, probably due to their phagocytic action.

At present many workers are studying the isolation of sporozoites from infected mosquitoes and, if this proves to be successful, then the in vitro cultivation of the sporogonic phase of *Plasmodium* may be of scientific interest only.

## F. Conclusions

The culture techniques developed for *P. falciparum* since 1976 have been remarkable for their success. With the current knowledge it should be possible to study the complete cycle of this parasite and develop further the techniques for drug testing, immunology and biochemistry. Strenuous efforts should also be made to achieve the same results with *P. vivax*.

## References

Aikawa M, Beaudoin RL (1970) *Plasmodium fallax:* high resolution autoradiography of exoerythrocytic stages treated with primaquine in vitro. Exp Parasitol 27:454–463

Alger NE (1968) In vitro development of *Plasmodium berghei* ookinetes. Nature 218:774

Anfinsen CB, Geiman QM, McKee RW, Ormsbee RA, Ball EG (1946) Studies on malaria parasites VIII: factors affecting the growth of *P. knowlesi* in vitro. J Exp Med 84:607–621

Ball EG, Anfinsen CB, Geiman QM, McKee RW, Ormsbee RA (1945) In vitro growth and multiplication of the malaria parasite *Plasmodium knowlesi*. Science 101:542–544

Ball GH, Chao J (1971) The cultivation of *Plasmodium relictum* in mosquito cell lines. J Parasitol 57:391–395

Bass CC, Johns JM (1912) The cultivation of malaria plasmodia (*Plasmodium vivax* and *Plasmodium falciparum*) in vitro. J Exp Med 16:567–579

Beaudoin RL, Pacheco ND (1980) Cultivation of exoerythrocytic stages of malaria parasites. The in vitro cultivation of pathogens of tropical diseases. In: Rowe DS, Hirumi H (eds) Proceedings of the workshop held in Nairobi, Kenya, 4–9 February 1979. Tropical diseases research series No. 3. Schwabe, Basel, pp 16–27

Beaudoin RL, Strome CPA, Clutter WG (1969) A tissue culture system for the study of drug action against the tissue phase of malaria. Milit Med 134:979–985

Campbell CC, Chin W, Collins WE, Moss DM (1980) Infection of *Anopheles freeborni* by gametocytes of cultured *Plasmodium falciparum*. Trans R Soc Trop Med Hyg 74/5:668–669

Carter R, Beach RF (1977) Gametogenesis in culture by gametocytes of *Plasmodium falciparum*. Nature 270:240–241

Carter R, Miller LH (1979) Evidence for environmental modulation of gametocytogenesis in *Plasmodium falciparum* in continuous culture. Bull WHO [Suppl] 57:37–52

Chen PH (1981) Preliminary study on the in vitro cultivation of ookinetes of rodent malarial parasites. Chin J Zool 1:1–10

Cohen S, Butcher GA (1971) Serum antibody in malarial immunity. Trans R Soc Trop Med Hyg 65:125–135

Cohen S, Butcher GA, Crandall RB (1969) Action of malarial antibody in vitro. Nature 223:368–371

Cox FEG (1977) Gametes of malaria parasites. Nature 270:204

Davis AG, Huff CG, Palmer TT (1966) Procedures for maximum production of exoerythrocytic stages of *Plasmodium fallax* in tissue culture. Exp Parasitol 19:1–8

De Oliveira MX, Meyer H (1955) *Plasmodium gallinaceum* in tissue culture. Observations after one year of cultivation. Parasitology 45:1–4

Doby JM, Barker R (1976) Essais d'obtention in vitro des formes pré-érythrocytaires de *Plasmodium vivax* en cultures de cellules, hépatiques humaines inoculées par sporozoites. C R Soc Biol (Paris) 170(3):661–665

Foley DA, Kennard J, Venderberg JP (1978) *Plasmodium berghei:* infective exoerythrocytic schizonts in primary monolayer cultures of rat liver cells. Exp Parasitol 46:166–178

Gavrilov W, Bobkoff G, Laurencin S (1938) Essai de culture en tissus de *Plasmodium gallinaceum*. Ann Soc Belg Med Trop 18:429–438

Geiman QM, Anfinsen GB, McKee RW, Ormsbee RA, Ball EG (1946) Studies on malarial parasites. Methods and techniques for cultivation. J Exp Med 84:583–606

Geiman QM, Siddiqui WA, Schnell JV (1966) In vitro studies on erythrocytic stages of plasmodia: medium improvement and results with several species of malaria parasites. Milit Med [Suppl] 131:1015–1025

Gomperts BD (1967) Metabolic changes in human red cells during incubation of whole blood in vitro. Biochem J 102:782–790

Gutteridge WE, Trigg PI (1970) Incorporation of radioactive precursors into DNA and RNA of *Plasmodium knowlesi* in vitro. J Protozool 17:89–96

Gutteridge WE, Trigg PI (1971) Action of pyrimethamine and related drugs against *Plasmodium knowlesi* in vitro. Parasitology 62:431–444

Haut A, Tudhope GR, Cartwright GE, Wintrope MM (1962) Studies on the osmotic fragility of incubated normal and abnormal erythrocytes. J Clin Invest 39:1818

Hawking F (1945) Growth of protozoa in tissue culture. I. *Plasmodium gallinaceum* exoerythrocytic forms. Trans R Soc Trop Med Hyg 39:245–263

Haynes JD, Diggs CL, Hines FA, Desjardins RE (1976) Culture of human malaria parasites, *Plasmodium falciparum*. Nature 263:767–769

Holbrook TW, Palczuk NC, Stauber IA (1974) Immunity to exoerythrocytic forms of malaria III: stage-specific immunization of turkeys against exoerythrocytic forms of *Plasmodium fallax*. J Parasitol 60:348–354

Holbrook TW, Spitalny GL, Palczuk NC (1976) Stimulation of resistance in mice to sporozoite induced *Plasmodium berghei* malaria by injections of avian exoerythrocytic forms. J Parasitol 62:670–675

Hollingdale MR, Leef JL, McCullough M, Beaudoin RL (1981) In vitro cultivation of the exoerythrocytic stage of *Plasmodium berghei* from sporozoites. Science 213:1021–1022

Huff CG, Bloom W (1935) A malarial parasite infecting all blood and blood-forming cells of birds. J Infect Dis 57:315–336

Ifediba T, Vanderberg JP (1981) Complete in vitro maturation of *Plasmodium falciparum* gametocytes. Nature 294:364–366

Jensen JB (1979) Observations on gametogenesis in *Plasmodium falciparum* from continuous culture. J Protozool 26:129–132

Kaushal DC, Carter R, Miller LH, Krishna G (1980) Gametocytogenesis by malaria parasites in continuous culture. Nature 490–492

McKee RW, Ormsbee RA, Anfinsen CB, Geiman QM, Ball EG (1946) Studies on malarial parasites: the chemistry and metabolism of normal and parasitized (*Plasmodium knowlesi*) monkey blood. J Exp Med 84:569–582

Meyer H, Musacchio MO (1959) *Plasmodium gallinaceum* in tissue cultures: results obtained during 4 years of uninterrupted cultivation of the parasite in vitro. Proceedings of the sixth international congressess on tropical medicine and malaria. Anais Inst Med Trop 16:Suppl. II 7:10–13

Pasvol G, Weatherall DJ, Wilson RJM, Smith DH, Gilles HM (1976) Fetal haemoglobin and malaria. Lancet 1:1269–1272

Phillips RS, Trigg PI, Scott-Finnigan TJ (1972) Culture of *Plasmodium falciparum* in vitro; a subculture technique used for demonstrating antiplasmodial activity in serum from some Gambians resident in an endemic malarious ares. Parasitology 65:525–535

Polet H (1966) In vitro cultivation of erythrocytic forms of *Plasmodium knowlesi* and *Plasmodium berghei*. Milit Med [Suppl] 131:1026–1031

Polet H, Conrad ME (1969) In vitro studies on the amino acid metabolism of *Plasmodium knowlesi* and the antiplasmodial effect of the isoleucine antagonists. Milit Med 134:939–944

Ponnudurai T, Meuwissen TJHE, Verhave JP, Leeuwenberg ADEM (1980) Functional maturity of gametocytes of *Plasmodium falciparum* produced in continuous in vitro cultures. WHO/MAL 80:921 WHO, Geneva

Richards WHG, Williams SG (1973) The removal of leucocytes from malaria infected blood. Ann Trop Med Parasitol 67/2:169–178

Richards WHG, Williams GG (1975) Malaria studies in vitro. III: the protein synthesising activity of *Plasmodium falciparum* in vitro after drug treatment in vivo. Ann Trop Med Parasitol 69/2:135–140

Richards WHG, Haynes JD, Scheibel LW, Sinden R, Desjardins RE, Wernsdorfer WH (1980) New developments in malaria chemotherapy using in vitro cultures. Current chemotherapy and infectious disease. Proceedings of the 11th ICC and the 19th ICAAC American Society of Microbiology 1980. American Society of Microbiologists, Washington, DC, pp 10–13

Rieckmann KH, Sax LJ, Campbell GH, Mrema JE (1978) Drug sensitivity of *Plasmodium falciparum*. An in vitro technique. Lancet 1:22–23

Rosales-Ronquillo MC, Silverman PH (1974) *Plasmodium berghei* ookinete formation in vector and non-vector cells substrates. In: Proceedings of the 3rd international congress of parasitology. München. Facta Publication, Vienna, vol 1, pp 124–125

Rosales-Ronquillo MC, Neinaber G, Silverman PH (1974) *Plasmodium berghei* ookinete formation in non-vector cell line. J Parasitol 60:1039–1040

Row R (1929) On some observations on the malarial parasites grown aerobically in simple cultures with special reference to the evolution and degeneration of the crescents. Indian J Med Res 16:1120–1125

Schneider I (1968a) Cultivation of in vitro *Plasmodium gallinaceum* oocysts. Exp Parasitol 22:178–186

Schneider I (1968b) Cultivation of *Plasmodium gallinaceum* oocysts in Grace's cell strain of *Aedes aegypti* (L.). In: Proceedings of the second international colloquium on invertebrate tissue culture. Tremezzo. Academic, London, pp 247–253

Siddiqui WA, Schnell JV (1973) Use of various buffers for in vitro cultivation of malaria parasites. J Parasitol 59:516–519

Siddiqui WA, Schnell JV, Geiman QM (1970a) In vitro cultivation of *Plasmodium falciparum*. Am J Trop Med Hyg 19:586–591

Siddiqui WA, Schnell JV, Geiman QM (1970b) Use of a commercially-available culture medium to test the susceptibility of human malarial parasites to antimalarial drugs. J Parasitol 56/1:188–189

Sinden RE, Smalley ME (1979) Gametocytogenesis of *Plasmodium falciparum* in vitro: the cell cycle. Parasitology 79:277–296

Sinden RE, Smith J (1980) Culture of the liver stages (exoerythrocytic schizonts) of rodent malaria parasites from sporozoites in vitro. Trans R Soc Trop Med Hyg 74:134–136
Smalley ME (1976) *Plasmodium falciparum* gametocytogenesis in vitro. Nature 264:271–272
Smalley ME, Brown J (1981) *Plasmodium falciparum* gametocytogenesis stimulated by lymphocytes and serum from infected Gambian children. Trans R Soc Trop Med Hyg 75: 316–317
Strome CPA, De Santis PL, Beaudoin RL (1979) The cultivation of the exoerythrocytic stages of *Plasmodium berghei* from sporozoites in vitro. In Vitro 15:531–536
Theakston RDG, Fletcher KA (1971) The use of isotopic tracer techniques for examining the preference of *Plasmodium berghei* for a particular age group of erythrocytes and for studying the dynamics of haemolysis in malaria. Ann Trop Med Parasitol 64:441–450
Trager W (1950) Studies on the extra-cellular cultivation of an intra-cellular parasite (avian malaria). Development of the organism in erythrocytes extracts, and the favouring effect of adenosine triphosphate. J Exp Med 92:349–365
Trager W (1952) Studies on the extra-cellular cultivation of an intra-cellular parasite (avian malaria). The effects of malate and of co-enzyme A concentrates. J Exp Med 96:465–474
Trager W (1971) A new method for intraerythrocytic cultivation of malaria parasites (*Plasmodium coatneyi* and *P. falciparum*). J Protozool 18:239–242
Trager W (1976) Prolonged cultivation of malaria parasites (*Plasmodium coatneyi* and *P. falciparum*). In: Van Den Bossche H (ed) Biochemistry of parasites and host-parasite relationships. North Holland, Amsterdam, pp 427–434
Trager W (1980) Cultivation of erythrocytic stages of malaria. In: Roweth DS, Hirumi H (eds) The in vitro cultivation of the pathogens of tropical diseases. Tropical diseases research series. Schwabe, Basel, pp 3–13
Trager W, Jensen JB (1976) Human malaria parasites in continuous culture. Science 193:673–675
Trager W, Jensen JB (1978) Cultivation of malarial parasites. Nature 273:621–622
Trigg PI (1968) A new continuous perfusion technique for the cultivation of malaria parasites in vitro. Trans R Soc Trop Med Hyg 62:371–378
Trigg PI (1975) Invasion of erythrocytes by *Plasmodium falciparum* in vitro. Parasitology 71:433–436
Trigg PI, Gutteridge WE (1971) A minimal medium for the growth of *Plasmodium knowlesi* in dilution cultures. Parasitology 62:113–123
Trigg PI, Shakespeare PG (1976a) The effects of incubation in vitro on the susceptibility of monkey erythrocytes to invasion by *Plasmodium knowlesi*. Parasitology 73:149–160
Trigg PI, Shakespeare PG (1976b) Factors affecting the long term cultivation of the erythrocytic stages of *Plasmodium knowlesi*. In: Van Den Bossche H (ed) Biochemistry of parasites and host-parasite relationships. North Holland, Amsterdam, pp 435–440
Vernes A (1980) Phagocytosis of *Plasmodium falciparum* parasitised erythrocytes by peripheral monocytes. Lancet 1297–1298
Williams SG, Richards WHG (1972) A simple aseptic method for the rapid removal of samples from small-scale cultures of micro-organisms. WHO/MAL/72:758 WHO, Geneva
Yoeli M, Most H (1965) Studies on sporozoite-induced infections of rodent malaria I. The pre-erythrocytic tissue stage of *Plasmodium berghei*. Am J Trop Med Hyg 14:700–714
Yoeli M, Uppmanis RS (1968) *Plasmodium berghei* ookinete formation in vitro. Exp Parasitol 22:122–128

# Host Responses to Malaria

CHAPTER 4

# Immunity

G. H. MITCHELL

## A. Introduction

Of the four species of *Plasmodium* responsible for essentially all naturally acquired malaria in man, only *P. falciparum* is frequently the direct cause of fatal disease. In the absence of specific treatment, the lethality of this infection, and the morbidity of malaria in general, is considerably influenced by the extent of the individual's previous exposure to the malaria species in question. Other important factors influencing the outcome of infection, but not to be considered here, may include the size of infective inoculum, concurrent disease, nutritional status and the host's possession or lack of any of the innate characteristics which reduce his susceptibility (for example, sickle cell trait). The transmission of malaria in a population provides a potent evolutionary selection pressure for such characteristics, which disadvantageously alter the parasites' milieu within the host by mechanisms independent of the host's acquired immune response, even when a proportion of carriers of the gene in question suffer severe disease as a consequence of it (e.g. sickle cell anaemia). Such innate resistance mechanisms have been recently reviewed by MILLER and CARTER (1976) (see also Chaps. 2 and 15). It would be unjustified to suppose that the transmission of malaria in a population does not also select for efficiency at countering malaria in the acquired immune response itself. Immune response genes are associated with the major histocompatibility complex (HLA system, in man), and CEPPELLINI (1973) showed differential rates of expression of HLA D antigens between lowland (recently malarious) and highland village populations (climatically protected from malaria transmission) in Sardinia. The differences were less marked than those found in the frequencies of glucose-6-phosphate dehydrogenase (G6PD) deficiency and thalassaemia (for which malaria transmission markedly selects) between the same populations, but significant compared with twenty-two "neutral" polymorphisms studied.

Similarly, genetic differences in the control of the immune response may underlie the very different outcome of infection with the same malaria in two broadly susceptible host species (or, for laboratory animals, two lines of a single host species). Thus the kra monkey (*Macaca fascicularis*) is a natural host of *P. knowlesi*, suffering a clinically mild although chronic disease even on first exposure. This malaria can also infect a number of other monkeys, including the rhesus monkey (*Macaca mulatta*). This macaque is closely allied to the kra, with which it interbreeds freely, intermediate forms occurring in their common range (FOODEN 1964), but it does not encounter *P. knowlesi* in nature. In the laboratory the rhesus is exquisitely susceptible to *P. knowlesi*, with perhaps nine of ten infected animals dying with fulminating parasitaemia irrespective of the size of infective inoculum. Yet the red cells of the kra are, if anything, marginally more readily invaded by *P. knowlesi* in vitro than are those of the rhesus, and the normal sera of both species support cultures of infected cells well (BUTCHER et al. 1973). Moreover, for the first 5 or 6 days of blood-induced infection the parasites' multiplication rate in the two hosts is the same, and a very large infusion of infected blood into a kra (sufficient to cause immediate patency) will result in a fatal fulminating parasitaemia (BUTCHER and MITCHELL, unpublished results). However, after a smaller challenge inoculum ($10^4$–$10^5$ parasites) the naive kra will control its parasitaemia at a peak of less than 5% (MITCHELL et al. 1979) and antibody of wide specificity capable of inhibiting merozoite invasion of red cells becomes detectable in its serum (COHEN et al. 1977). The rhesus monkey fails to produce such antibody fast enough to control the infection and requires several experiences of drug-controlled infection with *P. knowlesi* before a similar protective response of broad specificity is detectable (BUTCHER and COHEN 1972).

In other host-parasite systems, the age of the host at the time of infection may influence the outcome. For instance *P. berghei* is more virulent in weanling rats than in those more than 7 weeks old. This is at least in part due to the maturation of the immune system (SMALLEY 1975).

Clearly the persistence of a parasitosis in a population is influenced by many factors, apart from host immunity, but in the case of the immune response a balance must often be struck between lethal consequences to the host and the extermination of parasites. The too frequent occurrence of either extreme outcome would extinguish the parasite species if, as for malaria in man, no reservoir of infection exists beyond the short-lived vectors. The continued existence of endemic human malaria and of other enzootic malarias is evidence of the balance. It follows that natural malaria infections generally do not excite sterilising immunity; the initial infection may persist in the individual by some evasion of the immune response or, after eventual recovery from one parasitaemia, the host may still provide an acceptable environment for a subsequently introduced infection. However, this balance is not reflected in the majority of laboratory host-parasite systems, where the partnerships are essentially artificial. Thus the rodent malaria *P. berghei* and *P. yoelii* are frequently studied, but in *Rattus* and *Mus*, not the natural host *Thamnomys*. Hence death (*P. berghei* in many laboratory mouse strains) or sterilising immunity with complete refractoriness to reinfection (*P. yoelii* 17X in CBA mice, for instance) are often the end points of laboratory infections. Such artificial systems are useful, however, for an exaggerated response may be easier to analyse, and the successful vaccination of exquisitely susceptible hosts may lead to very effective malaria vaccination in man. Moreover, the use of syngeneic laboratory rodents allows the use of cell transfer experiments and, by appropriate manipulations, the roles of immunocompetent cell types (particularly T-cell subclasses) may soon be analysed in mouse malaria infections.

Useful reviews of the literature on the immune response to malaria are by COGGESHALL (1943), BROWN (1969), BUTCHER (1974), and COHEN (1979). BROWN (1976) provides a critical treatment of many of the hypothesised protective mechanisms. VOLLER et al. (1980) review the serodiagnosis of malaria. COHEN (1976a) reviews the mechanisms by which parasites may persist in sensitised hosts and COHEN

(1976 b) the essentials of the immune effector mechanisms operating against parasites.

A fuller, but introductory, account of the immune system itself may be found in ROITT (1980), and notes on the production and use of monoclonal antibodies in investigating tropical disease have been produced by the WORLD HEALTH ORGANIZATION (1980).

## B. The Clinical Expression of Immunity to Malaria in Man

Where *P. falciparum* is endemic, placentae are often found heavily infected with parasites on delivery, yet congenital malaria is very rare (BRUCE-CHWATT 1963). Protective maternal IgG certainly circulates in the fetus (EDOZIEN et al. 1962), and the developing fetal immune system may also be stimulated to produce protective IgM by soluble malaria antigens crossing the placenta from the infected mother. However, MCGREGOR (1972), quoting unpublished work from The Gambia, noted that S antigens (see Sect. C.V.4, below) were absent from the sera of newborn infants whose mothers' sera were positive, and that fetal IgM levels were not unusually high. After birth, colostral antibody and a milk diet, deficient in para-amino benzoic acid, which *Plasmodium* requires, will confer some protection (KRETSCHMAR and VOLLER 1973) on the neonate. Moreover, fetal haemoglobin-containing erythrocytes have been shown not to support optimal parasite growth (PASVOL et al. 1977).

For infants the rate of termination of parasitaemic episodes is higher than in the 1- to 4-year-old age group, and their infection rate is much smaller than would be anticipated from the entomological inoculation rate (i.e. most sporozoites fail to lead to an apparent blood infection) (MOLINEAUX and GRAMMICIA 1980). However, the prevalence and density of asexual parasitaemia increases with age.

Frank disease is likely to occur by about 6 months of age, and very high mortality rates and much illness afflict the age group up to about 5 years. Later death from malaria is unlikely, but high parasitaemias may still be experienced, sometimes with rather trivial symptomatology. An antitoxic rather than antiparasitic immunity has been suggested to explain this tolerance of parasitaemia with reduced morbidity. Parasitaemia will still be experienced by adults, with the density in individuals decreasing faster than the prevalence in a population with increasing age. These relationships, long known, are well illustrated by the data from the Garki project (MOLINEAUX and GRAMMICIA 1980).

Splenic enlargement is usual in children, and indeed is exploited in measurement of endemicity [for details of this and other aspects of malaria epidemiology the collation of MACDONALD's work by BRUCE-CHWATT and GLANVILLE (1973) should be consulted]. The immunopathology of malaria is reviewed elsewhere in this book (Chap. 5), but amongst the notable features are autoimmune anaemia, which may be mediated by immune complex attachment to red cells (FACER et al. 1978), and the nephrotic syndrome of quartan (*P. malariae*) malaria in children, which is initiated by the deposition of malaria antigen-antibody complex on the kidney glomerular basement membrane (HOUBA et al. 1971).

Total immunoglobulin synthesis and turnover are elevated in exposed populations, but not all of this can be ascribed to malaria in an environment so rich in pathogens; indeed administration of antimalarials to Gambians reduces their rate of Ig synthesis from about thrice to about twice that of expatriate West Africans in the United Kingdom (COHEN et al. 1961). Moreover, it must be assumed that not all the antibody whose genesis is brought about by malaria infection is directed against malaria parasite antigens, since lymphocyte mitogen production (GREENWOOD and VICK 1975) may cause polyclonal activation following infection which may lead to the elaboration of irrelevant antibody specificities. The induction of responses to other antigens is hampered by malaria; tetanus toxoid immunisation, for example, is poorly effective where malaria is endemic (MCGREGOR and BARR 1962).

However, the eventual potency and relevance of the antibody reponse to malaria of the exposed adult population has been demonstrated by passive transfer of pooled IgG prepared from adults to infected children (COHEN and MCGREGOR 1963). Large doses were given, and a very marked suppression (but not cure) of parasitaemias of *P. falciparum* and *P. malariae* was brought about. This result has been confirmed in several model systems and the mode(s) of action of the antibody have been investigated in vitro. (See Sect. C.V, below).

## C. Malaria Antigens, the Induction of Immunity and Protective Mechanisms in Infection and Vaccination

### I. Specificity of Antimalarial Immune Responses

Protective immune responses to malaria are usually species specific, although some cross-protection is known, especially in rodent systems (COX 1970; NUSSENZWEIG et al. 1972b), and they may also be strain specific (but the term strain has been used loosely in malariology). Moreover, the effectiveness of the response to an early episode of parasitaemia may be limited to the intrastrain antigenic variant present during that episode, when this can be defined (BROWN 1974). However, malaria infection leads to an increase in the number of the host's cells (killer or K cells) capable of damaging foreign cells coated with antibody. The target cells may be quite irrelevant to the disease, e.g. chicken erythrocytes are lysed by K cells from *P. chabaudi*-infected mice (MCDONALD and PHILLIPS 1978) or *P. falciparum*-infected children (GREENWOOD et al. 1977) if they are first coated with anti-chicken red-cell antibody.

When parasites of a single stage in the life cycle are used to sensitise an animal, any protective response seen will be stage specific, except possibly in the case of gamete immunisation (see GWADZ et al. 1979). This suggests that the morphological plasticity of *Plasmodium* is paralleled by a diversity in those structural and functional macromolecules which the immune response is able to damage.

Serological tests indicate immune status rather poorly, but indicate prior exposure to malaria well. In general, the serologically detectable antibody response is not specific to the inducing malaria species, and material from other species may be used as target antigen (even avian parasites for human malaria: KIELMANN et al. 1970).

## II. Immune Response to Sporozoites

Sporozoites disappear rapidly from the circulation after introduction into skin capallaries, but their exact fate is unknown in both normal and immune hosts. If isolated rat liver is perfused with medium bearing sporozoites of *P. yoelii nigeriensis*, the sporozoites are rapidly removed from the perfusate (almost 80% after 1 min, and almost 95% after 15 min). Prior treatment of the liver with colloidal silica to disable Küpffer cells reduces the rate at which sporozoites are removed (59% after 15 min) (SMITH and SINDEN 1981). It seems then, that the Küpffer cell (the fixed macrophage of the liver) may be the distal point of entry for development in parenchyma cells. Peritoneal macrophages have been used as "models" of the Küpffer cells by DANFORTH et al. (1980). When sporozoites are incubated with them in the presence of normal serum, the sporozoites gain entry if the macrophage and serum donor species would normally be susceptible to the malaria in question. Following sporozoite entry the macrophage degenerates but the sporozoite within it remains intact. If serum from a sporozoite-vaccinated host is used, then the macrophage remains morphologically normal and the sporozoite within it is destroyed.

Mice are readily protected against subsequent *P. berghei* sporozoite challenge by i.v. vaccination with X-irradiated sporozoites (NUSSENZWEIG et al. 1967). Large serum doses transferred from such animals into normal mice confer some protection on challenge, but this protection is not absolute, and all such passively protected mice eventually develop parasitaemia. However, they have many fewer liver schizonts on challenge than do controls, and viable sporozoites are rapidly cleared from their circulation, as judged by the inoculation of sequential blood samples into clean animals (NUSSENZWEIG et al. 1972a). The incubation of sporozoites with sera from vaccinated animals results in their losing infectivity (VANDERBERG et al. 1969) and there is some correlation of this effect with the titre of an antibody which precipitates around sporozoites, the circumsporozoite precipitin (CSP). In the CSP reaction surface antigen is capped and shed (COCHRANE et al. 1976), but only the exterior face of the plasma membrane is disorganised as judged by freeze-fracture studies (AIKAWA et al. 1979). A *P. berghei* sporozoite antigen of 44 kilodaltons is precipitated by sera from vaccinated mice, and a monoclonal antibody reactive with this "Pb44" antigen has been produced by a hybridoma derived from a vaccinated mouse spleen cell and myeloma cell fusion. This monoclonal antibody mediates a CSP reaction, immunofluorescence and neutralisation of sporozoite infectivity (YOSHIDA et al. 1980).

CSP antibody (and an immunofluorescence-detected antibody) has been found in an endemically infected human population (NARDIN and NUSSENZWEIG 1979) and it must be likely that antisporozoite protective antibody also arises under the circumstances of repeated natural inoculation. When fully viable sporozoites of *P. berghei* are inoculated into drug covered rodents a protective response is mounted, resulting in sterilisation of sporozoite inocula; this is demonstrated when the withdrawal of the drug followed by sporozoite inoculation fails to lead to parasitaemia (VERHAVE 1975). In common with hosts vaccinated with attenuated sporozoites, these animals remain susceptible to a challenge of asexual erythrocytic parasites.

Vaccination with variously irradiated or otherwise attenuated sporozoites has been effective in many systems, including avian malarias (MULLIGAN et al. 1941;

RICHARDS 1966) and human malarias (CLYDE 1975). The immunity engendered in man to *P. falciparum* and *P. vivax*, following repeated bites of irradiated infected mosquitoes, was, however, rather short lived (about 6 months), and the mechanisms involved remain unknown. BRAY (1976) found isolated irradiated sporozoites ineffective in protecting two Gambian children against natural challenge with *P. falciparum*.

## III. Immune Response to the Exoerythrocytic Phase

As will be clear from elsewhere in this book (Chap. 1), the extent, nature, and pathology of exoerythrocytic (EE) schizogony varies amongst the subgenera of *Plasmodium*.

Free EE merozoites of the avian malaria *P. fallax* have been used as immunogen in turkeys (HOLBROOK et al. 1974). Although liver schizonts in mammals may be found surrounded by phagocytes (BROWN 1969) there is as yet little evidence of protective immune responses in mammalian malaria against either transient EE schizonts or the more persistent hypnozoite forms (see Chap. 1). It is safer to assume that this reflects the paucity of data and present difficulty of observing these stages rather than a deficiency in the hosts' immune response.

However, whereas immunity engendered by sporozoite vaccination in rodents was found by FOLEY and VANDERBERG (1977) not to protect against challenge by intraperitoneal injection of immature exoerythrocytic schizonts, BAFORT et al. (1978) reached the opposite conclusion in the same rat-*P. berghei* model, suggesting that immunity to liver stages was a consequence of sporozoite vaccination. Antisera obtained from sporozoite-vaccinated mice and from mice infected with or recovered from blood stage parasites will react with EE forms as judged by IFAT. EE stages from 14–42 h post sporozoite inoculation were studied by DANFORTH et al. (1978), who found the reactivity of antisporozoite serum decreased against parasites older than 24 h postinoculation, and the reactivity of the anti-blood-stage serum increased against parasites older than 16 h postinoculation.

## IV. Immune Response to the Sexual Stages

The immune response to gametocytes, like that to pre-erythrocytic stages, remains relatively unstudied. Gametocytes may be observed to persist in the circulation following the near clearance of asexual blood forms, but their infectivity for mosquitoes may decline (HAWKING et al. 1966). Gametocyte production in vitro may be stimulated by lymphocytes and serum from infected donors (SMALLEY and BROWN 1981).

Immune sera react with gametocytes, but not gametes, as judged by IFAT (SINDEN et al. 1978). The vertebrate hosts of *Plasmodium* spp. do not experience gametes during infection, as gametogenesis occurs in the vector. However, several immunisation experiments have utilised gamete-enriched preparations as immunogen, following the argument that antibody directed against gametes might effectively block transmission when taken up by the vector with the infective blood meal, by combining with the nascent gametes and preventing fertilisation. This has been substantiated in *P. gallinaceum* (GWADZ 1976), *P. yoelii* (MENDIS and TAR-

GETT 1979), and *P. knowlesi* (GWADZ et al. 1979). In the latter two cases, the vaccinated hosts, when challenged (so that mosquitoes might feed on them), were found to be largely protected against asexual parasitaemia. This may have resulted from the contamination of vaccines with asexual parasites or may suggest some similarity of antigen; if there are common antigens then the lack of antigamete activity in the sera of exposed populations, or of either sporozoite or blood-stage parasite-vaccinated hosts (GWADZ et al. 1979) is surprising.

Of a panel of monoclonal antibodies raised against *P. gallinaceum* gametes, two specific types were found to act synergistically in blocking transmission by preventing proper microgamete exflagellation through agglutination. Neither antibody was effective when used alone (RENER et al. 1980).

## V. Immune Response to Asexual Erythrocytic Parasites

The pathology of malaria in mammals is a consequence of the cyclical proliferation of asexual erythrocytic parasites, and the immune responses they engender have, quite properly, attracted considerable attention. It follows that the present work can be no more than a synopsis of the immense literature that has resulted.

### 1. Recognition of Infected Cells

For most of its development a parasite within a red cell may be insulated from direct effects of antibody because of the impermeability to antibody of the intact red-cell membrane, but the parasites' activities lead to the appearance of antigens on the external membrane of the red cell, sometimes associated with observable anatomical structures. Thus excrescences on the surface of the *P. falciparum*-infected cell which function as anchorage points to associate the infected cell with the vascular endothelium during the sequestered phase of schizogony (AIKAWA and STERLING 1974) are stainable for electron microscopy by immunoferritin techniques with specific antibody (KILEJIAN et al. 1977). Caveolae (corresponding to Schüffners dots in vivax-type parasites) are sites of antigen deposition or introduction at the red-cell surface (AIKAWA et al. 1975).

Very late in merogony the integrity of the rhesus red-cell membrane is breached in a small proportion of *P. knowlesi* schizont-infected cells (as judged by permeability to ferritin), allowing the display of antigens of the parasitophorous vacuolar membrane. As rupture and merozoite release would normally follow rapidly, this may be immaterial (L. H. BANNISTER 1981, personal communication).

Since the permeability of the infected cell for a number of molecules is known to be altered (e.g. glucose into *P. berghei*-infected cells; HOMEWOOD and NEAME 1974) it has been suggested (HOLZ et al. 1977) that lipid is synthesised by the parasite and transported to the host-cell membrane to effect these alterations. Other components, more immunogenic than lipid, may also be incorporated to modify the infected cell's relationship with plasma nutrients. Isolation of infected cells' plasmalemmae for antigenic analysis is difficult; nitrogen cavitation disruption of *P. knowlesi*-infected rhesus cells yields membrane preparations with at least three components precipitable by immune sera which cannot be found in uninfected rhesus cells or isolated schizonts (SCHMIDT-ULLRICH et al. 1979). If, in the same host-parasite system, intact schizont-infected cells are radio-iodinated with lactoperoxidase as catalyst, then four precipitable antigens are labelled, out of six antigens found when bulk membrane is prepared from infected cells by passage through a Stanstead cell disruptor. These four may be taken as being available on the exterior of the intact schizont-infected red cell (DEANS and COHEN 1979). It is noteworthy that similar radio-iodination techniques applied to red cells from *P. berghei*-infected mice indicate that four novel components arise on the surface of uninfected cells as well as infected cells in the circulation (HOWARD et al. 1980a), and that comparable changes induced on the surface of normal and parasitised cells of *P. yoelii*-infected mice vary according to the duration of parasitaemia (HOWARD et al. 1980b).

## 2. Effector Mechanisms Directed Against Infected Cells

The antigenicity of infected cells is shown by their agglutination, opsonisation, and possible sensitisation for destruction by antibody-dependent lymphocytes, when exposed to antibody of appropriate specificity, and by their recognition and probable direct killing by splenic immunocytes.

For *P. knowlesi* infections in rhesus monkeys, the antigens involved in both agglutination and opsonisation are variant specific (see Antigenic Variation, Sect. C.VI.2, below). Thus antibody in serum taken early in a (drug-controlled) infection will, in vitro, both agglutinate and opsonise for macrophage engulfment parasites of the same stabilate as that used to infect the monkey, but will be relatively inactive against a population of parasites isolated later on in the monkey's infection (BROWN and HILLS 1974). The dynamics of the two antibodies (agglutinin and opsonin) vary somewhat as different specificities or subclasses are involved. The biological importance to the host of the agglutinin response is obscure but, in vivo, opsonisation is undoubtedly an important component of the protective immune response as judged, for instance, by the histology of the spleen. Specific phagocytic activity is not confined to macrophages; TOSTA and WEDDERBURN (1980) showed that mouse erythrocytes parasitised by *P. yoelii* were opsonised for eosinophils (taken from normal mice) by serum from *P. yoelii*-recovered mice. Avian as well as mammalian malarias promote opsonins (CANNON and TALIAFERRO 1931; ZUCKERMAN 1945).

Evidence is relatively sparse for the intraerythrocytic killing of parasites by immunocytes dependent for their targeting on specific antibody (antibody-dependent cellular cytotoxicity: ADCC) COLEMAN et al. (1975) labelled *P. berghei*-infected cells with $^{51}Cr$ and incubated with immune or normal spleen cells and immune or normal mouse serum for 18 h. Whilst higher $^{51}Cr$ counts were obtained in immune preparations than normal (taken to indicate immune lytic release of label) all supernatants were rich in chromate. This form of experiment is difficult to interpret because of the ultimate release of $^{51}Cr$ on schizont rupture, the association of label with red cell rather than parasite, and the "discomfiture" of parasites in cultures heavily laden with effector cells. BROWN and SMALLEY (1980) employed the multiplication rates of *P. falciparum* cultured over 2 days to assess the ADCC due to peripheral blood lymphocytes and sera from acutely, chronically or non-infected individuals. The only killing demonstrated was antibody dependent and, in general, required a high lymphocyte : parasite ratio (50:1). At low ratios, growth-promoting effects were noted.

An assay system using parasite multiplication rates over 24 h was employed by LANGHORNE et al. (1978) to examine immune cells capable of killing *P. knowlesi* in the absence of antibody. Parasite multiplication was depressed by immune spleen cells from vaccinated rhesus or chronically infected kra monkeys but not by normal peripheral blood or spleen mononuclear cells. Cells separable by erythrocyte rosetting and lacking surface immunoglobulin were most active. The mode of action remains unknown.

### 3. The Immunological Relationships of the Extracellular Merozoite

The free erythrocytic merozoite is an important target for protective antibody. The clinical immunity of rhesus monkeys suffering repeated infections of *P. knowlesi* correlates quite well with the ability of their serum to inhibit red cell invasion in vitro (BUTCHER and COHEN 1972). Test cultures initiated with trophozoites and maintained through a single asexual cycle employ two parameters to measure inhibitory antibody: the microscopically determined parasite multiplication rate and the incorporation of a radio-labelled amino acid into parasite protein. The latter allows an assessment of parasite growth which is unaffected by the agglutination of parasitised cells in some immune sera; such agglutination vitiates microscopic counts. The system has demonstrated the complement independence, classes (IgG, IgM) and species specificity of antibody involved, and the activity of $F(ab^1)_2$ fragments (COHEN et al. 1969).

The very synchronous and rapid development of *P. knowlesi* lent itself to demonstrating the free merozoite as target; for *P. falciparum* this is less certain (MITCHELL et al. 1976), but a modified technique has been used in the field for assessing the antibody in exposed populations to a panel of local parasite isolates (WILSON and PHILLIPS 1976).

During merogony the merozoite acquires a surface coat of bifurcated filaments about 20 nm long, covering its surface apart from the apical prominence (BANNISTER et al. 1975). This is retained by the parasite during its brief period in the plasma, and mediates the initial adherence to a red cell (BANNISTER et al. 1977), but is shed as the red cell is invaded (LADDA 1969; BANNISTER et al. 1975). Combination of antibody with the merozoite coat of *P. knowlesi* has been demonstrated by electron microscopy, and the inhibition of invasion related in part to agglutination of merozoites by antibody to their coat material (MILLER et al. 1975); however, agglutination is not a prerequisite of the inhibition of invasion, as shown by film sequences made by BUTCHER and COHEN (1970).

Observations of the cardinal role of the merozoite in protective immunity have led to the development of techniques for merozoite isolation, using agglutinins or lectins (MITCHELL et al. 1973, 1975; DAVID et al. 1978) or cell-sieving techniques (DENNIS et al. 1975) to allow, for instance, antigenic analysis (DEANS and COHEN 1979), and vaccination studies. Merozoite preparations, relatively uncontaminated with other cell types but including some infected cells and debris, have been successfully used to protect rhesus and kra monkeys against *P. knowlesi* (MITCHELL 1977; MITCHELL et al. 1979), and owl (douroucouli) monkeys (*Aotus trivirgatus*) against *P. falciparum* (MITCHELL et al. 1977). Preparations of late merogonic stages freed from schizonts by saponin lysis and partially purified on sucrose gradients (SIDDIQUI et al. 1978) have similarly been used to vaccinate owl-monkeys (SIDDIQUI

1977). In contrast to sporozoite vaccination, merozoite vaccination requires potent immunological adjuvants (see Sect. D, below).

It is noteworthy that merozoite inhibitory antibody, whilst frequently engendered by merozoite vaccination, may be insufficient to explain the clinical immunity observed in vaccinated rhesus monkeys, (BUTCHER et al. 1978). However, of a panel of monoclonal antibodies produced by hybridomas formed on the fusion of spleen cells from recovered *P. yoelii*-infected mice with myeloma cells, only those antibodies found uniquely reactive with free merozoites in a fluorescent antibody test were effective in passively conferring protection against *P. yoelii* challenge (FREEMAN et al. 1980). This result seems to confirm the importance of antimerozoite antibody, and potentially such monoclonal antibodies may be used to isolate the functionally important antigens of the merozoite.

### 4. Further Antigens Associated with Erythrocytic Parasites

Many antigens other than those discussed above may be recognised by reaction with sera from appropriately sensitised hosts.

Antigens of *P. falciparum,* prepared by Hughes press disruption of infected cells, have been fractionated and categorised by temperature sensitivity by WILSON et al. (1973). Of the five classes recognised, only S antigens are commonly found free in the plasma of malarious Africans, and these are also detected in supernatants of cultured *P. falciparum* taken at (but not before) the time of schizont rupture (WILSON and BARTHOLOMEW 1975). Following cultivation of *P. knowlesi* in medium containing [$^3$H]isoleucine, antibody precipitable labelled material is released during schizont rupture and merozoite reinvasion. A third of this material is antigenically distinct from known membrane or cytoplasmic determinants (MCCOLM and TRIGG 1980).

Plasma from infected hosts has been used as an antigen source in the vaccination of chickens against *P. gallinaceum,* with some success (TODOROVIC et al. 1967), but is less effective in protecting rhesus monkeys against *P. knowlesi* (COLLINS et al. 1977).

Partial analyses of the antigenic material obtained from lysed or disrupted infected red cells have been performed for many species (see ZUCKERMAN and RISTIC 1968). For *P. knowlesi* it has been possible to identify a sequential development of parasite antigens by analysing lysates of infected cells from synchronous infections by crossed immunoelectrophoresis. Of the eleven antigens recognised, nine were stage independent, ring parasites lacked two and only segmented schizonts and free merozoites possessed one (DEANS et al. 1978). The pooled sera used to define these antigens were drawn from monkeys which had been vaccinated with merozoite preparations in Freund's complete adjuvant and then challenged with viable parasites; sera from animals repeatedly infected and cured, or suffering chronic drug suppressed infection, evince little or no precipitating antibody against these antigens.

PERRIN et al. (1981 a) have used sera from individuals in endemic areas and from patients suffering their first exposure to *P. falciparum* to examine antigen produced from lysed, synchronously culture-grown, radio-labelled parasites of this species. Stage-specific antigens were identified, of 115, 137, and 200 kilodaltons molecular weight, restricted to schizonts. These were not recognised by the single-exposure sera, but the stage-independent antigens were.

Crude antigen preparations of disrupted, lysed or attenuated infected red cells have been extensively used as vaccinating material. These have been reviewed by BROWN (1969) and COHEN and MITCHELL (1980), and very usefully tabulated by DESOWITZ and MILLER (1980). Physicochemical characterisation of the antigens involved has been limited. For instance, the elution characteristics from molecular sieve chromatography of a protective fraction of disrupted *P. knowlesi* were reported by SIMPSON et al. (1974). One antigen, derived from the unique inclusion bodies of *P. lophurae*, notable on light microscopy, has been more thoroughly investigated and proves to be a protein consisting of 73% histidine and with a calculated molecular weight of 37.5 kilodaltons (KILEJIAN 1974, 1978). This material is protective in ducklings, but they are rather unsuitable for vaccination studies because of the brief period between the onset of immunocompetence towards vaccination and the occurrence of natural age-immunity to the parasite. As it was considered that the antigen also occurred in *P. lophurae* merozoite rhoptry material, similar protein was sought in *P. falciparum* from merozoite-enriched preparations (KILEJIAN and OLSEN 1979).

Clearly the advent of hybridoma technology and burgeoning availability of monoclonal antibodies will rapidly advance the functional and chemical analysis of malaria antigens. Antigenic determinants may be located by fluorescence or immunoelectron microscopy, the biological effects of their combination with antibody assessed in vivo or in vitro and their retrieval from crude lysates by immunoaffinity chromatography achieved, for subsequent analysis, with uniquely reacting antibody. Initial experiments to these ends have been reported for *P. falciparum* blood stages (PERRIN et al. 1981 b), the sporozoites of *P. berghei* (YOSHIDA et al. 1980), and gametes of *P. gallinaceum* (RENER et al. 1980), as mentioned above.

## VI. Evasion of the Immune Response

### 1. Immunodepression

The chronicity of malaria infection in many instances implies that the parasites either avoid stimulating parasiticidal mechanisms or that they evade the consequences of such stimulation. Much of the foregoing emphasises that the former proposition is largely untenable. However, although some non-specific but potentially parasiticidal macrophage mechanisms such as phagocytosis are excited by malaria, other more specialised macrophage functions such as antigen presentation may be deranged by the disease (LOOSE et al. 1972). Furthermore, a lymphocyte mitogen has been identified (GREENWOOD and VICK 1975) which may interfere with specific responsiveness.

Sporozoite vaccination of mice is less effective than usual if instituted 4 days after a blood-induced *P. berghei* infection, and the immune response to vaccination is even more severely curtailed in mice vaccinated 7 days after infection. None of these animals mounts a secondary antibody response on reinoculation with sporozoites (ORJIH and NUSSENZWEIG 1979). Thus the immunodepression associated with malaria may encompass the response to the parasites themselves. Immunodepression in malaria has been reviewed by WEDDERBURN (1974) and GREENWOOD (1974).

Immunodepression notwithstanding, the evasion of the immune response remains an important facet of the biology of malaria parasites.

## 2. Antigenic Variation

Many protozoa possess the ability to vary antigens in such a way as to abrogate the effectiveness of previously stimulated antibody. This antigenic variation has been demonstrated in several *Plasmodium* species: *P. berghei* (BRIGGS and WELLDE 1969) following an earlier observation of COX (1959), *P. cynomolgi* (VOLLER and ROSSAN, 1969), and, with the greatest clarity, by BROWN and his colleagues in *P. knowlesi* (BROWN and BROWN 1965; BROWN and HILLS 1974; review by BROWN 1974). Whilst relatively cumbersome protection tests are at present required for the demonstration of antigenic variation in the other species, the agglutination of schizont-infected cells [used as a defining system – SICA test (BROWN and BROWN 1965)], in vitro opsonisation and merozoite inhibition may all be used to demonstrate antigenic variation in *P. knowlesi*.

It is clear in this species that each peak of parasitaemia in a chronically relapsing infection is associated with a parasite population serologically distinguishable from all preceding and subsequent populations. Two mechanisms of antigenic variation might be hypothesised, selection or induction. From the dynamics of a chronic relapsing infection, the two could not be distinguished. However, BROWN (1973) sensitised rhesus monkeys with *P. knowlesi* antigen in Freund's incomplete adjuvant, so producing a high agglutinin titre to the variant employed, but no protective response. On challenge with an accurately known small number of parasites of the sensitising variant, the sensitised monkey suffered an infection with essentially identical parasite multiplication to that in a naive control. The emergent parasite population in the sensitised monkey was of a different variant. It may be concluded that the new variant serotype was induced. Selection would have inevitably resulted in a delay in the dynamics of the infection whilst the selected minority population expanded after the loss of the major original population. Furthermore, BROWN (1973) suggested that the agglutinin was itself responsible for inducing variation in the parasites. Unfortunately attempts to induce variation in vitro with similar sera, rich in agglutinin but without detectable inhibitory effect, have been inconclusive (G. A. BUTCHER 1979, personal communication).

For laboratory strains of parasites, generally maintained by blood passage, the repertoires of variant antigens may be different from strain to strain (this appears to be true for *P. knowlesi* as judged by the paucity of cross-reactive schizont agglutinins; MITCHELL and BUTCHER, unpublished data), but sufficiently severe exposure to antigens of one strain (e.g. by merozoite vaccination and repeated challenge) will engender protection which transcends strains as well as intrastrain variants (MITCHELL et al. 1975). Similarly, repeated challenge of rhesus monkeys with defined variants of *P. knowlesi* induces clinical immunity and cross-reacting merozoite inhibitory antibody to variants of which the host has no experience, as judged by the absence of agglutinin to such variants at the time of challenge (BUTCHER and COHEN 1972).

*P. berghei* in rats typically results in chronic subpatent infection which follows the inital acute parasitaemia. Serum drawn when the subpatent infection is eventually sterilised is more effective in the passive transfer of protection than serum taken at any other time (PHILLIPS and JONES 1972). This may relate to the possession of antibody against most or all of the variants that the line of parasites is able to express.

The possibilities for the alteration of antigens by vector transmitted parasites (i.e. following exchange of genetic information on gamete fusion) remain to be studied, but merozoite antigen of one variant type has been successfully used to vaccinate against sporozoite challenge with a second strain of *P. knowlesi* (RICHARDS et al. 1977).

## VII. The Anatomical and Cellular Bases of Immunity to Malaria

The spleen is central to malaria immunity. Congenitally asplenic or splenectomised animals frequently suffer fatal infection when challenged with parasites that are more mildly pathogenic in intact animals [for instance, *P. yoelii* (17X non-lethal) or *P. chabaudi* in mice (OSTER et al. 1980)], and the passive transfer of immune serum is largely ineffective in protecting splenectomised rats against challenge with *P. berghei* (BROWN and PHILLIPS 1974). Similarly, splenectomy during the resolution of acute *P. berghei* in rats leads to relapse and death (QUINN and WYLER 1980), and unfractionated spleen cells from immunised rats are effective in the adoptive transfer of immunity to *P. berghei* (BROWN et al. 1976). In the case of the lethal and resolving lines of *P. yoelii* the rapidity of the splenic T-cell response to malaria antigen correlates with the outcome of infection (WEINBAUM et al. 1978). Interestingly, chronic *P. inui* infection is resolved by rhesus monkeys following splenectomy (WYLER et al. 1977), probably through the loss of a suppressor T-cell source. The spleen is not required for the induction or expression of immunity to sporozoites in the mouse (SPITALNY et al. 1976), and may be rivalled in importance by the liver in effecting immunity to blood stage *P. yoelii* in this host, since lymphocytes preferentially home there and Küpffer cells become activated (DOCKRELL et al. 1980).

This primacy of the spleen is to be expected in an organ in which both multiple affector and effector limbs of the immune response are sited. More subtle manipulations of the immune system than splenectomy are needed to dissect the requirements for a protective response. Similarly, neonatal thymectomy or congenital athymia derange both cellular and humoral functions, while adoptive T-cell transfer potentially augments both groups of functions.

In the light of this, B-cell deletion has been evaluated in several systems. For instance, RANK and WEIDANZ (1976) demonstrated that bursectomised chickens, if protected with drug during an initial parasitaemia of *P. gallinaceum*, were able to resist subsequent rechallenge with this malaria apparently independently of antibody-secreting cells. Mice made B-cell deficient by continual injection of anti $\mu$ chain antiserum nevertheless control and eradicate *P. chabaudi* infection and will subsequently resist *P. vinckei* (but die from *P. berghei* or the normally avirulent *P. yoelii*) (GRUN and WEIDANZ 1981). This contrasts with the response of similarly treated mice to *P. yoelii* (ROBERTS and WEIDANZ 1979). In this case, as in that of *P. gallinaceum*, initial control of parasitaemia is dependent on an effective B-cell population but, after a cure of initial infection, anti-$\mu$-treated mice control a challenge but suffer a prolonged patent infection.

It is to be expected in the complex of responses of each different host species to each different malaria that there may be some redundancy of effector mechanisms, allowing deletion of one mechanism without vitiating the whole, but it would be premature to conclude from these results that antibody is generally insignificant in controlling relapsing parasitaemia. Moreover, the loss of helper function in antibody production may be the most deleterious effect of athymia in the context of the response to malaria infection, since hyperimmune serum without T-cell transfer protects nude mice from death on infection with *P. yoelii* (ROBERTS et al. 1977). Against this may be set the finding of PLAYFAIR et al. (1977a) that, in *P. yoelii* vaccination, those vaccine doses which maximally primed helper T cells, were not protective, leading these authors to demonstrate the classical, delayed type hypersensitivity (DTH) T-cell response in this system (COTTRELL et al. 1978). DTH responses are also known from primate malaria vaccination (PHILLIPS et al. 1970; CABRERA et al. 1976).

EUGUI and ALLISON (1979) related the susceptibility of mouse strains to *P. chabaudi* (and the subsequent ability to control *P. yoelii*) to the levels of the natural killer (NK) cell activity possessed by the strain. Thus A mice (low NK activity) succumb to *P. chabaudi*, Balb/C, and B10A mice (intermediate NK activity) recover from *P. chabaudi* malaria but are not protected by such exposure against later *P. yoelii*, but C57BL and CBA mice (high NK activity) are protected against *P. yoelii* after recovery from *P. chabaudi*. They further suggested that a product of NK cells/macrophages killed parasites within circulating erythrocytes. There is other evidence of such intracellular damage to parasites, and disorganised or pyknotic ("crisis" form) parasites are often found in animals clearing a peak of parasitaemia. The effector mechanism(s) may be entirely non-specific with regard to parasite species; for instance, *P. knowlesi*-vaccinated rhesus remain susceptible to *P. fragile*, *P. cynomolgi*, and *P. coatneyi* but if, during one of these infections, they are challenged with and clear an infection of *P. knowlesi*, then damaged parasites of the other species are found, but the non-*P. knowlesi* infection, although temporarily depressed, is not cleared (MITCHELL 1977; BUTCHER et al. 1978). (See also Sect. D.I, below).

## D. Immunostimulants and Immunological Adjuvants in the Induction of Immune Responses to Malaria

Many of the antigen preparations used in experimental malaria vaccines require the addition of potent immunological adjuvants before they promote effective responses. This is not the case with attenuated sporozoites, nor with radiation-attenuated blood parasites, but is a notable feature of primate immunisation with dead or fractionated malaria antigen. It remains to be seen if the adjuvant requirements of isolated pure antigens (for instance, prepared by affinity chromatography with monoclonal antibodies) will be as severe as those of the heterogeneous preparations usually employed up to the time of writing. It is noteworthy that the histidine-rich protein antigen of *P. lophurae* (see Sect. C.V.4, above) is effective in ducks without adjuvant (KILEJIAN 1978).

Adjuvants are poorly understood in general, but characteristics that may be important are depot effects, recruitment of immunocompetent cell populations, direct interaction with cells involved in antigen processing and presentation, and the inhibition of feedback mechanisms or suppressor cells. WHITE (1976) usefully reviewed the adjuvant properties of microbial products. BOMFORD (1980a, b) has attempted to discriminate between the effectiveness in stimulating humoral or cell-mediated immune responses of a number of the principal adjuvants (Freund's, alhydrogel, *Corynebacterium parvum, Bordetella pertussis,* muramyl dipeptide, and saponin) which have, elsewhere, been employed in malaria vaccines.

## I. Differentiation Between Non-Specific Immunostimulant and Adjuvant Effects

Immunostimulants generate activity in cells of the immune system which is not specifically directed against the stimulating agent, but which may result in aggression towards foreign cells, or microbe-infected or other altered autochthonous cells (e.g. tumour cells). Immunological adjuvants modulate the specific responses directed against the immunogens they accompany. As might be expected, a number of substances exert both immunostimulant and adjuvant effects.

In the absence of malaria antigen, non-specific immunostimulants may induce responses protective against subsequent malaria challenge, but not specific for malaria. Such immunostimulants may not necessarily be effective adjuvants in malaria vaccine systems. For example, 1.4 mg of *C. parvum* suspension given i.p. to a mouse 3 h before challenge with *P. yoelii* is notably effective in depressing the consequent parasitaemia for several days, but by day 7 parasitaemias have risen to about 50% of those found in controls (COTTRELL et al. 1977). When similar doses were given to mice as adjuvant with a *P. yoelii* vaccine 3 weeks before challenge, the mice so treated were no better protected than were mice which had received antigen alone (parasite clearance in 10 days) (PLAYFAIR et al. 1977b). An apparent adjuvant effect of *C. parvum* was found in one of two kra monkeys receiving *P. knowlesi* merozoite vaccine (MITCHELL et al. 1979). However, *C. parvum* is very active as an adjuvant in some other systems, e.g. for ovalbumin in the delayed type hypersensitivity response of the mouse (BOMFORD 1980a) and, as judged by plaque-forming cell response in vitro, for antibody to sheep red cells (SLJIVIC and WATSON 1977). Since *C. parvum* activates macrophages (BOMFORD and CHRISTIE 1975), its non-specific effect against malaria, which is demonstrable in athymic as well as normal mice (CLARK 1976; cited by COTTRELL et al. 1977), is ascribed to a soluble macrophage secretion factor which kills parasites within red cells (CLARK et al. 1977).

Broadly similar, non-specific stimulation is induced by *Mycobacterium* spp. and *Bordetella pertussis,* and the former may be very active in stimulating a response capable of killing intracellular parasites (for instance, the activity of the attenuated mycobacterium bacille Calmette-Guerin, BCG, given i.v. to mice, demonstrated by CLARK et al. 1977). Mycobacteria are incorporated with a light mineral oil and emulsifier to form Freund's complete adjuvant (FCA); Freund's incomplete adjuvant (FIA) lacks the bacteria. The evidence from a number of malaria vaccination reports employing adjuvant-alone controls (e.g. RIECKMANN et al.

1979; SIDDIQUI 1977) is that mycobacteria given as FCA have no discernible effect on the course of a challenge parasitaemia. This may be a temporal relationship; challenge would normally be more than 2 weeks after adjuvant administration, by which time non-specific effects may have waned. The potentiation of specific responses to malaria antigen by FCA is thus a true adjuvant effect.

Of a panel of immunostimulants possessing more precisely defined activity, namely concanavalin A, adenine-uridine polymer (T-cell mitogens), *Escherichia coli* endotoxin lipopolysaccharide B(LPS – a B-cell mitogen), diethyl stilboestrol (DES – a stimulant of the reticuloendothelial system, especially of the liver), none was found to be uniformly effective in non-specifically protecting mice against *P. yoelii* and *P. vinckei* blood-stage challenge (COTTRELL et al. 1977). DES has little effect on subsequent *P. berghei,* whereas LPS, repeatedly administered for many days, does delay a *P. berghei* parasitaemia (MACGREGOR et al. 1969), and *Salmonella typhosa* endotoxin administration reduces the peak parasitaemia of *P. lophurae* in the fowl (BARRETT et al. 1971).

Three immunostimulants known to promote interferon production have been examined in the *P. berghei*-mouse model by JAHIEL et al. (1969): Newcastle disease virus, statolon, and a copolymer of polyriboinosinic and polyribocytidilic acids. Protection was marked when either of the first two agents was given shortly after sporozoite challenge, but none of the agents was effective prior to challenge with blood forms. The parasite within the Küpffer cell or liver parenchyma cell may therefore be affected by interferon.

## II. Mycobacteria and Synthetic Analogues of Their Cell Wall Components as Malaria Vaccine Adjuvants

Freund's complete adjuvant was developed in parallel with malaria vaccination attempts. In 1945 Freund and colleagues reported the use of mycobacteria and lanolin to adjuvate *P. lophurae* vaccine, and in 1947 the same group were using paraffin oil and emulsifier with mycobacteria for preparations from this species and *P. cathemerium* (FREUND et al. 1945; THOMSON et al. 1947). FCA had been applied to primate malaria vaccination by 1948 (FREUND et al. 1948). DESOWITZ and MILLER (1980) have tabulated the malaria vaccines which have employed FCA.

The complete adjuvant is clinically unacceptable. Severe local inflammation occurs at the depot site (especially if the antigen has lipase activity: WORLD HEALTH ORGANIZATION 1976), and is long lasting since the oil is not metabolised. The presence of the mycobacteria induces granulomata.

The replacement of FCA by an acceptable alternative in malaria vaccination and other applications has excited considerable interest. Dissection of the components of the mycobacterial cell wall responsible for immunoadjuvant effects led to the identification, by ELLOUZ et al. (1974), and synthesis, by MERSER et al. (1975), of the smallest active moiety, *N*-acetyl-muramyl-L-alanyl-D-isoglutamine (muramyl dipeptide: MDP), which effectively replaced whole mycobacteria when employed with protein antigen in water-in-oil emulsions. MDP and several related compounds have subsequently been investigated in primate malaria vaccination. REESE et al. (1978) employed saponised schizont antigen from long-term cultured *P. falciparum,* which failed adequately to protect owl monkeys (*Aotus trivirgatus*) when given with FCA, but apparently protected one out of three monkeys when presented with MDP in FIA. The relative failure of the antigen was attributed to the small dose size; equally possible is a loss of functionally important antigens occurring during maintenance of the parasite line for 1 year in vitro.

SIDDIQUI et al. (1979) reported the use of MDP in a groundnut-oil emulsion in the same host-parasite model but using antigen prepared ex vivo. One of three monkeys was protected. Similarly, MITCHELL et al. (1979) found groundnut oil could not reliably replace FIA when used as a carrier for *Mycobacterium butyricum* or for nor-MDP (*N*-acetylglucosamine-3-yl-acetyl-L-alanyl-D-isoglutamine) in merozoite vaccination of rhesus. FIA with nor-MDP was effective in two out of five vaccinated rhesus. A more promising system involved the lipid-soluble 6-0-stearoyl-substituted MDP, presented with liposomes, as adjuvant for a falciparum vaccine. Four out of four owl monkeys were protected from death by this preparation, although high parasitaemias were suffered (SIDDIQUI et al. 1978). However, squirrel monkeys (*Saimiri sciureus*) were not protected after vaccination with a lysed *P. knowlesi* schizont antigen and 6-0-stearoyl MDP-liposome adjuvant, and nor-MDP with aminobutyric acid substituted for alanine (to enhance lipid solubility) was ineffective with liposomes in merozoite vaccination of rhesus against *P. knowlesi* (MITCHELL et al. 1980). Nevertheless lipid-soluble MDP derivatives with liposomes may prove to be effective replacements for FCA.

## III. Non-Bacterial Adjuvants in Malaria Vaccines

Systematic investigation of adjuvants with common antigen preparations has been limited. DESOWITZ (1975) examined ten adjuvants in rats with *P. berghei* vaccine, of which five were fairly effective (including *B. pertussis,* but not FCA, which seems to be of limited use in rodent malaria vaccination). Of the effective non-bacterial adjuvants, two were surfactants (saponin and hexylamine), and the others levamisole (phenylimidothiazole), and polyinosinic-polycytidylic acid. Antigen precipitated with alum or given with vitamin A, *Serratia marcescens* endotoxin, or polyadenylic-polyuredilic acid was ineffective. The adjuvant activities of these preparations are not well enough characterised to allow a rational list of attributes of an effective adjuvant to be compiled, and the animals used were not immunologically mature (SMALLEY 1975). Therefore the efficacy of levamisole, for instance, may have derived from its stimulation of T-cell maturation [see review of levamisole activity by SYMOENS (1980)].

The adjuvant activity of saponin is particularly important, since it is often used in preparing (and may then remain to contaminate) malaria lysate antigens. Whilst "antigen alone" controls are usual in tests of novel adjuvants, a synergistic effect of saponin on the test adjuvant may not be excluded and should be borne in mind in appraising adjuvants used with such antigen. Apart from the work of DESOWITZ (1975), saponin marginally improved the already very effective dead *P. gallinaceum* sporozoite antigens of RICHARDS (1966), and was apparently effective with *P. knowlesi* merozoite vaccine in the kra monkey (MITCHELL et al. 1979). Saponin, a mixture of glycosides extracted from the bark of *Quillaia,* is established as a veterinary adjuvant in foot-and-mouth disease vaccine (with aluminium hydroxide gel), and defined fractions have been under investigation with this antigen (DALSGAARD et al. 1977). Bomford (1980 a, b) examined the adjuvant activity of saponin with soluble antigen (ovalbumin) and membrane-bound antigen (sheep red cells). Saponin was outstandingly the most effective adjuvant tested in promoting the antibody response (haemolysin) to sheep red cells in the mouse, but did not (in common with FCA) promote a cell-mediated (delayed type hypersensitivity – DTH) response in this animal to red cells, although it did promote DTH to ovalbumin.

Siddiqui et al. (1981) have successfully employed a novel synthetic lipoidal amine, *N,N*-dioctadecyl-$N^1$,$N^1$-bis (2-hydroxyethyl) propane diamine (CP-20, 961) as adjuvant with a saponin-freed merogonic stage vaccine of *P. falciparum* in *Aotus*. This adjuvant, developed as an interferon inducer, is known to increase antibody and DTH to sheep red cells in guinea pigs, and to enhance the specific cytotoxicity towards EL-4 tumour cells of spleen cells from mice sensitised using it with EL-4 cells (Niblack et al. 1979). A metabolisable soya bean oil emulsion is employed as carrier, which in mice is cleared from the injection site by 14 days postinoculation. However, macrophages laden with lipid degradation products persist by the regional lymph nodes, in which a pronounced modulation of lymphocyte traffic may be seen (Anderson and Reynolds 1979). Siddiqui et al. (1981) noted structural analogies between CP-20,961 and 6-0-stearoyl MDP, which similarly adjuvates this vaccine, as noted in Sect. D.II, above.

In extrapolating from success in vaccinating owl monkeys with *P. falciparum* to vaccinating man, it should be borne in mind that this monkey is more readily protected by drug-cured infection than is man [see, for instance, Voller et al. (1973) and Voller and Richards (1970)] and, moreover, routinely survives parasitaemias of 10% or more, an order of magnitude more intense than the levels that are clinically disturbing in man. Equally, another favoured primate model, *P. knowlesi* in *Macaca mulatta*, may represent a more demanding vaccination model than man and his malarias. Whilst the owl monkey is the only satisfactory experimental simian host for falciparum malaria, and its successful immunisation by any antigen-adjuvant vaccine combination intended for subsequent human trial would be imperative, the efficacy of the putative adjuvant with a *P. knowlesi* vaccine in the rhesus might also be considered a very worthwhile indicator of likely success in man.

## References

Aikawa M, Sterling CR (1974) Intracellular parasitic protozoa. Academic, New York

Aikawa M, Miller LH, Rabbege J (1975) Caveola-vesicle complexes in the plasmalemma of erythrocytes infected by *Plasmodium vivax* and *P. cynomolgi*. Unique structures related to Schüffner's dots. Am J Path 79:285–300

Aikawa M, Cochrane AH, Nussenzweig RS, Rabbege J (1979) Freeze-fracture study of malaria sporozoites: antibody-induced changes of the pellicular membrane. J Protozool 26:273–279

Anderson AO, Reynolds JA (1979) Adjuvant effects of the lipid amine CP-20, 961. J Retic Soc 26:667–680

Bafort JM, Pryor WH, Beaudoin RL (1978) Malaria vaccine: the effect of sporozoite induced immunity on exo-erythrocytic stages. Ann Soc Belge Med Trop 58:63–64

Bannister LH, Butcher GA, Dennis ED, Mitchell GH (1975) Structure and invasive behavior of *Plasmodium knowlesi* merozoites in vitro. Parasitology 71:483–491

Bannister LH, Butcher GA, Mitchell GH (1977) Recent advances in understanding the invasion of erythrocytes by merozoites of *Plasmodium knowlesi*. Bull WHO 55:163–169

Barret JT, Rigney MM, Breitenbach RP (1971) The influence of endotoxin on the response of chickens to *Plasmodium lophurae* malaria. Avian Dis 15:7–13

Bomford R (1980 a) The comparative selectivity of adjuvants for humoral and cell-mediated immunity I: effect on the antibody response to bovine serum albumin and sheep red blood cells of Freund's incomplete and complete adjuvants, alhydrogel, *Corynebacterium parvum, Bordetella pertussis,* muramyl dipeptide, and saponin. Clin Exp Immunol 39:426–434

Bomford R (1980 b) The comparative selectivity of adjuvants for humoral and cell-mediated immunity II: effect on delayed type hypersensitivity in the mouse and guinea pig, and cell mediated immunity in the mouse of Freund's incomplete and complete adjuvants, alhydrogel, *Corynebacterium parvum, Bordetella pertussis,* muramyl dipeptide, and saponin. Clin Exp Immunol 39:435–441

Bomford R, Christie GH (1975) Mechanisms of macrophage activation by *Corynebacterium parvum* II: in vivo experiments. Cell Immunol 17:150–155

Bray RS (1976) Vaccination against *Plasmodium falciparum:* a negative result. Trans R Soc Trop Med Hyg 70:258

Briggs NT, Wellde BT (1969) Some characteristics of *Plasmodium berghei* relapsing in immunised mice. Milit Med 134:1243–1248

Brown IN (1969) Immunological aspects of malaria infection. Adv Immunol 11:267–349

Brown IN, Phillips RS (1974) Immunity to *Plasmodium berghei* in rats: passive serum transfer and the role of the spleen. Infect Immun 10:1213–1218

Brown J, Smalley ME (1980) Specific antibody dependent cellular cytotoxicity in human malaria. Clin Exp Immunol 41:423–429

Brown KN (1973) Antibody induced variation in malaria parasites. Nature 242:49–50

Brown KN (1974) Antigenic variation in malaria. In: Porter R, Knight J (eds) Parasites in the immunised host: mechanisms of survival. Ciba Foundation Symposium 25 new series. Elsevier, North-Holland, Amsterdam, pp 35–46

Brown KN (1976) Resistance to malaria. In: Cohen S, Sadun EH (eds) Immunology of parasitic infections. Blackwell, Oxford, pp 268–295

Brown KN, Brown IN (1965) Immunity to malaria: antigenic variation in chronic infections of *Plasmodium knowlesi.* Nature 208:1286–1288

Brown KN, Hills LA (1974) Antigenic variation and immunity to *Plasmodium knowlesi:* antibodies which induce antigenic variation and antibodies which destroy parasites. Trans R Soc Trop Med Hyg 68:139–142

Brown KN, Hills LA, Jarra W (1976) Preliminary studies of artificial immunisation of rats against *Plasmodium berghei* and adoptive transfer of this immunity by splenic T and T+B cells. Bull WHO 54:149–154

Bruce-Chwatt LJ (1963) Congenital transmission of immunity to malaria. In: Garnham PCC, Pierce AE, Roitt I (eds) Immunity to protozoa. Blackwell, Oxford, p 89

Bruce-Chwatt LJ, Glanville VJ (1973) (eds) Dynamics of tropical disease. A selection of papers of the late George Macdonald. Oxford University Press, London

Butcher GA (1974) Immunological aspects of malaria. Guy's Hosp Rep 123:247–270

Butcher GA, Cohen S (1970) Schizogony of *Plasmodium knowlesi* in the presence of normal and immune serum (Abstract). Trans R Soc Trop Med Hyg 64:470

Butcher GA, Cohen S (1972) Antigenic variation and protective immunity in *Plasmodium knowlesi* malaria. Immunology 23:503–521

Butcher GA, Mitchell GH, Cohen S (1973) Mechanism of host specificity in malarial infection. Nature 244:40–42

Butcher GA, Mitchell GH, Cohen S (1978) Antibody mediated mechanisms of immunity to malaria induced by vaccination with *Plasmodium knowlesi* merozoites. Immunology 34:77–86

Cabrera EJ, Speer CA, Schenkel RH, Barr ML, Silverman PH (1976) Delayed dermal hypersensitivity in rhesus monkeys (*Macaca mulatta*) immunised against *Plasmodium knowlesi.* Z Parasitenkd 50:31–42

Cannon PR, Taliaferro WH (1931) Acquired immunity in avian malaria III. Cellular reactions in infection and superinfection. J Prevent Med 5:37

Cepellini R (1973) Specific immune response genes and defence against malaria (abstract) 9th Int Cong Trop Med Malaria, Athens 1:267
Clark IA (1976) Immunity to intra-erythrocyte protozoa in mice with specific reference to *Babesia* spp. PhD Thesis, University of London
Clark IA, Cox FEG, Allison AC (1977) Protection of mice against *Babesia* spp and *Plasmodium* spp with killed *Corynebacterium parvum*. Parasitology 74:9–18
Clyde DF (1975) Immunisation of man against falciparum and vivax malaria by use of attenuated sporozoites. Am J Trop Med Hyg 24:397–401
Cochrane AH, Aikawa M, Jeng M, Nussenzweig RS (1976) Antibody induced ultrastructural changes of malarial sporozoites. J Immunol 116:859–867
Coggeshall LT (1943) Immunity in malaria. Medicine (Baltimore) 22:87–102
Cohen S (1976a) Survival of parasites in the immunised host. In: Cohen S, Sadun EH (eds) Immunology of parasitic infections. Blackwell, Oxford, pp 35–46
Cohen S (1976b) Immune effector mechanisms. In: Cohen S, Sadun EH (eds) Immunology of parasitic infections. Blackwell, Oxford, pp 18–34
Cohen S (1979) Immunity to malaria. Proc R Soc Lond B 203:323–345
Cohen S, McGregor IA (1963) Gamma globulin and acquired immunity to malaria. In: Garnham PCC, Pierce AE, Roitt I (eds) Immunity to protozoa. Blackwell, Oxford, pp 123–159
Cohen S, Mitchell GH (1980) Prospects for immunisation against malaria. Curr Top Microbiol Immunol 80:97–137
Cohen S, McGregor IA, Carrington SC (1961) Gamma globulin and acquired immunity to human malaria. Nature 192:733–737
Cohen S, Butcher GA, Crandall RB (1969) Action of malarial antibody in vitro. Nature 223:368–371
Cohen S, Butcher GA, Mitchell GH, Deans JA, Langhorne J (1977) Acquired immunity and vaccination in malaria. Am J Trop Med Hyg 26:223–229
Coleman RM, Rencricca NJ, Stout JP, Brisette WH, Smith DM (1975) Splenic mediated erythrocyte cytotoxicity in malaria. Immunology 29:49–54
Collins WE, Contacos PG, Harrison AJ, Starfill PS, Skinner JC (1977) Attempts to immunise monkeys against *Plasmodium knowlesi* by using heat-stable serum-soluble antigens. Am J Trop Med Hyg 26:373–376
Cottrell BJ, Playfair JHL, de Sousa B (1977) *Plasmodium yoelii* and *Plasmodium vinckei:* the effects of non-specific immunostimulation on murine malaria. Exp Parasitol 43:45–53
Cottrell BJ, Playfair JHL, de Sousa B (1978) Cell mediated immunity in mice vaccinated against malaria. Clin Exp Immunol 34:147–158
Cox FEG (1970) Protective immunity between malaria parasites and piroplasms in mice. Bull WHO 43:325–336
Cox HW (1959) A study of relapse *Plasmodium berghei* infection isolated from white mice. J Immunol 82:209–214
Dalsgaard K, Jensen MH, Sorensen KJ (1977) Saponin adjuvants IV: evaluation of the adjuvant Quil A in the vaccination of cattle against foot and mouth disease. Acta Vet Scand 18:349–360
Danforth HD, Orjih AU, Nussenzweig RS (1978) Immunofluorescent staining of exoerythrocytic schizonts of *Plasmodium berghei* with stage specific immune serum. J Parasitol 64:1123–1125
Danforth HD, Aikawa M, Cochrane AH, Nussenzweig RS (1980) Sporozoites of mammalian malaria: attachment to, interiorization, and fate within macrophages. J Protozool 27:193–202
David PH, Hommel M, Benichou J-C, Eisen HA, Pereira de Silva LH (1978) Isolation of malaria merozoites: relase of *Plasmodium chabaudi* merozoites from schizonts bound to immobilised concanavilin A. Proc Nat Acad Sci USA 75:5081–5084
Deans JA, Cohen S (1979) Localisation and chemical characterisation of *Plasmodium knowlesi* schizont antigens. Bull WHO [Suppl] 57:93–100
Deans JA, Dennis ED, Cohen S (1978) Antigenic analysis of sequential erythrocytic stage of *Plasmodium knowlesi:* Parasitology 77:333–344

Dennis ED, Mitchell GH, Butcher GA, Cohen S (1975) *In vitro* isolation of *Plasmodium knowlesi* merozoites using polycarbonate sieves. Parasitology 71:475–481
Desowitz RS (1975) *Plasmodium berghei:* immunogenic enhancement of antigen by adjuvant addition. Exp Parasitol 38:6–13
Desowitz RS, Miller LH (1980) A perspective on malaria vaccines. Bull WHO 58:897–908
Dockrell HM, de Souza JB, Playfair JHL (1980) The role of the liver in immunity to blood stage murine malaria. Immunology 41:421–430
Edozien JC, Gilles HM, Udeozo IOK (1962) Adult and cord blood gamma globulin and immunity to malaria in Nigerians. Lancet II:951
Ellouz F, Adam A, Ciorbarn R, Lederer E (1974) Minimal structural requirements for adjuvant activity of bacterial peptidoglycan derivatives. Biochem Biophys Res Comm 59:1317–1325
Eugui EM, Allison AC (1979) Malaria infections in different strains of mice and their correlation with natural killer activity. Bull WHO [Suppl] 57:231–238
Facer CA, Bray RS, Brown J (1978) Direct Coombs antiglobulin reactions in Gambian children with *Plasmodium falciparum* malaria. Clin Exp Immunol 35:119–127
Foley DA, Vanderberg JP (1977) *Plasmodium berghei:* transmission by intraperitoneal inoculation of immature exoerythrocytic schizonts from rats into rats, mice, and hamsters. Exp Parasitol 43:69–81
Fooden J (1964) Rhesus and crab-eating macaques: intergraduation in Thailand. Science 143:363–365
Freeman RR, Trejdosiewicz AJ, Gross GAM (1980) Protective monoclonal antibodies recognising stage specific merozoite antigens of a rodent malaria parasite. Nature 284:366–368
Freund J, Sommer HE, Walter AW (1945) Immunisation against malaria vaccination of ducks with killed parasites incorporated with adjuvants. Science 102:200–202
Freund J, Thomson KJ, Sommer HE, Walter AW, Pisani TM (1948) Immunisation of monkeys against malaria by means of killed parasites with adjuvants. Am J Trop Med 28:1–22
Greenwood BM (1974) Immunosuppression in malaria and trypanosomiasis. In: Porter R, Knight J (eds) Parasites in the immunised host: mechanisms of survival. (Ciba Foundation Symposium 25 new series). Elsevier, North Holland, Amsterdam, pp 137–146
Greenwood BM, Vick RM (1975) Evidence for a lymphocyte mitogen in human malaria. Nature 257:592–594
Greenwood BM, Oduloju AJ, Stratton D (1977) Lymphocyte changes in acute malaria. Trans R Soc Trop Med Hyg 71:408–410
Grun JL, Weidanz WP (1981) Immunity to *Plasmodium chabaudi adami* in the B-cell-deficient mouse. Nature 290:143–145
Gwadz RW (1976) Malaria: successful immunisation against the sexual stages of *Plasmodium gallinaceum*. Science 193:1150–1151
Gwadz RW, Carter R, Green I (1979) Gamete vaccines and transmission-blocking immunity in malaria. Bull WHO [Suppl] 57:175–180
Hawking F, Worms MJ, Gammage K, Goddard PA (1966) The biological purpose of the blood cycle of the malaria parasite *Plasmodium cynomolgi*. Lancet II:422–424
Holbrook TW, Palczuk NC, Stauber LA (1974) Immunity to exoerythrocytic forms of malaria. III: stage specific immunisation of turkeys against exoerythrocytic forms of *Plasmodium fallax*. J Parasitol 60:348–354
Holz GG, Beach DH, Sherman IW (1977) Octadecanoic fatty acids and their association with haemolysis in malaria. J Protozool 24:566–574
Homewood CA, Neame KD (1974) Malaria and the permeability of the host erythrocyte. Nature 252:718–719
Houba V, Allison AC, Adeniyi A, Houba JE (1971) Immunoglobulin classes and complement in biopsies of Nigerian children with the nephrotic syndrome. Clin Exp Immunol 8:761–764
Howard RJ, Smith PM, Mitchell GF (1980a) Characterisation of surface proteins and glycoproteins on red blood cells from mice infected with haemosporidia: *Plasmodium berghei* infections of BALB/c mice. Parasitology 81:273–298

Howard RJ, Smith PM, Mitchell GF (1980b) Characterisation of surface proteins and glycoproteins on red blood cells from mice infected with haemosporidia: *Plasmodium yoelii* infections of BALB/c mice. Parasitology 81:299–314

Jahiel RI, Nussenzweig RS, Vilcek J, Vanderberg J (1969) Protective effect of interferon inducers on *Plasmodium berghei* malaria. Am J Trop Med Hyg 18:823–835

Kielmann A, Sarasin G, Bernhard A, Weiss N (1970) Further investigations on *Plasmodium gallinaceum* as an antigen in the diagnosis of human malaria. Bull WHO 43:617–622

Kilejian A (1974) A unique histidine rich polypeptide from the malaria parasite, *Plasmodium lophurae*. J Biol Chem 249:4650–4655

Kilejian A (1978) Histidine rich protein as a model malaria vaccine. Science 201:922–924

Kilejian A, Olson J (1979) Proteins and glycoproteins from human erythrocytes infected with *Plasmodium falciparum*. Bull WHO [Suppl] 57:101–107

Kilejian A, Abati A, Trager W (1977) *Plasmodium falciparum* and *Plasmodium coatneyi*: immunogenicity of knob-like protrusions on infected erythrocyte membranes. Exp Parasitol 42:157–164

Kretschmar W, Voller A (1973) Suppression of *Plasmodium falciparum* malaria in *Aotus* monkeys by milk diet. Z Tropenmed Parasit 24:51–59

Ladda RL (1969) New insights into the fine structure of rodent malaria parasites. Milit Med 134:825–865

Langhorne J, Butcher GA, Mitchell GH, Cohen S (1978) Preliminary investigations of the role of the spleen in immunity to *Plasmodium knowlesi* malaria, In UNDP World Bank WHO Tropical Disease research series no. 1: Role of the spleen in the immunology of tropical disease. Schwabe, Basel, pp 205–225

Loose LD, Cook JA, DiLuzio NR (1972) Malarial immunosuppression – a macrophage mediated effect. Proc Helm Soc Wash 39:484–493

MacGregor RR, Sheagren JN, Wolff SM (1969) Endotoxin induced modification of *Plasmodium berghei* infection in mice. J Immunol 102:131–139

McColm AA, Trigg PI (1980) Release of radio-isotope labelled antigens from *Plasmodium knowlesi* during merozoite re-invasion in vitro. Parasitology 81:199–209

McDonald V, Phillips RS (1978) Increase in non-specific antibody mediated cytotoxicity in malarious mice. Clin Exp Immunol 34:159–163

McGregorIA (1972) Immunology of malarial infection and its possible consequences. Br Med Bull 28:22–27

McGregor IA, Barr M (1962) Antibody response to tetanus toxoid immunisation in malarious and non-malarious Gambian children. Trans R Soc Top Med Hyg 56:364

Mendis KN, Targett GAT (1979) Immunisation against gametes and asexual erythrocytic stages of a rodent malaria parasite. Nature 277:389–391

Merser C, Sinay P, Adam A (1975) Total synthesis and adjuvant activity of bacterial peptidoglycan derivatives. Biochem Biophys Res Comm 66:1316–1322

Miller LH, Carter R (1976) Innate resistance in malaria. Exp Parasitol 40:132–146

Miller LH, Aikawa M, Dvorak JA (1975) Malaria (*Plasmodium knowlesi*) merozoites immunity and the surface coat. J Immunol 114:1237–1242

Mitchell GH (1977) A review of merozoite vaccination against *Plasmodium knowlesi* malaria. Trans R Soc Trop Med Hyg 71:281–282

Mitchell GH, Butcher GA, Cohen S (1973) Isolation of blood-stage merozoites from *Plasmodium knowlesi* malaria. Int J Parasitol 3:443–445

Mitchell GH, Butcher GA, Cohen S (1975) Merozoite vaccination against *Plasmodium knowlesi* malaria. Immunology 29:397–407

Mitchell GH, Butcher GA, Voller A, Cohen S (1976) The effect of human immune IgG on the in vitro development of *Plasmodium falciparum*. Parasitology 72:149–162

Mitchell GH, Richards WHG, Butcher GA, Cohen S (1977) Merozoite vaccination of douroucouli monkeys against falciparum malaria. Lancet I:1335–1338

Mitchell GH, Richards WHG, Voller A, Dietrich FM, Dukor P (1979) Nor-MDP, saponin, corynebacteria, and pertussis organisms as immunological adjuvants in experimental malaria vaccination of macaques. Bull WHO [Suppl] 57:189–197

Mitchell GH, Cohen S, Black CDV, Voller A, Dietrich FM, Dukor P (1980) Novel adjuvants in malaria vaccination. In: Van den Bossche H (ed) The host-invader interplay. 3rd International Symposium on the biochemistry of parasites and host parasite relationships. Elsevier, North Holland, Amsterdam, pp 629–632 (abstract)

Molineaux L, Grammicia G (1980) The Garki project. World Health Organization, Geneva

Mulligan HW, Russell PF, Mohan BN (1941) Active immunisation of fowls against *Plasmodium gallinaceum* by injections of killed homologous sporozoites. J Mal Inst Ind 4:25–34

Nardin EH, Nussenzweig RS (1979) Antibodies to sporozoites: their frequent occurrence in individuals living in an area of hyperendemic malaria. Science 206:597–599

Niblack JF, Otterness IG, Hemsworth GR, Wolff JS, Hoffman WW, Kraska AR (1979) CP-20,961: a structurally novel synthetic adjuvant. J Retic Soc 26:655–666

Nussenzweig RS, Vanderburg J, Most H, Orton C (1967) Protective immunity produced by the injection of X-irradiated sporozoites of *Plasmodium berghei*. Nature 216:160–162

Nussenzweig RS, Vanderberg JP, Sanabria Y, Most H (1972a) *Plasmodium berghei:* accelerated clearance of sporozoites from blood as part of immune mechanism in mice. Exp Parasitol 31:88–97

Nussenzweig RS, Vanderburg J, Spitalny G, Rivera I, Orton C, Most H (1972b) Sporozoite induced immunity in mammalian malaria – a review. Am J Trop Med Hyg 21:722–728

Orjih AU, Nussenzweig RS (1979) *Plasmodium berghei:* suppression of antibody response to sporozoite stage by acute blood stage infection. Clin Exp Immunol 38:1–8

Oster CN, Koontz LC, Wyler DJ (1980) Malaria in asplenic mice: effects of splenectomy, congenital asplenia, and splenic reconstitution on the course of infection. Am J Trop Med Hyg 29:1138–1142

Pasvol G, Weatherall DJ, Wilson RJM (1977) Effects of foetal haemoglobin on susceptibility of red cells to *Plasmodium falciparum*. Nature 270:171–173

Perrin LH, Dyal R, Rieder H (1981a) Characterisation of antigens from erythrocytic stages of *Plasmodium falciparum* reacting with human immune sera. Trans R Soc Med Trop Hyg 75:163–165

Perrin LH, Ramirez E, Lambert PM, Miescher PA (1981b) Inhibition of *P. falciparum* growth in human erythrocytes by monoclonal antibodies. Nature 289:301–303

Phillips RS, Jones VE (1972) Immunity to *Plasmodium berghei* in rats: maximum levels of protective antibody activity are associated with eradication of the infection. Parasitology 64:117–127

Phillips RS, Wolstencroft RA, Brown IN, Brown KN, Dumonde DC (1970) Immunity to malaria. III. Possible occurrence of a cell-mediated immunity to *Plasmodium knowlesi* in chronically infected and Freund's complete adjuvant sensitised monkeys. Exp Parasitol 28:339–355

Playfair JHL, de Souza B, Cottrell BJ (1977a) Reactivity and cross reactivity of mouse helper T cells to malaria parasites. Immunology 32:681

Playfair JHL, de Souza B, Cottrell BJ (1977b) Protection of mice against malaria by a killed vaccine: differences in effectiveness against *P. yoelii* and *P. berghei*. Immunology 33:507–515

Quinn TC, Wyler DJ (1980) Resolution of acute malaria (*Plasmodium berghei* in the rat): reversibility and spleen dependence. Am J Trop Med Hyg 29:1–4

Rank RG, Weidanz WP (1976) Non-sterilising immunity in avian malaria: an antibody independent phenomenon. Proc Soc Exp Biol Med 151:257–259

Reese RT, Trager W, Jensen JB, Miller DA, Tantravahi R (1978) Immunisation against malaria with antigen from *Plasmodium falciparum* cultivated in vitro. Proc Nat Acad Sci USA 75:5665–5668

Rener J, Carter R, Rosenberg Y, Miller LH (1980) Anti-gamete monoclonal antibodies synergistically block transmission of malaria by preventing fertilisation in the mosquito. Proc Nat Acad Sci USA 77:6797–6799

Richards WHG (1966) Active immunisation of chicks against *Plasmodium gallinaceum* by inactivated homologous sporozoites and erythrocytic parasites. Nature 212:1492–1494

Richards WHG, Mitchell GH, Butcher GA, Cohen S (1977) Merozoite vaccination of rhesus monkeys against *Plasmodium knowlesi* malaria; immunity to sporozoite (mosquito-transmitted) challenge. Parasitology 74:191–198

Rieckmann KH, Cabrera EJ, Campbell GH, Jost RC, Miranda R, O'Leary TR (1979) Immunisation of rhesus monkeys with blood-stage antigens of *Plasmodium knowlesi*. Bull WHO [Suppl] 57:139–151

Roberts DW, Weidanz WP (1979) T-cell immunity to malaria in the B-cell deficient mouse. Am J Trop Med Hyg 28:1–3

Roberts DW, Rank RG, Weidanz WP, Finerty JF (1977) Prevention of recrudescent malaria in nude mice by thymic grafting or by treatment with hyperimmune serum. Infect Immun 16:821–826

Roitt IM (1980) Essential immunology. 4th edn. Blackwell, Oxford

Schmidt-Ullrich R, Wallach DFH, Lightholder J (1979) Fractionation of *Plasmodium knowlesi*-induced antigens of rhesus monkey erythrocyte membranes. Bull WHO [Suppl] 57:115–121

Siddiqui WA (1977) An effective immunisation of experimental monkeys against a human malaria parasite, *Plasmodium falciparum*. Science 197:388–389

Siddiqui WA, Kramer K, Richmond-Crum SM (1978) *In vitro* cultivation and partial purification of *Plasmodium falciparum* antigen suitable for vaccination studies in *Aotus* monkeys. J Parasitol 64:168–169

Siddiqui WA, Taylor DW, Kan SC, Kramer K, Richmond-Crum SM, Kotani S, Shiba T, Kasumoto S (1979) Immunisation of experimental monkeys against *Plasmodium falciparum:* use of synthetic adjuvants. Bull WHO [Suppl] 57:199–203

Siddiqui WA, Kan SC, Kramer K, Case S, Palmer K, Niblack JF (1981) Use of a synthetic adjuvant in an effective vaccination of monkeys against malaria. Nature 289:64–66

Simpson GL, Schenkel RH, Silverman PH (1974) Vaccination of rhesus monkeys against malaria by use of sucrose density gradient fractions of *Plasmodium knowlesi* antigens. Nature 274:304–305

Sinden RE, Canning EU, Bray RS, Smalley ME (1978) Gametocyte and gamete development in *Plasmodium falciparum*. Proc R Soc Lond B 201:375–399

Sljivic VS, Watson SR (1977) The adjuvant effect of *Corynebacterium parvum:* T-cell dependence of macrophage activation. J Exp Med 145:45–57

Smalley ME (1975) The nature of age immunity to *Plasmodium berghei* in the rat. Parasitology 71:337–347

Smalley ME, Brown J (1981) *Plasmodium falciparum* gametocytogenesis stimulated by lymphocytes and serum from infected Gambian children. Trans R Soc Trop Med Hyg 75:316–317

Smith J, Sinden RE (1981) Studies on the uptake of sporozoites of *Plasmodium yoelii nigeriensis* by perfused rat liver. Trans R Soc Trop Med Hyg 75:188–189 (abstract)

Spitalny GL, Rivera-Ortiz C, Nussenzweig RS (1976) *Plasmodium berghei:* the spleen in sporozoite induced immunity to mouse malaria. Exp Parasitol 40:179–188

Symoens J (1980) Prospects for immunotherapy of parasitic diseases. In: Van den Bossche H (ed) The host invader interplay. 3rd International symposium on the biochemistry of parasites and host parasite relationships. Elsevier, North Holland, Amsterdam, pp 615–627

Thomson KJ, Freund J, Sommer HE, Walter AW (1947) Immunisation of ducks against malaria by means of killed parasites with or without adjuvants. Am J Trop Med 27:79–105

Todorovic R, Ferris D, Ristic M (1967) Immunogenic properties of serum antigens from chickens acutely infected with *Plasmodium gallinaceum*. Ann Trop Med Parasitol 61:117–124

Tosta CE, Wedderburn N (1980) Immune phagocytosis of *Plasmodium yoelii*-infected erythrocytes by macrophages and eosinophils. Clin Exp Immunol 42:114–120

Vanderberg JP, Nussenzweig RS, Most H (1969) Protective immunity produced by the injection of X-irradiated sporozoites of *Plasmodium berghei*. V. In vitro effects of immune serum on sporozoites. Milit Med 134:1183–1190

Verhave JP (1975) Immunisation with sporozoites. PhD thesis. Katholieke Universiteit te Nijmegen
Voller A, Richards WHG (1970) Immunity to *Plasmodium falciparum* in owl monkeys (*Aotus trivirgatus*). Z Tropenmed Parasitkd 21:160–166
Voller A, Rossan RN (1969) Immunological studies with simian malarias. I. Antigenic variants of *Plasmodium cynomolgi bastianellii*. Trans R Soc Trop Med Hyg 63:46–56
Voller A, Green DI, Richards WHG (1973) Cross immunity studies with East and West African strains of *Plasmodium falciparum* in owl monkeys (*Aotus trivirgatus*). J Trop Med Hyg 76:135–139
Voller A, Meuwissen JHETh, Verhave JP (1980) Methods for measuring the immunological response to plasmodia. In: Kreier JP (ed) Malaria, Vol 3. Academic, New York, pp 67–109
Wedderburn N (1974) Immunodepression produced by malarial infection in mice. In: Porter R, Knight J (eds) Parasites in the immunised host: mechanisms of survival. Ciba foundation Symposium 25 new series. Elsevier, North Holland, Amsterdam, pp 121–135
Weinbaum FI, Weintraub J, Nkrumah FK, Evans CB, Tigelaar RE, Rosenberg YJ (1978) Immunity to *Plasmodium berghei yoelii* in mice. II. Specific and non-specific cellular and humoral responses during the course of infection. J Immunol 121:629–636
White RG (1976) The adjuvant effect of microbial products on the immune response. Ann Rev Microbiol 30:579–600
Wilson RJM, Bartholomew RK (1975) The release of antigens by *Plasmodium falciparum*. Parasitology 71:183–192
Wilson RJM, Phillips RS (1976) Method to test inhibitory antibodies in human sera to wild populations of *Plasmodium falciparum*. Nature 263:132–134
Wilson RJM, McGregor IA, Wilson ME (1973) The stability and fractionation of malarial antigens from the blood of Africans infected with *Plasmodium falciparum*. Int J Parasitol 3:511–520
World Health Organization (1976) Immunological adjuvants. Technical Report series 595. WHO, Geneva
World Health Organization (1980) Hybridoma technology with special reference to parasitic diseases. UNDP/World Bank/WHO, Geneva
Wyler DJ, Miller LH, Schmidt LH (1977) Spleen function in quartan malaria (due to *Plasmodium inui*) evidence for both protective and suppressive roles in host defence. J Infect Dis 135:86–93
Yoshida N, Nussenzweig RS, Potocnjak P, Nussenzweig V, Aikawa M (1980) Hybridoma produces protective antibodies directed against the sporozoite stage of malaria parasite. Science 207:71–73
Zuckerman A (1945) In vitro opsonic tests with *Plasmodium gallinaceum* and *Plasmodium lophurae*. J Infect Dis 77:28
Zuckerman A, Ristic M (1968) Blood parasite antigens and antibodies. In: Weinman D, Ristic M (eds) Infectious blood diseases of man and animals vol 1. Academic, New York, pp 80–122

CHAPTER 5

# Clinical Pathology

V. BOONPUCKNAVIG, T. SRICHAIKUL, and S. PUNYAGUPTA

## A. Introduction

Malaria has always been considered as one of the most important and deadly diseases of man. In 1955 a short-lived hope of malaria eradication was created when a global programme was initiated by the World Health Organization (WHO 1955, 1956). Twenty years later, because of the development of resistance to DDT by the mosquitoes and to chloroquine by *Plasmodium falciparum*, as well as financial problems, the programme was declared a failure (WHO 1975).

In recent years the prevalence of malaria has been noted to be rising sharply in many countries (McCABE 1966; KIEL 1968; HEINEMAN 1972; O'HOLOHAN 1976), particularly in Southeast Asia, where the incidence is almost three and a half times higher than that in 1972 (WERNSDORFER 1980). The authors have experienced many hundreds of malaria cases in Thailand during the past 25 years and, only recently, we find that disease due to *Plasmodium falciparum* is becoming more severe in terms of clinical complications, with high morbidity and mortality (PUNYAGUPTA et al. 1974). One may try to correlate this change to the development of strains of *P. falciparum* resistant to the standard antimalarial drugs, chloroquine, and quinine. Another explanation is based on the remarkable change in the parasite density seen in the severe cases with multi-organ involvement. In the past it was uncommon to find serious cases with a parasite density of 10% or more. Recent observations of surprisingly heavy parasite density, for example over 90% of erythrocytes infected and frequently with double or triple infections in a single erythrocyte, are both interesting and disturbing.

We must therefore take a new and cautious look into various aspects of malaria, particularly the clinical disease, pathogenesis, and pathology, which may be of benefit to the therapeutic approaches. Moreover, experimental studies of malarial infection in animals have contributed to our understanding of the mechanism of the disease processes in man. The importance of work in animal models has been emphasised by BRUCE-CHWATT (1978).

This chapter is intended to give the reader a short review of the pathogenesis and clinical features, as well as pathological information, and to add some newer aspects of human malaria, particularly falciparum infection, by arranging the data by specific organ systems.

## B. Pathogenesis

The life cycle of malaria parasites in the human host consists of three phases, the sporozoite, the tissue phase and the erythrocytic phase. The pathological changes in malarial infection occur mostly during the erythrocytic phase. The disease processes may be similar to those caused by other infective agents in which factors from both parasites and host are involved.

## I. The Parasites

In all four species of human malaria, the exoerythrocytic and erythrocytic phases are similar in most aspects. However, the clinicopathological manifestations are different. The difference in the degree of merozoite production as well as the capability of the merozoites of each species to invade the erythrocytes probably is one of the main factors which determines the degree of host response. Recently more severe clinical cases of *P. falciparum* infection with multisystem involvement have been encountered. At the same time, some changes in the parasites have been observed, namely the development of resistance to the effective chemotherapeutic agents and the finding of unexpected hyperparasitaemia (Deaton 1970; Dennis et al. 1967; Punyagupta et al. 1974; Srichaikul 1973a). The relationship between the parasite density and the mortality has been well documented by Field (1949), i.e. the greater the density the higher the mortality.

## II. Host-Parasite Interaction

During the complex life cycle in man, the malaria parasites enter the red cells and undergo rapid growth and development. The release of merozoites gives rise to new infection in other red cells. This asexual phase is critical to both host and parasites. In man it is responsible for the clinical manifestations and complications. As for the parasites, only during this stage can they be eradicated. Both specific and non-specific host responses to malaria can occur. The specific changes are mainly related to the red-cell alterations, whereas the non-specific changes involve various systems of the host. All of the systems which are involved in these changes are briefly reviewed in this section.

### 1. Red Blood Cells

The protective mechanism of erythrocytes depends on several factors. These are the age of the cells, the cellular membrane structure and intracellular biochemical composition including enzymes, as well as the various changes in haemoglobin (Pasvol and Weatherall 1980).

It is well known that *P. falciparum* attacks red cells of all ages although the younger population are more susceptible, whereas *P. vivax* and *P. ovale* infect only young red cells and *P. malariae* involves only older cells. Recently many studies have shown that specific receptors on the red-cell membrane may be needed for the invasion of certain malaria species, e.g. Duffy-positive cells would be susceptible to *P. vivax* whereas this selectivity was not observed in *P. falciparum* (Miller et al. 1975, 1976, 1977). On the other hand, experimental study has indicated that a sialoglycopeptide might act as a receptor for *P. falciparum* (Pasvol and Weatherall 1980). It has been shown that *P. falciparum* invasion of the red cells from heterozygotes and homozygotes with sickle cell anaemia is decreased, and the subsequent intraerythrocytic growth retarded. The aggregates of haemoglobin S which occur under low oxygen tensions were proposed as a factor responsible for the retarded growth of the parasites (FRIEDMAN 1978; PASVOL et al. 1978). Furthermore, the decrease in parasite growth or density was also demonstrated in various other red-cell disorders, i.e. in homozygotes with haemoglobin C (FRIEDMAN et al. 1979; THOMPSON 1963), in persistent high haemoglobin F (PASVOL et al. 1976, 1977) and in female heterozygotes for glucose-6-phosphate dehydrogenase (G6PD) deficiency (EATON et al. 1976; BIENZLE et al. 1972). A mechanism for the resistance in G6PD-deficient red cells has been proposed recently (PASVOL and WEATHERALL 1980).

The subsequent pathological changes in the host can be induced by various changes of the red cells. During parasite metabolism, haemozoin or malaria pigment is derived from the utilisation of haemoglobin in the infected erythrocytes (FLETCHER and MAEGRAITH 1972). The role of this substance in cellular injury is still unclear. However, malaria pigment in unbound form is toxic to cell metabolism. Furthermore, massive intravascular haemolysis which occurs in certain individuals with G6PD deficiency or hyperparasitaemia would produce haemoglobinaemia and haemoglobinuria. Massive breakdown of the red cells commonly gives rise to the most two serious complications, namely acute renal failure and disseminated intravascular coagulation (DIC). Excessive haemolysis can also cause hypoxia of many vital organs.

Previous studies demonstrated that there was an increase in stickiness and rigidity, and a decrease in deformability of the erythrocytes infected by *P. falciparum*. These changes possibly cause agglutination of these infected red cells and subsequently lead to the so-called plugging phenomenon of the microcirculation (LUSE and MILLER 1971; MILLER et al. 1971, 1972). The obstruction of the blood flow in the microcirculation by these agglutinated erythrocytes which contain mostly the late schizonts is the consistent pathological finding described in the brains of patients dying from falciparum infection.

## 2. Reticuloendothelial System and Immune Response

The non-specific host defence mechanism against malarial infection involves reticuloendothelial (RE) cell hyperplasia and various leucocytic responses. Eradication of malaria parasites may be achieved through the phagocytic activity of macrophages in spleen and bone marrow, and also by the specific antibodies produced during the infection. It is well known that in a malarial host without a spleen, the infection spreads very rapidly. In case of such a hyperparasitaemia, severe systemic complications followed by a very high mortality rate are usually observed unless prompt, effective treatment is given.

In the presence of a highly virulent infection the immune responses are very obvious. One interesting pathological finding was unusual proliferation of the lymphoid and reticulum (histiocytic) cells in the walls of the splenic vessels. The proliferation of these cells sometimes protruded from the walls into the lumen of the blood vessels, causing partial obstruction of the blood flow. This phenomenon was first described in bird and duck malaria and was also mentioned in a few falciparum cases (RIGDON 1944a). Autopsy findings by our group in cases of severely complicated *P. falciparum* infection strongly support RIGDON'S earlier observation.

Previous immunological studies showed that the antibodies produced consisted of IgG, IgM, IgA, and IgD during malarial infection (COHEN and BUTCHER 1972). In the presence of highly virulent infections which loaded the body with malarial antigen, insoluble immune complexes consisting of both IgG and IgM were formed. These complexes in certain situations became pathogenic. So far, they have been demonstrated in the kidney, causing acute glomerulonephritis in *P. falciparum* and a nephrotic syndrome in *P. malariae* infection in man. These complexes also contribute to the destruction of red cells and platelets (FACER et al. 1979; ROSENBERG et al. 1973; NEVA et al. 1970; WOODRUFF et al. 1979). Complement activation, especially C3, also participates in the pathogenesis of lesions of both kidneys and blood cells.

### 3. Endogenous Mediators

Activation of the complement system by both classical and alternative pathways has been demonstrated during *P. falciparum* infection (PETCHCLAI et al. 1977; SRICHAIKUL et al. 1975). The causal relationship between the activation of C3 and the severity of clinical complications, namely anaemia, thrombocytopaenia, and DIC, has also been demonstrated. Along with the activation of the complement system various endogenous mediators of acute inflammation are released. The fall of kininogen with a simultaneous rise of kininogenases, as well as an increase in blood histamine, has been demonstrated in experimental animals infected with *P. knowlesi* (MAEGRAITH and ONABANJO 1970; ONABANJO and MAEGRAITH 1971). Recently, the increase in blood histamine has been demonstrated in man infected with *P. falciparum*, and a correlation between the blood histamine level, degree of parasitaemia, severity of complications, reduction of C3 and platelets, and finally DIC has also been found (SRICHAIKUL et al. 1976a). The increase in blood histamine during the acute phase of infection was most likely to be a factor responsible for the development of clinical complications. It can cause vasodilatation and increase in vascular permeability followed by hypovolaemia and circulatory stasis. Experimental studies also indicated the role of histamine in the occurrence of DIC (MCKAY et al. 1971).

### 4. Microcirculation

An alteration in the microcirculation is probably the most important change in the malarial host. Various mechanisms are responsible for this alteration. In experimental animals infected with *P. knowlesi*, it was shown that there was a generalised vasoconstriction of the vessels to the visceral organs. Simultaneously, an abnormal increase in the permeability of small vessels, particularly in the brain, was observed. Leakage of plasma from the vascular lumen caused hypovolaemia. Both hypovolaemia and vasoconstriction subsequently induced a severe reduction of blood flow to various organs and stasis of the microcirculation would then follow (MAEGRAITH 1974; MAEGRAITH and FLETCHER 1972). In man, a decrease in blood volume as well as a reduction of blood flow was demonstrated in certain cases of falciparum infection with heavy parasitaemia (CHONGSUPHAJAISIDHI et al. 1971). The occlusion of capillaries and venules by the agglutinated infected erythrocytes, as well as the formation of fibrin thrombi, probably occurred at this critical point when the rate of blood flow was severely retarded. Subsequently, injury of the endothelial cells due to local anoxia would develop and lead to further increase in permeability of the vessels. The most harmful vicious cycle could then occur.

## C. Clinicopathological Correlation

The distribution and frequency of human infection by *P. falciparum*, *P. vivax*, *P. malariae*, and *P. ovale* differ in various parts of the world (WHO 1969). The major differences in the clinical diseases, namely the pattern of fever, the incubation period and the severity of clinical symptoms are well known and need not be mentioned in detail here. As *P. falciparum* is the most significant species of all in terms of prevalence, morbidity, and mortality it will be described in more detail as a representative of the other types of infection.

Infection of man with non-human primate malaria such as *P. cynomolgi* has been reported as a laboratory accident or as experimental infections (COATNEY et al. 1971; CROSS et al. 1973; MOST 1972).

The clinicopathological description will be classified into uncomplicated and complicated malaria, and the latter will be further subdivided according to the organ systems affected.

### I. Uncomplicated Malaria

Following a variable incubation period according to the species, the patients will experience some constitutional symptoms of malaise, headache, and myalgia prior to the development of high fever with chills. Some may experience aches and pains in the chest, abdomen or joints. At this stage malaria parasites may not be detected in the peripheral blood examination. The classical features of a sudden rise of temperature and shaking chills described as the cold period because of vasoconstriction is most striking, followed by the hot phase when the temperature will rise to as high as 41 °C and remain there for a few hours. These features which are characteristic of endotoxaemia occur at the time that merozoites emerge from infected erythrocytes. During the attack tachypnoea, tachycardia, extreme headache, body ache, nausea, vomiting, profound sweating, and sensorial disturbances are the usual symptoms. Symptoms and signs of orthostatic hypotension are prominent features (BUTLER and WEBER 1973). Between each attack patients may be asymptomatic. In classical textbook cases, which are infrequently seen nowadays, paroxysms of fever with associated symptoms occur at intervals of less than 48 h for *P. falciparum*, 48 h for *P. vivax*, and *P. ovale*, and 72 h for *P. malariae*.

In everyday practice while malaria cases may present with any type of fever, low-grade or high sustained temperature with or without rigors, the most constant associated symptoms are severe headache and vomiting, followed by an afebrile stage during which the patient feels reasonably well.

In the early stage of acute malaria we have found hepatomegaly with or without tenderness to be more frequent than splenomegaly whereas, in the chronic stage, splenomegaly is more prominent. A variable degree of jaundice with slight to moderate anaemia is most commonly noted, particularly in areas where haemolytic diseases such as haemoglobinopathy and G6PD deficiency are prevalent. Minute petechiae and subconjunctival haemorrhages may be observed. Lymph node enlargement is insignificant.

In chronic malaria the symptoms are less severe. Anaemia with splenomegaly and fever are the main complaints. In *P. vivax* and *P. ovale* the relapses may occur many months or even years later because of the persistence of the hepatic stages (see Chap. 1).

## II. Complicated Malaria

Of the four human species, *P. falciparum* is the only species that is notorious for causing complications. The reasons are as follows: firstly, one sporozoite of *P. falciparum* yields as many as 40000 merozoites to invade the erythrocytes as compared with 1:10000 in *P. vivax*, 1:15000 in *P. ovale*, and 1:2000 in *P. malariae;* secondly, the high capability of *P. falciparum* merozoites to invade all ages of erythrocytes and the high rate of reproduction of asexual erythrocytic forms. Parasitaemia in *P. falciparum* therefore may reach as high as 90% of total erythrocytes, compared with less than 1% in the other species.

**Table 1.** Maximum level of parasitaemia recorded in 51 falciparum malaria cases and mortality in each group

| No. of infected erythrocytes per 100 erythrocytes | No. of cases | No. of deaths | (%) |
|---|---|---|---|
| Below 5 | 27 | 2 | (7) |
| 6–10 | 11 | 3 | (26) |
| 11–30 | 5 | 3 | (60) |
| 31–50 | 4 | 2 | (50) |
| 51–70 | 1 | 1 | (100) |
| 71–90 | 2 | 2 | (100) |
| Over 91 | 1 | 1 | (100) |
| Total | 51 | 14 | (28) |

**Table 2.** The clinical complications in 51 falciparum malaria cases and associated mortality

| Clinical manifestations | No. of cases | No. of deaths | (%) |
|---|---|---|---|
| Cerebral complications | 42 | 14 | (33) |
| Non-oliguric renal failure | 18 | 1 | (6) |
| Oliguric renal failure (<20 ml/h) | 13 | 13 | (100) |
| Pulmonary complications | 20 | 14 | (70) |
| Cardiac involvement | 9 | 4 | (44) |
| Shock | 4 | 3 | (75) |
| Skin and mucous membrane bleeding only | 12 | 5 | (42) |
| Massive gastrointestinal bleeding | 9 | 9 | (100) |
| Hepatomegaly with abnormal transaminases (>100 units) | 13 | 2 | (15) |
| Haemoglobinuria | 9 | 6 | (67) |

**Table 3.** Multiple organ complications in 51 falciparum malaria patients

| Organ involved | No. of cases | No. of deaths | Number of cases with other organs also involved | | | | | |
|---|---|---|---|---|---|---|---|---|
| | | | Brain | Kidney | Lung | Heart | Massive gastro-intestinal bleeding | Liver |
| Brain | 42 | 14 (33) | – | 27 | 20 | 7 | 9 | 9 |
| Kidney | 31 | 14 (45) | 27 | – | 20 | 9 | 9 | 11 |
| Lung | 20 | 14 (70) | 20 | 20 | – | 9 | 9 | 6 |
| Heart | 9 | 4 (44) | 8 | 9 | 9 | – | 2 | 4 |
| Massive gastrointestinal bleeding | 9 | 9 (100) | 9 | 9 | 9 | 2 | – | 1 |
| Liver | 13 | 2 (15) | 10 | 11 | 6 | 4 | 1 | – |

From 1969 to 1975 the authors studied in detail 51 clinical cases of complicated falciparum malaria at Ramathibodi University Hospital in Bangkok. There were 39 males and 12 females aged 17–45 years. The clinical data from these 51 cases are summarised in Tables 1–3.

As regards pathological data, autopsy specimens of malaria cases already available in the Department of Pathology, Ramathibodi University Hospital, were restudied in detail. A total of 22 cases were reviewed and the pertinent pathological findings in brain, lungs, and kidneys are summarised in Tables 4 and 5. Cases 1–7 were among the same group of patients recorded in Tables 1–3. Cases 11–22 were sent from provincial hospitals and had no accompanying clinical information. Specimens from major organs were submitted for pathological study.

The maximum levels of parasitaemia in each case and the outcome of patients are presented in Table 1. Those who had more than 50% of erythrocytes infected by *P. falciparum* never survived, while those with between 10% and 15% parasite density had a 50% chance of survival. In this series of 51 cases about half had a parasitaemia of over 5% of total erythrocytes, and one-fourth had over 10%. These findings may explain the high mortality of 28% in the whole group.

## 1. Haematology Complications

Haematological complications, which are the most common of all complications in malaria, have long been an interesting subject of extensive investigations. Changes of the erythroid and leucocytic series along with the RE cell hyperplasia are well-known manifestations. Recently thrombocytopaenia, coagulopathy, and bleeding have been increasingly common problems in complicated falciparum infections (Borochovitz et al. 1970; Neva et al. 1970; Punyagupta et al. 1974). The haematological complications are important because most of them reflect the defence mechanisms of the hosts to malarial infection, as well as the prognosis.

The present review attempts to summarise the haematological complications of human malarial infections. The discussion will be devoted to the complications of various systems including erythroid, leucocytic, and haemostatic changes. Mech-

**Table 4.** Autopsy findings[a] in 22 cases of *P. falciparum* infection

| Case No. | Sex/ age | Histopathology findings | | | | | | | | | |
|---|---|---|---|---|---|---|---|---|---|---|---|
| | | Brain | | | Lung | | | Kidneys | | | Others |
| | | PE in vessels | Haemor- rhage | Granu- loma | Oedema | Membrane formation | Haemor- rhage | Haemo- globin casts | Tubular necrosis | Tubular degeneration | Demonstration of fibrin thrombi in |
| 1 | M 36 | +++ | – | – | – | + | – | + | – | + | ND |
| 2 | M 24 | + | – | – | + | ++ | – | + | – | +++ | Glomeruli |
| 3 | M 19 | ++++ | Petechiae | + | + | – | + | + | – | ++ | Brain, lungs, skin, adrenal |
| 4 | M 53 | ++ | Ring | + | + | – | + | + | – | ++ | Brain, lungs |
| 5 | M 35 | ++ | Ring | + | + | + | + | + | ++ | – | Brain, lungs |
| 6 | M 35 | – | – | – | + | – | + | + | ++ | – | ND |
| 7 | M 25 | ++ | Massive & old | – | – | – | ++ | – | – | ++ | Lungs, skin |
| 8 | M 20 | + | Ring | – | + | – | + | + | ++ | + | Brain |
| 9 | M 49 | – | – | – | + | – | – | + | ++ | – | ND |
| 10 | M 30 | – | – | – | + | – | – | + | ++ | – | ND |
| 11 | M 44 | – | Petechiae | – | – | + | + | + | + | + | Brain, lungs |
| 12 | M 35 | ++ | Ring & old | + | – | + | + | + | ++ | – | Brain |
| 13 | M 20 | ++ | Ring | + | + | – | + | + | + | + | Brain |
| 14 | M 35 | – | – | – | ++ | – | + | + | ++ | + | ND |
| 15 | F 30 | ++ | Petechiae | + | ++ | – | – | + | + | + | Brain |
| 16 | M 25 | ++ | Ring | + | ++ | + | + | + | ++ | – | Brain |
| 17 | M 19 | + | Ring | – | ++ | – | + | + | ++ | – | Brain |
| 18 | M 18 | ++ | Petechiae | – | ++ | – | – | – | – | ++ | ND |
| 19 | M 28 | – | – | – | + | – | – | + | ++ | – | ND |
| 20 | F 24 | ++ | – | – | – | – | + | + | – | ++ | ND |
| 21 | M 30 | ++ | – | – | + | – | – | + | ++ | + | ND |
| 22 | M 22 | + | – | – | + | – | – | + | ++ | + | ND |

[a] Clinical data on cases 1–10 are summarized in Table 5

+, ++, +++, ++++: mild, moderate, severe, very severe; –, negative; PE, parasitised erythrocytes; ND, not detectable

Cases 1–7 are in the same series as Tables 1–3

**Table 5.** Clinical data on ten autopsy cases with complications

| Case No. | Parasitaemia max % | Parasitaemia at death | PE in cerebral vessels | Duration of illness | Clinical mani-festation | Laboratory evidence of DIC | Pathological evidence of fibrin thrombi | Use of heparin |
|---|---|---|---|---|---|---|---|---|
| 1 | 2 | neg | +++ | 15 | BRPGL | Yes | No | Yes |
| 2 | 7 | pos | + | 9 | BRP | Yes | Yes | Yes |
| 3 | 90 | pos | ++++ | 6 | BRPGC | Yes | Yes | Yes |
| 4 | 40 | neg | ++ | 10 | BRPGS | Yes | Yes | Yes |
| 5 | 40 | pos | ++ | 7 | BRPG | Yes | Yes | Yes |
| 6 | 5 | neg | − | 9 | BRPGC | Yes | No | Yes |
| 7 | 30 | neg | ++ | 21 | BRPG | Yes | Yes | No |
| 8 | 40 | pos | + | 10 | BRPG | Yes | Yes | Yes |
| 9 | 10 | neg | − | 19 | BRPCL | Yes | No | Yes |
| 10 | 8 | pos | − | 7 | BRP* | NR | No | No |

B, brain complication; C, cardiac arrest; G, gastrointestinal bleeding; L, liver failure; NR, no record; P, pulmonary complication; P*, secondary bacterial pneumonia; R, acute renal failure; S, shock

**Table 6.** Mechanisms of anaemia in malaria

| Major mechanisms | Evidence presented | Manifestations |
|---|---|---|
| 1. Bone marrow suppression | 1. Decreased erythroid proliferation<br>2. Suppression of erythropoietin | Erythroid hypoplasia, mostly in acute malaria |
| | 3. Dyserythropoiesis and defective maturation of normoblasts | Ineffective erythropoiesis mostly in chronic malaria |
| | 4. Defect in haem synthesis<br>5. Iron excess and dysutilisation | Hypochromic anaemia |
| | 6. Folate deficiency | Megaloblastic anaemia |
| 2. Haemolysis | 1. Parasitised red cells | |
| | 1.1 In RE organs | Extravascular haemolysis |
| | 1.2 In circulation | Intravascular haemolysis |
| | 2. Non-parasitised red cells by: | |
| | 2.1 Membrane changes<br>2.2 Increased Na influx<br>2.3 Immunological effects | Extravascular haemolysis |
| | 2.4 Interaction of drug and G6PD deficiency | Intravascular haemolysis |
| | 2.5 Hyperactivity of reticulo-endothelial system | Extravascular haemolysis and/or hypersplenism |

anisms inducing these complications, their clinical significance regarding treatment, and prognosis particularly of *P. falciparum* infection are also briefly reviewed.

### a) Anaemia

Anaemia is the most common hematological complication. It occurs in every species of malarial infection, and is always present in complicated malaria. The mechanisms of anaemia in malaria are complex and are listed in Table 6. Bone marrow suppression as a causative mechanism of anaemia has two major manifestations, first, erythroid hypoplasia in the majority of acute malaria patients (SRICHAIKUL et al. 1967) and, second, ineffective erythropoiesis found mostly in chronic cases (SRICHAIKUL et al. 1969). The mechanisms inducing the above abnormalities are still unclear at present. However, marked suppression of erythropoietin during malarial infection (T. SRICHAIKUL et al., unpublished data) and a decreased proliferation and/or increased destruction of normoblasts during their development in bone marrow have been found (SRICHAIKUL et al. 1973). In the group having an increased destruction of normoblasts, a defect in haem synthesis was also observed (STRICHAIKUL et al. 1976b). Recently, a picture of dyserythropoiesis as indicated by an abnormal nuclear structure of normoblasts in the bone marrow has been noted. However, an attempt to demonstrate invasion of malarial parasites into these abnormal normoblasts by electron microscopy was unsuccessful (ABDALLA et al. 1980). Iron overloading with hypochromic anaemia indicating iron dysutilisation was also demonstrated (SRICHAIKUL et al. 1976b, 1969, 1979). Megaloblastic anaemia caused by folate deficiency has been noted in a few cases (STRICKLAND et al. 1970; SULLIVAN 1969). The megaloblastic erythropoiesis was quite prominent in the majority of our *P. falciparum* patients who presented with severe hyperparasitaemia and multisystem complications. Although these changes were observed transiently, they also contributed to the more severe degree of anaemia which had already occurred from haemolysis resulting from the infection.

Haemolysis, observed in all species of malaria, was most prominent in acute falciparum infection (ABDALLA et al. 1980). Numerous evidence indicated that haemolysis occurred in both parasitised erythrocytes and, probably, a greater number of non-parasitised red cells. Most of the parasitised red cells are destroyed in the spleen by the selective, so-called "pitting" mechanism of the splenic macrophages (BALCERZAK et al. 1972; SCHNITZER et al. 1972; SCHNITZER et al. 1973). The non-parasitised red cells which have membrane defects as a result of injury from previous parasitisation lose their deformability, and finally are captured by macrophages in the spleen (BALCERZAK et al. 1972; SCHNITZER et al. 1972; SCHNITZER et al. 1973). Changes of membrane lipids, ATP, and sodium content in the red cells as a consequence of the membrane defects were demonstrated (AREEKUL 1973; CONRAD 1969, 1971; VARAVITHYA et al. 1972). The attachment of complement containing immune complexes of both IgM and IgG antibodies (FACER et al. 1979; ROSENBERG et al. 1973; WOODRUFF et al. 1979) also causes haemolysis of these cells in the RE organs. All of the above changes produce the picture of extravascular haemolysis which generally occurs in malaria patients. Intravascular haemolysis of mainly parasitised cells was only a minor mechanism except in patients with G6PD deficiency or hyperparasitaemia.

The hyperplasia of the reticuloendothelial system which is always observed during malaria infection causes yet more erythrocytic destruction in the spleen (ABDALLA et al. 1980; SHEAGREN et al. 1970). In chronic malaria the patient's spleen may be very large, producing the clinical syndrome of "hypersplenism" or "big spleen syndrome." These patients usually have a huge spleen accompanied by pancytopaenia and hyperplasia of all the haematopoietic precursors. Erythrophagocytosis is a consistent finding in the spleen and sometimes in the bone marrow.

b) Leucocytic Response

Peripheral leucocytic changes during the malaria infection vary according to the stages of the disease. Usually there is a mild lymphocytosis with low normal, white blood counts in chronic malaria. However, in acute malaria, slight leucocytosis with predominant neutrophilia is observed (DALE and WOLFF 1973; REILEY and O'NEIL 1971). In acute, severely ill falciparum patients, we have observed leucaemoid blood pictures with occasional young forms of neutrophils. Atypical lymphocytes are noted occasionally in both uncomplicated and complicated cases, but more young cells are seen only in severe complicated *P. falciparum*. Recent studies have shown that, during acute malarial infection, there is a defect of T-lymphocytes as indicated by a decrease in total T cells and depressed blastoid transformation with PHA and con A (OSUNKOYA et al. 1972; GILBREATH et al. 1978, 1979; WELLS et al. 1979). Accompanying these findings, lymphocytotoxic antibodies of T-lymphocytes in serum have been demonstrated (GILBREATH et al. 1978, 1979). The abnormalities of the T-lymphocytes during malarial infection indicate a defective cell-mediated immune response (CMIR) in malaria patients. How this defective CMIR could play a significant role in the pathogenesis and the occurrence of high incidence of Burkitt's lymphoma in falciparum endemic areas is still unknown (EDITORIAL 1970; FEORINO and MATHEWS 1974; STEWART 1970; WEDDERBURN 1970; ZIEGLER et al. 1972).

Hyperplasia of lymphocytes and plasma cells has been demonstrated in the bone marrow of the patients infected with *P. vivax* and mild *P. falciparum* (SRICHAIKUL 1967; Srichaikul et al. 1969). Similar findings were found in spleen and lymph nodes together with hyperplasia of the phagocytes (TALIAFERRO and MULLIGAN 1937).

The results of our autopsy studies of falciparum-infected patients who presented with high parasitaemia and multisystem complications were somewhat different from the previous findings. Bone marrow in certain cases revealed a marked decrease of myeloid cell precursors. About 50% of marrow tissue was replaced by lymphoid cells including mature lymphocytes, small and large transformed lymphocytes, with occasional immunoblasts (Fig. 1). Migration of these cells into the sinusoids was noted. Large numbers of mononuclear, phagocytic cells with very active phagocytosis of infected red cells, malaria pigment, and occasional normoblasts were observed throughout the bone marrow (Fig. 2).

The proliferation of lymphoid cells and histiocytes was unusually striking in spleen and lymph nodes. Approximately half of the cells were small lymphocytes, the remaining cells being small and large transformed, cleaved and non-cleaved lymphocytes (Fig. 3). Immunoblasts, transitional plasma cells and plasmocytoid cells were prominent (Fig. 4). These cells appeared also in the red pulp of spleen, paracortical, and medullary areas of the lymph nodes in smaller numbers. There was diffuse and nodular proliferation of lymphoid cells in the subendothelial layer of the trabecular vein of the spleen (Fig. 5). Similar findings were described in the spleens of birds and ducks with malarial infection, and this was believed to be a cause of splenic infarction (RIGDON 1944a). An unusual proliferation of lymphoplasma cells and phagocytic cells in the capsules of lymph nodes and accessory spleen were observed. Moreover, in one of our cases, an active, peculiar penetration of these cells from an accessory spleen into the nearby pancreatic tissue was

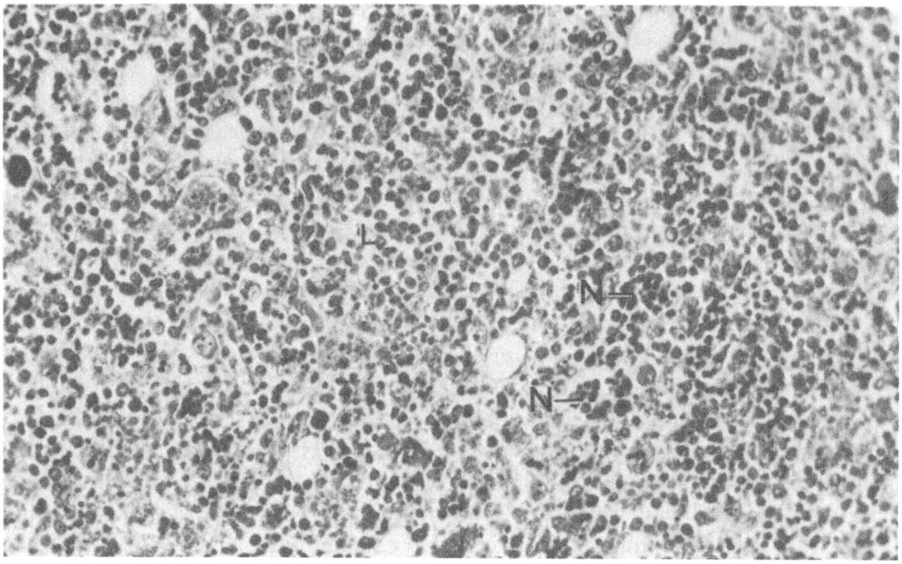


**Fig. 1.** Bone marrow demonstrating the proliferation of lymphoid and histiocytic cells. *L*, island of lymphoid cells; *N*, clumps of normoblasts. HE, × 368

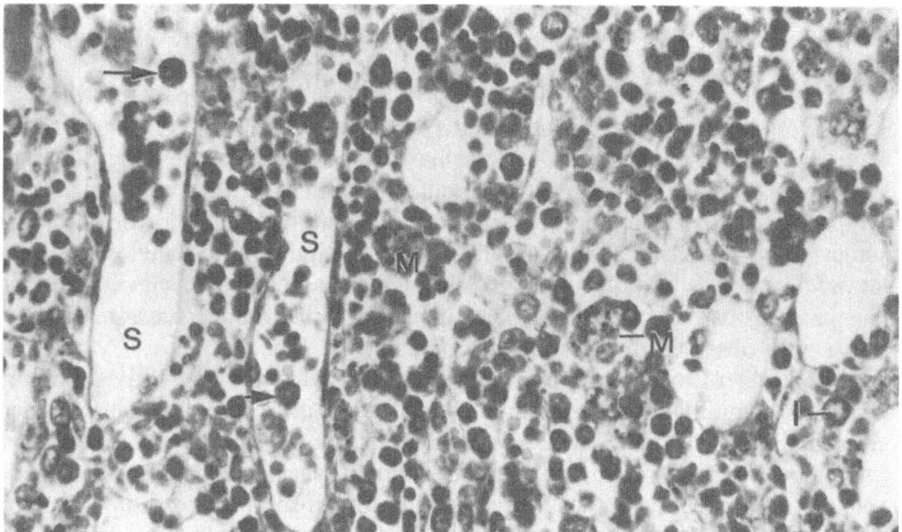


**Fig. 2.** Bone marrow showing active phagocytosis by macrophages (*M*) and migration of small and large transformed lymphocytes (*arrows*) into the sinusoids (*S*). *I*, immunoblast. HE, × 928

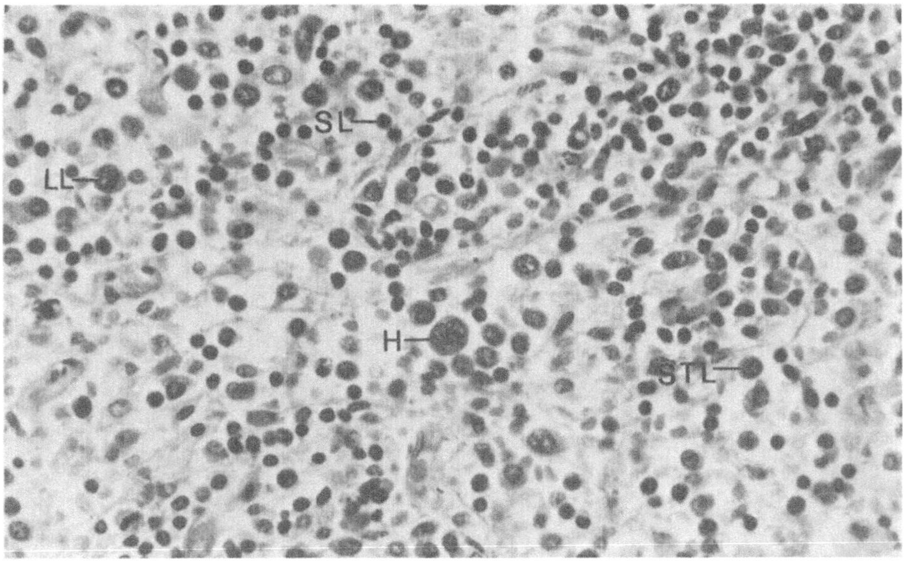


**Fig. 3.** Proliferation of lymphoid cells and histiocytes in a lymph node. *SL*, small lymphocyte; *STL*, small transformed lymphocyte; *LL*, large lymphocyte; *H*, histiocyte. HE, ×928

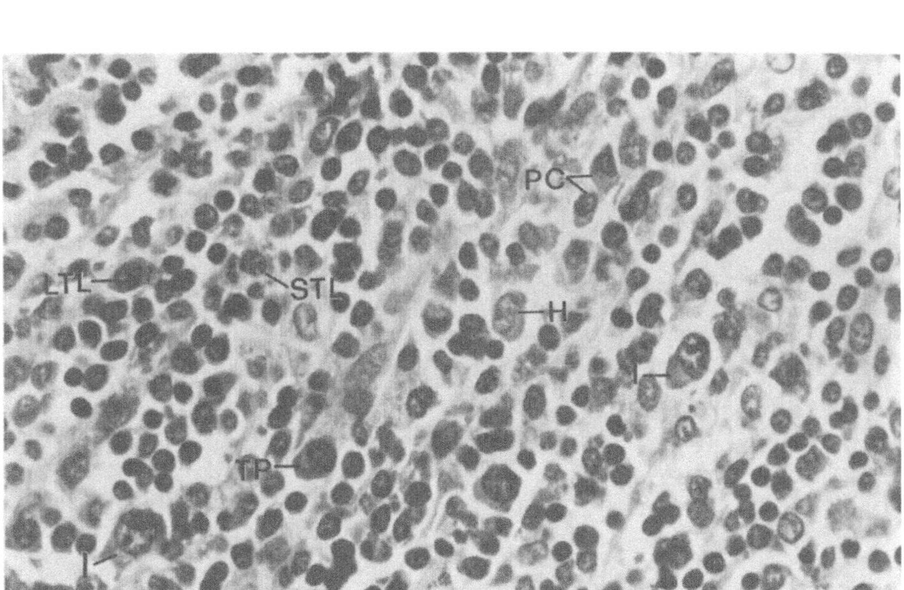


**Fig. 4.** Spleen is densely infiltrated with cells in the lymphocytic system. *PC*, plasmocytoid cells; *LTL*, large transformed lymphocyte; *STL*, small transformed lymphocyte; *TP*, transitional plasma cell; *I*, immunoblasts; *H*, histocyte. HE, ×1470

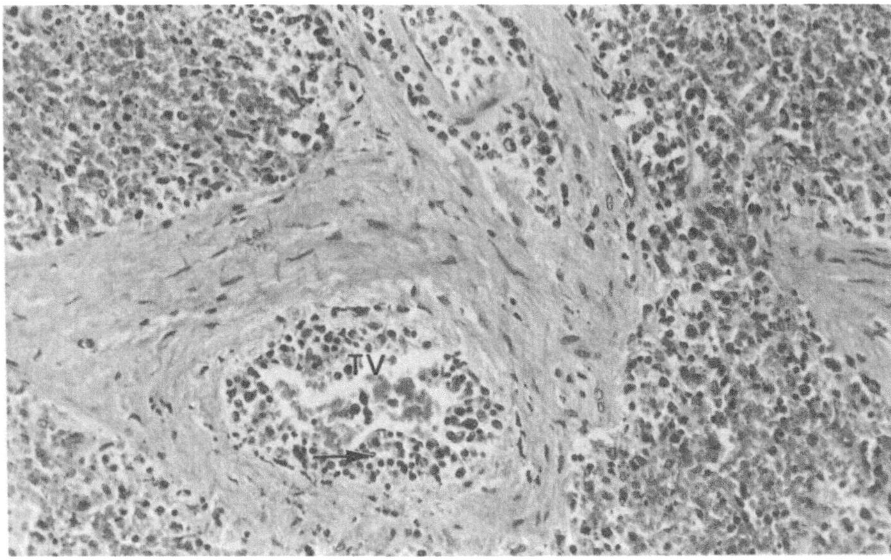


**Fig. 5.** Spleen in case with severe parasitaemia (90%) DIC and multiorgan involvement demonstrating proliferation of lymphoid cells (*arrow*) in the subendothelium of the trabecular vein (*TV*) with migration of these cells into the vascular lumen. Note the splenic sinusoids are congested with infected erythrocytes. HE, ×464

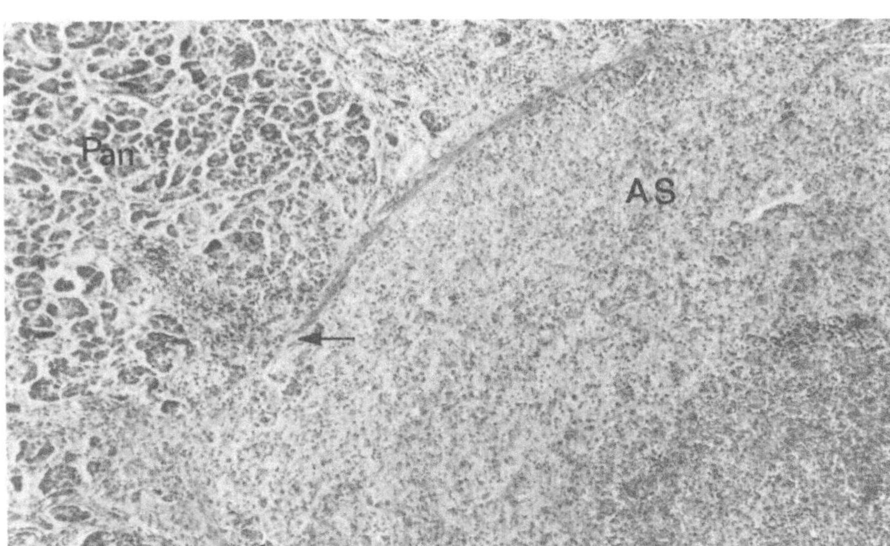


**Fig. 6.** Accessory spleen (*AS*) embedded in the tail of the pancrease (*Pan*), showing hyperplastic lymphoid cells penetrating through (*between arrows*) the splenic capsule into the pancreatic tissue. HE, ×928

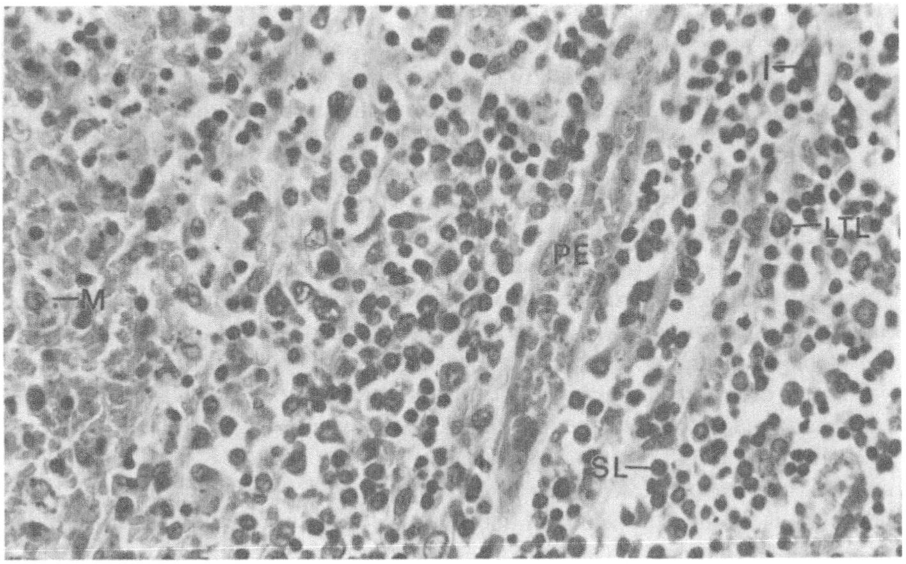


**Fig. 7.** Spleen showing lymphocytic cell hyperplasia. Splenic sinusoids and vessel are congested with parasitised erythrocytes (*PE*). *I*, immunoblast; *LTL*, large transformed lymphocyte; *SL*, small lymphocyte; *M*, macrophage. HE, ×928

noted (Fig. 6). Active phagocytosis of infected red cells, malaria pigment by macrophages and occlusion of small vessels by infected erythrocytes (Fig. 7) were also found. Evidence of extramedullary haematopoiesis, mostly of normoblastic erythropoiesis, was also present in the spleen.

c) Thrombocytopaenia and Coagulopathy

Thrombocytopaenia in malaria infection was observed by Hill et al. (1964) and was found in both *P. vivax* and *P. falciparum* (Fajardo and Rao 1971; Beale et al. 1972; Skudowitz et al. 1973). Two major mechanisms induce thrombocytopaenia in malaria, namely the increased destruction of platelets either by hyperactivity of RE cells and/or by immune destruction (Neva et al. 1970; Skudowitz et al. 1973), and disseminated intravascular coagulation (DIC) (Dennis et al. 1967). The latter was more severe and was believed to be more important clinically (Bergin 1967; Borochovitz et al. 1970; Punyagupta et al. 1974).

Coagulopathy has been observed in both falciparum and vivax malaria. However, in mild falciparum and vivax infection a mild coagulopathy, as reflected by either a prolongation of partial thromboplastin time or prothrombin time, without thrombocytopaenia and clinical bleeding was observed (Butler and Weber 1973; Jaroonvesama et al. 1975). It was believed that hepatic involvement during malaria infection caused this abnormality (Butler and Weber 1973). On the contrary, coagulopathy found in complicated falciparum infection was more severe, as indicated by the significant coagulation abnormalities accompanied by thrombocytopaenia and clinical bleeding. DIC was the most important mechanism for this abnormality.

d) Disseminated Intravascular Coagulation

DEVAKUL et al. (1966) considered that the disappearance of injected $^{125}I$-labelled fibrinogen in human falciparum malaria was most likely to be associated with intravascular coagulation. Subsequently the results from various investigations in man and animal models supported the evidence for DIC (BERGIN 1967; DENNIS et al. 1967; DENNIS and CONRAD 1968; BOROCHOVITZ et al. 1970; STONE et al. 1972; JAROONVESAMA 1972; REID and NKRUMAH 1972; GOODALL 1973; PUNYAGUPTA et al. 1972, 1974; JAROONVESAMA et al. 1975; JOHNSON et al. 1977). Massive intravascular haemolysis of the infected erythrocytes with their released thromboplastic substances was postulated to be an accelerated mechanism of intravascular coagulation. Furthermore, the activation of the complement system and massive releasing of blood histamine in severe falciparum-infected cases also initiated the development of DIC and other complications (SRICHAIKUL et al. 1975, 1976). On the other hand many studies have revealed negative evidence against the occurence of DIC (BEALE et al. 1972; BUTLER and WEBER 1973; SKUDOWITZ et al. 1973; VREEKEN and CREMER-GROOTE 1978; HOWARD and COLLINS 1972; REID and SUCHARIT 1972). However, it should be noted that the negative results were obtained from studies in mild or uncomplicated malaria. In our study of 51 severe falciparum malaria cases, DIC was observed in 33 cases (Table 7). The criteria used in the diagnosis of DIC were the concomitant findings of thrombocytopaenia, coagulopathy, increase in fibrin degradation products and the clinical evidence of multisystem involvement. It is also interesting to note that fibrin thrombi were found in 12 out

**Table 7.** Observed complications during the clinical course of 33 DIC[a] and 18 non-DIC cases among 51 complicated falciparum patients

| Manifestations | DIC (33 cases) | Non-DIC (18 cases) |
|---|---|---|
| Clinical | No. (%) | No. (%) |
| Cerebral complications | 31 (93) | 11 (61) |
| Non-oliguric renal failure | 11 (33) | 7 (39) |
| Oliguric renal failure (<20 ml/h) | 13 (39) | 0 (0) |
| Pulmonary complications | 20 (60) | 0 (0) |
| Cardiac involvement | 9 (27) | 0 (0) |
| Shock | 3 (9) | 1 (6) |
| Skin and mucous membrane bleeding only | 10 (30) | 2 (11) |
| Massive gastrointestinal bleeding | 9 (27) | 0 (0) |
| Hepatomegaly with abnormal transaminase (>100 units) | 7 (21) | 6 (33) |
| Haemoglobinuria | 8 (21) | 1 (6) |
| Mortality | 14 (42) | 0 (0) |
| Laboratory | Range/mean (%)[b] | Range/mean (%)[b] |
| Number of infected erythrocytes/100 erythrocytes | 5–100/ 20 (100) | 5–20/ 4 (100) |
| Platelets ($\times 10^3/mm^3$) | 20–50/ 38 (100) | 50–90/65 (80) |
| Partial thromboplastin time (s) | 50–88/ 78 (100) | 35–55/48 (22) |
| Fibrin degradation products (μg %) | 40–160/120 (100) | 0–20/15 (45) |

[a] Criteria for the diagnosis of DIC: see text. [b] Percent of abnormal results in each group

of 22 autopsy specimens (Tables 4, 5). The evidence of intravascular fibrin deposition lacking at autopsies reported previously (MAEGRAITH 1974) might be due to technical problems. To be able to demonstrate fibrin thrombi in the histopathological material a thorough search is essential, including multiple sections of various organs, and serial sections of the suspected areas which must be stained with special fibrin stain.

e) Bleeding

This complication has been observed only in falciparum infection. In general, petechiae, and purpura of the skin are the early manifestations. Subsequently, epistaxis, gum, and conjunctival haemorrhages are noted. Massive bleeding from the gastrointestinal tract is the terminal event. Nineteen out of the 33 DIC patients had bleeding from haemostatic failure, and nine presented massive, fatal, gastrointestinal bleeding (Table 7). This is in contrast to the non-DIC patients, of whom only two experienced milder bleeding. Furthermore, there was a definite correlation between the severity of bleeding and degree of coagulopathy.

The interrelations of DIC and bleeding could be demonstrated by histopathological study of the skin obtained from our autopsy specimens from falciparum-infected cases who had had bleeding. Grossly, the haemorrhage in the skin ranged from petechiae to ecchymoses and even diffuse hemorrhages. Microscopically, several specimens of skin obtained from small haemorrhagic spots showed arterial fibrin thrombi. The arteries and arterioles of subcutaneous tissue were the most common place to find the thrombosis (Fig. 8). Usually, large amounts of malarial pigment and nuclear debris were included in the thrombi. Thrombus was rarely detectable in the capillaries in the dermal papillae. Necrosis of the thrombosed arterial walls was an additional finding occurring together with haemorrhage and necrosis in the surrounding soft tissue (Fig. 9).

## 2. Water and Electrolyte Complications

The results of studies of the blood volume in acute malaria are contradictory, probably depending on the stage, the severity of the disease and the groups of individuals concerned (FELDMAN and MURPHY 1945; KEAN and TAYLOR 1946; MALLOY et al. 1967; SITPRIJA et al. 1967; CHONGSUPHAJAISIDHI et al. 1971). However, in mild to moderately severe cases increased plasma volume, water retention, and hyponatraemia are usually recognised (MALLOY et al. 1967), while in more severe cases a reduction in blood volume has been observed (CHONGSUPHAJAISIDHI et al. 1971). In some cases dehydration due to severe vomiting, inability to drink and marked perspiration from high fever are found. In such instances, hypovolaemia and hypotension may be observed and the increase in capillary permeability may lead to the stage of shock.

a) Hyponatraemia

In some severe cases inappropriate secretion of antidiuretic hormone may be the mechanism of production of hyponatraemia (MILLER et al. 1967). In severe hyponatraemic patients, the intravenous infusion of a moderate amount of fluid may lead to serious pulmonary complications. In our series moderate to marked hyponatraemia was a constant finding.

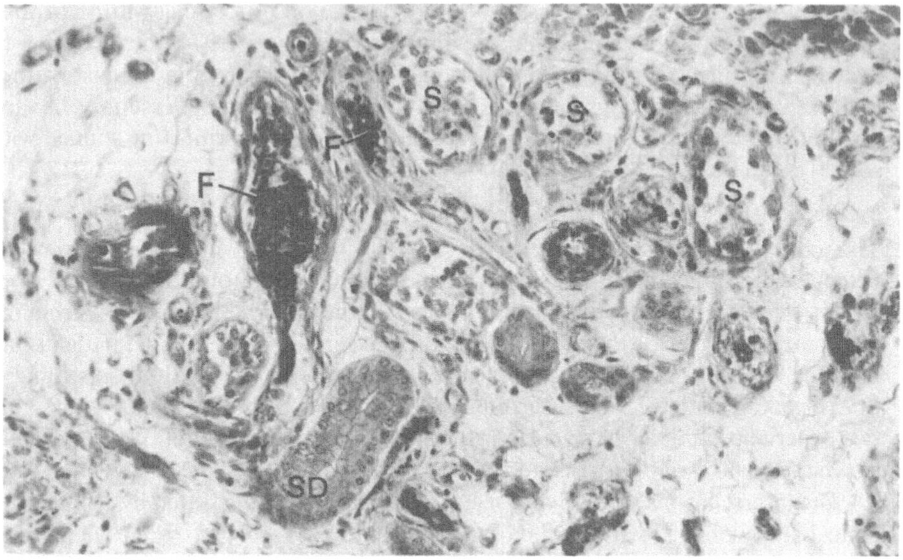


**Fig. 8.** Skin demonstrating fibrin thrombi (*F*) in arteries of subcutaneous tissue. Note necrosis of sweat gland (*S*). *SD*, sweat duct. PTAH, ×464

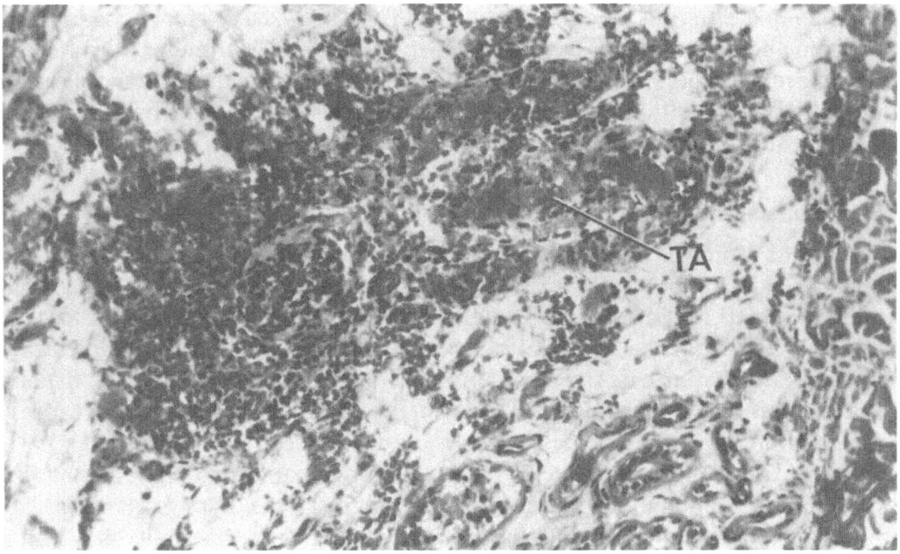


**Fig. 9.** Skin (same case as Fig. 8) showing necrosis of thrombosed arteries (*TA*) with diffuse haemorrhage. HE, ×464

b) Hypoproteinaemia

Diminished serum protein and albumin and slightly elevated globulin are observed in acute malaria. Only mild proteinuria is found. The increase in serum protein catabolism and probable decrease in albumin synthesis from liver dysfunction may be the responsible factors. Leakage of serum protein, particularly of albumin, due

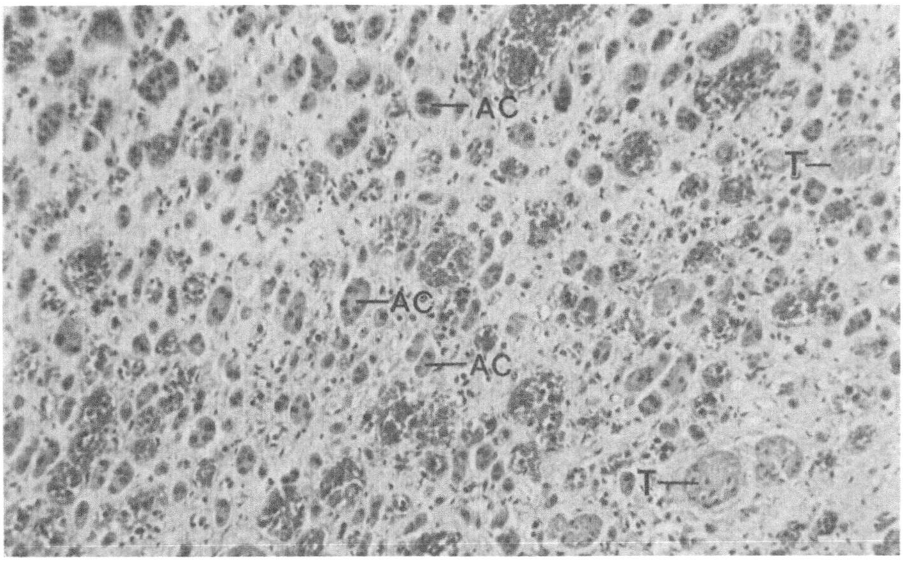


**Fig. 10.** Adrenal gland showing thrombosis (*T*) of the cortical vessels and severe atrophy of cortical cells (*AC*) with fibrosis. HE, × 232

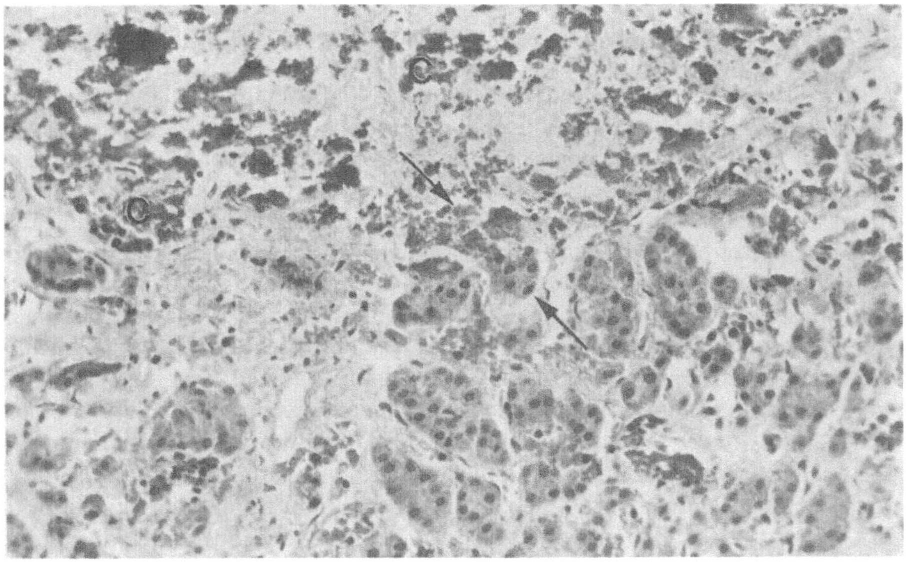


**Fig. 11.** Adrenal gland (same case as Fig. 10) demonstrating necrosis and calcification of cortical cell cord (*between arrows*). *C*, diffuse calcification in necrotic areas, HE, × 464

to the increase in vascular permeability has been considered. However, MALLOY et al. (1967) found that no marked loss of albumin across capillaries occurred. In our series hypoalbuminaemia and hypoproteinaemia were constant and, in some serious cases, the serum albumin was as low as 1 g/100 ml during the acute stage. This probably leads to further serious complications, particularly pulmonary oedema. Oedema in malaria may be due to a combination of increase in vascular permeability and fluid retention.

The symptom complex of hyponatraemia, diarrhoea, vomiting, and hypotension are characteristic evidence for adrenal cortical insufficiency. Pathological studies of adrenal glands have shown some changes, namely lipid depletion, of the adrenal cortices with some degree of oedema, haemorrhagic necrosis, degeneration, thrombosis, and cellular infiltration. BROOKS et al. (1969), however, found an increase in plasma 17-hydroxy corticosteroids, but a decrease in urinary steroids, probably reflecting decreased hepatic conjugation, and they concluded that the pituitary-adrenal function was normal.

The adrenals were studied microscopically in all our postmortems. In general the sinusoids were engorged with malaria pigment-laden macrophages (MPLM) and small numbers of infected red cells. In about 50% of cases, there were mild to severe degrees of cortical cell degeneration and lipid depletion, particularly of the zona fasciculata. In some cases, cells in this zone showed foamy and cystic degeneration, and necrosis. Each cord of these cells was replaced by mononuclear leucocytes and macrophages. Interestingly enough, one case in our series (case 3, Table 4) showed diffuse sinusoidal occlusion with fibrin-platelet thrombi associated with severe diffuse cortical cell atrophy (Fig. 10), with diffuse necrosis and calcification (Fig. 11). This case died in shock.

### 3. Liver Complication

Even though hepatomegaly is commonly encountered in acute or chronic malaria, serious liver complications are unusual (DELLER et al. 1967; RAMACHANDRAN and PERERA 1976). Jaundice is frequently observed and haemolysis may be the significant mechanism. In this study liver complications were much less frequent than those of brain, kidney or lungs (Tables 2, 3). Significant hepatic enlargement associated with hypertransaminasaemia of over 100 units was found in only 13 of the 51 cases. Liver function tests may be abnormal, increased liver enzymes indicating some degree of liver-cell injuries. Increased alkaline phosphatase is probably correlated to the Kupffer cell hyperplasia and the reduction in serum protein as already discussed. On microscopic examination of liver biopsy or autopsy specimens, the most specific feature of malaria infection is the presence of malaria pigment in the Kupffer cells. In SRICHAIKUL'S (1959) correlative study of liver function, degree of parasitaemia and liver biopsies, malaria pigment was present in Kupffer cells as early as the 6th day after the beginning of clinical symptoms, and would disappear between 3 and 6 months later. Although malarial pigment is an end product of the digestion of haemoglobin by the parasite, the amount of malaria pigment in the liver is not related to the degree of parasitaemia but depends on the duration or chronicity of the disease. In *P. falciparum*-infected *Aotus* monkeys, the pigment was first seen in the perilobular Kupffer cells, while later on the midzonal and centrolobular Kupffer cells were involved (AIKAWA et al. 1980). In experimental *P. lophurae* infections in young ducks, RIGDON (1944b) demonstrated phagocytic activity of the Kupffer cells beginning as early as the 2nd day of infection. Ultrastructurally, malaria pigment appears in two forms, a rectangular crystalloid formed in mammalian malaria, and a uniform electron-dense mass in avian and reptilian malaria (AIKAWA 1971). Some additional information on liver histopathology

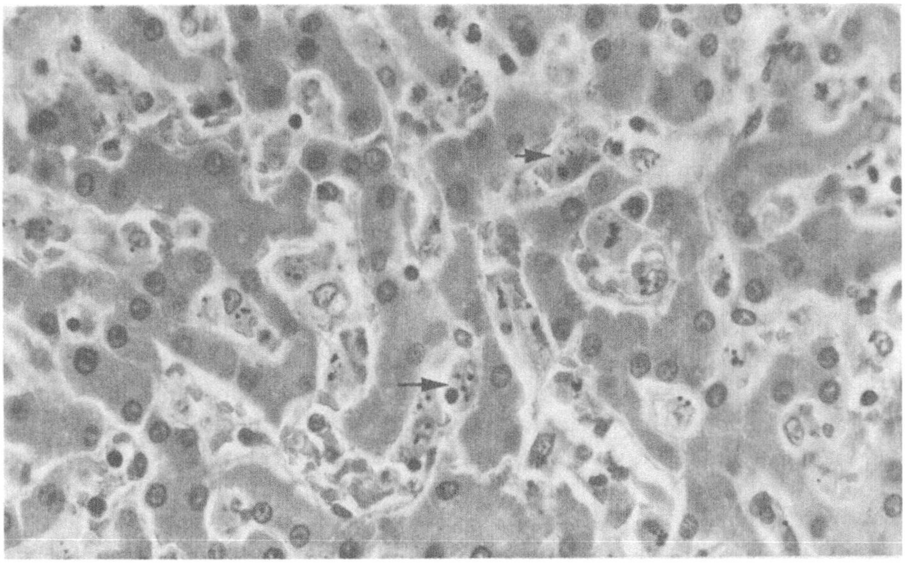

**Fig. 12.** Malarial pigment in Kupffer cells. Parasitised erythrocytes and mononuclear cells are also phagocytosed by Kupffer cells (*arrow*). HE, ×928

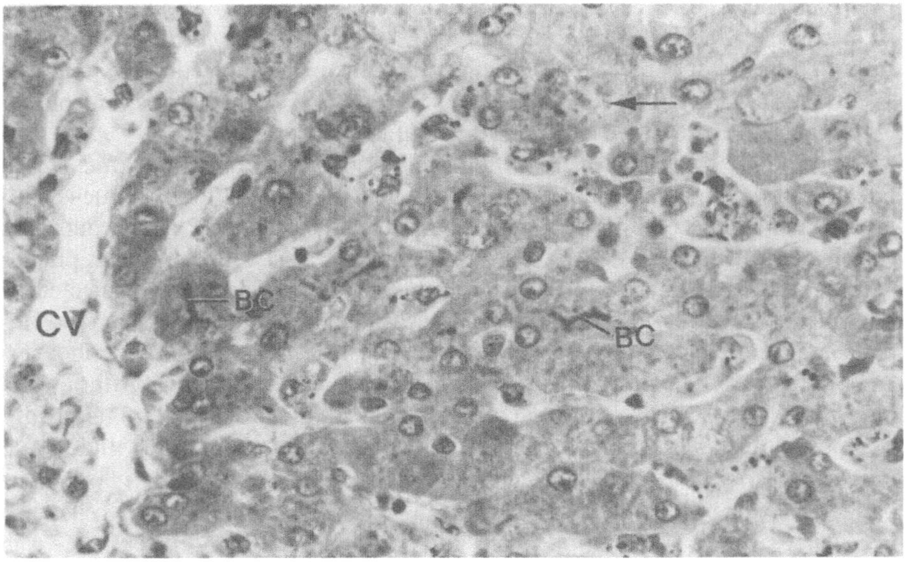


**Fig. 13.** Bile stasis in bile canaliculi (*BC*). Necrosis of certain liver cells is demonstrated (*arrow*). *CV*, central vein. HE, ×928

emerged from a series of liver biopsy studies. For instance, pre-erythrocytic forms of *P. vivax* were demonstrated in a liver biopsy obtained from a patient receiving treatment by mosquito-induced malaria on the 7th day after the first mosquito feed (SHORTT et al. 1948). In general, microscopic abnormalities of liver parenchyma were demonstrable in almost all biopsies from patients who had hepatitis associated with *P. vivax* (MCMAHON et al. 1954) and *P. falciparum* (DELLER et al. 1967) infection. In addition to hyperplasia and hyperactive phagocytosis by Kupffer cells, the liver cells showed mild to severe degeneration with necrosis of individual cells. Mitosis of liver cells was prominent. Acute and chronic inflammatory cell infiltration and non-specific granulomata were found randomly in the hepatic sinusoids and portal areas, and were most prominent in patients with hepatomegaly and jaundice (RAMACHANDRAN and PERERA 1976). On the contrary, WHITE and DOERNER (1954) found no hepatocellular lesions in a series of biopsies on *P. falciparum* or *P. vivax*-infected patients, although all of them had abnormal liver function tests. An electron microscopic study was made of a liver section taken 15 min postmortem from a patient with falciparum malaria associated with multiple complications. It showed plasma membrane disruption and mitochondrial dense bodies in liver cells. Kupffer cells or sinusoidal lining cells were vacuolated and contained parasitised or non-parasitised erythrocytes, and malaria pigment. This pigment appeared as membrane-bound osmiophilic bodies in which rectangular or trapezoidal areas were incorporated (ROSEN et al. 1967). Gross characteristics of autopsy liver in acute falciparum infection are enlargement and diffuse slate-grey discoloration of both capsular and cut surfaces. Microscopic lesions include all of the above-mentioned features as well as dense, mononuclear cell infiltration in the portal areas. Occasional presentation of small, round, hyaline material in the liver cells and Kupffer cells associated with necrosis of the liver cells has been described (SPITZ 1946). Centrolobular necrosis may be caused by portal venous constriction as a result of an adrenergic effect in acute malaria infection (MAEGRAITH 1974). In experimental studies by RAY and SHARMA (1958), the hepatic centrolobular lesions can be prevented in thoracic sympathectomised animals.

In our autopsy studies, histopathological lesions of the liver in *P. falciparum* infection could be divided into two main groups, the first without hepatic-cell alteration, and the second showing definite hepatocellular damage. Both groups had similar general characteristics of Kupffer cell hyperplasia with prominent phagocytic activity. The phagocytosed material included malaria pigment, infected or non-infected red cells, nuclear debris and occasional mononuclear leucocytes. Hepatic sinusoids were engorged with distorted erythrocytes, MPLM, lymphocytes and plasma cells. The liver cells of the first group were well preserved without definite mitotic change (Fig. 12). Local atrophic changes of the liver cells in this group were detectable and attributed to increased pressure in the sinusoids. Individual liver cell necrosis was rarely detectable. This group comprised the majority of patients who had moderate parasitaemia. In the second group, the liver cells were irregularly swollen with multiple nuclei and occasional patchy necrosis. There was centrolobular bile stasis in bile canaliculi (Fig. 13). The cytoplasm of these liver cells was clouded with small, round, hyaline masses, and occasional haemosiderin pigment. The patients in the second group had high parasitaemia and severe jaundice associated with other serious complications.

### 4. Brain Complication

The incidence of cerebral involvement in *P. falciparum* malaria is between 0.25% and 2.3% (DAROFF et al. 1967). The mortality varies greatly from none to as high as 50%. In our study cerebral complications were the most commonly encountered in 42 out of 51 complicated cases and the mortality was 33% (Table 3). In *P. vivax* infection cerebral complication is rarely observed (DHAYAGUDE and PURANDARE 1943) and it has never been recognised in *P. malariae* or *P. ovale* infection.

The change in the sensorium is usually progressive from confusion, disorientation, and lethargy to deep coma. Some may present with abrupt personality changes or frank psychosis. Others may experience focal neurological signs of tremor, twitching, chorea, myoclonus or hemiparesis. Those who recover will recover fully without residual neurological signs except in some rare instances.

Cerebral malaria is usually observed in patients with high parasitaemia but it may be found in cases with low parasite blood levels. Jaundice, anaemia, and renal impairment are frequently noted at the time of cerebral involvement. With effective therapy patients may recover rapidly within the first 24 h, but some may take a few days to regain consciousness. Some may not recover at all and die with cerebral as well as other complications.

There are various yet inconclusive explanations for the mechanism of cerebral malaria. Normally the cerebral vessels are permeable only to specific substances such as small carbohydrate molecules. Malaria infection induces some vasoactive substances which may cause the endothelium of the cerebral vessels to dysfunction, allowing a leakage of water and protein into the brain tissue. This leads to an increase in plasma viscosity, stasis of the cerebral circulation, and packing of erythrocytes, particularly those containing late schizogonic stages in the cerebral capillaries (MAEGRAITH 1969; MAEGRAITH and FLETCHER 1972).

It has been observed that, following the administration of quinine and chloroquine, the recovery of cerebral symptoms is very rapid in spite of the fact that parasitaemia may still be noted. MAEGRAITH and his colleagues at Liverpool showed that the protein leakage in the brain can be inhibited by anti-inflammatory drugs including chloroquine and corticosteroids.

In falciparum malaria deep schizogony occurs in various visceral organs (LUSE and MILLER 1971). The changes in the erythrocytic membrane which attaches to the endothelium may enhance the agglutination and trapping of erythrocytes to the small vessels, the so-called stickiness. Thus plugging of the vessels may contribute to the cerebral damage (AIKAWA et al. 1975). Investigation in rodent *P. berghei* malaria disclosed the fact that immune mechanisms may cause agglutination of infected red cells (WRIGHT 1968) and cerebral lesions can be prevented by antithymocyte antiserum (WRIGHT et al. 1971).

Studies in human falciparum infection have shown that involvement of the brain is associated with the presence of fibrin degradation products in the circulation (REID and NKRUMAH 1972; JAROONVESAMA 1972); yet the role of DIC in the pathogenesis of cerebral malaria is still inconclusive. A direct effect of "malarial toxin" on the blood vessel walls has not been proven. A role for malaria pigment in the production of cerebral thrombi was demonstrated in monkeys infected with *P. knowlesi* or by intravenous injection of disodium ferrihaemate (ANDERSON and MORRISON 1942). Of particular interest, BOONPUCKNAVIG et al. (1973) demonstrated by electron microscopy a focal injury of the glomerular capillary wall at the site of attachment of the sequestrated, parasitised erythrocyte in *P. berghei*-infected mice. They suggested that the lesion may represent a direct injury of

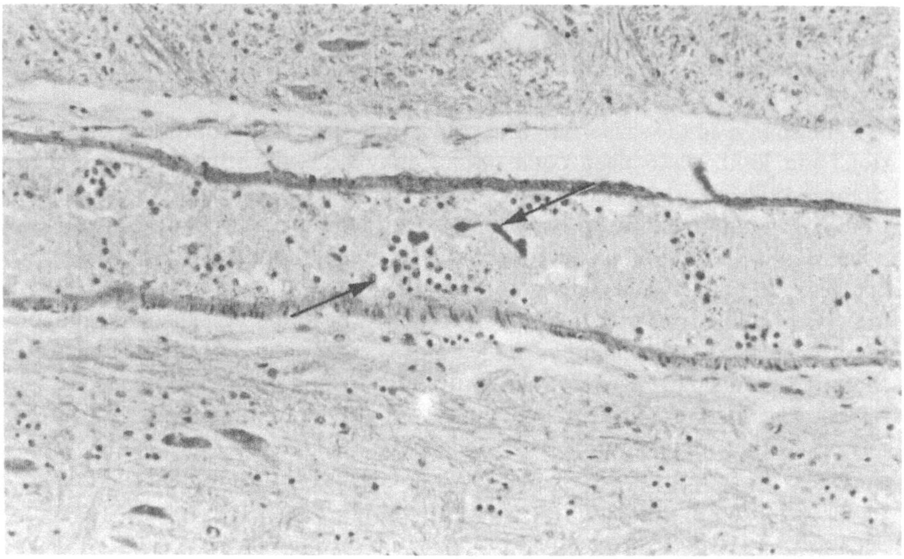

**Fig. 14.** Groups of infected erythrocytes, macrophages, mononuclear leucocytes, and fibrin thrombi (*between arrows*) circulating in an artery of the brain stem. HE, × 232

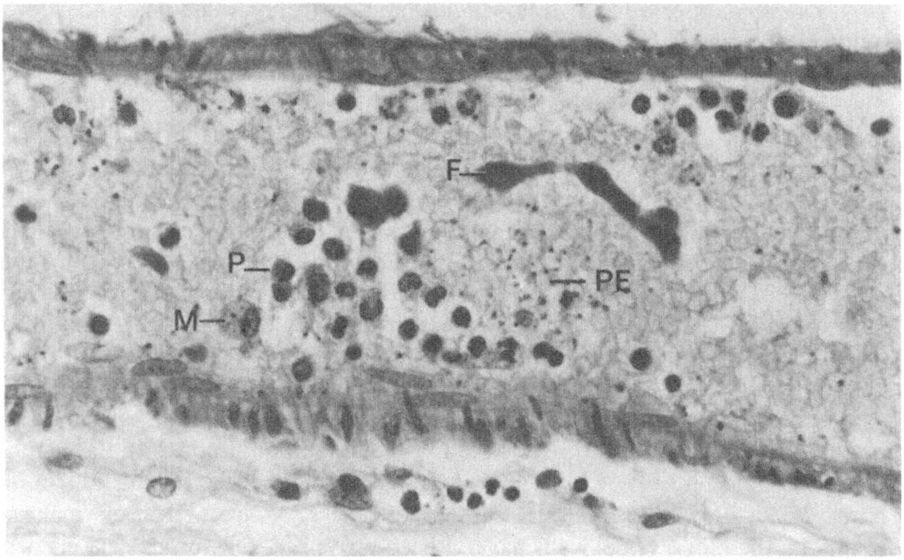


**Fig. 15.** Higher magnification of Fig. 14 showing details of the cells. *PE*, group of parasitised erythrocytes; *F*, fibrin thrombi; *M*, macrophage containing malaria pigment; *P*, plasma cell. HE, × 928

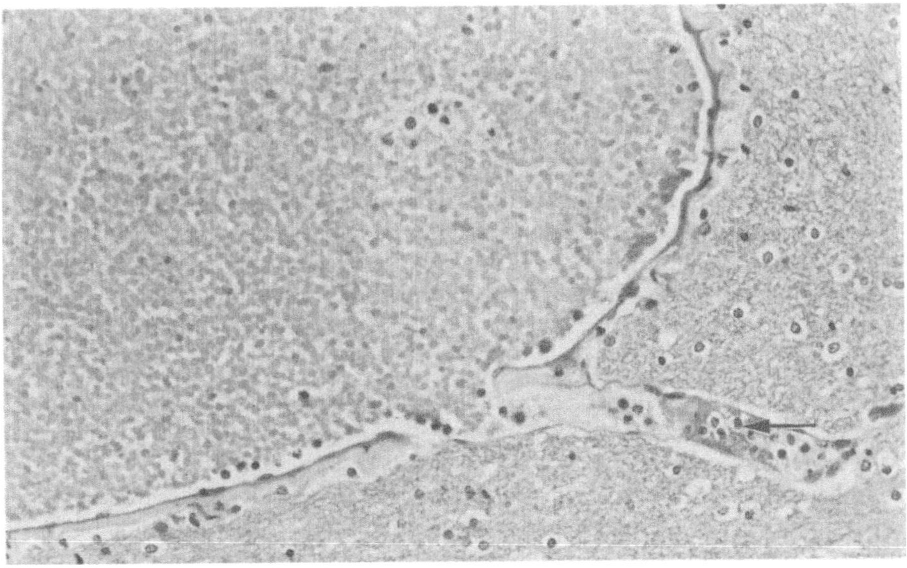

**Fig. 16.** Brain showing cystic dilatation of an arteriole. The outflow capillary is occluded (*arrow*). HE, ×464

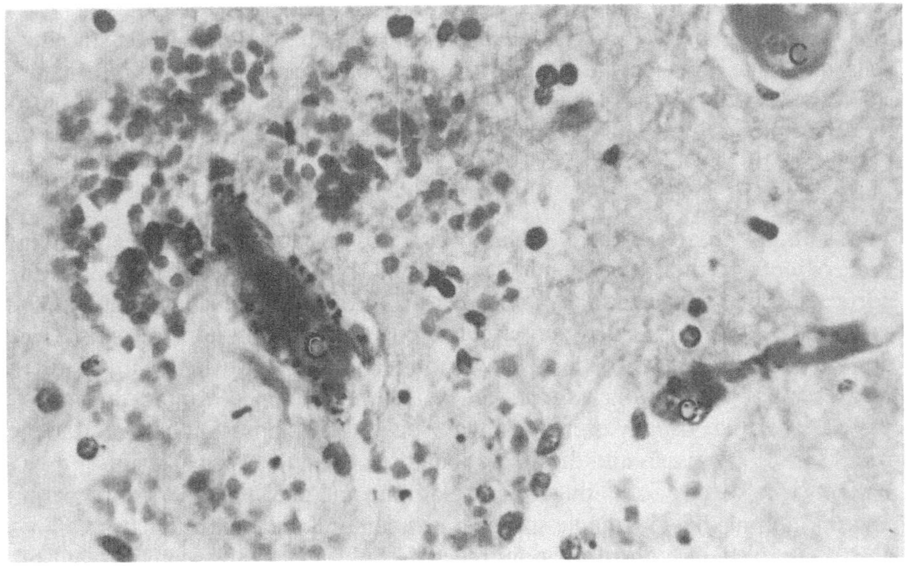

**Fig. 17.** Early developed ring haemorrhage and demyelinisation of brain tissue around a thrombosed capillary. Note all three capillaries (*C*) are occluded by fibrin thrombi. HE, ×928

glomerular capillary walls by malaria parasites or their metabolites. There have been several reviews of brain pathology in falciparum infection (Dhayagude and Purandare 1943; Spitz 1946; Winslow et al. 1975; Aikawa et al. 1980). Others are primarily concerned with the clinicopathological correlations (Thomas 1971) and pathogenesis (Maegraith 1948; Maegraith and Fletcher 1972). Grossly, brain may show only severe oedema and congestion. However, the striking characteristics of brains in cerebral malaria are distinct slate-grey discoloration due to the deposition of malaria pigment and numerous petechiae, usually seen in the meninges and on the cut surface of the cerebrum, cerebellum, and brain stem. In our study, specific microscopic lesions of the brain in the fulminating cases of falciparum infection which were fatal in the comatose stage of cerebral malaria are:

a) Vascular Occlusion

Most of the capillaries are congested with parasitised erythrocytes. The numbers and distribution of these infected erythrocytes are not correlated with the degree of antimortem parasitaemia.

Moreover, parasitised erythrocytes remained to be seen in the cerebral vessels in certain cases which had negative parasitaemia before death (see Table 5). In practice, almost all levels of capillaries in the brain and spinal cord are involved. In our study, cerebral vessels were also occluded by thrombi composed of fibrin, and a small amount of malaria-pigmented granules. This association of agglutinated, infected, red cells and fibrin thrombi was seen in 12 out of 22 patients (see Table 4). In the large calibre vessels, the infected red cells frequently rim the periphery of the lumen, and this has been called a margination effect.

Occasionally, in well-preserved specimens of brain, clumps of parasitised red cells, mononuclear phagocytic cells, lymphocyte, and plasma cells with fibrin masses are seen in the arteries (Figs. 14, 15). Consequently, cystic dilatation of the artery that may well be caused by a blockage of capillary outflow by these groups of cells and fibrin is observed (Fig. 16).

b) Haemorrhage

In our autopsy material there are many patterns of haemorrhage in cerebral malaria. Minute haemorrhages can be seen around thrombosed capillaries in the subcortical cerebral tissue and they are rather profuse in the cerebellum. The extravasated red cells in the dilated perivascular spaces are mostly non-parasitised with few infected cells. Haemorrhages that are discussed frequently in the literature, the ring haemorrhages, in our experience are always developed around thrombosed vessels. There has usually been a distinct zone of demyelinisation between the central thrombosed vessels and the area of hemorrhage in this type of lesion (Fig. 17). Patients who survive for a longer period of time and die with other complications present multiple haemorrhagic spaces in the cerebral and cerebellar tissue. These spaces are filled with ghosts of non-infected erythrocytes plus some infected cells (Fig. 18). Blood vessels of larger calibre than capillaries containing no agglutinated erythrocytes or fibrin thrombi are in the centre. However, adjacent to the vessel walls there are accumulations of fibrin and a few microglial cells.

c) Inflammatory Lesions

A variety of cellular reactions within the brain tissue have been described in cases of falciparum infection. The most common lesion, the so-called malarial or Durck's granuloma, occurs frequently in the white matter of all parts of the brain.

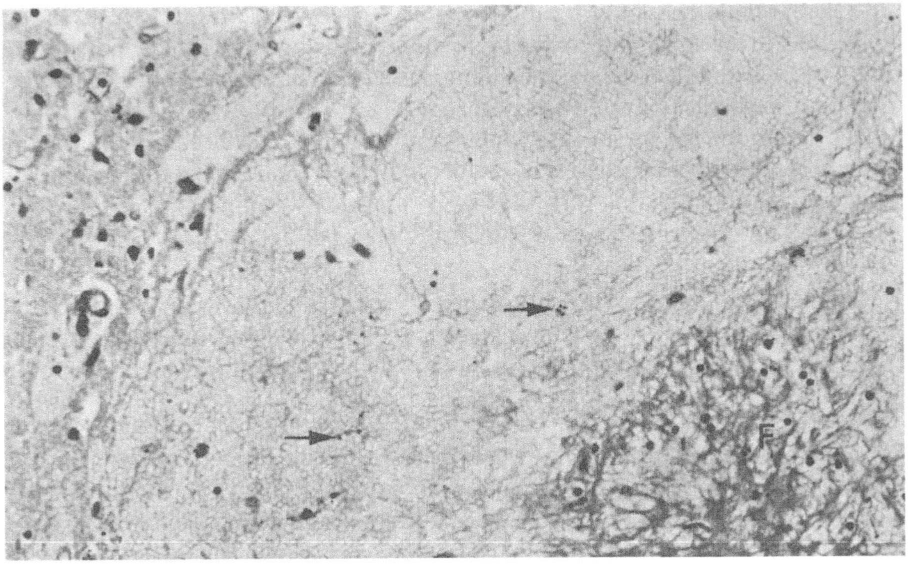


**Fig. 18.** A part of well-circumscribed space in brain containing ghost red blood cell and fibrin exudate (*F*). Small numbers of infected erythrocytes (*arrows*) are noted. HE, × 464

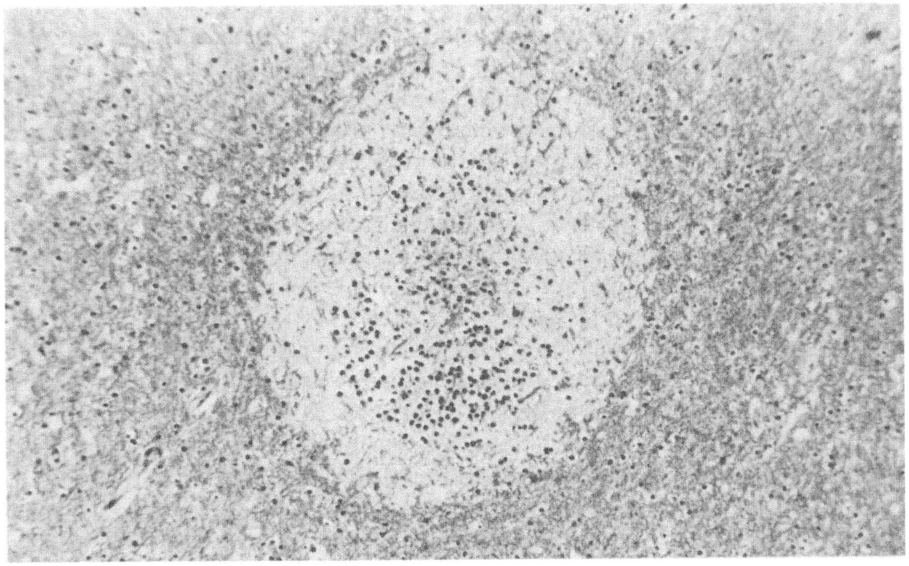

**Fig. 19.** A well-developed malarial granuloma in brain. HE, × 464

The lesions consist of a centrally located, thrombosed capillary, surrounded by necrotic brain tissue and small numbers of extravasated red cells, with accumulated glial cells. Necrotic neurones with glial reaction may present at the periphery of newly formed lesions. Glial cells and a few mononuclear leucocytes are more condensed in the well-developed lesions, which appear as light-staining, reticulated areas with a dark-staining centre (Fig. 19).

Glial granulomata have been interpreted as part of the repair process (SPITZ 1946). Extravasation of infected red cells, malaria pigment, fibrin, and possibly the free parasites stimulate the normal inflammatory cell, mainly mononuclear phagocyte, reaction in the brain and other organs.

Furthermore, the nerve cells in almost every region of the brain and spinal cord show some degree of degeneration and necrosis, with enlargement of the pericellular spaces (RIGDON and FLETCHER 1945).

## 5. Kidney

The kidney is an organ commonly involved in malaria, both in acute and chronic infections. Proteinuria of varying degrees is consistently observed. Azotaemia may be found even in uncomplicated cases, probably due to the hypercatabolism.

### a) Acute Renal Failure

Renal failure as demonstrated by oliguria, and rarely anuria, as well as increased blood urea nitrogen (BUN) and creatinine, occurs in less than 1% of cases (SHEEHY and REBA 1967). This complication is usually associated with a high level of parasitaemia, haemoglobinuria, and rapidly progressive anaemia (CANFIELD et al. 1968; CANFIELD 1969), liver and cerebral involvement and consumptive coagulopathy. Non-oliguric renal failure may also be observed in acute falciparum malaria. Recently, the pathogenetic mechanism of acute renal failure in malaria has been reviewed (BOONPUCKNAVIG and SITPRIJA 1979). In our clinical study of 51 complicated falciparum cases, 31 developed acute renal failure. Eighteen cases were non-oliguric in type and DIC was clinically detectable in 11 of these. DIC was evident in all 13 oliguric patients. The overall mortality rate of both oliguric and non-oliguric types was 45% and 100% in oliguric renal failure (Tables 2, 3). However, with early haemodialysis the mortality of oliguric patients was reduced to 40% (UBOLWATRA et al., personal communication). In 42 cases of acute renal failure reported by STONE et al. (1972) 67% died of pulmonary insufficiency. The oliguric phase may last from a few days to a few weeks with dialysis treatment. During recovery diuresis occurs, but not to the marked degree observed in classical, acute, tubular necrosis.

Blackwater fever is a well-known complication in acute *P. falciparum* malaria. This condition does not necessarily indicate any renal abnormality. Associated azotaemia and oliguria may be seen in some cases. It occurs as a result of rapid and massive intravascular haemolysis. The haemoglobin and its derivatives are successively excreted in the urine (MAEGRAITH 1944). In falciparum malaria haemolysis usually occurs extravascularly. Intravascular haemolysis may occur spontaneously, or it may relate to some therapeutic agents, particularly quinine. In areas where G6PD deficiency is prevalent this complication is commonly encountered (BENJAPONGSH 1966). Blackwater fever may be seen in cases with minimal parasitaemia. DUKES et al. (1968) have pointed out the important effect of a hypersensitivity state resulting from a partial loss of immunity which may cause a severe intravascular haemolysis upon reinfection. The histological changes of the kidney in patients who had clinical evidence of acute renal insufficiency vary from degeneration to tubular necrosis and, in some instances, tubulorhexis may occur. Renal biopsy obtained from patients with non-oliguric renal failure showed only focal vacuolisation of the proximal convoluted tubules without other abnormalities (SITPRIJA et al. 1967). On the other hand, STONE et al. (1972) reported that in the microscopic renal lesion of 42 cases, tubular degeneration and regeneration were the essential findings in biopsy specimens. The autopsy material showed patchy tubular necrosis and pigmented casts. In addition, these changes included tubular dilatation that was conspicuous in the distal and collecting tubules. The mitotic activity of regenerating cells was more pronounced in the macula densa than it appeared to be in other parts of the distal tubules (BOONPUCKNAVIG and SITPRIJA 1979). Significant tubular necrosis was also described in renal biopsies from patients with acute renal failure, jaundice, and anaemia (MUKHERJEE et al. 1971). Histological and electron microscopic findings in a renal biopsy in blackwater fever included tubular atrophy accompanied by lymphocytic infiltration, the demonstration of iron pigment within fibroblasts and atrophied tubular epithelium, while hyaline and eosinophilic casts in the tubules were reported (ROSEN et al. 1968). In an autopsy study SPITZ (1946) demonstrated deeply pigmented casts in the distal convoluted and collecting tubules associated with necrosis and regeneration of tubular epithelium in 14% of cases with clinical evidence of renal insufficiency. The amount of haemoglobin casts was reported to be greater in those cases with evidence of blackwater fever (WINSLOW et al. 1975).

Our study of fatal cases of acute renal failure concomitant with other severe complications, revealed various degrees of tubular damage ranging from minimal, non-specific degeneration to marked tubular necrosis involving most of the distal tubules, collecting and certain proximal tubules. Patients who recovered from the acute phase of renal failure and subsequently died with other complications have also shown regeneration of tubular epithelial cells, in approximately 80% the tubules containing eosinophilic, granular, haemoglobin casts, and necrotic epithelial cells (Fig. 20). Additionally special stains for haemoglobin and haemosiderin have revealed dense haemoglobin casts occluding the collecting tubules in the renal medulla (Fig. 21). These findings may explain the local severe dilatation of the tubule in the proximal portion (Fig. 22). Moreover, there were haemoglobin and traces of haemosiderin granules in the epithelial lining of the proximal convoluted tubules. By electron microscopy, these proximal tubules were seen to contain dense bodies in their cytoplasm (Fig. 23). Mononuclear phagocytic cells and chronic inflammatory cells were infiltrated in the interstitial tissue in association with severe tubular necrosis and tubulorhexis. Occasionally, these cells infiltrated round peritubular vessels which were occluded by parasitised red cells.

### b) Glomerulonephritis

Recently HOUBA (1979) has divided glomerulonephropathy associated with malarial infection into two main groups: (a) acute, transient, and reversible nephritis and (b) chronic, progressive renal lesions.

The first group developed in human falciparum infection (BERGER et al. 1967; HARTENBOWER et al. 1972; BHAMARAPRAVATI et al. 1973; FUTRAKUL et al. 1974), *P. falciparum* in *Aotus* monkeys (HOUBA 1975; HUTT et al. 1975), *P. cynomolgi* in rhesus monkeys (WARD and CONRAN 1966), and *P. berghei* in rodents (BOONPUCKNAVIG et al. 1972; V. BOONPUCKNAVIG et al. 1973; SUZUKI 1974; GEORGE et al. 1976).

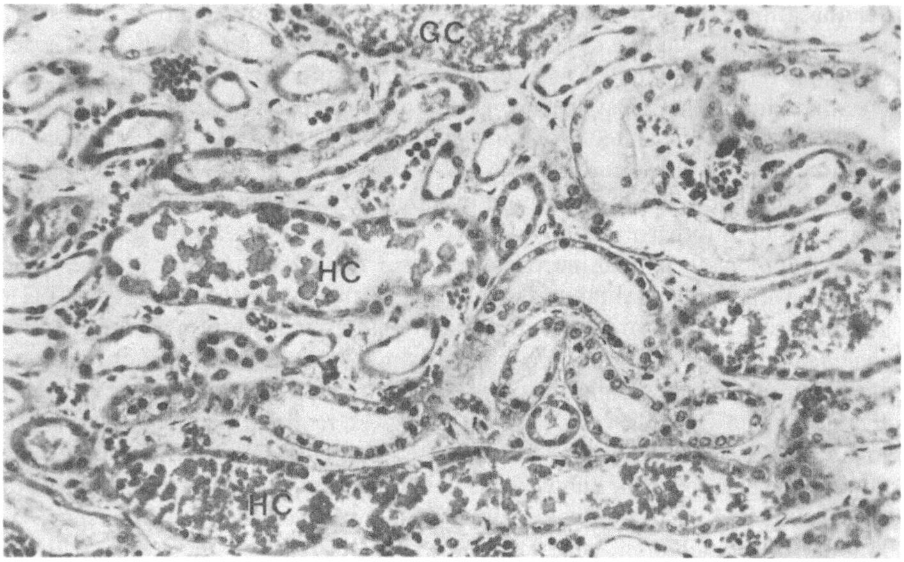


**Fig. 20.** *P. falciparum* infection with acute renal failure showing haemoglobin casts (*HC*) and granular cast (*GC*) in the convoluted and collecting tubules. HE, × 464

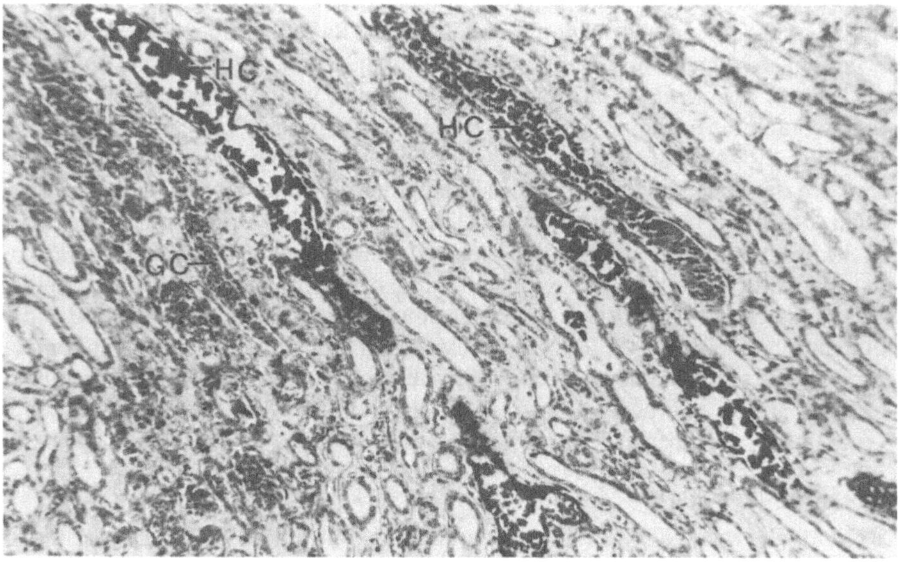


**Fig. 21.** Renal medulla showing dense collection of haemoglobin casts (*HC*) and granular cast (*GC*) in collecting ducts. Stained for haemoglobin, × 232

In patients with *P. falciparum* infection, urinary abnormality and glomerular pathology could be detected on about the 7th day after patent infection (BHAMARAPRAVATI et al. 1973). Light microscopy of renal biopsy tissue revealed mild hypercellularity of all glomeruli and irregular thickening of certain capillary walls. In our studies on autopsy kidneys, the pathological changes did not always

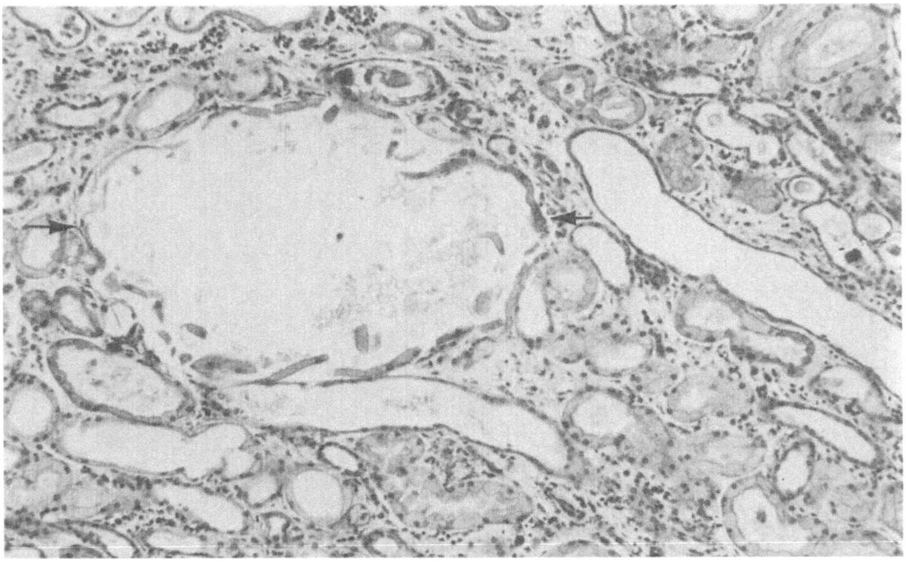

**Fig. 22.** Same cases as Fig. 21 showing cystic dilatation of a tubule (*between arrows*) in renal cortex. *P. falciparum* infection with acute renal failure. HE, ×232

correlate with the severity of the disease. There was no difference between glomerular alterations in DIC and non-DIC patients.

Glomerular hypercellularity is mainly due to the engorgement of capillary lumens with MPLM and mononuclear leucocytes, together with slight mesangial cell hyperplasia and increased mesangial matrix. A considerable amount of eosinophilic homogeneous or granular material is deposited along the capillary walls and in the mesangial areas (Fig. 24). Special stains show no definite thickening of the basement membrane. It should be added, however, that fibrin deposition in the glomeruli is very rare when compared with findings in the cerebral vessels. This may be explained by the fibrinolytic activity of kidney tissue (MYRHE-JENSEN 1971; SRAER et al. 1973). Fluorescent microscopy of both renal biopsy and autopsy specimens revealed granular deposits of immunoglobulins, complement and, in rare instances, malarial antigen in glomeruli during the 2nd and 3rd weeks of disease. The pattern of deposition is similar in all the cases. The complexes are confined mainly to mesangial areas and extend along certain contiguous loop walls (Fig. 25). IgM and BlC are most commonly deposited, together with IgG and IgA in a few cases. Eluates of immunoglobulin from autopsy kidneys have shown to be antimalarial antibody. Moreover, serum-soluble antigen was detected in cases with high parasitaemia (MCGREGOR et al. 1968; WILSON et al. 1969, 1975a, 1975b). Electron microscopy showed that lesions included electron-dense deposits in the subendothelial and paramesangial areas. Entrapment of deformed or fragmented erythrocytes in the spaces formed by folds of endothelium and subendothelial deposits of granular and amorphous particles were demonstrated (BHAMARAPRAVATI et al. 1973; BOONPUCKNAVIG and SITPRIJA 1979).

The evolution of the glomerular lesions was observed in mice infected with *P. berghei* (BOONPUCKNAVIG et al. 1972; V. BOONPUCKNAVIG et al. 1973). By im-

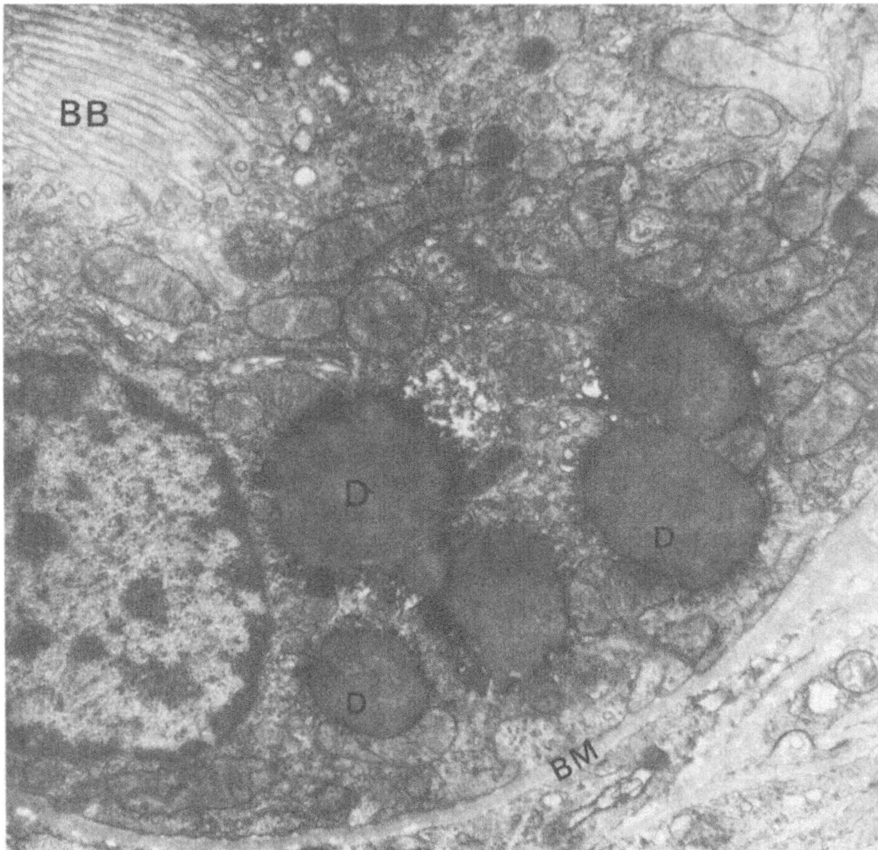


**Fig. 23.** Electron dense bodies (*D*) in an epithelial cell of proximal tubule in *P. falciparum* infection. *BB*, brush border; *BM*, tubular basement membrane. Electron micrograph, × 15400

munofluorescent microscopy, malarial corpuscular antigen in erythrocytes was detected in vessels on day 3 of the infection (S. BOONPUCKNAVIG et al. 1973). At the same time, either free-floating parasitised erythrocytes or groups of cells including infected erythrocytes, mononuclear phagocytic cells and lymphocytes appeared within the glomerular capillaries (Fig. 26) as was shown also in the cerebral vessels by light microscopy (Figs. 14, 15).

During the 2nd week of infection granular formed antigen, mouse globulin and C3 were diffusely deposited in mesangial areas and distributed along certain glomerular capillary walls. The eluated gammaglobulin from the kidneys proved to be anti-*P. berghei* antibody. Electron-dense deposits were demonstrated in the glomeruli from the 2nd week of infection onwards (V. BOONPUCKNAVIG et al. 1973). On day 10 of the infection serum-soluble malarial antigen and antimalarial antibody were detected (BOONPUCKNAVIG et al. 1976). By light microscopy proliferative lesions of glomeruli were most severe on day 14 of the infection. The sever-

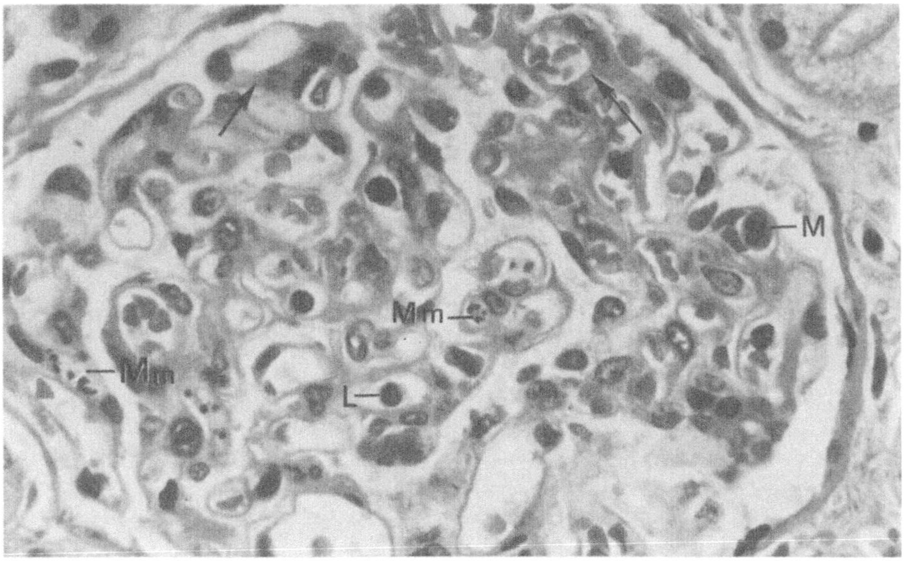


**Fig. 24.** *P. falciparum* infection, autopsy kidney. A glomerulus showing mild hypercellularity and irregular deposits of homogeneous, eosinophilic material (*arrows*) in mesangial areas. *M*, monocyte; *Mm*, malaria pigment-laden macrophages; *L*, lymphocyte. HE, × 1470

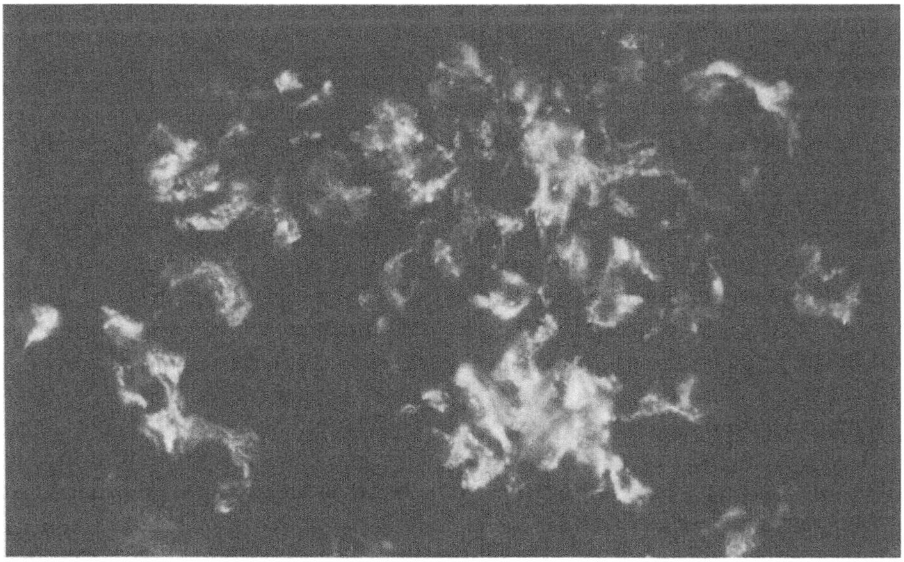

**Fig. 25.** Same case as Fig. 24 showing granular deposits of IgM in mesangial areas and along certain capillary walls. Fluorescent anti-human IgM, × 1470

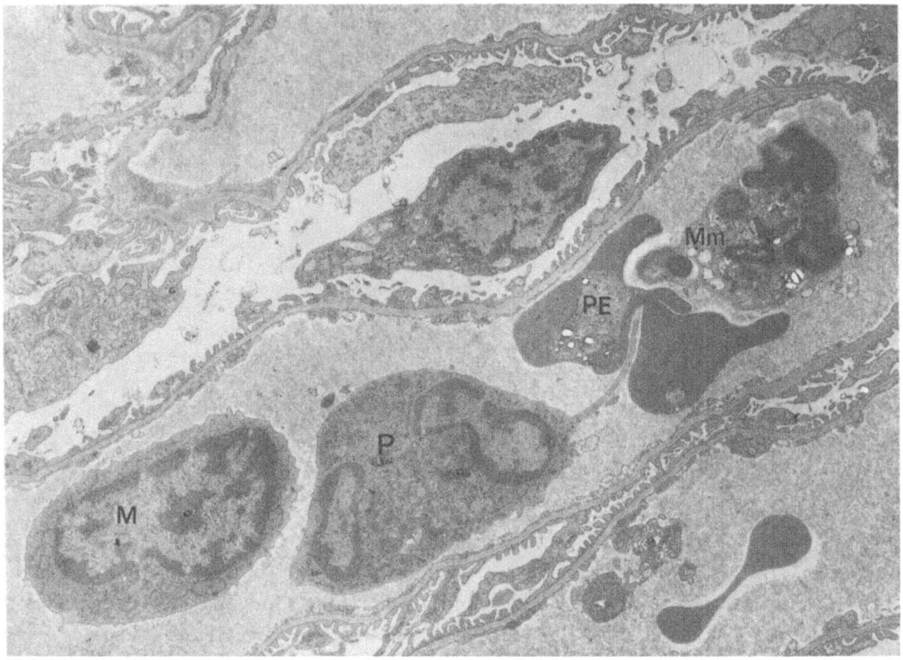


**Fig. 26.** Kidney in *P. berghei*-infected mouse, day 3 of infection, showing phagocytic activity of macrophage in the circulation. Note a parasitised erythrocyte (*PE*) is about to be phagocytosed by a phagocytic cell (*P*). Glomerular structures appear normal. *Mm*, malaria pigment-laden macrophage; *M*, monocyte. Electron micrograph, ×9165

ity of glomerular pathology, immunopathology, and course of disease could be modified in this experimental model.

The amount of granular antigen and intensity of immune complex deposits on the glomeruli are reduced in mice receiving an injection of colloidal carbon before or during the *P. berghei* infection (S. BOONPUCKNAVIG et al. 1979). Furthermore, malarial immune complexes were not detected in the glomeruli of *P. berghei*-infected mice which were treated with an immunosuppressive drug (cyclophosphamide) on day 5 of the infection (ENDARDJO et al. 1978). Recently V. BOONPUCKNAVIG et al. (1979) reported a different pattern of glomerular lesions in *P. berghei*-infected mice that received a suboptimal dose of the antimalarial drug chloroquine. The hyperimmune animals showed focal, immune complex, glomerular lesions. Recently PARBTANI and CAMERON (1979) reported detailed clinical information on this experimental animal model.

The special feature of this type of malaria glomerulonephropathy is the good response of the disease to treatment by antimalarial drugs.

The second group of glomerulonephropathy is associated with *P. malariae* in children and adults (GILLES and HENDRICKSE 1960, 1963; KIBUKAMUSOKE et al. 1967; KIBUKAMUSOKE 1968; ALLISON et al. 1969) and in the *Aotus* monkey (VOLLER et al. 1971, 1973; HOUBA 1975). KIBUKAMUSOKE and HUTT (1967) reported the histological findings in renal biopsies from 77 nephrotic patients in Uganda. Twenty-nine of the 31 cases, both children and adults, in whom *P. malariae* was found showed various types of proliferative glomerular lesions, including minimal, focal, lobular, and chronic forms. The most common glomerular alteration in adults was reported to be proliferative glomerulonephritis characterised by proliferation of endothelial cells and occasional lobulation. Severe glomerulosclerosis appeared in a few adolescent patients.

HENDRICKSE et al. (1972) presented the results of light and immunofluorescent microscopic studies on renal biopsies in their collaborative clinicopathological study of 63 Nigerian children. Early in the course of the disease, there was thickening of the glomerular capillary walls. This change appeared to be segmental and affected only a few glomeruli. Special stains showed double contours of plexiform arrangements and fibrillary thickening of the basement membrane. Later on, more capillaries were involved and narrowing of some capillary lumens was prominent. Eventually, the whole glomerulus was hyalinised and sclerosed accompanied by extensive tubular atrophy and interstitial mononuclear cell infiltration. The severity of the histopathological lesions was divided into three grades which could be correlated with the results of treatment. Immunofluorescent examination showed glomerular, granular deposits of immunoglobulins in almost all the renal biopsy specimens (SOOTHILL and HENDRICKSE 1967; HOUBA et al. 1970, 1971; HENDRICKSE et al. 1972). There were certain differences in the sizes and patterns of the deposits (WARD and CONRAN 1969). The most common finding was of coarse, granular deposits distributed along the capillary walls. Very fine granules, uniformly distributed along the capillary walls, were found in a minority of cases. A mixed pattern was also observed. The relationship between the pattern of immunoglobulin deposits and response to treatment has been documented (HENDRICKSE et al. 1972). IgG and IgM may be detected together, or either of them may deposit alone. C3 can be detected in certain specimens but less extensively than immunoglobulin deposits. In about one-third of cases, *P. malariae* granular antigen was detected. Soluble antigen of *P. malariae* could be detected only by sensitive radioisotopic techniques in sera of man and monkeys with this infection (HOUBA et al. 1976).

Electron microscopic studies of biopsy specimens showed localisation of the electron-dense material within the glomerular basement membranes (HOUBA et al. 1970; ALLISON and HOUBA 1976). Irregular thickening of the basement membranes was very pronounced. The presence of small, lacunae scattered throughout the basement membrane appeared to be a constant finding in quartan malarial nephritis as described by HENDRICKSE and ADENIYI (1979).

In conclusion, studies in man and experimental animal models indicate that immune complexes play an important role in the pathogenesis of both groups of glomerulonephropathies associated with malaria. However, glomerular injury in the first group is reversible after antimalarial drug therapy. On the other hand, glomerulonephropathy in the second group is progressive and does not respond to antimalarial drugs. Several factors that promote chronicity of the latter group of glomerular disease have been proposed and these hypotheses are well summarised in WHO (1972) and HOUBA (1979).

## 6. Gastrointestinal Tract

In acute malaria, while gastrointestinal symptoms of anorexia, nausea, vomiting, abdominal pain, and diarrhoea are frequently observed, the true mechanism has not been elucidated. Olsson and Johnston (1969) and Karney and Tong (1972) reported abnormal D-xylose and other absorptive tests as well as abnormal biopsies of the small intestine in falciparum malaria. Ischaemic changes of the mucosa may in part be responsible for this abnormality (Maegraith and Fletcher 1972). Vasoconstriction of the intestinal arterioles has been demonstrated, which may be explained on the basis of hyperexcitation of the sympathetic nervous system (Skirrow et al. 1964).

Gastrointestinal bleeding has been observed in severe falciparum malaria with evidence of DIC. Some patients may present with melaena. In our study of 33 falciparum cases with evidence of DIC, nine experienced massive gastrointestinal bleeding and all of these died (Table 7). Bleeding was observed on admission in four cases, was noted during the clinical course in five, and three of these five received heparin administration for the treatment of DIC.

Postmortem examination of the gastrointestinal tract has shown multiple foci of mucosal haemorrhage in the stomach, small intestine and, occasionally, in the colon. Histopathological changes in non-haemorrhagic areas include dense accumulations of parasitised erythrocytes, MPLM, lymphocytes, and plasma cells in the oedematous lamina propria. Fibrin thrombi are demonstrable in submucosal arterioles (Fig. 27) in one case (case No. 3, Tables 4, 5). These changes are more pronounced in the jejunum than in the other parts of the gastrointestinal tract.

## 7. Cardiopulmonary System

Of all the complications in falciparum malaria cardiopulmonary involvement is considered the most serious that usually leads to a fatal outcome.

Cardiac dysfunction has been noted clinically, particulary in the terminal stage of malaria; yet pathological changes of the myocardium have rarely been specified in previous studies. Acute myocardial infarction complicating falciparum infection has only been documented in a few cases reported by Merkel (1946).

In our autopsy study of falciparum infection, dilatation of the myocardial capillaries was remarkable. These vessels were distended with both infected and non-infected red cells as well as groups of mononuclear phagocytes, lymphocytes, and plasma cells (Fig. 28). Extravasation of infected and uninfected red cells accompanied by cellular inflammatory responses appeared locally in the interstitial tissue.

In spite of the fact that fibrin thrombi could be detected in several organs in severe cases complicated by DIC, none of these had fibrin thrombi in the coronary arteries and their branches. Acute myocardial infarction was not discovered in our study although cardiac arrest had been the immediate cause of death in three cases.

In recent years pulmonary complications have been noted more frequently than previously. They may be divided into two categories, acute pulmonary oedema and acute respiratory insufficiency.

In cases with acute pulmonary oedema the clinical features simulate those of classical pulmonary congestion of cardiac origin, namely evidence of fluid overload caused either by excessive intravenous infusion or oral intake or both, high central venous pressure, congestive hepatomegaly with hepatojugular refluxes, engorgement of the neck veins and congestive rales in both lungs. In most instances

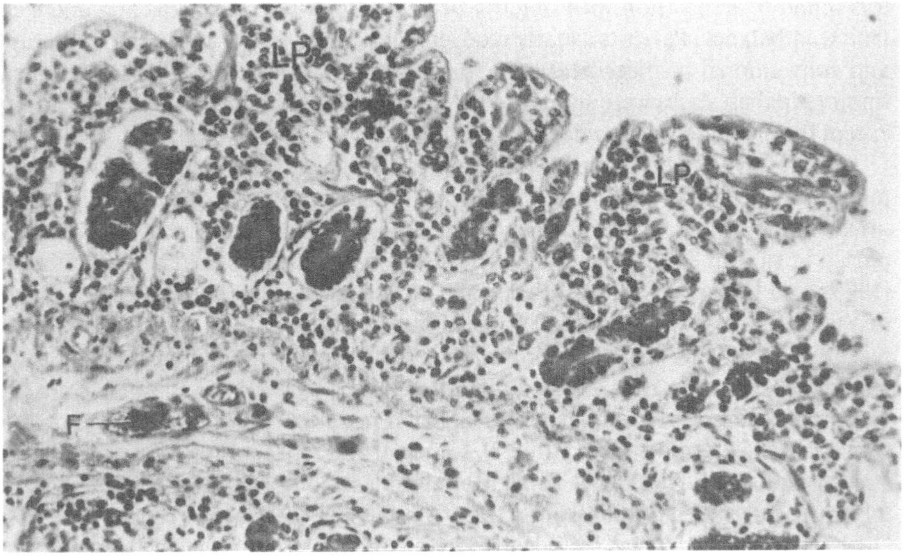


**Fig. 27.** Jejunum, showing dense infiltration of lymphocytes, plasma cells and malaria pigment-laden macrophages in the lamina propria (*LP*). Fibrin thrombus (*F*) is within the lumen of an arteriole. HE, × 464

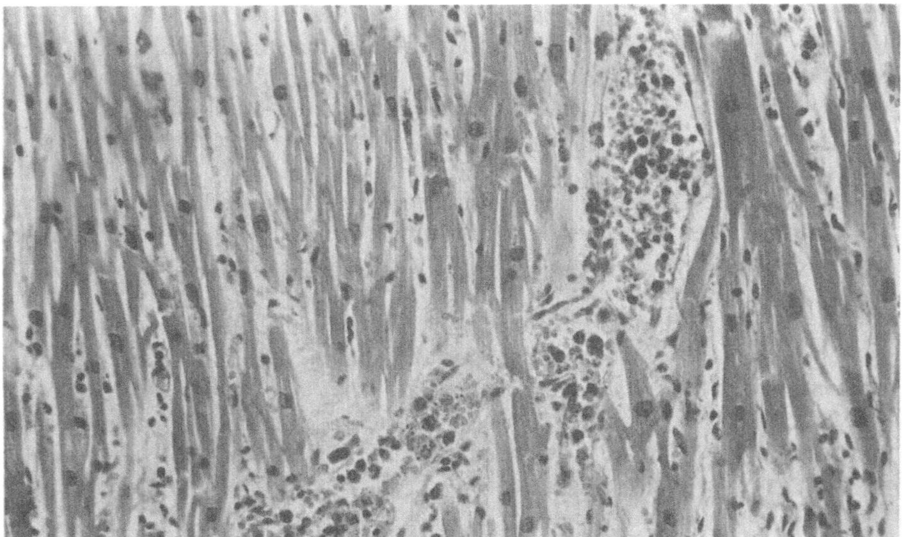

**Fig. 28.** Left ventricle showing myocardial vessels congested with parasitised erythrocytes and clusters of lymphoid cells and macrophages. HE, × 464

it is found in association with oliguria or anuria with hypoproteinaemia and electrolyte imbalance. Patients usually recover following effective antimalarial therapy and conventional medical treatment for pulmonary congestion. The pathological findings in these cases were similar to those of pulmonary oedema of cardiac origin, except for the evidence of malaria infection.

Another type of pulmonary complication, the so-called malarial lungs or acute pulmonary insufficiency is most serious, least understood and only recently recognised. In fact this is the "adult acute respiratory distress syndrome" (ARDS) reported in various severe bacterial or viral infections. Brooks et al. (1968), Sheehy (1975), and Deaton (1970) have reported a total of ten cases of American soldiers in Vietnam, all of whom died in spite of intensive therapy. In Thailand we have reported 12 patients with acute pulmonary insufficiency in falciparum malaria of whom nine died (Punyagupta et al. 1974).

In our series of 51 complicated falciparum malaria, 20 cases had lung complications, with 70% mortality (Table 2). Cerebral and renal complications were constantly associated with them (Table 3). Pulmonary complications in *P. falciparum* infection were also reported from Africa (Marks et al. 1977; Martell et al. 1979). Other pulmonary changes included reversible interstitial pulmonary oedema (Godard and Hansen 1971), and bilateral pleural effusion (Al-Ibrahim and Holzman 1975). Haemodynamic studies by Fein et al. (1978) suggested that pulmonary oedema was the result of a change in capillary membrane permeability. Tong et al. (1972) studied the pulmonary function in pulmonary complications of falciparum malaria and found a decrease in arterial oxygen tension, pulmonary shunting and increase in total and resistive work.

This complication of acute pulmonary insufficiency, or ARDS, in malaria is a separate entity from pulmonary oedema, even though in some cases evidence of fluid overload may also be found. The classical features are as follows:

1. It is found in the 1st week or early 2nd week of acute falciparum malaria with heavy parasitaemia.

2. Other complications, particularly of cerebral, renal, and haematological involvement, are recognised prior to the lung complications. In some cases, fluid overload may be the precipitating factor. Central venous pressure is usually low at the time of attack.

3. Patients develop abrupt respiratory distress, namely tightness in the chest, orthopnoea, cyanosis, severe cough, and tachycardia. Laboratory tests show hypoxaemia in spite of intensive oxygen therapy. The disease runs a rapidly progressive course and the patient usually succumbs during the first 24 h or soon afterwards. Extensive respiratory care including a peep ventilator may be life saving if malarial parasites can be eradicated in time, and other complications, particularly those of electrolyte and haematological abnormalities and renal involvement, can be corrected.

Pathologically, in general congestion, oedema, and haemorrhage are among the common gross findings. Microscopically, the pulmonary lesions appear in many forms. Throughout most of both lungs there is distention of alveolar capillaries due to the accumulation of clusters of cells including infected red cells, MPLM, lymphocytes, and plasma cells (Fig. 29). Increased pulmonary reticuloendothelial activity has been demonstrated by the increased lung uptake of technetium 99M-sulphur colloid (Ziessman 1976).

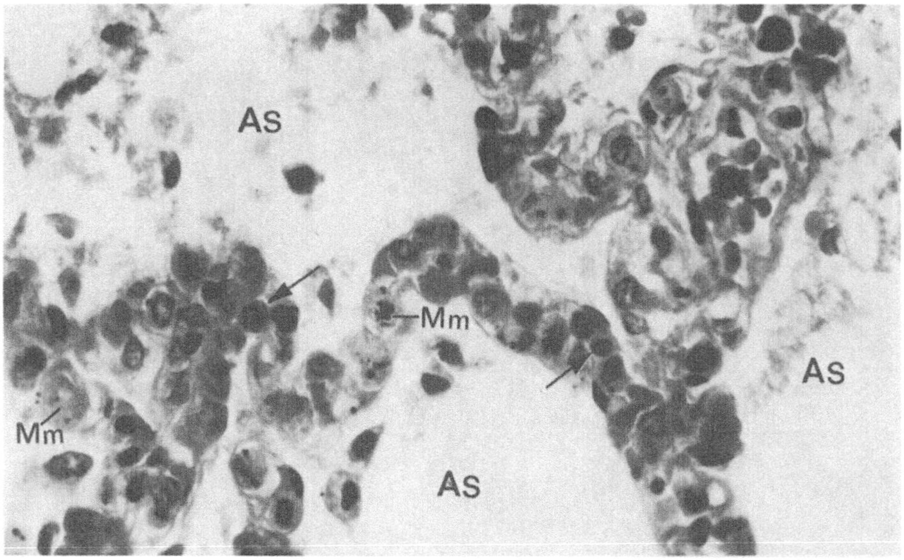


**Fig. 29.** Pulmonary alveolar capillaries congested with malaria pigment-laden macrophages (*Mm*), lymphocytes and plasma cells (*arrows*). *AS*, alveolar space. HE, × 1470

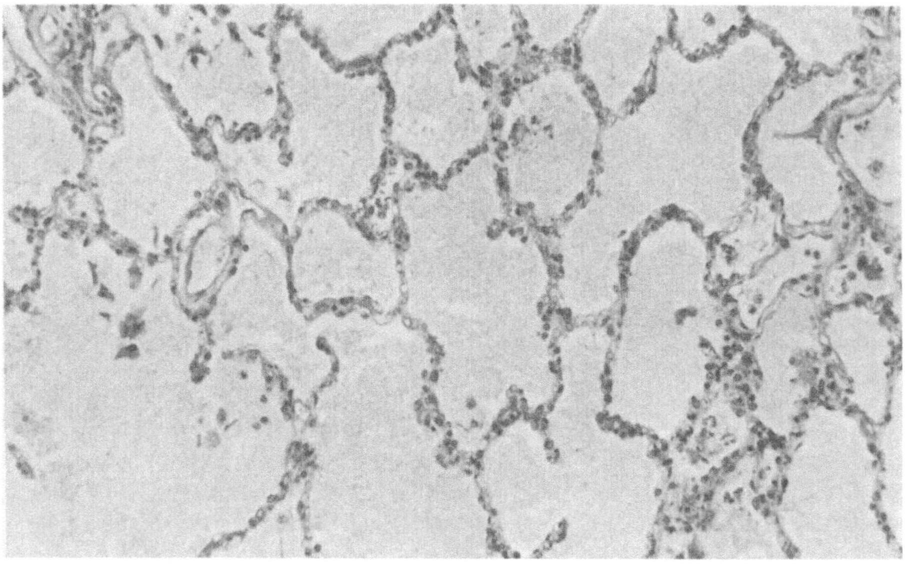

**Fig. 30.** Showing severe oedema of lung. HE, × 368

In addition, our postmortem examinations of lungs from falciparum-infected patients who had terminal pulmonary complications have shown three distinct histological features. In the majority of cases (see Tables 4, 5) the alveoli and alveolar ducts contain pale, eosinophilic, proteinaceous fluid (Fig. 30) with scattered, small, haemorrhagic foci. Changes are similar in both lungs in all cases except for

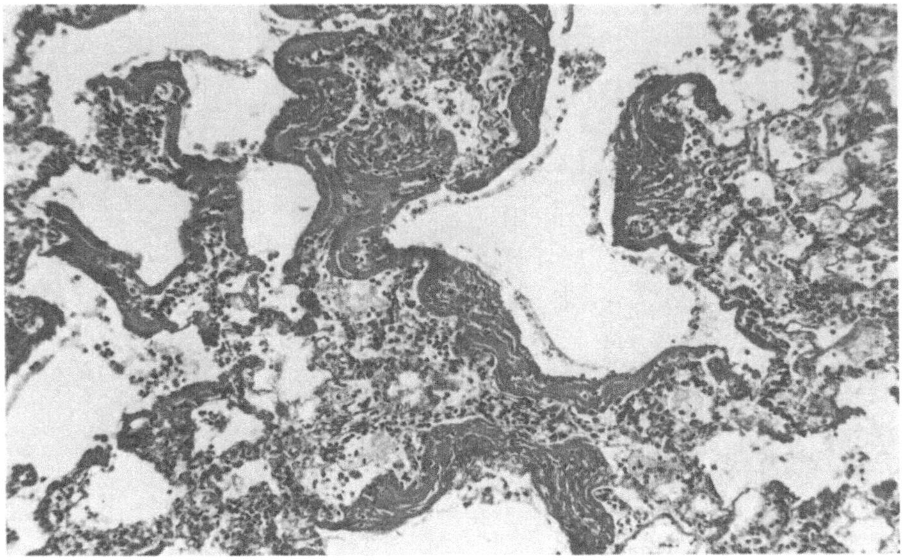

**Fig. 31.** The inner surface of the pulmonary alveoli is coated with a laminated membrane. HE, ×232

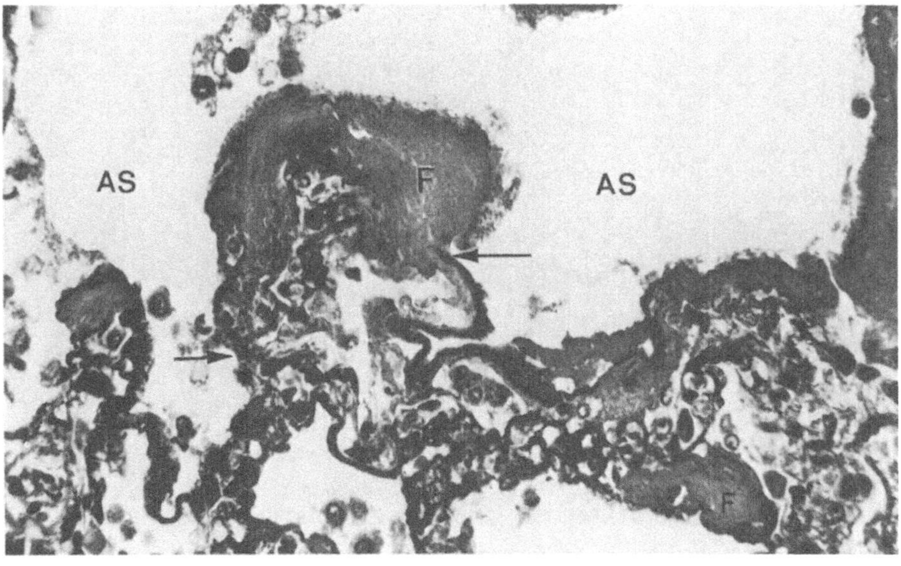


**Fig. 32.** Fibrin component of the pulmonary alveolar membrane. *Arrows* indicate points of rupture of alveolar basement membrane. *F*, fibrin; *AS*, alveolar space. PTAH, ×928

the degree of severity. Interlobular septae are severely oedematous. Fibrin thrombi can be demonstrated in certain alveolar capillaries. The second group of patients have no or slight pulmonary oedema, but show prominent membrane coating on the inner surface of alveoli, alveolar ducts, and the terminal bronchioles. These

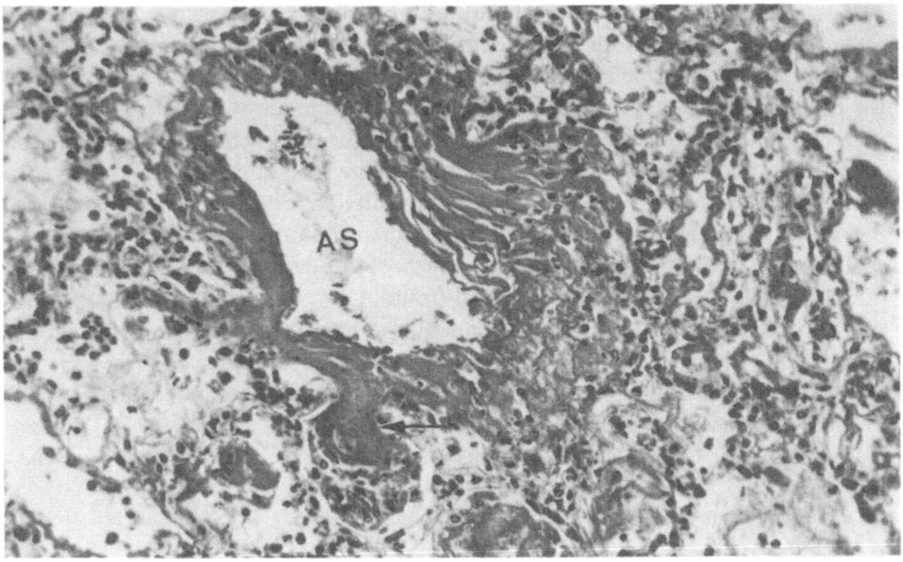


**Fig. 33.** Severe destruction of pulmonary alveoli by laminated membrane and cellular inflammatory reaction. Note the membrane contains malaria pigment (*arrow*) and cell debris. *AS*, alveolar space. HE, ×464

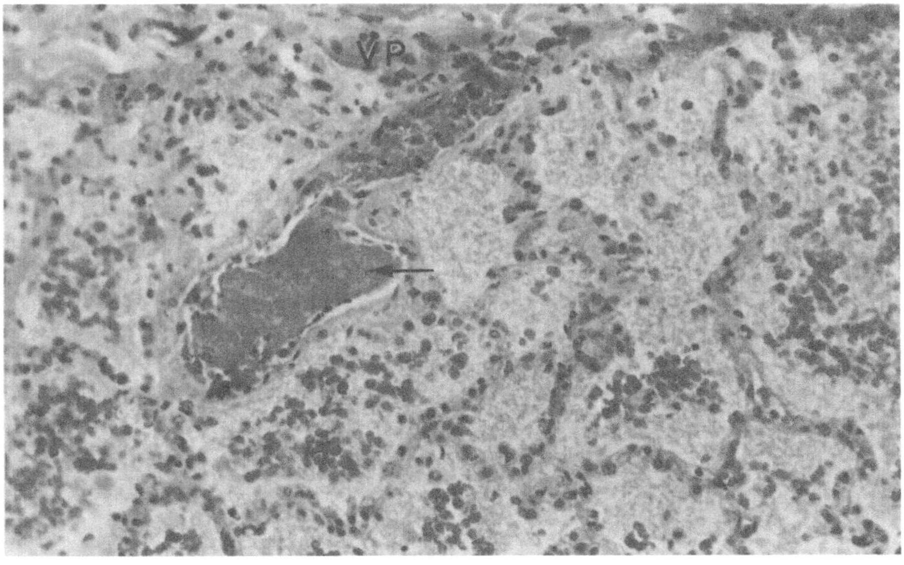


**Fig. 34.** Oedema and haemorrhage with fibrin platelets thrombus (*arrow*) in a septal vessel of lung. *VP*, visceral pleura. HE, ×464

membranes may be uniformly or irregularly distributed in some pulmonary lobules. Although they have been called "hyaline membrane" by several investigators, according to our observations these membranes have a different histological architecture from the membranes in typical hyaline membrane disease. The outstanding features of the membrane found in malarial lung include the laminated appearance and the finding of nuclear debris, malaria pigment, and mononuclear leucocytes between each layer of the membranes (Fig. 31). Special stains show that the membranes are composed mainly of fibrin and mucopolysaccharide material, with traces of haemosiderin pigment. Neutral fats and haemoglobin are not present. Occasionally, membranes are prominently located at the junction of the alveolar ducts and alveolar sacs (Fig. 32). Eventually they become thickened, destroy the underlying alveolar walls, and induce cellular inflammatory reactions (Fig. 33). Another group of pulmonary lesions consists of lobular or extensive haemorrhages that are always developed together with pulmonary oedema and the appearance of fibrin thrombi in the vessels of larger calibre than the capillaries. These thrombi may not be seen in areas of haemorrhage (Fig. 34).

Furthermore, SPITZ (1946) has described secondary bacterial infection of the lungs in 42% of patients. Other types of pneumonitis, including atypical pneumonia, were described by APPLEBAUM and SHRAGER (1944). In our series, this type of complication developed in 3 out of 22 cases.

## 8. Multiple Organ Complication and Concluding Remarks

In complicated falciparum malaria usually more than one of the major organs are involved (Table 3). Cerebral complication is the most frequent and has been detected the earliest. About one-half of all patients with brain involvement also showed renal and pulmonary complications. Renal failure of oliguric or non-oliguric type was the second most common complication, and about two-thirds of them experienced concomitant cerebral manifestations. Lung, liver, and cardiac involvement and gastrointestinal bleeding were also recognised at the same time or later. Almost all cases with pulmonary oedema or pulmonary insufficiency, as well as those with massive gastrointestinal haemorrhages and cardiac involvement, experienced preceding brain and renal complications. Some other complications such as pancreatitis (JOHNSON et al. 1977), nephrotic syndrome (BERGER et al. 1967) and renal failure due to acute glomerulonephritis were not observed in our patients with *P. falciparum* infection.

All falciparum cases with massive gastrointestinal bleeding died in spite of intensive treatment. All of them presented laboratory evidence of DIC. Pulmonary complications produce a very high mortality of 70% followed by cardiac, pulmonary, and renal complications with about 45%. About one-third of patients with cerebral malaria died. Liver involvement offers the best prognosis. However, the cause of death is the result of multiorgan rather than single organ involvement. The overall mortality in these 51 complicated cases of *P. falciparum* malaria was 28%. Table 7 shows clearly the bad prognosis in cases with laboratory evidence of DIC, where the mortality rate was 42%, compared with nil in the non-DIC group.

# References

Abdalla S, Weatherall DJ, Wickramasinghe SN, Hughes M (1980) The anaemia in *P. falciparum* malaria. Br J Haematol 46:171–183

Aikawa M (1971) Parasitological review: *Plasmodium:* the fine structure of malarial parasites. Exp Parasitol 30:284–320

Aikawa M, Miller LH, Rabbege JR (1975) Caveola-vesicle complexes in the plasmalemma of erythrocytes infected by *Plasmodium vivax* and *P. cynomolgi*. Am J Pathol 79:285–300
Aikawa M, Suzuki M, Gutierrez Y (1980) Pathology of malaria. In: Kreier JP (ed) Malaria, vol 2. Academic, New York, pp 47–102
Al-Ibrahim MS, Holzman RS (1975) Bilateral pleural effusions with *Plasmodium falciparum* infection. Am J Trop Med Hyg 24:910–912
Allison AC, Houba V (1976) Immunopathology due to complexes of antigen and antibody (Type III reactions), in parasitic infections. In: Cohen S, Sadun E (ed) Immunology of parasitic infections. Blackwell Scientific, Oxford, pp 436–447
Allison AC, Houba V, Hendrickse RG, de Petris S, Edington GM, Adeniyi A (1969) Immune complexes in the nephrotic syndrome of African children. Lancet I:1232–1238
Anderson WAD, Morrison DB (1942) Role of parasite pigment (ferrihemic acid) in the production of lesions in malaria. Arch Pathol 33:677–686
Applebaum IL, Shrager J (1944) Pneumonitis associated with malaria. Arch Intern Med 74:155–162
Areekul S (1973) Rigidity of red cell during malarial infection. J Med Assoc Thai 56:163–166
Balcerzak SP, Arnold JD, Martin DC (1972) Anatomy of red cell damage by *Plasmodium falciparum* in man. Blood 40:98–104
Beale PJ, Cormack JD, Oldrey TBN (1972) Thrombocytopenia in malaria with immunoglobulin (IgM) changes. Br Med J 1:345–347
Benjapongsh W (1966) Clinical studies of blackwater fever with erythrocyte glucose-6-phosphate dehydrogenase deficiency. J Dep Med Serv 17:128–133
Berger M, Birch LM, Conte NF (1967) The nephrotic syndrome secondary to acute glomerulonephritis during falciparum malaria. Ann Intern Med 67:1163–1171
Bergin J (1967) Malaria and the lung. Milit Med 132:522–526
Bhamarapravati N, Boonpucknavig S, Boonpucknavig V, Yaemboonruang (1973) Glomerular changes in acute *Plasmodium falciparum* infection: An immunopathologic study. Arch Pathol 96:289–293
Bienzle U, Ayeni O, Lucas AO, Luzzatto L (1972) Glucose-6-phosphate dehydrogenase and malaria, greater resistance of females heterozygous to enzyme deficiency and of males with non-deficient variant. Lancet I:107–110
Boonpucknavig S, Boonpucknavig V, Bhamarapravati N (1972) Immunopathological studies of *Plasmodium berghei*-infected mice. Immune complex nephritis. Arch Pathol 94:322–330
Boonpucknavig S, Benchachai P, Boonpucknavig V, Bhamarapravati N (1973) *Plasmodium berghei:* Detection in organs of infected mice by means of immunofluorescence. Trans R Soc Trop Med Hyg 67:410–415
Boonpucknavig S, Wongsawang S, Boonpucknavig V, Bhamarapravati N (1976) Serum-soluble malarial antigens and immune complex nephritis in *Plasmodium berghei berghei* infected mice. J Trop Med Hyg 79:116–119
Boonpucknavig S, Bandaso R, Boonpucknavig V, Bhamarapravati N (1979) Immunopathological studies of *Plasmodium berghei* infected mice (effect of carbon particles). J Trop Med Hyg 82:79–83
Boonpucknavig V, Sitprija V (1979) Renal disease in acute *Plasmodium falciparum* infection in man. Kidney Int 16:44–52
Boonpucknavig V, Boonpucknavig S, Bhamarapravati N (1973) *Plasmodium berghei* infection in mice: An ultrastructural study of immune complex nephritis. Am J Pathol 70:89–108
Boonpucknavig V, Boonpucknavig S, Bhamarapravati N (1979) *Plasmodium berghei*-infected mice: Focal glomerulonephritis in hyperimmune state. Arch Pathol Lab Med 103:567–572
Borochovitz D, Crosley AL, Metz J (1970) Disseminated intravascular coagulation with fatal haemorrhage in cerebral malaria. Br Med J 2:710
Brooks MH, Kiel FW, Sheehy TW, Barry KG (1968) Acute pulmonary edema in falciparum malaria: A clinicopathological correlation. N Engl J Med 279:732–737
Brooks MH, Barry KG, Cirksena WJ, Malloy JP, Bruton J, Gilliland PF (1969) Pituitary-adrenal function in acute falciparum malaria. Am J Trop Med Hyg 18:872–877

Bruce-Chwatt (1978) Introduction. In: Killick-Kendrick R, Peters W (ed) Rodent malaria. Academic, London, pp. XI–XXV
Butler T, Weber DM (1973) On the nature of orthostatic hypotension in acute malaria. Am J Trop Med Hyg 22:439–442
Canfield CJ (1969) Renal and hematologic complications of acute falciparum malaria in Vietnam. Bull NY Acad Med 45:1043–1057
Canfield CJ, Miller LH, Batelloni PH, Eichler P, Barry KG (1968) Acute renal failure in *Plasmodium falciparum* malaria: Treatment by peritoneal dialysis. Arch Intern Med 122:199–203
Chongsuphajaisiddhi T, Kasemsuth R, Tejavanija S, Harinasuta T (1971) Changes in blood volume in falciparum malaria. Southeast Asian J Trop Med Public Health 2:344–350
Coatney GR, Collins WE, Warren McW, Contacos PG (1971) The primate malarias. U.S. Dept of Health, Education and Welfare, NIH, NIAID, Bethesda, Maryland
Cohen S, Butcher GA (1972) The immunologic response to *Plasmodium*. Am J Trop Med Hyg 21:713–721
Conrad ME (1969) Pathophysiology of malaria: Hematologic observations in human and animal studies. Ann Intern Med 70:134–141
Conrad ME (1971) Hematologic manifestations of parasitic infections. Semin Hematol 8:267–303
Cross JH, Hsu-Kuo M, Lien JC (1973) Accidental human infection with *Plasmodium cynomolgi bastianellii*. Southeast Asian J Trop Med Public Health 4:481–483
Dale DG, Wolff SM (1973) Studies of the neutropenia of acute malaria. Blood 41:197–206
Daroff RB, Deller JJ Jr, Kastl AJ, Blocker WW Jr (1967) Cerebral malaria. JAMA 202:119–122
Deaton JG (1970) Fatal pulmonary edema as a complication of acute falciparum malaria. Am J Trop Med Hyg 19:196–201
Deller JJ Jr, Cifarelli PS, Berque S, Buchanan R (1967) Malaria hepatitis. Milit Med 132:614–620
Dennis LH, Conrad ME (1968) Anticoagulant and antimalarial action of heparin in simian malaria. Lancet I:769–771
Dennis LH, Eichelberger JW, Inman MM, Conrad ME (1967) Depletion of coagulation factors in drug-resistant *Plasmodium falciparum* malaria. Blood 29:713–721
Devakul K, Harinasuta T, Reid HA (1966) $^{125}$I-labelled fibrinogen in cerebral malaria. Lancet II:886–888
Dhayagude RG, Purandare NM (1943) Autopsy study of cerebral malaria with special reference to malarial granuloma. Arch Pathol 36:550–558
Dukes DC, Sealey BJ, Forbes JI (1968) Oliguric renal failure in blackwater fever. Am J Med 45:899–903
Eaton JW, Eckman JR, Berger E, Jacob HS (1976) Suppression of malaria infection by oxidant-sensitive host erythrocytes. Nature 264:758–760
Editorial (1970) Burkitt lymphoma and malaria. Lancet II:300–301
Endardjo S, Boonpucknavig S, Boonpucknavig V, Bhamarapravati N (1978) Immunopathological studies of *Plasmodium berghei berghei*-infected mice: Effect of cyclophosphamide. J Trop Med Hyg 81:25–31
Facer C, Bray RS, Brown J (1979) Direct Coombs antiglobulin reaction in Gambian children with *P. falciparum* malaria, I. Incidence and classes specificity. Clin Expt Immunol 35:119–127
Fajardo LF, Rao S (1971) Platelet enlargement in malaria. 136:463–464
Fein A, Rackow EC, Shapiro L (1978) Acute pulmonary edema in *Plasmodium falciparum* malaria. Am Rev Respir Dis 118:425–429
Feldman HA, Murphy FD (1945) The effect of alterations in blood volume on the anemia and hypoproteinemia of human malaria. J Clin Invest 24:780–792
Feorino PM, Mathews HM (1974) Malarial antibody levels in patients with Burkitt's lymphoma. Am J Trop Med Hyg 23:574–576
Field JW (1949) Blood examination and prognosis in acute falciparum malaria. Trans R Soc Trop Med Hyg 43:33–48

Fletcher A, Maegraith B (1972) The metabolism of the malarial parasite and its host. Adv Parasitol 10:31–48

Friedman MJ (1978) Erythrocyte mechanism of sickle cell resistance to malaria. Proc Natl Acad Sci USA 75:1994–1997

Friedman MJ, Roth EF, Nagel RL, Trager W (1979) The role of hemoglobin C, S, and N Balt in the inhibition of malarial parasite development in vitro. Am J Trop Med Hyg 28:777–780

Futrakul P, Boonpucknavig V, Boonpucknavig S, Mitrakul C, Bhamarapravati N (1974) Acute glomerulonephritis complicating *Plasmodium falciparum* infection. Clin Pediatr (Phila) 13:281–283

George CRP, Parbtani A, Cameron JS (1976) Mouse malaria nephropathy. J Pathol 120:235–249

Gilbreath MT, Pavanand K, Phisphumvidhi P, Kongchareon S, Wimonwattrawatee T (1978–1979) Partial characterization of mitogenesis inhibiting factor in malarial serum. AFRIMS Annual Progress Report, pp 367–369. Available from Armed Forces Research Institute of the Medial Sciences, Bangkok, Thailand

Gilles HM, Hendrickse RG (1960) Possible aetiological role of *Plasmodium malariae* in "nephrotic syndrome" in Nigerian children. Lancet I:806–807

Gilles HM, Hendrickse RG (1963) Nephrosis in Nigerian children: Role of *Plasmodium malariae*, and effect of antimalarial treatment. Br Med J 2:27–31

Godard JE, Hansen RA (1971) Interstitial pulmonary edema in acute malaria: Report of a case. Radiology 101:523–524

Goodall HB (1973) Giant nuclear masses in the lungs and blood in malignant malaria. Lancet II:1124–1126

Hall AP (1976) The treatment of malaria. Br Med J 1:323–328

Hartenbower DL, Kantor GL, Rosen VJ (1972) Renal failure due to acute glomerulonephritis during falciparum malaria: case report. Milit Med 137:74–76

Heineman HS (1972) The clinical syndrome of malaria in the United States. A current review of diagnosis and treatment for American physicians. Arch Intern Med 129:607–616

Hendrickse RG, Adeniyi A (1979) Quartan malarial nephrotic syndrome in children. Kidney Int 16:64–74

Hendrickse RG, Adeniyi A, Edington GM, Glasgow EF, White RHR, Houba V (1972) Quartan malarial nephrotic syndrome: collaborative clinico-pathologic study in Nigerian children. Lancet I:1143–1148

Hill GJ II, Knight V, Jeffery GM (1964) Thrombocytopenia in vivax malaria. Lancet I:240–241

Houba V (1975) Immunopathology of nephropathies associated with malaria. Bull WHO 52:199–207

Houba V (1979) Immunologic aspects of renal lesions associated with malaria. Kidney Int 16:3–8

Houba V, Allison AC, Hendrickse RG, de Petris S, Edington GM, Adeniyi A (1970) Immune complex in the nephrotic syndrome of Nigerian children. In: Bonomo L, Turk JL (eds) Proceedings of the international symposium of immune complex diseases, pp 23–35. Available from Carlo Erba Foundation Milan

Houba V, Allison AC, Adeniyi A, Houba JE (1971) Immunoglobulin classes and complement in biopsies of Nigerian children with the nephrotic syndrome. Clin Exp Immunol 8:761–774

Houba V, Lambert PH, Voller A, Soyanwo MAO (1976) Clinical and experimental investigation of immune complexes in malaria. Clin Immunol Immunopathol 6:1–12

Howard WA, Collins WE (1972) Heparin therapy in simian *Plasmodium knowlesi* malaria. Lancet II:738–739

Hutt MRS, Davies DR, Voller A (1975) Malarial infections in *Aotus trivirgatus* with special reference to renal pathology: II *P. falciparum* and mixed malaria infections. Br J Exp Pathol 56:429–438

Jaroonvesama N (1972) Intravascular coagulation in falciparum malaria. Lancet I:221–223

Jaroonvesama N, Harinasuta T, Muangmanee L, Asawapokee N (1975) Coagulation studies in falciparum and vivax malaria. Southeast Asian J Trop Med Public Health 6:419–424

Johnson RC, de Ford JW, Carlton PK (1977) Pancreatitis complicating falciparum malaria. Case report. Postgrad Med 61:181–183

Karney WW, Tong MJ (1972) Malabsorption in *Plasmodium falciparum* malaria. Am J Trop Med Hyg 21:1–5

Kean BH, Taylor CE (1946) Medical shock in the pathogenesis of algid malaria. Am J Trop Med 26:209–219

Kibukamusoke JW (1968) Malaria prophylaxis and immunosuppressant therapy in management of nephrotic syndrome associated with quartan malaria. Arch Dis Child 43:598–600

Kibukamusoke JW, Hutt MSR (1967) Histological features of the nephrotic syndrome associated with quartan malaria. J Clin Pathol 20:117–123

Kibukamusoke JW, Hutt MSR, Wilks NE (1967) The nephrotic syndrome in Uganda and its association with quartan malaria. Q J Med 36:393–408

Kiel FW (1968) Malaria in Vietnam. In: Sommers SC (ed) Pathology annual, vol III. Appleton-Century-Crofts, New York, pp 1–27

Luse SA, Miller LH (1971) *Plasmodium falciparum* malaria: Ultrastructure of parasitized erythrocytes in cardiac vessels. Am J Trop Med Hyg 20:655–660

Maegraith BG (1944) Blackwater fever anuria. Trans R Soc Trop Med Hyg 38:1–23

Maegraith BG (1948) Pathological processes in malaria. Trans R Soc Trop Med Hyg 41:687–699, 702–704

Maegraith BG (1969) Complication of falciparum malaria. Bull NY Acad Med 45:1061–1064

Maegraith BG (1974) Other pathological processes in malaria. Bull WHO 50:187–193

Maegraith BG, Fletcher A (1972) The pathogenesis of mammalian malaria. Adv Parasitol 10:49–57

Maegraith BG, Onabanjo AO (1970) The effects of histamine in malaria. Br J Pharmacol 39:755–764

Malloy JP, Brooks MH, Barry KG (1967) Pathophysiology of acute falciparum malaria. II. Fluid compartmentalization. Am J Med 43:745–750

Marks SM, Holland S, Gelfand M (1977) Malarial lung: Report of a case from Africa successfully treated with intermittent positive pressure ventilation. Am J Trop Med Hyg 26:179–180

Martell RW, Kallenbach J, Zwi S (1979) Pulmonary oedema in falciparum malaria. Br Med J 1:1763–1764

McCabe ME (1966) Malaria-A military medical problem yet with us. Med Serv J Can 22:313–332

McGregor IA, Turner MW, Williams K, Hall P (1968) Soluble antigens in the blood of African patients with severe *Plasmodium falciparum* malaria. Lancet I:881–884

McMahon AE, Kelsey JE, Derauf DE (1954) Hepatitis of malarial origin: clinical and pathologic study of fifty four Korean veterans. Arch Intern Med 93:379–386

McKay DG, Linder MM, Cruse VK (1971) Mechanisms of thrombosis in the microcirculation. Am J Pathol 63:231–254

Merkel WC (1946) *Plasmodium falciparum* malaria: the coronary and myocardial lesions observed at autopsy in two cases of acute fulminating *P. falciparum* infection. Arch Pathol 41:290–298

Miller HL, Makaranond P, Sitprija V, Suebsanguan C, Canfield CJ (1967) Hyponatraemia in malaria. Ann Trop Med Parasitol 61:265–279

Miller LH, Usami S, Chien S (1971) Alteration in the rheologic properties of *Plasmodium knowlesi*-infected red cells. A possible mechanism for capillary obstruction. J Clin Invest 50:1451–1455

Miller LH, Chien S, Usami S (1972) Decreased deformability of *Plasmodium coatneyi*-infected red cells and its possible relation to cerebral malaria. Am J Trop Med Hyg 21:133–137

Miller LH, Shiroishi T, Dvorak JA, Durocher JR, Schrier BK (1975) Enzymatic modification of the erythrocyte membrane surface and its effect on malarial merozoite invasion. J Mol Med 1:55–63
Miller LH, Mason SJ, Clyde DF, McGinniss (1976) The resistance factor to *Plasmodium vivax* in blacks. The Duffy-blood-group genotype, Fy Fy. N Engl J Med 295:302–304
Miller LH, Haynes JD, Mc Auliffe FM, Shiroishi T, Durocher JR, Mc Ginniss MH (1977) Evidence for differences in erythrocyte surface receptors for the malarial parasites, *P. falciparum* and *P. knowlesi*. J Exp Med 146:277–281
Most H (1972) *Plasmodium cynomolgi* malaria: Accidental human infection. Am J Trop Med Hyg 22:157–158
Mukherjee AP, White JC, Lau KS (1971) Falciparum malaria associated with jaundice, renal failure, and anaemia. Trans R Soc Trop Med Hyg 65:808–814
Myrhe-Jensen O (1971) Localization of fibrinolytic activity in the kidney and urinary tract of rats and rabbits. Lab Invest 25:403–411
Neva FA, Sheagren JN, Shulman NR, Canfield CJ (1970) NIH conference, malaria: Host-defense mechanisms and complications. Ann Intern Med 73:295–306
O'Holohan DR (1976) Clinical and laboratory presentation of malaria: An analysis of one thousand subjects with malaria parasitemia. J Trop Med 79:191–196
Olsson RA, Johnston EH (1969) Histopathologic changes and small-bowel absorption in falciparum malaria. Am J Trop Med Hyg 18:355–359
Onabanjo AO, Maegraith BG (1971) Circulating plasma kinins in malaria. Trans R Soc Trop Med Hyg 65:5
Osunkoya BO, Williams AO, Reddy S (1972) Spontaneous lymphocyte transformation in leukocyte culture of children with falciparum malaria. Trop Geogr Med 25:157–161
Parbtani A, Cameron JS (1979) Experimental nephritis associated with *Plasmodium* infection in mice. Kidney Int 16:53–63
Pasvol G, Weatherall DJ (1980) The red cell and the malarial parasite. Br J Haematol 46:165–170
Pasvol G, Weatherall DJ, Wilson RJM, Smith DH, Gilles HM (1976) Fetal hemoglobin and malaria. Lancet I:1269–1272
Pasvol G, Weatherall DJ, Wilson RJM (1977) Effects of fetal hemoglobin on susceptibility of red cells to *Plasmodium falciparum*. Nature 270:171–173
Pasvol G, Weatherall DJ, Wilson RJM (1978) Cellular mechanism for the protective effect of hemoglobin S against *P. falciparum* malaria. Nature 274:701–703
Petchclai B, Chutanonh R, Hiranras S, Benjapongs W (1977) Activation of classical and alternative complement pathways in acute falciparum malaria. J Med Assoc Thai 60:172–176
Punyagupta S, Srichaikul T, Akarawong K (1972) The use of heparin in fatal pulmonary edema. J Med Assoc Thai 55:121–131
Punyagupta S, Srichaikul T, Nitiyanant P, Petchclai B (1974) Acute pulmonary insufficiency in falciparum malaria: Summary of 12 cases with evidence of disseminated intravascular coagulation. Am J Trop Med Hyg 23:551–559
Ramachandran S, Perera MVF (1976) Jaundice and hepatomegaly in primary malaria. J Trop Med Hyg 79:207–210
Ray AP, Sharma GK (1958) Experimental studies on liver injury in malaria. II. Pathogenesis. Indian J Med Res 46:367–376
Reid HA, Nkrumah FK (1972) Fibrin degradation products in cerebral malaria. Lancet I:218–221
Reid HA, Sucharit P (1972) Ancrod, heparin, and ε-aminocaproic acid in simian knowlesi malaria. Lancet II:1110–1112
Reiley CG, O'Neil B Jr (1971) Leukocyte response in acute malaria. Am J Med Sci 262:153–158
Rigdon RH (1944a) A consideration of the mechanism of splenic infarcts in malaria. Am J Trop Med 24:349–354
Rigdon RH (1944b) A pathological study of the acute lesions produced by *Plasmodium lophurae* in young white Pekin ducks. Am J Trop Med 24:371–377

Rigdon RH, Fletcher DE (1945) Lesions in the brain associated with malaria. Pathology in man and on experimental animals. Arch Neurol Psychiatry 53:191–198

Rosen S, Roycroft DW, Hano JE, Barry KG (1967) The liver in malaria: Electron microscopic observations on a hepatic biopsy obtained 15 minutes post mortem. Arch Pathol 83:271–277

Rosen S, Hano JE, Inman MM, Gilliland PF, Barry KG (1968) The kidney in blackwater fever: Light and electron microscopic observation. Am J Clin Pathol 49:358–370

Rosenberg EB, Strickland GT, Yang S, Whalen GE (1973) IgM antibodies to red cells and autoimmune anemia in patients with malaria. Am J Trop Med Hyg 22:146–152

Schnitzer B, Sodeman T, Mead ML, Contacos PG (1972) Pitting function of the spleen in malaria; ultrastructural observations. Science 177:175–177

Schnitzer B, Sodeman TM, Mead ML, Contacos PG (1973) An ultrastructural study of the red pulp of the spleen in malaria. Blood 41:207–218

Sheagren JM, Tobie JE, Fox LM, Wolff SM (1970) Reticuloendothelial system phagocytic function in naturally acquired human malaria. J Lab Clin Med 75:481–487

Sheehy TW (1975) Disseminated intravascular coagulation and severe falciparum malaria. Lancet I:516

Sheehy TW, Reba RC (1967) Complications of falciparum malaria and their treatment. Ann Intern Med 66:807–809

Shortt HE, Garnham PCC, Covell G, Shute PG (1948) The preerythrocytic stage of human malaria, *Plasmodium vivax*. Br Med J:547

Sitprija V, Indraprasit S, Pochanugool C, Benyajati C, Piyarath P (1967) Renal failure in malaria. Lancet I:185–188

Skirrow MB, Chongsuphajaisiddhi T, Maegraith BG (1964) The circulation in malaria: II. Portal angiography in monkeys (*Macaca mulatta*) infected with *Plasmodium knowlesi* and in shock following manipulation of the gut. Ann Trop Med Parasitol 58:502–510

Skudowitz RB, Katz J, Lurie A, Levin J, Metz J (1973) Mechanisms of thrombocytopenia in malignant tertian malaria. Br Med J 2:515–518

Soothill JF, Hendrickse RG (1967) Some immunological studies of nephrotic syndrome of Nigerian children. Lancet I:629–632

Spitz S (1946) The pathology of acute falciparum malaria. Milit Surg 99:555–572

Sraer JD, Boelaert J, Mimoune O, Morel-Maroger L, Hornych H (1973) Quantitative assessment of fibrinolysis on isolated glomeruli. Kidney Int 4:350–352

Srichaikul T (1959) A study of pigmentation and other changes in the liver in malaria. Am J Trop Med Hyg 8:110–118

Srichaikul T (1967) The significance of plasmocytosis in bone marrow of human malaria in correlation with gamma globulin. Annual Report of SEATO Laboratory Medical Research Center, Rajvithi Road, Bangkok, Thailand

Srichaikul T (1973) Hematologic changes in human malaria. J Med Assoc Thai 56:658–663

Srichaikul T, Panikbutr N, Jeumtrakul P (1967) Bone marrow change in human malaria. Ann Trop Med Parasitol 8:40–50

Srichaikul T, Wasanasomsithi M, Poshyachinda V, Panikbutr N, Rabieb T (1969) Ferrokinetic studies and erythropoiesis in malaria. Arch Intern Med 124:623–628

Srichaikul T, Siriasawakul T, Poshyachinda M, Poshyachinda V (1973) Ferrokinetics in patients with malaria: Normoblasts and iron incorporation *in vitro*. Am J Clin Pathol 59:166–174

Srichaikul T, Puwasatien P, Karnjanajetanee J, Bokisch VA (1975) Complement changes and disseminated intravascular coagulation in *Plasmodium falciparum* malaria. Lancet I:770–772

Srichaikul T, Archararit N, Siriasawakul T, Viriyapanich Y (1976a) Histamine changes in *Plasmodium falciparum* malaria. Trans R Soc Trop Med Hyg 70:36–38

Srichaikul T, Siriasawakul T, Poshyachinda M (1976b) Ferrokinetics in patients with malaria: Haemoglobin synthesis and normoblasts *in vitro*. Trans R Soc Trop Med Hyg 70:244–246

Srichaikul T, Noyes W, Chaisiripaumkeeree W, Choawanakul V (1979) Serum ferritin and iron binding capacity in malaria. Mahidol University Annual Research Abstract, Mahidol University, Bangkok, Thailand, p 265

Stewart AM (1970) Burkitt lymphoma and malaria. Lancet I:771
Stone WJ, Hanchett JE, Knepshield JH (1972) Acute renal insufficiency due to falciparum malaria. Arch Intern Med 129:620–628
Strickland GT, Kostivas JE (1970) Folic acid deficiency complicating malaria. Am J Trop Med Hyg 19:910–915
Sullivan LW (1969) Of men, malaria, and megaloblasts. N Engl J Med 280:1354–1355
Suzuki M (1974) *Plasmodium berghei:* Experimental rodent model for malarial renal immunopathology. Exp Parasitol 35:187–195
Taliaferro WH, Mulligan HW (1937) The histopathology of malaria with special reference to the function and origin of the macrophages in defense. Indian Med Res Mem 29:1–138
Thomas JD (1971) Clinical and histopathological correlation of cerebral malaria. Trop Geogr Med 23:232–238
Thompson GR (1963) Malaria and stress in relation to haemoglobins S and C. Br Med J 2:976–978
Tong MJ, Ballantine TVN, Youel DB (1972) Pulmonary function studies in *Plasmodium falciparum* malaria. Am Rev Respir Dis 106:23–29
Varavithya W, Chongsuphajaisiddhi T (1972) Erythrocyte composition in *P. falciparum* infection in man. Southeast Asian J Trop Med Public Health 3:175–181
Voller A, Draper CC, Shwe T, Hutt MSR (1971) Nephrotic syndrome in monkey infected with human quartan malaria. Br Med J 4:208–210
Voller A, Davies DR, Hutt MSR (1973) Quartan malarial infections in *Aotus trivirgatus* with special reference to renal pathology. Br J Exp Pathol 54:457–468
Vreeken J, Cremer-Groote TLM (1978) Hemostatic effect in non-immune patients with falciparum malaria: No evidence of diffuse intravascular coagulation. Br Med J 2:532–534
Ward PA, Conran PB (1966) Immunopathologic studies of simian malaria. Milit Med 131:1225–1232
Ward PA, Conran PB (1969) Immunopathology of renal complications in simian malaria and human quartan malaria. Milit Med 134:1228–1236
Wedderburn N (1970) Effect of concurrent malarial infection on development of virus-induced lymphoma in Balb-c mice. Lancet II:1114–1116
Wells RA, Pavanand K, Zolyom S, Permpanich B, MacDermott RP (1979) Loss of circulating T lymphocytes with normal levels and B and null lymphocytes in Thai adults with malaria. Clin Exp Immunol 35:202–209
Wernsdorfer WH (1980) The importance of malaria in the world. In: Kreier JP (ed) Malaria, vol 1. Academic, New York, p 68–69
White LG, Doerner AA (1954) Functional and needle biopsy study of the liver in malaria. JAMA 155:637–639
Wilson RJM, Mc Gregor IA, Hall P, Williams K, Bartholomew R (1969) Antigens associated with *Plasmodium falciparum* infections in man. Lancet I:201–205
Wilson RJM, Mc Gregor IA, Williams K, (1975a) Occurrence of S-antigens in serum of *Plasmodium falciparum* infections in man. Trans R Soc Trop Med Hyg. 69:453–459
Wilson RJM, Mc Gregor IA, Hall PJ (1975b) Persistence and reoccurrence of S-antigens in *Plasmodium falciparum* infections in man. Trans R Soc Trop Med Hyg. 69:460–467
Winslow DJ, Conner DH, Sprinz H (1975) Malaria. In: Marcial-Rojas RA (ed) Pathology of protozoal and helminthic disease. Williams and Wilkins, Baltimore, pp 195–224
Woodruff AW, Ansdell VE, Pettitt LE (1979) Cause of anaemia in malaria. Lancet I:1055–1057
World Health Organization (1955) Resolution WHA 8.30. Off Rec WHO 63:31
World Health Organization (1956) Resolution WHA 9.61. Off Red WHO 71:43
World Health Organization (1969) Parasitology of malaria. WHO Tech Rep Ser 433:5–35
World Health Organization (1972) Immunopathology of nephritis in Africa (Memorandum). Bull WHO 46:387–396
World Health Organization (1975) The malaria situation in 1974. WHO Chron 29:474–481
Wright DH (1968) The effect of neonatal thymectomy on the survival of golden hamsters infected with *Plasmodium berghei.* Br J Exp Pathol 46:379–384

Wright DH, Masembe RM, Bazier ER (1971) The effect of antithymocyte serum on golden hamsters and rats infected with *Plasmodium berghei*. Br J Exp Pathol 52:465–477
Ziegler JL, Bluming AZ, Morrow RH Jr (1972) Burkitt's lymphoma and malaria. Trans R Soc Trop Med Hyg 66:285–291
Ziessman HA (1976) Lung uptake of $^{99M}$Tc-sulfur colloid in falciparum malaria: Case report. J Nucl Med 17:794–796

# Experimental Models

CHAPTER 6

# In Vitro Techniques for Antimalarial Development and Evaluation

R. E. DESJARDINS

## A. Introduction

With the recent development of techniques for the continuous in vitro cultivation of *Plasmodium falciparum* we are on the threshold of a new era in malaria research. This new technology provides unprecedented opportunities for advancing the search for new antimalarial drugs and for elucidating the mechanisms of action of existing drugs. It is reasonable to anticipate that the application of these methods in laboratories throughout the world will lead to novel approaches to the chemotherapy and chemoprophylaxis of malaria.

Interest in short-term cultivation of plasmodia for chemotherapeutic research antedates the development of methods for continuous cultivation of the parasite by many years. BASS and JOHNS first reported in vitro maturation of the asexual stages of *Plasmodium falciparum* and *Plasmodium vivax* in 1912.

Though continuous cultivation techniques had to await the landmark discovery by TRAGER and JENSEN (1976) and independently by HAYNES et al. (1976) of the microaerophilic property of the erythrocytic stage of the parasite, a great deal of information was obtained in earlier studies using short-term cultures, without which the present potential for advantageous use of the new technology could not be realised.

The present chapter reviews the current state of development of the methods for continuous in vitro cultivation of *Plasmodium falciparum* as they have been applied to antimalarial chemotherapeutic research. An effort has been made, in this context, to set the stage for the many anticipated advances made possible by these developments.

## B. The Role of In Vitro Methods in Antimicrobial Drug Research

In a review of the early work with short-term cultures of malaria parasites (BERTAGNA et al. 1972) the authors made the following observation: "The advantages of in vitro methods for studying micro-organisms apply equally to the study of plasmodia." It is the availability of methods for cultivation of individual species of bacteria that has led to a plethora of useful antibacterial drugs with a wide variety of specificities (BUSHBY 1964). Furthermore, the availability of bacteria in abundant supply from in vitro cultures has contributed greatly to the present detailed knowledge of the mechanisms of action of most of these drugs. The development of cell culture techniques for harvesting and studying viruses promises similar advances against these subcellular organisms in the foreseeable future (COLLINS and BAUER 1979). The lack of similar technology for plasmodia has, on the other hand, greatly hampered progress in antimalarial drug development and in understanding the specific mode of action of most existing antimalarial drugs.

## I. Advantages

Application of in vitro techniques can greatly improve the overall efficiency and precision of a chemotherapeutic research programme. It is, therefore, worthwhile to consider in detail the inherent advantages of in vitro methods as they pertain in general and in particular to antimalarial drug development. In contrast to experimental models requiring laboratory animals, in vitro methods are inexpensive because of their relatively conservative requirements for space, equipment, and manpower. The ability to obtain information with small quantities of a new chemical entity may also represent a considerable saving in the earliest stages of development, i.e. screening and analogue selection. Results are generally obtained rapidly, requiring only a few generation cycles of the organism. As a consequence of these factors, the efficiency of in vitro methods is high, making it possible to process and evaluate large numbers of compounds. Most antimalarial drug development work in recent years has employed large-scale screening and lead-directed chemical synthesis (PETERS 1974a; ROZMAN and CANFIELD 1979). The potential value of in vitro methods to this approach is self-evident.

Similarly, because of the greater efficiency of in vitro methods, a larger variety of isolates of the microorganism can be studied with the same compound, providing a broader range of information with respect to the pathogen. By selecting isolates of plasmodia with known in vivo and in vitro antimalarial drug susceptibilities and resistance patterns, it is possible to draw inferences regarding similarities in mode of action and to evaluate cross-resistance characteristics. Novel approaches to chemotherapeutic activity may also be suggested by the application of in vitro techniques. The more precise quantitation possible with properly designed experiments may provide suitable data for detailed structure-activity determinations with a variety of analogues in relation to a known or putative drug receptor. Detailed information regarding possible drug-interactions is also readily obtainable, i.e. synergism and antagonism. Likewise, antagonism of drug effect by nutrients and metabolic precursors can be precisely determined and may yield valuable information with respect to the mechanism of drug action.

Certain characteristics of in vitro methods, exclusive of their greater precision and efficiency, provide opportunities for observations which cannot be readily obtained from in vivo models. For example, they permit control of variables such as inoculum size and medium composition. Similarly, by eliminating host factors such as drug metabolism and host immunity, a better assessment of intrinsic drug activity is obtained. It is, furthermore, possible to evaluate in vitro certain host factors such as erythrocyte receptor specificities (MILLER et al. 1975) and serum factors in a controlled manner. Finally, it is possible in vitro to evaluate parent compounds and known or putative metabolites of parent compounds separately, especially since only small quantities of each are required.

## II. Limitations

There are also important limitations associated with the use of in vitro models and these should be recognised. Perhaps the most frequently cited limitation is the inability to detect the potential antimicrobial activity of compounds which require in vivo metabolism to an active state. Though examples of this phenomenon are uncommon, among these are the antimalarial drug proguanil and the trypanocidal drug tryparsamide. It is, therefore, an important consideration. Similarly, certain compounds which require some form of host interaction, such as protein binding for suramin (WILLIAMSON and SCOTT-FINNIGAN 1978) and enhancement of host immunity for levamisole (HADDEN et al. 1975), may be inactive when assessed in vitro.

Another limiting characteristic of in vitro methods as they are commonly applied is the artificial time-course of drug exposure, which is usually at a constant level of concentration for a relatively short period of time. Techniques have been developed which permit in vitro approximation of the time-concentration kinetics of a drug to anticipated in vivo exposure (BERGAN et al. 1980; MURAKAWA et al. 1980). These, however, are combersome and not readily adaptable to the culture requirements of *Plasmodium falciparum*. This characteristic (i.e. constant drug concentration over time) may, however, permit in vitro detection of antimicrobial activity for drugs which are too rapidly metabolised to provide measurable activity in vivo. It may then be possible to generate analogues with more favourable pharmacokinetic characteristics and a level of antimicrobial activity similar to the initial compound.

Though in vitro methods permit simultaneous measurement of many different parameters of potential drug activity, such as growth in numbers or size, morphological maturation, incorporation of metabolic precursors or generation of measurable metabolites, none of these are universally applicable to all modes of potential drug action. It is, therefore, possible that improper selection of measured parameters will result in a failure to detect a particular drug activity (GUTTERIDGE and TRIGG 1970).

Finally, certain problems inherent in the use of in vitro techniques must be acknowledged. By their nature, they will tend to be broadly selective in screening compounds, tending to identify many which will ultimately prove too toxic to mammalian cells for active consideration as new drugs. Many compounds will also prove to be highly insoluble in the aqueous electrolyte media generally employed to support life in vitro. Others will be subject to artefacts peculiar to in vitro systems such as adherence to the glass or plastic vessel in which the experiment is carried out.

The above considerations lead to the conclusion that, while the availability of in vitro cultivation techniques is an important and welcome addition to the investigative resources of antimalarial drug research, they are neither a substitute nor a replacement for in vivo or basic biochemical methods. A well-designed drug development programme must carefully integrate these varied approaches, recognising their respective advantages and limitations and their mutual potential contributions towards the goal of identifying and characterising useful new antimalarial drugs.

## III. Specific Applications to Malaria

### 1. Qualitative Aspects

It may be worthwhile, before exploring the methods and applications which have so far been developed, to review the desirable characteristics of a hypothetical in vitro model for general use in the evaluation of potential antimalarial drug activity. Clearly, no one system will be all-encompassing because of the many intrinsic variables and varied goals of different investigations. Nevertheless, broad guidelines can be suggested in the interests of optimum breadth of sensitivity and efficiency.

The first consideration is the requirement for an abundant, continuous and stable source of parasites, which the pioneering work and discoveries of TRAGER and his colleagues have at last provided. Techniques for in vitro drug evaluation should be designed with maximum efficiency and minimum use of costly and scarce resources. At the same time, the methods should be versatile and thereby adaptable to special purposes and applications, such as the ability to measure simultaneously more than one parameter of drug action and the ability to assess drug interactions such as synergism and antagonism.

It is perhaps unnecessary, but important, to point out the requirements for precision, accuracy and the greatest possible specificity. The goals of accuracy and precision can be readily achieved by careful design of an experimental in vitro system. However, as pointed out earlier, lack of specificity is a limitation associated with in vitro methods which must always be recognised in the interpretation of results obtained from such a model.

An in vitro model for the evaluation of antimalarial drugs should also be capable of providing data with a variety of drug-susceptible and multidrug-resistant isolates of the parasite. Fortunately, there is now sufficient experience with many isolates of *P. falciparum* with varying drug-susceptibility characteristics (JENSEN and TRAGER 1978; DESJARDINS et al. 1979) to be confident that this objective is attainable.

In the interest of maximising the breadth of sensitivity of an in vitro model, the culture methods should employ a defined minimal growth medium to reduce as much as possible potential interference with drug action by nutrients in the medium. This important objective is, unfortunately, seldom achieved, and certainly has yet to be realised for *P. falciparum*, though work is proceeding towards that goal (SIDDIQUI and RICHMOND-CRUM 1977; ZHENGREN et al. 1980).

### 2. Quantitative Aspects

In addition to these qualitative aspects of the design of an in vitro experimental model for the evaluation of antimalarial drug activity, it is important to consider the quantitative value of the data obtained. In vitro methods, by their nature, permit the greatest possible precision in defining intrinsic drug activity. The data generated by such a model may be quantitated classically in a number of different ways (TALLARIDA and JACOB 1979). Perhaps the simplest method, and the one most commonly employed in bacteriology, is to determine by serial dilution the minimum concentration of drug necessary to suppress effectively some measured parameter of growth or life function, i.e. minimum inhibitory concentration (MIC). This method has been employed in the development of an extremely valuable technique for use in epidemiological studies to identify chloroquine-resistant isolates of *P. falciparum* in the field (RIECKMANN et al. 1978).

It is often of value to determine the killing activity as well as the suppressive activity of a measured concentration of drug, i.e. minimum cidal concentration (MCC). Depending on the specific mechanism of action of a particular drug and the parameter measured, this may or may not be higher than the minimum inhibitory concentration. A difference between the MIC and MCC for a given drug in relation to the pharmacokinetics of the drug in vivo may be of considerable importance with respect to anticipated efficacy. This distinction, as well as the importance of duration of drug exposure, was clearly recognised and evaluated in the method described by RICHARDS and MAPLES (1979).

A more precise definition of the activity of an antimicrobial drug can be achieved by generating data based on measurements of activity at a series of concentrations and fitting these data to a generalised concentration-response curve. In this way statistical comparisons can be made, usually based on the estimated theoretical 50% suppressive concentration ($IC_{50}$), which is the least variate point in a classical concentration-response relation. This method is also capable of providing additional information with respect to intrinsic activity by analysis of the characteristic slope generated by the particular drug. This will tend to vary for different modes of action. Though, as a general rule, more data are required for application of these analytic methods, DESJARDINS et al. (1979) described a semiautomated computer-assisted graphic technique for rapid and efficient generation and analysis of concentration-response data for potential antimalarial drugs.

## C. Short-Term In Vitro Cultures

Many investigators applied in vitro methods to the study of antimalarial drugs prior to the development of continuous culture techniques. Substantial contributions to current knowledge of the metabolism of plasmodia have been made by experiments with short-term in vitro cultures. Various species of plasmodia were employed in these studies. The parasites were obtained in each case from a suitable infected host, i.e. *P. gallinaceum* and *P. lophurae* from fowl, *P. berghei* from rodents, *P. knowlesi* and *P. cynomolgi* from monkeys, and *P. falciparum* from owl monkeys and from man. Short-term cultures of these parasites have also been used to investigate the kinetics and mechanisms of action of known antimalarial drugs.

A method was described by GEIMAN et al. in 1946 for cultivation of malaria parasites which was subsequently used to demonstrate the antimalarial activity of chloroquine in vitro (GEIMAN 1948). Drug effect was measured by decrements in glucose utilisation, lactate production and parasite multiplication. In this system chloroquine was active only at very high concentrations (1.612 μg/ml). An automated system was described by CENEDELLA and SAXE (1966) for assessment of drug effect based on glucose consumption, lactate production, and the release of free amino acids during a 1-h incubation of *P. berghei*-parasitised rat erythrocytes. This method, too, proved relatively insensitive for use in detecting activity with known antimalarial drugs. Observations based on the effect of drugs on the morphology of the parasite have also been reported (LADDA and ARNOLD 1966; TRAGER 1967).

The use of radioisotope label techniques to evaluate antimalarial activity of drugs in vitro was described as early as 1952 by CLARKE (1952).

The requirement for a suitable infected host as a source of parasites, and the fact that short-term cultures permitted observations to be made during only a single intraerythrocytic maturation cycle in most cases, limited the utility of these methods in antimalarial chemotherapeutic research. Attempts to apply these techniques to large-scale screening for potential new drugs have, therefore, not been very successful. The use of existing in vivo models, primarily in rodents (OSDENE et al. 1967) and monkeys (SCHMIDT 1978), has proved to be more efficient and productive. Nevertheless, a great deal of useful information regarding the activity of known antimalarial drugs has been obtained with short-term in vitro models. This work has been thoroughly reviewed by BERTAGNA et al. (1972) and, more recently, by TRIGG (1976). The reader is encouraged to consult these authoritative reviews for a detailed description of the use of in vitro techniques with short-term cultures of plasmodia in antimalarial drug research.

A number of important contributions will be considered here because they exemplify some of the applications which can now be anticipated with continuous cultivation techniques. These will be presented according to the species of plasmodia employed in each investigation.

## I. *Plasmodium knowlesi*

### 1. Studies on Mode of Drug Action

POLET and BARR (1968a) described the preparation of cultures of *P. knowlesi* obtained from infected rhesus monkeys and a method for radioisotopic labelling of the nucleic acids and proteins of these parasites in vitro with tritium labelled orotic acid and uniformly carbon-14 labelled isoleucine. These cultures were synchronised within one growth cycle, enabling the investigators to make observations in relation to the morphological stage of development of the parasite at specific points in time during a 20-h incubation period. With these techniques they were later able to demonstrate (POLET and BARR 1968b) that both chloroquine and dihydroquinine inhibited nucleic acid synthesis earlier than they did protein biosynthesis, and that this effect was relatively more pronounced against the more mature form of the intraerythrocytic parasite. They were also able to demonstrate in this in vitro model, using radiolabelled chloroquine and dihydroquinine, that both drugs were considerably more concentrated by parasitised red blood cells than by normal erythrocytes, suggesting that the antimalarial effect of both drugs was attributable to their selective accumulation in parasitised cells. The same observation, of selective accumulation of chloroquine in parasitised erythrocytes, was also reported using short-term in vitro cultures of *P. berghei* from infected mice (FITCH 1969) and *P. falciparum* from infected owl monkeys (FITCH 1970). This work will be described in more detail later.

A dilution method and a continuous membrane perfusion method for short-term in vitro cultivation of *P. knowlesi* were also described by TRIGG (1968), which permitted segmentation and reinvasion of fresh erythrocytes to begin a second cycle of intraerythrocytic maturation. These techniques have been used extensively by TRIGG and his colleagues to study the kinetics and mechanisms of action of a variety of antimalarial drugs. Pyrimethamine, a potent inhibitor of plasmodial dihydrofolate reductase (FERONE et al. 1969), was shown by GUTTERIDGE and TRIGG (1971) to be stage specific in its activity in vitro against *P. knowlesi*. This observation was consistent with the early in vivo observations of McGREGOR and SMITH (1952) with this drug. The explanation for this phenomenon, the stage specificity of antimalarial activity, remains to be determined (FERONE 1977).

TRIGG et al. (1971) also evaluated the activity of cordycepin, a naturally occurring purine nucleoside antibiotic, using the *P. knowlesi* in vitro model. Marked inhibition of growth and maturation were observed at a concentration of $10^{-5}$ *M*. Kinetic studies using radiolabelled amino acids and nucleic acid precursors and lactate production demonstrated that the earliest effect of the drug was on DNA and RNA synthesis. This demonstration exemplifies the use of simultaneous measurements of multiple parameters over time as a method for gaining information relevant to the mechanism of action of a particular drug. A similar "lag period" between the inhibition of DNA and RNA synthesis and subsequent incorporation of amino acids into protein was observed with chloroquine (GUTTERIDGE et al. 1972). There was also a good correlation in this study between inhibition of growth, as determined by morphological assessment, and suppression of macromolecular biosynthesis with respect to the concentration of the drug.

## 2. Use in Drug Screening

The use of short-term in vitro cultures as a screen for potential new antimalarial drugs has been described by a number of investigators. One such system using *P. knowlesi* from infected rhesus monkeys was described by CANFIELD et al. (1970). Parasites harvested at a density of 10%–20% were diluted in Eagle's medium with Hank's salts, L-glutamine and amino acids supplemented with human serum (10%), sodium bicarbonate buffer and antibiotics (penicillin and streptomycin). Antimalarial drug activity was assessed during 18–22 h of incubation by observing morphological maturation (percent of parasites in schizogony), lactic acid production and the incorporation of $^{14}$C-methionine into trichloroacetic acid precipitable protein. By measuring these parameters for each drug at a variety of concentrations these investigators were able to construct concentration-response curves for active compounds. They demonstrated similarity of the concentration-response characteristics of chloroquine assessed by the three different parameters. It should be stressed, however, that the variable time was not included in the design of these studies. In this important respect, these experiments differed from those of GUTTERIDGE et al. (1972). cited previously in which the effect of chloroquine on amino acid incorporation preceded the effect on lactic acid production. A variety of antimalarial drugs were evaluated in this in vitro screen and most, but not all, were active. As also reported previously (GUTTERIDGE and TRIGG 1971) the activity of the diaminopyrimidines, trimethoprim, and pyrimethamine was not detected in this system, which was limited to a single intraerythrocytic maturation cycle. However, in a system with folate-deficient medium supplemented with fetal bovine serum and incorporation of $^{14}$C-orotic acid into DNA as an indicator, these investigators were able to demonstrate the antimalarial activity of folic acid inhibitors (McCORMICK et al. 1971) and the synergistic effect of trimethoprim and sulphalene in vitro (McCORMICK and CANFIELD 1972). Other combinations, such as quinine with pyrimethamine and quinine with chloroquine, were not potentiating. The ability of this in vitro system to provide useful data for structure activity correlations was further demonstrated by MCCORMICK et al. (1974) with the evaluation of a large number of purine analogues.

### 3. Advantages and Disadvantages

Despite the apparent utility and versatility of the short-term culture of *P. knowlesi* as an in vitro model, it has not become a major part of the effort to discover new antimalarial drugs. It has, in fact, proved to be too expensive and cumbersome to serve as a large-scale screen, requiring a population of infected rhesus monkeys as a source of parasites and technically demanding laboratory techniques. The lack of available drug-resistant isolates of the parasite is another limitation of this system. Nevertheless, its use in experienced hands has continued to provide important information relevant to the mechanisms of action of a variety of antimalarial drugs. The fact that it remains synchronous for short-term in vitro application has been advantageous for certain applications. Recently MCCOLM et al. (1980) and HOMMEL et al. (1979) demonstrated that prior treatment of erythrocytes with certain membrane active drugs and with chloroquine or quinine prevented subsequent invasion by *P. knowlesi* in vitro, suggesting a novel mechanism of action for the latter two antimalarial drugs. Use of *P. knowlesi* in vitro will doubtless remain an important resource in antimalarial drug research, especially since it is now possible to maintain this parasite continuously in vitro (BUTCHER 1979). The potential opportunity to combine in vitro studies with in vivo studies in rhesus monkeys has unfortunately been rendered difficult because of the extreme shortage of available monkeys.

## II. *Plasmodium berghei*

### 1. Studies on Mode of Drug Action

Early experiments with *P. berghei* in vitro were limited to very brief periods of incubation (CENEDELLA and SAXE 1967). The antimalarial activity of mepacrine was demonstrated by inhibition of uptake and incorporation of radiolabelled adenosine by *P. berghei*-parasitised mouse erythrocytes during a 30-min incubation at 37 °C in Krebs buffer (VAN DYKE and SZUSTKIEWICZ 1969). Use of this technique as an in vitro screen for antimalarial drugs was proposed by VAN DYKE et al. (1970), and a later application of this method led to demonstration of the importance of hypoxanthine as the substrate for exogenous purine uptake by the parasite (VAN DYKE et al. 1977).

Major contributions to current concepts of the mechanisms of action of existing antimalarial drugs have also been made with the use of short-term in vitro experiments with *P. berghei*. Demonstration of high-affinity chloroquine receptors associated with *P. berghei*-infected red blood cells by FITCH (1969) and their absence when the parasite is resistant to chloroquine provided strong support for an emerging new concept (MACOMBER et al. 1966). This observation, later confirmed with *P. falciparum* from experimentally infected owl monkeys (FITCH 1970), is presently regarded as a key factor in the chemotherapeutic selectivity of the 4-

aminoquinolines and perhaps other quinoline-based antimalarial drugs as well (FITCH et al. 1979). Further evaluation of this phenomenon has led to the identification by FITCH and his colleagues of ferriprotoporphyrin IX, a constituent of malaria pigment, as the chloroquine receptor of erythrocytes infected with chloroquine-sensitive strains of *P. berghei* (CHOU et al. 1980). The lack of production of malaria pigment by chloroquine-resistant strains of *P. berghei* is consistent with this hypothesis. However, since both sensitive and resistant isolates of *P. falciparum* accumulate malaria pigment, the relevance of this distinction and the mechanism described remain to be demonstrated for this species. (See also Part II, Chap. 1.)

Evaluation of antimalarial drug activity by induced changes in malaria pigment has been vigorously pursued with *P. berghei* in vitro (WARHURST et al. 1972). At micromolar concentrations chloroquine causes the accumulation of pigment-laden autophagic vacuoles during brief (60- to 70-min) periods of exposure in *P. berghei* (WARHURST et al. 1974). This "pigment clumping" induced by therapeutic concentrations of chloroquine was first described by HOMEWOOD et al. (1971) and has been used to investigate the activity of a large number of known and potential antimalarial agents (WARHURST and THOMAS 1975; PORTER and PETERS 1976; PETERS et al. 1977a) as well as various specific metabolic inhibitors (WARHURST and THOMAS 1978). Antimalarial drugs such as quinine, mefloquine (WR 142490) and halofantrine (WR 171669) are potent inhibitors of the chloroquine-induced pigment-clumping phenomenon in *P. berghei*. This observation is regarded as presumptive evidence of a partially shared mechanism of action of these drugs. (See also Chap. 10).

An important aspect of the work of these investigators with short-term in vitro cultures of *P. berghei* has been the correlation of in vitro with in vivo observations which are readily obtainable with the murine model. Important questions remain, though, regarding the relevance of these phenomena to the human parasite, *P. falciparum*. This is an urgent consideration in view of the relative ease with which mefloquine resistance has been induced in *P. berghei* (PETERS et al. 1977b; KAZIM et al. 1979). It is noteworthy, in this regard, that chloroquine-resistant strains of *P. berghei* are generally less sensitive to quinoline methanols (such as mefloquine) and phenanthrene alcohols (such as halofantrine) than are chloroquine-sensitive strains. This is not true of *P. falciparum*, at least with the small number of isolates which have been evaluated to date (DESJARDINS et al. 1979).

## 2. Improved Technique for Drug Screening and Evaluation

Seeking to extend the time during which *P. berghei*-infected erythrocytes could be maintained in vitro, WILLIAMS and RICHARDS (1973) reported that considerable improvement could be achieved by separating the infected red blood cells from leucocytes present in freshly obtained specimens. This technique consisted of a series of columns of cellulose powder (Whatmann, CF11) through which diluted fresh blood from an infected rat was filtered. The leucocytes remained adherent in the columns while the erythrocytes passed through without adversely affecting the viability of the parasites which were still infective in vivo and metabolically active in vitro. Nearly linear uptake of radiolabelled L-leucine was observed during a 24-h incubation of these leucocyte-free preparations in Trigg's minimal medium (TRIGG and GUTTERIDGE 1971).

With the leucocyte-free *P. berghei* culture technique, the experimental methods which had been applied chiefly with *P. knowlesi* in vitro were feasible with parasites from rats, which are less expensive and easier to handle than rhesus monkeys. It was then possible to correlate drug effect as measured by various parameters in vitro with parasite viability determined by inoculation in mice. RICHARDS and WILLIAMS (1973) were thus able to demonstrate that inhibition of incorporation of [$^3$H]leucine into protein of *P. berghei*-infected rat erythrocytes in vitro was, indeed, indicative of loss of viability. The in vitro antimalarial concentration-response curves for chloroquine and pyrimethamine were evaluated in this way, yielding 50% inhibitory concentrations of 7.0 μg/ml (22 μ*M*) and 18 μg/ml (72 μ*M*) respectively. As was pointed out by the authors, the inhibitory concentrations of both drugs in these experiments were considerably higher than expected based on previous results with chloroquine against *P. knowlesi* (GUTTERIDGE et al. 1972) and the binding constant of pyrimethamine to the dihydrofolate reductase of *P. berghei* (FERONE et al. 1969). Nevertheless, the concentration-response curves were reproducible with this technique, and it provided a convenient in vitro model for assessing antimalarial drug activity with *P. berghei.*

As was also pointed out by the authors, this new in vitro model with *P. berghei* provided the following advantages over other existing in vitro and in vivo screens employed at that time (RICHARDS and WILLIAMS 1973):

1. Drug activities could be assessed more rapidly and economically.
2. Higher concentrations of drugs could be evaluated than might be possible in vivo.
3. Host factors such as metabolism, excretion, and drug toxicity were eliminated.
4. Very small quantities of compound were needed.
5. Rodents were inexpensive and easier to handle than monkeys.
6. A wide range of drug-resistant isolates of *P. berghei* were available.
7. There is no known health risk associated with laboratory handling of rodent blood or *P. berghei.*

Further refinement of short-term culture techniques for *P. berghei* were described by SMALLEY and BUTCHER (1975). Instead of the series of cellulose columns described by WILLIAMS and RICHARDS (1973) for removing leucocytes from infected rat blood, the newer method consisted of centrifugation (450 g for 6 min, 30 °C) and a subsequent wash with 9 volumes of bicarbonate buffered culture medium. Following removal of the supernatant and buffy coat layers, the infected red blood cells were resuspended in culture medium supplemented with fetal calf serum. When incubated in an orbital incubator at 37 °C for 24 h only 37%–48% of the parasites survived. However, when incubated in a shaking water bath at 15 °C there was apparent reinvasion of new erythrocytes with an increase in parasite density by a factor of 1.2–3.0. Widespread enthusiasm for this improved short-term culture technique for *P. berghei* in antimalarial drug research was apparently interrupted by the discovery a year later of continuous cultivation techniques for *P. falciparum* (TRAGER and JENSEN 1976; HAYNES et al. 1976). However, the potential advantage of *P. berghei* associated with the opportunity for parallel in vivo and in vitro experiments remains.

## III. *Plasmodium falciparum*

### 1. Early Experiences in Laboratory Studies

Interest in the possibility of assessing antimalarial drug activity in vitro with the human pathogen, *P. falciparum* has flourished since the parasite was first identified by LAVERAN (1880). The earliest report of in vitro observations of antimalarial drug (quinine) effect on *P. falciparum* was that of BASS (1922), who had earlier reported the first short-term cultivation of the parasite (BASS and JOHNS 1912). Morphological changes induced by various antimalarial drugs in *P. falciparum* developing in vitro were described in detail by BLACK in 1946.

An early attempt to maintain this species of *Plasmodium* in complex media was reported in 1929 by HOROVITZ and SAUTET as essentially unsuccessful. However, with the development of a medium for the cultivation of mammalian plasmodia during World War II (ANFINSEN et al. 1946), and with the resurgence of interest in fundamental malaria research in the early 1960s, GEIMAN et al. (1966) reported excellent growth of *P. falciparum* in vitro from early ring forms to mature segmented schizonts. Further adaptation of this technique by SIDDIQUI et al. (1972) provided an excellent in vitro model for the assessment of antimalarial drug activity. Parasites obtained from experimentally infected owl monkeys were incubated at 37 °C in a complex bicarbonate buffered culture medium under an atmosphere of 5% $CO_2$ and 95% air for a period of 24 h. Since the infection in the monkeys was synchronous it was possible to select the specimen for initiating cultures when the parasites were predominantly in the "ring" stage. In the absence of effective drugs these would normally mature to segmented schizonts during the 24-h incubation. When an effective drug was added to the culture medium the maturation process was impaired and this could be assessed by morphologically enumerating the parasites at various stages during the incubation period. In this way the investigators evaluated the susceptibility of five characterised isolates of *P. falciparum* to several different antimalarial drugs. The in vitro results were reported to correlate well with clinical and in vivo experimental results reported for the five isolates tested (SIDDIQUI et al. 1972).

### 2. Development of Drug Sensitivity Tests for Field Use

#### a) Original Macrotest

Though SIDDIQUI et al. (1970) showed that a commercial culture medium could readily be substituted for the complex "Harvard medium" used in their work, a simpler technique developed by RIECKMANN et al. (1968) has been applied more readily for field use. The method, as described originally, required small samples of venous blood with patent parasitaemia. After defibrination the blood was aliquoted in volumes of 1.0 ml and placed in small flat-bottomed glass vials to which a solution containing 5 mg glucose had previously been added and dried. The vials were then incubated at 38–40 °C for 24 h without agitation. Cultures were initiated with blood specimens from patients infected with *P. falciparum*, with parasites in the late ring or early trophozoite stage of development. During the incubation period, in samples without added drug, approximately 70% of the parasites matured beyond binucleated schizonts. Drug effect was assessed by comparing the relative proportion of parasites which matured beyond that stage in a vial to which the drug had been added, to a simultaneous control vial without drug added. With this technique chloroquine-sensitive and -resistant isolates were readily distinguishable (RIECKMANN 1971).

This method of assessing the susceptibility of an isolate of *P. falciparum* to chloroquine has been used extensively throughout the world in epidemiological studies. Results with this short-term in vitro method correlate well, in fact, with the standard in vivo procedure for assessing the susceptibility of a particular isolate of *P. falciparum* to chloroquine (RIECKMANN 1980; RICHARDS et al. 1980). As an experimental tool, this method was not used extensively for screening. However, it did provide important information with respect to the activity of many potential new antimalarial drugs, including mefloquine (WORLD HEALTH ORGANIZATION 1973). Lack of cross-resistance with chloroquine was demonstrated by RIECKMANN in vitro with chloroquine-resistant strains of *P. falciparum* which were subsequently used in the initial human volunteer studies with mefloquine (TRENHOLME et al. 1975). The method was also used to demonstrate the long duration of antimalarial activity in the serum of human volunteers after a single oral dose of the drug (RIECKMANN et al. 1974).

b) Microtest for Field Use

A later refinement of the technique described above, with the object of reducing the amount of blood required to perform the assay, was also described by RIECKMANN et al. (1978). The newer method, which was conducted in microtitration plates, required less than 1.0 ml blood and was less sensitive to variations attributable to high parasitaemia and predominance of very early ring forms in the specimen obtained. The microcultures were incubated with 10 volumes of HEPES and bicarbonate buffered RPMI 1640 culture medium in a sealed candle jar as described by TRAGER and JENSEN (1976), thus permitting better maturation of early intraerythrocytic forms to mature schizonts. These microtitration plates can be prepared by addition of solutions containing known amounts of chloroquine or other antimalarial drugs (LOPEZ ANTUÑANO and WERNSDORFER 1979), which are then dried for subsequent field use.

### 3. Use for Drug Screening

Though the short-term cultivation of *P. falciparum* has not been used extensively in the search for potential new antimalarial drugs, the availability of a variety of drug-resistant isolates of the human pathogen has made this an attractive possibility. The obstacle to this application has, of course, been the requirement for infected blood from humans or owl monkeys to initate the cultures. Nevertheless, a number of investigators have employed short-term cultures of *P. falciparum* in the evaluation of experimental compounds of particular interest. TRAGER (1966, 1971) reported the use of an in vitro culture technique with *P. falciparum* obtained from infected owl monkeys to evaluate a class of drugs, antipantothenates, under development at that time as potential new antimalarial drugs.

A somewhat different use of short-term in vitro cultures of *P. falciparum* to measure the antimalarial activity of chloroquine and a new compound, an amidinourea, was reported by RICHARDS and WILLIAMS (1975). In this case, blood specimens were obtained from a group of infected owl monkeys 18 h after they had been treated with various doses of chloroquine or the amidinourea. These specimens were then diluted and incubated in a manner similar to that described earlier by these investigators for *P. berghei* (WILLIAMS and RICHARDS 1973). At multiple time points during a 24-h incubation, samples of these cultures were obtained to assess the incorporation of [$^3$H]leucine by the parasites into trichloroacetic acid precipitable protein. As expected, the parasites from the treated monkeys failed to incorporate the radioactive label as well as those of the control monkey. Perhaps a major contribution of this study was the demonstrated feasibility of using radioisotope incorporation techniques in conjunction with short-term in vitro culture of *P. falciparum* to evaluate antimalarial drug effect. This was also shown by IBER et al. (1975) in a modified application of the RIECKMANN et al. (1968) method using microtitration techniques and measuring incorporation of [$^{14}$C]isoleucine to evaluate chloroquine sensitivity of human isolates of *P. falciparum* in vitro. The incorporation of [$^{14}$C]isoleucine by *P. falciparum* and *P. knowlesi* during short-term in vitro cultures as well as its inhibition by the antibiotics puromycin and cycloheximide had also been demonstrated previously by SCHNELL and SIDDIQUI (1972).

## D. Continuous Culture Technology for *Plasmodium falciparum*

The development of techniques for the continuous cultivation of *P. falciparum* has already contributed to research on the chemotherapy of malaria in two important general respects:

1. Continuous stock cultures provide a reliable source of parasites.
2. Drug effect can be assessed over a longer period of time.

### I. Improved Evaluation and Monitoring of Drug Responses

Non-human species of *Plasmodium* have been used for in vitro studies partly because of the difficulty in obtaining fresh specimens of *P. falciparum* in the laboratory and in some cases because in vitro and in vivo results could be compared more readily. The latter consideration will continue to justify the use of murine and simian parasites for many purposes. For others, though, the availability of the human parasite is a long-awaited laboratory resource. The ability to assess drug activity over a longer period of time with parasites which are presumably growing and multiplying in a more physiological mode is an important technical improvement. The antimalarial activity of some drugs such as pyrimethamine is more readily apparent over more than a single intraerythrocytic maturation cycle.

The benefits of the new technique became apparent early with the improved method for evaluating chloroquine susceptibility of field isolates of *P. falciparum* in microtitration plates described previously (RIECKMANN et al. 1978). When incubation was extended to 26–30 h in this system, reinvasion of new erythrocytes and an increase in parasitaemia were observed in control wells (RIECKMANN 1980). Taking further advantage of the opportunity to evaluate drug effect during longer periods of incubation, NGUYEN-DINH and TRAGER (1980) described a new 48-h test system. Infected red blood cells, either from cultures or from clinical specimens (NGUYEN-DINH et al., 1981) were diluted in a 50% suspension of fresh red blood cells in culture medium to obtain a parasite density of 0.1%–0.8%. The resulting parasitised erythrocyte suspension was then further diluted in culture medium, with or without drug added, to a 2% erythrocyte suspension. Following incubation in a candle jar at 37 °C for 48 h the parasites were counted in Giemsa-stained thin smears. An increase in parasite density from 0.5%–0.6% to 2.8%–3.7% was observed in control cultures during the period of incubation. Characteristic concentration-response curves for chloroquine were observed. Growth and multiplication of chloroquine-susceptible isolates were completely inhibited at a concentration of 0.01 μg/ml. Complete inhibition of a chloroquine-resistant isolate required 0.10 μg/ml. This 48-h test has also been successfully applied to similar studies with mefloquine and quinine (Nguyen-Dinh, personal communication) and pyrimethamine (NGUYEN-DINH and PAYNE, 1980).

A similar in vitro test system was described by KRAMER and SIDDIQUI (1981), in which drug effect was assessed over a period of 72 h. In this case the parasites were incubated in a 5% suspension of erythrocytes with an initial parasite density of 1%–2% at 37 °C. A sealed incubation chamber, continuously gassed with a mixture of 2% $O_2$, 8% $CO_2$, and 90% $N_2$, was used rather than the candle jar technique. Susceptibility of two previously characterised strains and one newly isolated strain of culture adapted *P. falciparum* was assessed with chloroquine, amodiaquine, quinine, and pyrimethamine. Increase in the proportion of infected red blood cells was assessed at the end of the 72-h incubation period in control specimens and at various concentrations of each drug. Chloroquine completely inhibited growth and multiplication of the known susceptible strain (Uganda-Palo Alto) at a concentration of 0.01 μg/ml. The known resistant strain (Vietnam-Oak Knoll) and the newly isolated strain (from the Philippines) were completely inhibited at concentrations of 0.03 μg/ml and 0.1 μg/ml respectively. All three strains were completely inhibited at a concentration of 0.01 μg/ml of amodiaquine, and all were inhibited by quinine at a concentration of 0.10 μg/ml. The three strains appeared resistant to pyrimethamine in vitro, requiring greater than 1.0 μg/ml for suppression, despite the fact that one of these (Vietnam-Oak Knoll) was sensitive to pyrimethamine in vivo.

The in vitro methods for assessment of drug susceptibility of RIECKMANN et al. (1978), NGUYEN-DINH and TRAGER (1980), and KRAMER and SIDDIQUI (1981) all rely on a morphological criterion of response and all report a single concentration as the end point. In each case this end point is the concentration of drug in the first sample showing complete inhibition of growth. This measurement, the minimum inhibitory concentration (MIC), while imprecise and dependent on the concentrations selected for testing, is suitable for distinguishing susceptible and resistant isolates. It may also, as suggested by RIECKMANN (1980), be influenced somewhat by the inoculum size and therefore requires standardisation for interpretation. An important characteristic of the test system proposed by NGUYEN-DINH and TRAGER (1980) is that it lends itself well to standardisation of the inoculum size.

The application of longer-duration in vitro cultures for field use has been hampered by the lack of available non-immune human serum or plasma in tropical areas. It would, therefore, be of great interest if a suitable substitute for that constituent of the culture medium could be identified. SAX and RIECKMANN (1980) suggested pooled rabbit serum and SIDDIQUI (1981) suggested calf serum plus proteose peptone as alternatives. Successful continuous cultures were maintained in both cases, but application to field use with clinical specimens remains to be demonstrated.

Despite acknowledged limitations, the original in vitro macrotest of RIECKMANN et al. (1968) has been the most successfully applied diagnostic test for chloroquine resistance and was designated the WHO Standard Test in 1979. Recent field evaluation of the newer microtest (RIECKMANN et al. 1978), however, indicates that it offers many advantages and may replace the macrotest (WERNSDORFER 1980). Further evaluation of the 48-h test of NGUYEN-DINH and TRAGER (1980), with possible substitution of rabbit or calf serum for non-immune human serum in the culture medium, may provide an even more versatile system for field use. A preliminary trial has been successfully conducted with chloroquine and pyrimethamine in Honduras (NGUYGEN-DINH et al., 1981).

Investigation of the kinetics of antimalarial activity in vitro requires more sophisticated methods than those developed for diagnostic purposes. It may, as is the case for many antibacterials, be important to distinguish between the MIC and the minimum cidal concentration (MCC) for a particular compound. The slope of the concentration-response curve for a potential drug may also provide useful information with respect to the mechanism of action and anticipated therapeutic ratio of a potential new drug. Parallelism between the effect of an active compound alone and in the presence of potential antagonists (e.g. sulphonamides and para-aminobenzoic acid) can also help to identify mechanisms of action. Comparisons of potency among selected compounds of a related chemical structure also requires greater precision than can be offered by techniques which depend on selected concentrations for assessment of activity. At the same time, techniques which are developed for use in the context of a drug development programme must remain as simple and efficient as possible.

## II. Studies on Mode of Action and Kinetics

RICHARDS and MAPLES (1979) described a technique for evaluating the effect of chloroquine and pyrimethamine on parasite growth and viability using *P. falciparum* from continuous cultures. The isolate, which originated from Nigeria, was previously evaluated and found to be susceptible to both drugs in the owl monkey. It was subsequently adapted to in vitro culture by the technique of TRAGER and JENSEN (1976). The method for assessment of drug effect was designed to provide information relative to the viability of the parasites following a period of drug exposure sufficient to suppress growth. It is analogous to techniques employed in assessing bactericidal effects of antibacterial drugs.

Cultures were initiated in 3.5-cm Petri dishes with a parasite density of approximately 1.0% in a 6.6% suspension of erythrocytes in RPMI 1640 supplemented with bicarbonate, HEPES buffer and 10% human serum. When incubated for 96 h at 37 °C in a candle extinction jar with daily changes of culture medium the parasite density regularly increased from 1.0% to approximately 10%. When chloroquine

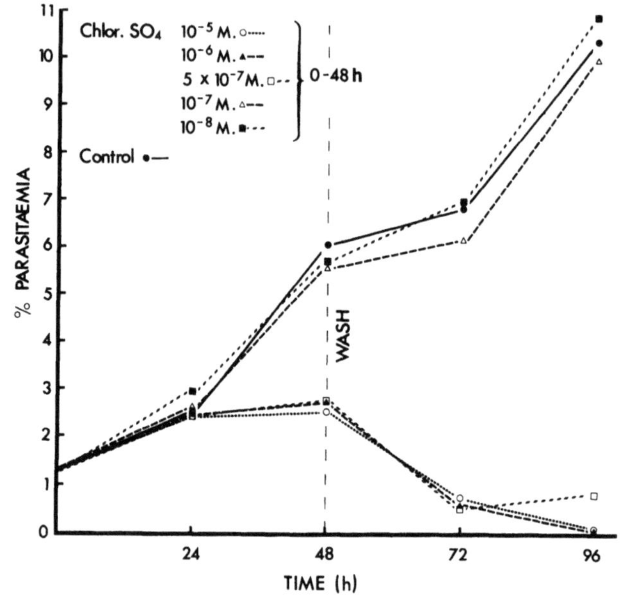


**Fig. 1.** The effect of various concentrations of chloroquine on the growth and viability of *P. falciparum* was assessed in vitro. Chloroquine was present in the culture medium during the initial 48 h. Following a wash the parasites were incubated for an additional 48 h in culture medium without chloroquine. There was no difference between the suppressive and cidal concentrations of the drug in this case. After Richards and Maples (1979)

or pyrimethamine were added to the culture medium a clear concentration-response relationship was apparent. Chloroquine at a concentration of $5 \times 10^{-7}$ *M* completely inhibited multiplication of the parasites when assessed at 48 h. The culture medium was then changed to one containing no active drug in all cultures for the remaining 48 h of incubation. As demonstrated by the graphs in Fig. 1, parasites exposed to concentrations of $5.0 \times 10^{-7}$ *M* or greater were no longer viable when the drug was subsequently removed. Those exposed to concentrations of $1.0 \times 10^{-7}$ *M* or less continued to grow and multiply and remained viable when the drug was subsequently removed. It is apparent, then, that within the limits of the concentrations selected for testing, there is no difference in a 48-h exposure between the inhibitory and cidal concentrations of chloroquine.

A similar experiment with pyrimethamine (Fig. 2) showed that at a concentration of $1.0 \times 10^{-9}$ *M* a slight inhibitory effect was apparent at 48 h but the parasites remained viable and grew in parallel with the control when the drug was removed for the subsequent 48 h. At $1.0 \times 10^{-8}$ *M* or greater concentrations pyrimethamine was both inhibitory and cidal. This difference between inhibitory and cidal concentrations of pyrimethamine may be related to the rapidity and ease with which plasmodia manifest resistance to this drug in clinical use. Insufficient doses of the drug may result in a suppressive but not a cidal effect in vivo, during which survival of viable but non-replicating parasites of a resistant subpopulation of organisms could occur. As the drug concentration decreases the remaining parasites, now re-

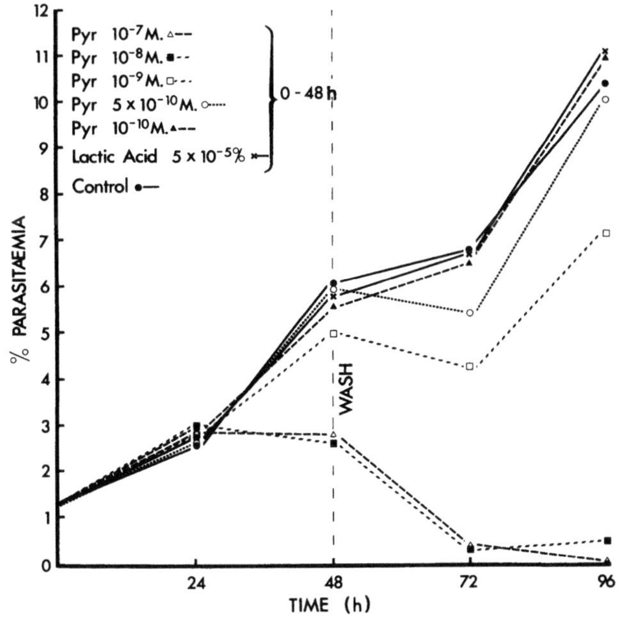


**Fig. 2.** The effect of various concentrations of pyrimethamine on the growth and viability of *P. falciparum* was assessed in vitro. Pyrimethamine was present in the culture medium during the initial 48 h. Following a wash the parasites were incubated for an additional 48 h in culture medium without pyrimethamine. There was apparent suppression of growth at $10^{-9}$ *M*, but a cidal effect was not seen until a concentration of $10^{-8}$ *M* was used. After RICHARDS and MAPLES (1979)

sistant to the drug, are free to resume multiplication, thus establishing a whole population of resistant plasmodia in the host. Conversely, resistance might not be expected to emerge as readily with a drug, such as chloroquine, which has a negligible difference between inhibitory and cidal concentrations. Resistance to chloroquine was, however, successfully induced in vitro in a previously susceptible isolate of *P. falciparum* by continuous cultivation at subinhibitory concentrations of the drug for a period of 1 month (NGUYEN-DINH and TRAGER 1978). The resistance was of high degree (>0.1 μg/ml) and stable during subsequent maintenance in vitro for 1 year.

## III. A Semiautomated Technique of Antimalarial Evaluation

Further characterisation of the antimalarial kinetics of effective compounds can be accomplished by quantitative analysis of the concentration-response relationship. DESJARDINS et al. (1979) described a semiautomated technique for assessment of antimalarial drug activity using continuous cultures as a source of known resistant and susceptible isolates of *P. falciparum*. This technique, which employs standard microtitration equipment and radioisotope uptake as an indicator of parasite growth and multiplication, was designed with maximum efficiency and precision for use in an experimental antimalarial drug development programme. Microtitra-

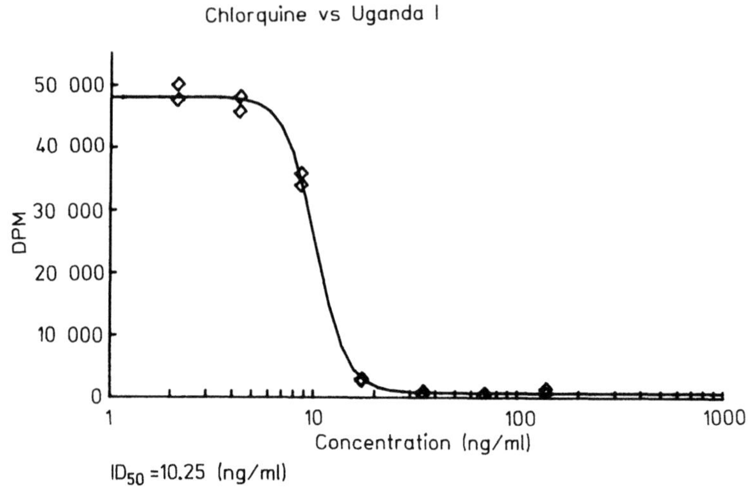


**Fig. 3.** A logistic-logarithmic analysis of the effect of chloroquine at various concentrations on the uptake of [G-$^3$H]hypoxanthine in vitro by erythrocytes parasitised with a chloroquine-sensitive isolate (African-Uganda I) of *P. falciparum*. After DESJARDINS et al. (1979)

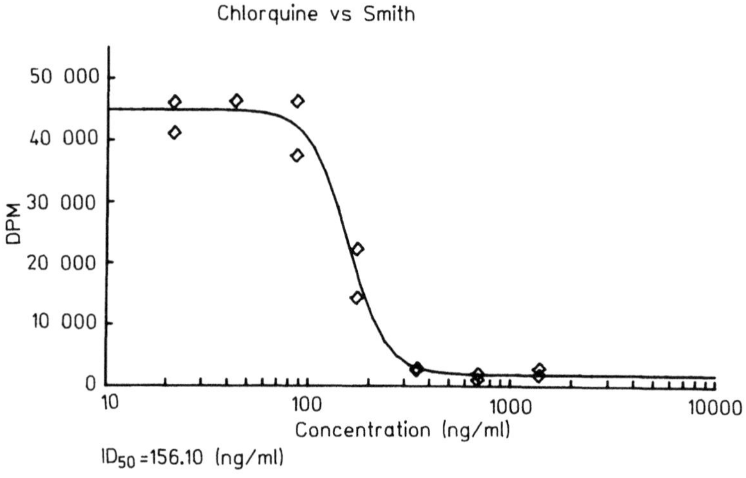


**Fig. 4.** A logistic-logarithmic analysis of the effect of chloroquine at various concentrations on the uptake of [G-$^3$H]hypoxanthine in vitro by erythrocytes parasitized with a chloroquine-resistant isolate (Vietnam-Smith) of *P. falciparum*. After DESJARDINS et al. (1979)

tion plates were prepared with serial twofold dilutions of the test compounds. Specimens of parasitised erythrocytes obtained from stock cultures with a parasite density of 0.25%–0.5% in a 1.5% red blood cell suspension in culture medium were prepared for addition to the wells of the plate. The culture medium was RPMI 1640 supplemented with bicarbonate and HEPES buffer and 10% human plasma. Two sets of control wells consisting of parasitised erythrocytes without drug added and non-parasitised erythrocytes were included. The microtitration plate was then covered and placed in an airtight box which was flushed with a gas mixture of 5%

**Table 1.** The in vitro antimalarial activity of chloroquine, amodiaquine, quinine, mefloquine (WR 142490) and pyrimethamine expressed as the concentration (ng/ml) causing 50% inhibition ($IC_{50}$) of the uptake of [G-$^3$H] hypoxanthine by *Plasmodium falciparum*

| Drug | Parasite strain | |
|---|---|---|
| | African (Uganda I) | Vietnam (Smith) |
| Chloroquine | 9.5±0.78[a] ($n$=12) | 182 ±23.4 ($n$=12) |
| Amodiaquine | 9.8±0.45 ($n$=2) | 23.7± 5.15 ($n$=2) |
| Quinine | 26.1±5.57 ($n$=12) | 109 ± 8.5 ($n$=12) |
| Mefloquine (WR 142490) | 6.7±1.00 ($n$=12) | 7.8± 1.41 ($n$=12) |
| Pyrimethamine | 4.7±0.40 ($n$=2) | >1500 ($n$=2) |

[a] All values are the mean ±1 SE of $n$ separate determinations of the $IC_{50}$

$O_2$, 5% $CO_2$, and 90% $N_2$ and incubated at 37 °C for 24 h. A small volume of culture medium containing [G-$^3$H]hypoxanthine was then added to each well of the plate, which was then returned to the box, flushed as previously and incubated at 37 °C for an additional 18–20 h.

At the end of the 42- to 44-h incubation period the plates were harvested on a MASH II automated cell harvester. This device deposited the particulate contents of each well (erythrocytes) on a small disc of filter paper which was then washed with copious volumes of distilled water. The discs were then dried and placed in scintillation vials for counting. The resulting DPM (disintegrations per minute) for each well, representing the uptake of [G-$^3$H]hypoxanthine, were entered by paper punch tape with the corresponding concentration of drug in a digital computer with a graphic display. In this way, concentration-response data for six compounds in duplicate were obtained from each microtitration plate.

Analysis of the resulting data over a 64-fold range of concentration required application of non-linear curve fitting techniques. The data for each active compound were fitted to a generalised logistic-logarithmic function which included the $IC_{50}$ (50% inhibitory concentration) as one of its parameters. The output from the computer programme included a graph such as those in Figs. 3 and 4, which show the activity of chloroquine against a sensitive (African-Uganda I) and resistant (Vietnam-Smith) isolate of *P. falciparum* respectively. Also included in the output were the respective estimates of the $IC_{50}$ and slope of the curve with corresponding 95% confidence limits. These estimates proved to be very precise and reproducible as demonstrated by the results of many separate determinations of the $IC_{50}$ for chloroquine, amodiaquine, quinine, pyrimethamine, and mefloquine against these two isolates of the parasite shown in Table 1.

Correlation of the results of this in vitro method with in vivo activity for one class of compounds is illustrated in Table 2. Early in vitro data (RIECKMANN 1971) suggested that amodiaquine, a 4-aminoquinoline, was more active than chloroquine itself against chloroquine-resistant *P. falciparum*. This difference is not of sufficient magnitude to support the use of amodiaquine clinically for cases of resistant falciparum malaria. However, it did lead to the development of a number of amodiaquine analogues of which the four compounds in Table 2 are representa-

**Table 2.** The in vitro and in vivo antimalarial activity of four amodiaquine analogues

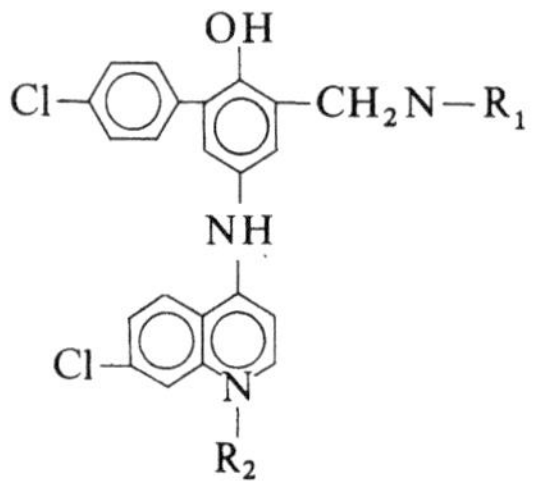

| WR number | 219744 | 225449 | 228258 | 228979 |
|---|---|---|---|---|
| $R_1$ | $(C_2H_5)_2$ | $(C_2H_5)_2$ | $HC(CH_3)_3$ | $HC(CH_3)_3$ |
| $R_2$ | – | = 0 | – | = 0 |
| Mouse $CD_{50}$[a] *P. berghei* | 15.2 | 19.7 | 25.3 | 23.2 |
| *Aotus* $CD_{50}$[b] *P. falciparum* | 2.9 | 4.0 | 1.4 | 4.0 |
| In vitro $IC_{50}$[c] *P. falciparum* | | | | |
| Uganda I | 2.5 | > 12 | 0.80 | 11.4 |
| Smith | 2.4 | > 12 | 0.65 | 11.7 |

[a] The 50% curative dose (mg/kg) in mice infected with *P. berghei* estimated by probit analysis (ARBA AGAR, University of Miami)
[b] The 50% curative dose (mg/kg) in owl monkeys (*Aotus trivirgatus*) infected with *P. falciparum* estimated by probit analysis (R. N. ROSSAN, Gorgas Memorial Laboratory)
[c] Concentration in vitro (ng/ml) causing 50% inhibition ($IC_{50}$) of the uptake of [G–$^3$H] hypoxanthine by chloroquine-sensitive (Uganda I) and resistant (Smith) strains of *P. falciparum*

tive. The results of the in vitro assessment of these compounds show excellent concordance with the results of their assessment in the owl monkey (ROSSAN, personal communication) and show no cross-resistance with chloroquine in two cases. The precision of this in vitro system, therefore, permits selection of the compound with the greatest intrinsic antimalarial activity from a class of compounds of similar structure. This characteristic, as well as efficiency for use as a primary screen, makes the system described by DESJARDINS et al. (1979) particularly suitable for use in a drug development programme. The in vitro activity of several antimalarial compounds under active consideration as potential new drugs are shown in Table 3. One of these, WR 171669 (halofantrine), has been evaluated in non-immune volunteers infected with chloroquine-resistant *P. falciparum* with very promising results (CANFIELD, personal communication).

## IV. Other Applications

Other investigators have recently identified compounds of potential interest as antimalarial drugs using *P. falciparum* maintained in continuous culture (TRAGER et al. 1978; UDEINYA and VAN DYKE 1980; SCHEIBEL et al. 1979). The unique opportunity afforded the investigators working with *P. falciparum* in vitro to explore in detail the mechanism of action of a potential antimalarial drug is illustrated by

**Table 3.** The in vitro antimalarial activity of several potential new antimalarial drugs expressed as the concentration (ng/ml) causing 50% inhibition ($IC_{50}$) of the uptake of [G-$^3$H]hypoxanthine by *Plasmodium falciparum*

| Compound | Parasite strain | |
|---|---|---|
| | African (Uganda I) | Vietnam (Smith) |
| WR 184806[a] | 10.0 | 7.7 |
| WR 180409[b] | 35.4 | 48.5 |
| WR 172435[c] | 7.9 | 3.2 |
| WR 171669[d] | 2.5 | 3.9 |
| WR 194965[e] | 4.6 | 6.5 |
| WR 99210[f] | 1.4 | 1.8 |
| WR 158122[g] | 52.0 | 171 |

[a] WR 184806 DL-2,8-Bis(trifluoromethyl)-4-[1-hydroxy-3-(*N*-*t*-butylamino)propyl] quinoline phosphate
[b] WR 180409 DL-Threo-α-(2-piperidyl)-2-trifluoromethyl-6-(4-trifluoromethylphenyl)-4-pyridine-methanol phosphate
[c] WR 172435 3-Di-*n*-butylamino-1-[2,6-bis(4-trifluoromethylphenyl)-4-pyridyl]-propanol methanesulfonate
[d] WR 171669 1-[1,3-Dichloro-6-trifluoromethyl-9-phenanthryl]-3-di(*n*-butyl)aminopropanol hydrochloride (=halofantrine)
[e] WR 194965 4-(*t*-Butyl)-2-(*t*-butylaminomethyl)-6-(4-chlorophenyl) phenol phosphate
[f] WR 99210 6,6-Diamino-1,2-dihydro-2,2-dimethyl-1-[γ-(2′,4′,5′-trichlorophenoxy)-propyloxy]-s-triazine hydrochloride
[g] WR 158122 2,4-Diamino-6-(2-naphthylsulfonyl) quinazoline

these recent investigations. SCHEIBEL et al. (1979) in exploring the activity of diethyldithiocarbamate, a metal chelating agent, demonstrated inhibition of parasite glycolysis by the drug and commented on the implications of their findings relative to oxidative metabolic processes of potential importance to the parasite. UDEINYA and VAN DYKE (1980), in exploring the activity of tunicamycin as an antimalarial drug, observed that inhibition of membrane glycoprotein synthesis by the drug apparently resulted in loss of essential recognition sites on the merozoite for erythrocyte reinvasion.

## E. The Future Role of In Vitro Techniques

The lessons of the past 30 years with respect to the adaptive capabilities of the *Plasmodium* when confronted with a new drug have hopefully been learned well. It is now clear that the search for new and potentially novel antimalarial drugs must be a continuing process. The experimental induction of resistance to mefloquine by *P. berghei* in mice is a sobering development (PETERS et al. 1977b; KAZIM et al. 1979) in the pursuit of this drug as the agent of choice for chloroquine-resistant falciparum malaria. The appearance of *P. falciparum* isolates resistant to mefloquine is an event anticipated by many with great concern.

It is reasonable with the newly available technology for cultivation of *P. falciparum* and its maintenance in the laboratory to expect a marked acceleration of progress in understanding the metabolism of the organism at a biochemical level. Use of in vitro screening techniques such as those described by RICHARDS and MAPLES (1979) and DESJARDINS et al. (1979) should also greatly accelerate the process of identification of new classes of potential antimalarial drugs and selection within those classes of compounds with the greatest intrinsic activity. The in vitro model must, however, be properly integrated with available in vivo models in the most efficient way possible.

The use of multidrug-resistant isolates of *P. falciparum* in an in vitro model affords the opportunity to seek compounds which are not cross-resistant with existing antimalarial drugs. In this regard a mefloquine-resistant isolate of *P. falciparum* would be an extremely valuable resource. It is not possible to predict with confidence the likelihood of emergence of resistance to mefloquine in the near future. Successful induction of resistance in *P. berghei* in vivo, while discomforting, is of uncertain significance. It is important to note that one of the strains of *P. berghei* which was made resistant to mefloquine by PETERS et al. (1977b) was initially resistant to chloroquine and manifested some cross-resistance to mefloquine at the onset of the experiment. This cross-resistance between chloroquine and mefloquine is generally the case with *P. berghei*, but not with *P. falciparum* (DESJARDINS et al. 1979).

The use of drug combinations has been suggested in the interest of delaying the emergence of resistance (PETERS 1974b). In this regard, it is important to distinguish between the goals of achieving a synergistic antimalarial effect and delaying the emergence of resistance. These may or may not be related characteristics of a particular combination, depending on the respective components and their modes of action. Evaluation of potential drug interactions for synergism, antagonism or indifference by in vitro techniques may suggest possibly favourable or unfavourable combinations. This is now quite feasible with the in vitro model for *P. falciparum*.

Another potential application of the in vitro model is the development of a relevant bioassay. Evaluation of the pharmacokinetics and pharmacodynamics of a new drug is an important early step in modern drug development. The lack of a suitable assay for the drug in biological fluids can cause serious delays. A reliable bioassay for antimalarial activity in blood following single and multiple doses of a potential new drug would add considerable confidence at the critical point in the drug development process when it is necessary to proceed from evaluations in noninfected volunteers (phase I) to initial therapeutic trials (phase II) in patients with malaria. Though such an assay would not distinguish between active metabolites and the parent compound, the kinetics of antimalarial activity itself is more relevant information for optimisation of proposed dosage regimens. Development of a bioassay based on existing techniques is feasible, but will require additional modifications to correct for potential serum effects on the growing parasites.

The greater precision of in vitro methods for assessing intrinsic antimalarial activity will allow better selection of potential new compounds based on structure-activity correlations. In the traditional approach, based on lead-directed synthesis, data such as $IC_{50}$ with defined confidence limits are extremely valuable. The amodiaquine analogues of Table 2 are an illustration of that approach. Newer techniques of drug design based on conformational analysis of three-dimensional molecular models (GUND et al. 1980) are even more dependent on precise estimates of activity for a group of related compounds. Such an approach is now feasible based on properly designed in vitro methods.

Additional foreseeable goals in the further development of in vitro models for research in malaria chemotherapy include:

1. Definition of a minimal essential medium
2. Synchronisation of cultured parasites for stage-specific studies of activity
3. Increase in the volume and production of parasites for biochemical studies
4. Development of methods for the cultivation of other species of *Plasmodium*, especially *P. vivax*
5. Determination of the mechanism for induction of gametogenesis in vitro.

These and many other objectives are being vigorously pursued in a growing number of laboratories around the world now that it is possible to maintain the parasite of greatest concern, *P. falciparum*, continuously in vitro. It is likely that significant progress in many of these laboratories will have been reported by the time this volume reaches the library shelves of those same institutions. It can be predicted, with confidence, that this new technology will result in major contributions to our knowledge of the molecular biology of the asexual life cycle of *P. falciparum* leading to truly novel approaches to the chemotherapy of malaria.

## References

Anfinsen CB, Geiman QM, McKee RW, Ormsbee RA, Ball EG (1946) Studies of malarial parasites. VIII. Nutrition of *Plasmodium knowlesi*. Factors affecting the growth of *Plasmodium knowlesi* in vitro. J Exp Med 84:607–621

Bass CC (1922) Some observations on the effects of quinine upon the growth of malarial plasmodia in vitro. Am J Trop Med Hyg 2:289–292

Bass CC, Johns FM (1912) The cultivation of malarial plasmodia (*Plasmodium vivax* and *Plasmodium falciparum*) *in vitro*. J Exp Med 16:567–579

Bergan T, Carlsen IB, Fuglesang JE (1980) An in vitro model for monitoring bacterial responses to antibiotic agents under simulated in vivo conditions. Infection [Suppl] 1:96–110

Bertagna P, Cohen S, Geiman QM, Haworth J, Königk E, Richards WHG, Trigg PI (1972) Cultivation techniques for the erythrocytic stages of malaria parasites. Bull WHO 47:357–373

Black RH (1946) The effect of antimalarial drugs on *Plasmodium falciparum* (New Guinea strains) developing in vitro. Trans R Soc Trop Med Hyg 40:163–170

Bushby SRM (1964) Chap. XX. Chemotherapy. In: Cochrane RG, Davey TF, McRobert G (eds) Leprosy in theory and practice. Wright, Bristol, p 344

Butcher GA (1979) Factors affecting the in vitro culture of *Plasmodium falciparum* and *Plasmodium knowlesi*. Bull WHO (Suppl 1) 57:17–26

Canfield CJ, Altstatt LB, Elliot Van B (1970) An in vitro system for screening potential antimalarial drugs. Am J Trop Med Hyg 19:905–909

Cenedella RJ, Saxe LH (1966) Automation in analytical chemistry. I. Automated mass screening of compounds for antimalarial activity. Mediad White Plains, NY, pp 281–293

Cenedella RJ, Saxe LH (1967) Automated mass screening of compounds for antimalarial activity. Technicon Symposium Mediad, New York, p 281

Chou AC, Chevli R, Fitch CD (1980) Ferriprotoporphyrin IX fulfills the criteria for identification as the chloroquine receptor of malaria parasites. Biochemistry 19:1543–1549

Clarke DH (1952) The use of phosphorus-32 in studies on *Plasmodium gallinaceum*. I. The development of a method for quantitative determination of parasitic growth and development in vitro. J Exp Med 96:439–450

Collins P, Bauer DJ (1979) The activity in vitro against herpes virus of 9-(2-hydroxyethoxymethyl)guanine (acycloguanosine), a new antiviral agent. J Antimicrob Chemother 5:431–436
Desjardins RE, Canfield CJ, Haynes JD, Chulay JD (1979) Quantitative assessment of antimalarial activity in vitro by a semiautomated microdilution technique. Antimicrob Agents Chemother 16:710–718
Ferone R (1977) Folate metabolism in malaria. Bull WHO 55:291–298
Ferone R, Burchall JJ, Hitchings GH (1969) *Plasmodium berghei* dihydrofolate reductase. Isolation, properties, and inhibition by antifolates. Mol Pharmacol 5:49–59
Fitch CD (1969) Chloroquine resistance in malaria: a deficiency of chloroquine binding. Proc Natl Acad Sci USA 64:1181–1187
Fitch CD (1970) *Plasmodium falciparum* in owl monkeys: Drug resistance and chloroquine binding capacity. Science 169:289–290
Fitch CD, Chan RL, Chevli R (1979) Chloroquine resistance in malaria: Accessibility of drug receptors to mefloquine. Antimicrob Agents Chemother 15:258–262
Geiman QM (1948) Cultivation and metabolism of malarial parasites. Proceedings IV th international congress on tropical medicine and malaria, Washington, pp 618–628
Geiman QM, Anfinsen CB, McKee RW, Ormsbee RA, Ball EG (1946) Studies on malarial parasites. VII. Methods and techniques for cultivation. J Exp Med 84:583–606
Geiman QM, Siddiqui WA, Schnell JV (1966) In vitro studies on erythrocytic stages of plasmodia; medium improvement and results with seven species of malarial parasites. Milit Med 131:1015–1025
Gund P, Andose JD, Rhodes JB, Smith GM (1980) Three-dimensional molecular modeling and drug design. Science 208:1425–1431
Gutteridge WE, Trigg PI (1970) Incorporation of radioactive precursors into DNA and RNA of *Plasmodium knowlesi*. J Protozool 17:89–96
Gutteridge WE, Trigg PI (1971) Action of pyrimethamine and related drugs against *Plasmodium knowlesi* in vitro. Parasitology 62:431–444
Gutteridge WE, Trigg PI, Bayley PM (1972) Effects of chloroquine on *Plasmodium knowlesi* in vitro. Parasitology 64:37–45
Hadden JW, Coffey RG, Hadden EM, Lopez-Corroles E, Sunshine GH (1975) Effects of levamisole and imidazole on lymphocyte proliferation and cyclic nucleotide levels. Cell Immunol 20:98–106
Haynes JD, Diggs CL, Hines FA, Desjardins RE (1976) Culture of human malaria parasites *Plasmodium falciparum*. Nature 263:767–769
Homewood CA, Warhurst DC, Baggaley VC (1971) Incorporation of radioactive precursors into *Plasmodium berghei* in vitro [laboratory demonstration]. Trans R Soc Trop Med Hyg 65:10
Hommel M, McColm AA, Trigg PI (1979) *Plasmodium knowlesi:* inhibition of invasion by pretreatment of erythrocytes with chloroquine and quinine. Ann Microbiol (Paris) 130B:287–293
Horovitz A, Sautet J (1929) Remarques sur la culture des parasites du paludisme. Ann Parasitol Hum Comp 7:151–160
Iber PK, Pavanand K, Wilks NE, Colwell EJ (1975) Evaluation of in vitro drug sensitivity of human *Plasmodium falciparum* by incorporation of radioactive isoleucine. J Med Assoc Thai 58:559–566
Jensen JB, Trager W (1978) *Plasmodium falciparum* in culture: Establishment of additional strains. Am J Trop Med Hyg 27:743–746
Kazim M, Puri SK, Dutta GP (1979) Chemotherapeutic studies with mefloquine and selection of a mefloquine-resistant strain of *Plasmodium berghei*. Indian J Med Res 70:95–102
Kramer KJ, Siddiqui WA (1981) A strain of *Plasmodium falciparum* from the Phillippines: Continuous in vitro cultivation and drug susceptibility studies. Tenth international congress on tropical medicine and malaria, Manila, Philippines Nov 9–15, 1980
Ladda R, Arnold J (1966) Morphologic observation on the effect of antimalarial agents on the erythrocytic forms of *Plasmodium berghei* in vitro. Milit Med 131:993–1008

Laveran A (1880) Note sur un nouveau parasite trouvé dans le sang de plusieurs malades atteints de fièvre palustre. Bull Acad Nat Méd (Paris) 9:1235–1236
Lopez-Antunano FJ, Wernsdorfer WH (1979) In vitro response of chloroquine-resistant *Plasmodium falciparum* to mefloquine. Bull WHO 57:663–665
Macomber PB, O'Brien RL, Hahn FE (1966) Chloroquine: Physiological basis of drug resistance in *Plasmodium berghei*. Science 152:1374–1375
McColm AA, Hommel M, Trigg PI (1980) Inhibition of malaria parasite invasion into erythrocytes pretreated with membrane active drugs. Mol Biochem Parasitol 1:119–127
McCormick GJ, Canfield CJ (1972) In vitro evaluation of antimalarial drug combinations. Proc Helminth Soc Wash 30:292–297
McCormick GJ, Canfield CJ, Willet GP (1971) *Plasmodium knowlesi:* In vitro evaluation of antimalarial activity of folic acid inhibitors. Exp Parasitol 30:88–93
McCormick GJ, Canfield CJ, Willet GP (1974) In vitro antimalarial activity of nucleic acid precursor analogs in the simian malaria *Plasmodium knowlesi*. Antimicrob Agents Chemother 6:16–21
McGregor IA, Smith DA (1952) Daraprim in the treatment of malaria. A study of its effects in falciparum and quartan infections in West Africa. Br Med J 1:730–732
Miller LH, Mason SJ, Dvorak JA (1975) Erythrocyte receptors for (*Plasmodium knowlesi*) malaria: Duffy blood group determinants. Science 189:561–563
Murakawa T, Sakamoto H, Hirose T, Nishida M (1980) New in vitro kinetic model for evaluating bactericidal efficacy of antibiotics. Antimicrob Agents Chemother 18:377–381
Nguyen-Dinh P, Trager W (1978) Chloroquine resistance produced in vitro in an African strain of human malaria. Science 200:1397–1398
Nguyen-Dinh P, Payne D (1980) Pyrimethamine sensitivity in *Plasmodium falciparum:* Determination in vitro by a modified 48-hour test. Bull WHO 58:909–912
Nguyen-Dinh P, Trager W (1980) *Plasmodium falciparum* in vitro: Determination of chloroquine sensitivity of three new strains by a modified 48-hour test. Am J Trop Med Hyg 29:339–342
Nguyen-Dinh P, Hobbs, JH, Campbell CC (1981) Assessment of chloroquine sensitivity of *Plamodium falciparum* in Choluteca, Honduras. Bull WHO 59:641–646
Osdene TS, Russel PB, Rane L (1967) 2,4,7-Triamino-6-ortho-substituted arylpteridines. A new series of potent antimalarial agents. J Med Chem 10:431–434
Peters W (1974a) Recent advances in antimalarial chemotherapy and drug resistance. Adv Parasitol 12:69–114
Peters W (1974b) Prevention of drug resistance in rodent malaria by the use of drug mixtures. Bull WHO 51:379–383
Peters W, Howells RE, Portus J, Robinson BL, Thomas S, Warhurst DC (1977a) The chemotherapy of rodent malaria, XXVII. Studies on mefloquine (WR 142,490). Ann Trop Med Parasitol 71:408–418
Peters W, Portus J, Robinson BL (1977b) The chemotherapy of rodent malaria, XXVIII. The development of resistance to mefloquine (WR 142,490). Ann Trop Med Parasitol 71:419–427
Polet H, Barr CF (1968a) DNA, RNA, and protein synthesis in erythrocytic forms of *Plasmodium knowlesi*. Am J Trop Med Hyg 17:672–679
Polet H, Barr CF (1968b) Chloroquine and dihydroquinine. In vitro studies of their antimalarial effect upon *Plasmodium knowlesi*. J Pharmacol Exp Ther 164:380–386
Porter M, Peters W (1976) The chemotherapy of rodent malaria, XXV. Antimalarial activity of WR 122,455 (a 9-phenanthrenemethanol) in vivo and in vitro. Ann Trop Med Parasitol 70:259–270
Richards WHG, Maples BK (1979) Studies on *Plasmodium falciparum* in continuous cultivation: I. The effect of chloroquine and pyrimethamine on parasite growth and viability. Ann Trop Med Parasitol 73:99–108
Richards WHG, Williams SG (1973) Malaria studies in vitro. II: The measurement of drug activities using leucocyte-free blood-dilution cultures of *Plasmodium berghei* and $^{3}$H-leucine. Ann Trop Med Hyg 67:179–190

Richards WHG, Williams SG (1975) Malaria studies *in vitro*. III. The protein synthesizing activity of *Plasmodium falciparum* in vitro after drug treatment in vivo. Ann Trop Med Parasitol 69:135–140

Richards WHG, Haynes JD, Scheibel LW, Sinden R, Desjardins RE, Wernsdorfer WH (1980) New developments in malaria chemotherapy using in vitro cultures. In: Nelson JD, Grassi C (eds) Current chemotherapy and infectious disease. American Society for Microbiology, Washington DC

Rieckmann KH (1971) Determination of the drug sensitivity of *Plasmodium falciparum*. J Am Med Assoc 217:573–578

Rieckmann KH (1980) Susceptibility of cultured parasites of *Plasmodium falciparum* to antimalarial drugs. In: Rowe DS, Hirumi H (eds) The in vitro cultivation of the pathogens of tropical diseases. Schwabe, Basel, pp 35–50

Rieckmann KH, McNamara JV, Frischer H, Stockert TA, Carson PE, Powell RD (1968) Effects of chloroquine, quinine, and cycloguanil upon the maturation of asexual erythrocytic forms of two strains of *Plasmodium falciparum* in vitro. Am J Trop Med Hyg 17:661–671

Rieckmann KH, Trenholme GM, Williams RL, Carson PE, Frischer H, Desjardins RE (1974) Prophylactic activity of mefloquine hydrochloride (WR 142,490) in drug-resistant malaria. Bull WHO 51:375–377

Rieckmann KH, Campbell GH, Sax LJ, Mrema JE (1978) Drug sensitivity of *Plasmodium falciparum:* An in vitro microtechnique. Lancet I:22–23

Rozman RS, Canfield CJ (1979) New experimental antimalarial drugs. Adv Pharmacol Chemother 16:1–43

Sax LJ, Rieckmann KH (1980) Use of rabbit serum in the cultivation of *Plasmodium falciparum*. J Parasitol 66:621–624

Scheibel LW, Adler A, Trager W (1979) Tetraethyliuram disulfide (Antabuse) inhibits the human malaria parasite *Plasmodium falciparum*. Proc Nat Acad Sci 76:5303–5307

Schmidt LH (1978) *Plasmodium falciparum* and *Plasmodium vivax* infections in the owl monkey (*Aotus trivirgatus*). III. Methods employed in the search for new blood schizonticidal drugs. Am J Trop Med Hyg 27:718–737

Schnell JV, Siddiqui WA (1972) The effects of antibiotics on $^{14}C$-isoleucine incorporation by monkey erythrocytes infected with malarial parasites. Proc Helminth Soc Wash 39:201–203

Siddiqui WA (1981) Continuous in vitro cultivation of *Plasmodium falciparum*. Replacement of human serum by calf serum and proteose peptone. Indian J Med Res 73:19–22

Siddiqui WA, Richmond-Crum SM (1977) Fatty acid-free bovine serum albumin as a plasma replacement for in vitro cultivation of *Plasmodium falciparum*. J Parasitol 63:583–584

Siddiqui WA, Schnell JV, Geiman QM (1970) Use of a commercially-available culture medium to test the susceptibility of human malarial parasites to antimalarial drugs. J Parasitol 56:188–189

Siddiqui WA, Schnell JV, Geiman QM (1972) A model in vitro system to test the susceptibility of human malarial parasites to antimalarial drugs. Am J Trop Med Hyg 21:392–399

Smalley ME, Butcher GA (1975) The in vitro culture of the blood stages of *Plasmodium berghei*. Int J Parasitol 5:131–132

Tallarida RJ, Jacob LS (1979) The dose-response relation in pharmacology. Springer, New York

Trager W (1966) Coenzyme A and the antimalarial action of antipantothenate against *Plasmodium lophurae*, *P. coatneyi*, and *P. falciparum*. Trans NY Acad Sci Ser II 28:1094–1108

Trager W (1967) The different effects of antimalarial drugs on *Plasmodium lophurae* developing intracellularly and extracellularly in vitro. Am J Trop Med Hyg 16:15–18

Trager W (1971) Further studies on the effects of antipantothenates on malaria parasites (*Plasmodium coatneyi* and *P. falciparum*) in vitro. J Protozool 18:232–239

Trager W, Jensen JB (1976) Human malaria parasites in continuous culture. Science 193:673–675

Trager W, Robert-Gero M, Lederer E (1978) Antimalarial activity of *S*-isobutyl adenosine against *Plasmodium falciparum* in culture. FEBS Lett 85:264–266

Trenholme GM, Williams RL, Desjardins RE, Frischer H, Carson PE, Rieckmann KH (1975) Mefloquine (WR 142,490) in the treatment of human malaria. Science 190:792–794

Trigg PI (1968) A new continuous perfusion technique for the cultivation of malaria parasites in vitro. Trans R Soc Trop Med Hyg 62:371–378

Trigg PI (1976) Parasite cultivation in relation to research on the chemotherapy of malaria. Bull WHO 53:399–406

Trigg PI, Gutteridge WE (1971) A minimal medium for the growth of *Plasmodium knowlesi* in dilution cultures. Parasitology 62:113–123

Trigg PI, Gutteridge WE, Williamson J (1971) The effects of cordycepin on malaria parasites. Trans R Soc Trop Med Hyg 65:514–520

Udeinya IJ, Van Dyke K (1979) Altered synthesis of membrane glycoproteins in cultured *Plasmodium falciparum* in the presence of tunicamycin. Proceedings of the 11 th international congress of chemotherapy, Boston 1–5 October 1979. Vol 2. Available from the American Society for Microbiology, Washington DC, pp 1098–1099

Van Dyke K, Szustkiewicz C (1969) Apparent new modes of antimalarial action detected by inhibited incorporation of adenosine-8-$^3$H into nucleic acids of *Plasmodium berghei*. Milit Med 134:1000–1006

Van Dyke K, Szustkiewicz C, Cenedella R, Saxe LH (1970) A unique antinucleic acid approach to the mass screening of antimalarial drugs. Chemotherapy 15:177–188

Van Dyke K, Trush MA, Wilson ME, Stealey PK (1977) Isolation and analysis of nucleotides from erythrocyte-free malarial parasites (*Plasmodium berghei*) and potential relevance to malaria chemotherapy. Bull WHO 55:253–264

Warhurst DC, Thomas SC (1975) Pharmacology of the malaria parasite – a study of dose-response relationships in chloroquine-induced autophagic vacuole formation in *Plasmodium berghei*. Biochem Pharmacol 24:2047–2056

Warhurst DC, Thomas SC (1978) The chemotherapy of rodent malaria, XXXI. The effect of some metabolic inhibitors upon chloroquine-induced pigment clumping (CIPC) in *Plasmodium berghei*. Ann Trop Med Parasitol 72:203–211

Warhurst DC, Homewood CA, Peters W, Baggaley VC (1972) Pigment changes in *Plasmodium berghei* as indications of activity and mode of action of antimalarial drugs. Proc Helminth Soc Wash 39:271–278

Warhurst DC, Homewood CA, Baggaley VC (1974) The chemotherapy of rodent malaria, XX. Autophagic vacuole formation in *Plasmodium berghei* in vitro. Ann Trop Med Parasitol 68:265–281

Wernsdorfer WH (1980) Field evaluation of drug resistance in malaria. *In vitro* micro-test. Acta Trop (Basel) 37:222–227

Williams SG, Richards WHG (1973) Malaria studies in vitro. I: techniques for the preparation and culture of leucocyte-free blood-dilution cultures of *Plasmodia*. Ann Trop Med Hyg 67:169–178

Williamson J, Scott-Finnigan TJ (1978) Trypanocidal activity of antitumor antibiotics and other metabolic inhibitors. Antimicrob Agents Chemother 13:735–744

World Health Organization (1973) Chemotherapy of malaria and resistance to antimalarials. WHO Tech Rep Ser 529:58

Zhengren C, Minxin G, Yuhua L, Shumin H, Nailin Z (1980) Studies on the cultivation of erythrocytic stage plasmodium in vitro. Chin Med J [Engl] 93:31–35

CHAPTER 7

# Use of Avian Malarias (In Vivo)

W. H. G. RICHARDS

## A. Introduction

To estimate the full impact that research into avian malaria has played in the development of knowledge of the parasite, its metabolism, malaria chemotherapy, and immunity can now be more fully appreciated than in the past. Although there is not the same number of species of malaria parasite in birds as in mammals, the host range is wider and at least 447 species of birds have been found infected with malaria parasites (COATNEY and ROUDABUSH 1949), spanning every continent in the world. It was fortunate that plasmodia in birds were found (DANILEWSKY 1885) so soon after LAVERAN described the causative organisms of human malaria in 1880, since the course of experimental observations in both types of parasites has proceeded side by side.

Avian malaria parasites are able to infect different invertebrate and vertebrate hosts and *Plasmodium gallinaceum* will develop in at least five different genera and in a great number of species of mosquitoes (GARNHAM 1966). Although there are many areas of similarity between avian and mammalian malaria there are three differences which differentiate between the two. The avian parasites infect nucleated erythrocytes whilst the mammalian species infect non-nucleated blood cells. The invertebrate vectors of avian species are usually mosquitoes of the genera *Aedes* or *Culex* and the mammalian species are confined to the *Anopheles* host. Most striking are the preerythrocytic stages of the avian parasites, which are found in the mesodermal tissues and require two generations in the host, whereas the mammalian species are found in the liver parenchyma cells with only one generation (see also Chap. 1).

Many distinguished scientists in the 1890 s and the early part of the next century contributed greatly to our knowledge. GRASSI and FELETTI (1890) isolated new species and made detailed comparative studies on the structural features of avian and mammalian malarias. LABBÉ (1893) directed his attentions towards the epidemiology, immunology, and evolution of the organisms. The endocorpuscular parasites of birds were not seriously considered in America until about 13 years after their discovery in Europe when Eugene OPIE (1898) studied parasites found in native birds and made careful observations on the morphology and physiology of the parasites. He described the displacement of the host-cell nucleus by the parasite and double infection of a single erythrocyte. He observed and reported the phenomenon of exflagellation and the subsequent union of gametes in the drawn blood of crows. This was later observed by MACCULLUM (1898) in *P. falciparum.* In the same year Ross (1898) described the role of mosquitoes as vectors of malaria. He had been stimulated by MACCULLUM'S earlier work and, when transferred to a region in India where human malaria was not common, he started to work with malaria-infected sparrows and *Culex* mosquitoes. Sporozoites were found in oocysts and traced to the salivary glands. Were it not for the use of birds as experimental hosts it is doubtful whether the mosquito transmission of malaria would have been established so early. While earlier workers confined their studies to vital but academic studies, the use of avian malaria for chemotherapy has been of paramount importance.

The effect of quinine on avian malaria was first reported by WASIELEWSKI in 1904, parasites being killed in vitro by a concentration as low as 1:10,000 at room temperature. KOPANARIS (1911) confirmed this work although tge concentration of quinine required to kill the parasites in vitro was found to be 1:1,200, while 1:2,000 was not parasiticidal. The SERGENTS (1921) conducted the first extensive series of experiments on the effects of quinine in vivo in bird malaria infections. Many others followed this work. The work of ROEHL (1926) using *P. relictum* and HEGNER and MANWELL (1927) using *P. cathemerium* demonstrated the successful use of pamaquine (plasmochin) on avian malaria with the later use of the drug to treat human malarias. This success stimulated the synthesis of many novel compounds, and their assay against *P. cathemerium*, including quinoline analogues, substituted phenyls, azo dye, and pyridines. Fifty-eight different chemicals were tested but it was found that members of the quinine series gave the best results. MANWELL (1930a, b, 1934) was the first to compare the effects of quinine and pamaquine on different species of bird malaria. KIKUTH'S report (1932) of the successful activity of mepacrine heralded the beginning of a new era of chemotherapy.

## B. Experimental Hosts and Methods

Most of the early experimental work on bird malaria was carried out in sparrows, chaffinches, pigeons, linnets, larks, and canaries. However, the utility of *P. gallinaceum* and *P. lophurae* as experimental models has led to young chickens and ducks becoming the hosts of choice. The techniques employed for both systems are similar but, for simplicity, only *P. gallinaceum* will be described.

Strains of *P. gallinaceum* may be maintained over many years by blood passage only, or by cyclical transmission through mosquitoes. Young chicks 5–7 days old are the most suitable, being susceptible, easy to handle and only weighing about 50 g, thus proving economical in drug demand.

### I. Transmission by Blood Inoculation

Direct inoculation by infected blood is usually employed for routine maintenance or to inoculate a number of animals for chemotherapy experiments. When only one or two birds need to be infected, a sufficient quantity of parasitised blood can be obtained from the leg vein or wing vein of an infected bird. The syringe and needle should be wetted with 0.1% heparin to prevent the blood from clotting. When a large number of chicks are to be infected from a single donor, blood is aspirated directly from the neck vein or from the heart. The blood is then diluted in glucose saline for use. The total number of parasitised erythrocytes used to infect experimental animals varies from 1 to 50 million and is dependent on the virulence of the strain and the route of inoculation. Infection given into the peritoneal cavity directly below the sternum, intramuscularly into the breast muscle, or subcutaneously in the neck region are slow, up to 7 days, to become patent. Infection given intravenously into the neck vein is easy, fast and gives great uniformity when large numbers of birds are used with more than 90% of the erythrocytes infected; death occurs between days 5 and 7.

### II. Drug Testing

Known and experimental drugs may be administered to chicks orally, intravenously, and intramuscularly; however, the oral route is the method used most frequently. The methods of ROLLO (1955) and RICHARDS (1966) used drugs maintained in solutions or suspensions and administered orally on a milligrams per kilogram basis. Experimental birds were infected intravenously and received the first dose of drug on the same day, then twice a day for the following 3 days. Blood films were made from all the birds on day 4. The parasitaemia in the untreated controls was between 70% and 95%, and the parasitaemias of the test birds were expressed as a percentage of the untreated controls. Whatever the test system used, the end result was achieved by comparing treated birds with a comparable group of untreated controls.

## C. Chemotherapy

Through time there have been many attempts to treat malarial fevers with the wearing of charms and bracelets. It is interesting to note that BARANGER and FILER (1953) using rings, bands or spirals of various metals placed around chicks infected with *P. gallinaceum* found some protective effects. Not only was there a prolonged survival time when compared with the untreated birds, but the asexual blood parasites were retarded. Even more intriguing was that removal of the band was followed by an increase in parasitaemia on the following day! Copper, iron or gold were the most effective.

### I. Quinine

The alkaloid quinine was recognised as having an effect against the fevers as long ago as 1630. This, the second of the antimalarials (the Chinese herb Qinghao is certainly older), acts as a blood schizontocide against the asexual parasites. Although quinine was known to alleviate the clinical signs of human malaria long before DANILEWSKY it was not until the avian malarias were discovered that an experimental host became available to test the effects of this and other chemical compounds. WASIELEWSKI (1904), KOPANARIS (1911), and LOURIE (1934a) reported on the action of the drug in vitro with suspensions of infected erythrocytes. LOURIE found that *P. cathemerium* parasites were still infective after 1 h incubation at 39 °C with quinine at a concentration of 1:500, while segmentation was delayed at the 1:5,000 level with exposures from 1 to 2 h. The author postulated that the action of quinine in vivo is not a direct one on the part of the drug since, he concluded, the very strong concentration of drug used in vitro could not be maintained as a blood level for any considerable length of time.

WAMPLER (1930) reported degenerative changes in the trophozoites and schizonts of *P. cathemerium* after treatment with quinine, and very similar changes were noted by MANWELL and HARING (1938) in *P. vaughani* infections treated with mepacrine.

It is interesting that, while quinine and related major alkaloids show significant schizontocidal activity against avian species of plasmodia, their relative potencies vary with the species (FINDLAY 1951; HILL 1963), viz:

*P. gallinaceum* in chicks: cinchonine > quinidine > cinchonidine > quinine
*P. lophurae* in ducks: quinine = quinidine > cinchonidine > cinchonine
*P. relictum* in canaries: quinine = quinidine > cinchonidine > cinchonine

This difference in response to quinine had been reported previously by MANWELL (1934) when he also examined the effect of pamaquine. Quinine had the greatest effect on *P. rouxi* with a decreasing activity through *P. relictum*, *P. cathemerium*, *P. circumflexum*, and *P. elongatum*. Pamaquine had equal activity against *P. rouxi* and *P. elongatum*, decreasing through *P. relictum*, *P. circumflexum*, and *P. cathemerium*. MANWELL concluded that the difference in response to drug treatment could be correlated with the differences in the reproductive rates at schizogony of the avian species. LOURIE (1934b) observed considerable differences in the response to quinine between strains of *P. relictum* but offers no explanation for the phenomenon. This was also reported by PETERS (1970) when, from collected reports, it appeared that a German strain of *P. relictum* was innately resistant to quinine. He also noted that resistance to quinine treatment could be induced in *P. relictum* and *P. gallinaceum* whilst, in *P. cathemerium*, workers were unable to develop any degree of tolerance.

HAAS et al. (1948) using quinine were able to demonstrate the complete suppression of erythrocytic schizogony in *P. gallinaceum*, whereas the exoerythrocytic cycle was completely unaffected.

A compound related to quinine, Endochine (3-*n*-heptyl-7-methoxy-2-methyl-4-quinolone), was synthesised in Germany and had marked activity against several avian malarias. STECK (1972), reviewing the data, found prophylactic and trophozoiticidal effects against *P. cathemerium* in canaries and gametocytocidal activity against *Haemoproteus* infection in finches. Further work demonstrated a lack of activity in mammalian species.

## II. 4-Aminoquinolines

Chloroquine and amodiaquine have established themselves as the drugs of choice, in the majority of the world, for the treatment of human malarias. Much of the chemical synthetic work was carried out in Germany, the original aim being to increase the efficacy of mepacrine, reduce the toxicity and eliminate the tissue-staining side effects of the drug. Comparatively little work was done in the avian malaria models and this was in comparison to mepacrine, with the results being expressed as quinine equivalents. The work, which was reported in WISELOGLE (1946), utilised *P. cathemerium* in canaries and ducks, *P. gallinaceum* in chicks, and *P. lophurae* in chicks and ducks. Chloroquine and amodiaquine were similar in activity and the most active. Oxychloroquine and bromoquine were next in activity followed by sontoquine.

COATNEY et al. (1953), analysing data on nearly 4000 compounds tested against *P. gallinaceum* at the National Institutes for Health, showed a rather low maximum tolerated dose for chloroquine of 30 mg/kg with an $ED_{75}$ of 1 mg/kg, whereas the writer has consistently used chloroquine at 100 mg/kg × 5 in 50-g chicks and found that 1 mg/kg × 5 demonstrated an $ED_{50}$. Also THOMPSON et al. (1953), using a method of including drug in the diet described by MARSHALL et al. (1942), examined a number of schizontocides against *P. lophurae* in chicks, and found that amodiaquine was 30 times more active than quinine and had curative activity when given at approximately 0.83 mg/kg per day. After more than a decade FINK and DANN (1967) used the Hartmann strain of *P. cathemerium* in a rather cumbersome test whereby compounds are given as a single intravenous bolus injection into the birds and the results are expressed as a delay in patency of blood-induced infections following the administration of the maximum tolerated dose of drug. Chloroquine at 20 mg base/kg was similar in activity to quinine at 50 mg base/kg.

It is interesting that in this system sulphadiazine at 250 mg/kg was without effect and pyrimethamine and proguanil at 12 mg/kg and 50 mg/kg had very low activity. It was suggested that this lack of activity was a direct result of the parasites being able to obtain ready formed folate from the canary host, although this would not appear to be so in *P. gallinaceum* and *P. lophurae*. The lack of activity of sulphadiazine was demonstrated by TAYLOR et al. (1952) against *P. gallinaceum* in vitro at more than 750 mg/litre but the drug had a minimum effective concentration of 34 mg/litre in vivo. In the same report chloroquine had a minimum effective concentration of 0.25 mg/litre in vitro and 0.2 mg/litre in vivo.

TERZIAN et al. (1949) examined the effect of drugs in a sugar solution supplied to *Aedes aegypti* after they had fed from chicks infected with *P. gallinaceum*. Eight days after infection some mosquitoes were dissected and sporozoite density was noted, while other mosquitoes were used to infect clean birds. As expected, proguanil at 0.001% and sulphadiazine at 0.1% were effective in arresting sporogony, whereas chloroquine at 0.03% and quinine at 0.05% were without effect.

The importance of the new drugs and the discovery from 1948 of rodent malaria saw a great deal of activity in testing the 4-aminoquinolines in simian models and *P. berghei*, with the avian models being largely ignored.

BEKHLI et al. (1977) and MOSHKOVSKIJ et al. (1978) reported on compound G-800, a 4-diethylaminoalkylaminobenzoquinoline (dabequine), a 4-aminoquinoline derivative synthesised in the Martsinovsky Institute of Medical Parasitology and Tropical Medicine in Moscow. Studies on *P. gallinaceum* in chicks and *P. berghei* in mice indicated that, although the drug had a lower intrinsic activity against the asexual parasites in the blood than chloroquine, it had a better therapeutic index. On an equivalent dose basis it had a more prolonged suppressive action than chloroquine. It was possible to induce drug resistance in dabequine and there was cross-resistance with chloroquine.

## III. 8-Aminoquinolines

The 6-methoxy-8-aminoquinoline antimalarials, of which pamaquine was the first to be synthesised, are the only compounds with sufficient activity against the exoerythrocytic, fixed tissue stages of the malarias to be of practical value in radical cure of the true relapsing infections (e.g. *P. vivax*). In some individuals these drugs have a profound toxic effect upon the erythrocytes, causing methaemoglobin formation and haemolysis. The history of the development of pamaquine, which found its beginnings in the work of GUTTMAN and EHRLICH (1891) with methylene blue, is well documented by STECK (1972). Minor modifications in the methylene blue structure, changes in the alkyl function and the introduction of a side chain gave an increased antimalarial activity. ROEHL (1926) demonstrated that pamaquine was 60 times more effective than quinine when tested against *P. relictum* in canaries. The therapeutic index was wider with pamaquine, although it was more toxic than quinine to canaries. ROEHL reported that a single, large dose of drug was able dramatically to reduce the parasitaemia, but recrudescences occurred. It is interesting to note that, while pamaquine was regarded as a poor schizontocide, when used in conjunction with quinine for clinical use it was effective in eliminating the gametocytes of *P. falciparum*. BISHOP and her two co-workers (BISHOP et al. 1947) compared the action of pamaquine with quinine and mepacrine against *P. relictum* in canaries infected either by sporozoite or by infected blood inoculation. Pamaquine had a prophylactic effect, preventing the development of pre-erythrocytic forms. In 1948 WALKER et al. also examined the same three compounds against *P. cathemerium* in ducklings. The animals were infected by $5 \times 10^8$ parasitised erythrocytes given intravenously and dosed either by giving the drug in the diet or by gavage. Blood films were monitored at 1 week and after 1 month. Birds with a negative parasitaemia after 1 month had blood withdrawn and inoculated into clean birds and the following day were challenged by reinfection. Pamaquine and mepacrine again showed suppressive and curative action, whereas quinine gave only a poor suppressive effect. Birds often failed to become infected after rechallenge and this was probably due to immunity developed from the first infection. In the same year WALKER and RICHARDSON (1948), using the same test system, examined possible potentiation between 8-aminoquinolines and selected naphthoquinones. The prophylactic action was unaffected but the curative action was potentiated. It was postulated that the two types of compounds had different types of activity against the exo- and erythrocytic stages of the parasite life cycle. Unacceptable levels of toxicity precluded the extensive use of pamaquine in man, and chickens were used to investigate the metabolism of the drug. The major metabolite proved to be 8-(4-diethylamino-1-methyl-butylamino)-5-hydroxy-8-methoxyquinoline. Quinoline-quinone precursors are recognised in the metabolism of pentaquine and isopentaquine. The drug isopentaquine, an isomer of pentaquine, is one of the most powerful 8-aminoquinolines that was produced from research in the United States in the World War II programme. The metabolism of the 8-aminoquinolines is interesting and the 6-hydroxy-8-(5-isopropylaminopentylamino) quinoline metabolite of pentaquine was as active as the parent compound against *P. gallinaceum* in vivo but more active in vitro (GREENBERG and RICHESON 1951). HANSON and TATUM (1951) drew some significant conclusions in their paper on their treatment of *P. cathemerium* infections in canaries with pentaquine. Using a schedule of 7.5 mg/kg of drug a cure could be obtained if the inoculum was small, but with larger inocula, $10^6$ parasitised erythrocytes or more intravenously, cures were not obtained. They concluded that inoculum size and host immunity played a part in the efficacy of the drug.

The most effective and acceptable 8-aminoquinoline synthesised in the United States during World War II was primaquine. This drug is very similar to pamaquine, which has a terminal diethylamine group on the side chain attached to the 8-position of the quinoline nucleus, whereas primaquine has a primary amino group. Even so, 20 years elapsed between synthesis of the two drugs. Primaquine, although a poor blood schizontocide, is a very effective gametocytocide and tissue schizontocide. COATNEY et al. (1953) studied the activity of four 8-aminoquinolines against *P. gallinaceum* in chicks. The maximum tolerated dose in milligrams base per kilogram was pentaquine 5.7, primaquine 6, isopentaquine 7.3, and pamaquine 8.9; and the corresponding $ED_{75}$ were 0.1, 0.2, 0.1, and 1.0. THOMPSON et al. (1953), examining the blood schizontocidal activity against *P. lophurae* in chicks by a drug diet method, found that primaquine at 0.17 mg/kg per day approximately gave a cure and was 150 times more active than quinine and more than twice as active as pamaquine at approximately 0.42 mg/kg per day.

NARAYANDAS and RAY (1954) allowed *Aedes aegypti* mosquitoes to feed on drug in a sugar solution after ingestion of a blood meal from *P. gallinaceum*-infected chicks. Even at concentrations up to 1% they were unable to demonstrate a definite sporontocidal activity for primaquine, pentaquine or pamaquine. TERZIAN et al. (1949), however, suggested that pamaquine inhibits infectivity by destroying the sporozoites. AIKAWA and BEAUDOIN (1968, 1969) in a series of detailed studies showed that primaquine had a specific effect on the mitochondria of *P. fallax* in tissue culture without damage to the host cell. There was pronounced swelling of the plasmodial mitochondria sufficient to affect the metabolic function and, the authors claimed, enough to establish this as the prime mode of action on the exoerythrocytic stages of malaria parasites.

There is no recorded testing in avian malaria models of the primaquine isomer quinocide, the drug which was preferred to primaquine in the USSR for human use.

## IV. Sulphonamides and Sulphones

The foundation for a biochemical approach to chemotherapy was probably initiated in 1935 with the advent of prontosil and the discovery by TRÉFOUËL et al. (1935) and COLEBROOK et al. (1936) that its action was not due to the dye but to the in vivo formation of an active metabolite, sulphanilamide. A description of the antimalarial activity of the sulphonamides soon followed, and DIAZ DE LEÓN (1937, 1938, 1940) claimed to have produced a clinical cure of *P. vivax* using Rubiazol (6-carboxy-4-sulphamide-2′-4′-diaminoazo-benzene) (see also Chap. 22).

COGGESHALL et al. (1941) examined the effectiveness of two new types of chemotherapeutic agents in malaria, promin, and sulphadiazine and then, with other workers ( COGGESHALL et al. 1944) studied the prophylactic and curative effects of certain sulphonamide compounds on the exoerythrocytic stages of *P. gallinaceum*. This work, corroborated by COATNEY and COOPER (1944), showed that sulphonamide compounds were prophylactic in chicks challenged with sporozoites of *P. gallinaceum* but, at that time, were shown to be relatively ineffective in man. TERZIAN (1947), feeding drug in a 4% sucrose solution to *Ae. aegypti* mosquitoes prior to and following their taking a blood meal from *P. gallinaceum*-

infected chicks, found that sulphadiazine from 0.1% to 0.4% inhibited oocyst development in the mosquito, and even at concentrations down to 0.01% led to less severe infections in chicks inoculated with mosquito suspensions. Later TERZIAN et al. (1949), using large batches of drug-treated mosquitoes, inoculated mosquito suspensions into clean chicks 10 days after taking an infective blood meal. Although *Anopheles quadrimaculatus* appeared to be more susceptible to the "toxic" action of the compounds than *Ae. aegypti*, the effects of the drug on *P. gallinaceum* in both vectors was comparable. Sulphadiazine, metachloridine, and proguanil were seen to suppress oocyst and sporozoite development if present for at least 4 days following an infective blood meal. However, if given later, the drugs had no effect on sporozoite formation, the inference being that, once the coding for the final nuclear division had been made, the drugs were no longer effective. In this series of experiments TERZIAN recognised that sulphonamides with their wide range of activity must interfere with some essential function and that this may be peculiar to the parasite and not essential to the host. WOODS (1940) was the first to mention that there was an antagonism between *p*-aminobenzoic acid (PABA) and a sulphonamide. MAIER and RILEY (1942) showed that the antimalarial action of many compounds is reversed by the addition of PABA. TERZIAN et al. (1949) were able to antagonise the effects of sulphadiazine and metachloridine by the concomitant administration of PABA while proguanil was unaffected by such treatment. A phenomenon reported by TERZIAN (1950) and TERZIAN et al. (1951) showed that various sulphonamides were able to increase the susceptibility of mosquitoes to infections with *P. gallinaceum*, a larger number of oocysts maturing in mosquitoes fed on sulphadiazine 1%; PABA 0.01% than in control groups of mosquitoes. Concentrations of drug greater or less than this were without effect. RAMAKRISHNAN et al. in 1963 demonstrated that the sulphone dapsone (DDS) and pyrimethamine potentiated each other's antimalarial action against the sporogonic cycle of *P. gallinaceum* in *Ae. aegypti* when administered to infected chicks before allowing the vectors to feed on the birds. A single dose of 210 mg/kg DDS plus 0.028 mg/kg pyrimethamine given 2 days before mosquitoes were fed on the birds completely inhibited sporozoite maturation. While this appears to be a rather high dose, neither DDS alone at 300 mg/kg nor pyrimethamine alone at 0.078 mg/kg were sporontocidal. Ten years earlier JASWANT SINGH et al. (1953) found that pyrimethamine at 0.7 and 2.0 mg/kg was sporontocidal.

Surprisingly the amount of data on sulphonamides or sulphones as schizontocides in an avian system is relatively restricted. COATNEY et al. (1953) found the $ED_{75}$ for sulphadiazine against a *P. gallinaceum* infection to be 62 mg/kg and for DDS 128 mg/kg.

Two groups of workers, COGGESHALL et al. (1944) and COATNEY and COOPER (1944) were able to show that sulphonamides act as true causal prophylactic drugs, and that sulphadiazine at 12.5 mg/kg produced a delay in the prepatent period while at 62.5 mg/kg was protective. COGGESHALL et al. (1944), using a rather inaccurate parameter of examining serial brain sections, were able to demonstrate that sulphadiazine, if given even when the exoerythrocytic forms of *P. gallinaceum* were developing, was able to produce an effect on their morphology. In retrospect it is possible to see how difficult it was to determine the activity of the sulpha compounds in the avian malaria systems, since MARSHALL et al. (1942) demonstrated a very marked difference in the kinetics of sulphanilamide in various species. Following an oral dose of 0.5 g/kg the blood level in all the animals studied reached a maximum between 17 and 27 mg% within the 1 st h but, after 6 h, it was virtually depleted in canaries, approximately 12 mg% in ducks, 17 mg% in chicks, and 17 mg% in pigeons. In mice, a maximum of 32 mg% was achieved in 1 h but the level was down to 14 mg% at 6 h. In the dog the blood level continued to rise, reaching a maximum of 38 mg% at 4 h and it was still 36 mg% at 6 h.

It is important therefore that, to demonstrate an effect with the short-acting sulphonamides, it is necessary to maintain an effective blood level by daily or, preferably, twice daily dosing. The disadvantage of the earlier sulphonamides and their rapid excretion was overcome with the introduction of the newer, long-acting sulphonamides that were able to sustain plasma concentrations for many days. Little work has been reported with these compounds; RICHARDS (1966) examined three sulphonamides against *P. gallinaceum* in chicks, 5-methyl-3-sulphonilamidoisoxazole (sulphamethoxazole), 2,6-dimethoxy-4-sulphonilamidopyrimidine (sulphadimethoxine), and 5,6-dimethoxy-4-sulphonilamidopyrimidine (sulphorthomidine; sulfadoxine, now known as Fanasil). After seven oral doses of drug beginning on the afternoon of the day of infection, followed by twice daily dosing for the next 3 days, the parasitaemia was estimated on the 4th day. The compounds had $ED_{50}$s respectively of 8 mg/kg, 14 mg/kg, and 20 mg/kg.

In the same test dapsone had an $ED_{50}$ of 100 mg/kg. The use of dapsone as an antimalarial has received comparatively little attention. Shortly after the antimalarial activity of the drug was discovered the drug was discarded as being too toxic for human use on its own (BUTTLE et al. 1937; COGGESHALL et al. 1941; LONG 1950). This was due, in part, to the assumption that the amount of sulphone required for treatment was comparable to that used with the sulpha drugs. Dapsone was used, however, by ARDIAS (1948) in the treatment of malaria, and 243 patients were treated with various doses of the drug. It was estimated that 9 g was the optimum dose where it had a marked effect on the developmental stages of the parasite, with the trophozoites being especially vulnerable. It was LEIKER (1956) who suggested that dapsone may have prophylactic properties against malaria, which he found to be absent from leprosarium patients treated with the drug, in contrast to the general population in a holoendemic area. RAMAKRISHNAN et al., however, in 1962, using *P. gallinaceum* and the simian malarias *P. knowlesi* and *P. cynomolgi*, concluded that dapsone did not possess any causal prophylactic, gametocytocidal or sporontocidal properties.

## V. Antifolates

The two most commonly used causal prophylactics in human malarias are the biguanide proguanil and 2,4-diaminopyrimidine pyrimethamine. The majority of screening tests for prophylactic activity have been conducted with the *P. gallinaceum-Aedes aegypti* system described by DAVEY in 1946. Using this model DAVEY (1946) showed that proguanil had definite causal prophylactic properties when the drug was given orally twice a day; at 1.74 mg/kg for 6 days death was delayed in some birds; at 4.3 mg/kg for 6 days death was delayed for some days; at 17.15 mg/kg for 5 days there was a marked delay in infection; at 34.3 mg/kg for

5 days there were some cures and, at 51.5 mg/kg for 5 days, there was cure but at this concentration there was a marked toxicity in the chicks. TERZIAN et al. (1949), studying the effects of various drugs on sporogony of *P. gallinaceum* in *Ae. aegypti*, allowed the mosquitoes to feed on infected chicks and then fed the insects on sugar solutions containing drugs. These mosquitoes were then used to infect clean birds. With proguanil at 0.01 mg% there was a reduced number of sporozoites in the mosquitoes compared with the untreated insects and a delayed parasitaemia in the birds although the mortality was the same as the controls. At 0.1 mg% no sporozoites were present in the mosquitoes and all the challenged birds survived.

The number of studies using avian malarias dropped markedly in the early 1950s when many laboratories adopted the mammalian-*P. berghei* model. ROLLO (1955), however, was one of the few who continued to use *P. gallinaceum* to produce valuable data on pyrimethamine. He demonstrated that the compound was very effective, seven doses of 0.015, 0.03, and 0.06 mg/kg orally inhibiting the parasitaemia, compared with the untreated controls, by 2%, 22%, and 99% respectively (ROLLO 1955). He described in the same paper the activity of proguanil where seven oral doses of drug at 0.5 mg/kg, 1.0 mg/kg, and 2.0 mg/kg gave 19%, 42%, and 89% inhibition respectively. The importance of the paper is in the careful work on the mode of action of sulphonamides, proguanil, and pyrimethamine. It was already recognised that sulphonamides containing an $NH_2$, $C_6H_4$, $SO_2$ or NH group act by competing with PABA. The antimalarial action of sulphonamides was postulated to have a similar action because PABA reverses it and because PABA is important for the metabolism of malaria parasites, as demonstrated in *P. berghei*, which is extremely sensitive to sulphadiazine (HAWKING 1953).

GREENBERG (1949) showed that the action of proguanil is potentiated by sulphadiazine and other antimalarials that are PABA competitors. ROLLO demonstrated a similar action with pyrimethamine and sulphadiazine, while pyrimethamine and proguanil were only additive in combination. The potentiation of pyrimethamine or proguanil by PABA antagonists was postulated and demonstrated as a phenomenon where the two components act at different points on the same metabolic pathway. The antagonism of sulphadiazine by both PABA and folic acid is competitive and was demonstrated in the *P. gallinaceum* model. The antagonism of pyrimethamine and proguanil by PABA and folic acid is less effective, although GREENBERG (1953), using high doses of PABA and folic acid in the *P. gallinaceum* system, showed that such antagonism was possible. Plasmodia are unable to utilise preformed folic or folinic acid and it is likely that they synthesise these from PABA (GOODWIN and ROLLO 1955) supplied by the breakdown of folic acid or of the folic acid antagonists. This potentiation of antimalarial activity between antifols and sulphonamides was known for many years and, although they had been used clinically, they were not extensively used in man. The advent of the longer-acting sulphonamides renewed interest in the possible use of combination therapy in man. RICHARDS (1966), using *P. gallinaceum*, studied a series of sulphonamides and the sulphone dapsone, and reported their intrinsic antimalarial activity together with potentiation of this activity when used in combination with pyrimethamine. They were assayed against normal and drug-resistant strains of *P. gallinaceum*. When infections with normal strains were treated with a seven-dose schedule, all the sulphonamides, the sulphone and pyrimethamine showed good antimalarial activity.

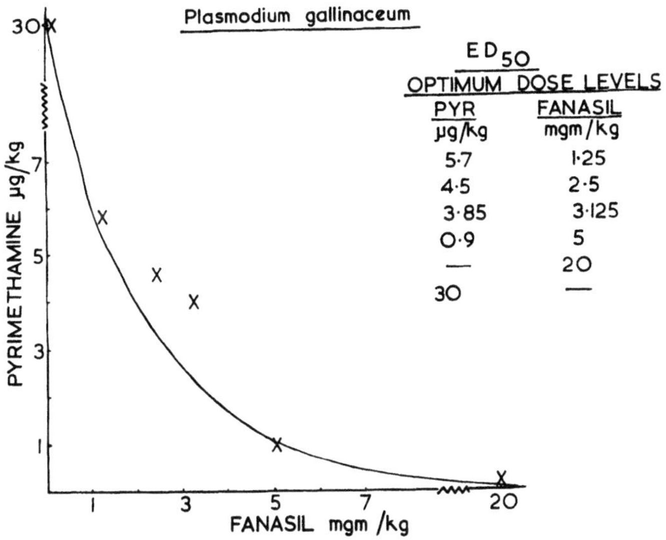


**Fig. 1.** Antimalarial activity of pyrimethamine and sulfadoxine (Fanasil) singly and in combination at levels required to give an $ED_{50}$ value. The $ED_{50}$ is the level where the parasitaemia is reduced to 50% of that of the untreated controls

**Table 1.** Antimalarial activity of pyrimethamine and sulfadoxine (Fanasil) against a normal and pyrimethamine-resistant isolate of *Plasmodium gallinaceum* in chicks. Results are expressed as the concentration of drug which reduces the parasitaemia to 50% of that of the untreated controls

| | *Plasmodium gallinaceum* $ED_{50}$ mg/kg × 7 orally | |
|---|---|---|
| | Normal | Pyrimethamine-resistant |
| Pyrimethamine | 0·0.3 | > 10 |
| Fanasil | 20 | 25 |
| Pyrimethamine + Fanasil | 0·004 + 2·6 | 0·02 + 5 |

When given in combination the optimum level of activity was about one-tenth of that when given alone (Fig. 1). The compounds were also tested against lines of *P. gallinaceum*, derived from the parent strain, made resistant to pyrimethamine and the triazine metabolite of proguanil, cycloguanil. The pyrimethamine-resistant line was unaffected by a dose of 10 mg/kg pyrimethamine, that is more than 300 times the dose effective against the normal strain. The other resistant line was resistant to 10 mg/kg cycloguanil, that is 25 times the dose effective against the normal parent strain. The sulphonamides and sulphone alone had comparable activity against both the normal and drug-resistant lines. Although the dose level of sulfadoxine or dapsone in combination with pyrimethamine was raised against the pyrimethamine-resistant line to produce the same antimalarial effect as against the normal strain, this was only by a factor of 2–5 (Table 1).

## VI. Amidinoureas

One group of compounds that never achieved widespread use in man is the amidinoureas. CURD et al. (1949) investigated the antimalarial activity of a series of 1-*N*-alkylamidino-3-phenylureas, but considered that they did not warrant further chemical or biological effort. In 1960, CHIN and his colleagues studied related compounds which lacked the *N*-alkyl substituent and found that 1-amidino-3-*p*-nitrophenylurea (nitroguanil) showed marked activity against *P. gallinaceum*. The required minimum effective antimalarial dose was four times that of proguanil, but the acute oral $LD_{50}$ in mice was about 25 times greater (CHIN et al. 1960a). Nitroguanil was subsequently used by CLYDE in Tanzania in more than 500 partially immune subjects with malaria infections (URBANSKI et al. 1964). The drug was shown to be active at high, yet well-tolerated doses, but showed no advantage over proguanil.

This writer's interest in the series was aroused by the isolation of L-amidino-3-*p*-cyanophenylurea in the course of other work. This substance, which is an analogue of nitroguanil, was tested against *P. gallinaceum* in chicks, and proved to be more active. From a wide range of compounds synthesised and tested the most active was the L-amidino-3-(3-chloro-4-cyanophenyl)urea (RICHARDS, unpublished work). This compound was tested against a normal, drug-sensitive strain of *P. gallinaceum* and six drug-resistant lines derived from the parent strain. Compared with chloroquine the amidinourea had about one-tenth of the activity against the drug-sensitive *P. gallinaceum*. The compound, although less active than pyrimethamine, had more powerful antimalarial activity than nitroguanil. The result (Tables 2, 3) show that the effective concentration of the novel compound was comparable with that needed for the sensitive parent strain, but not for isolates resistant to the pyrimethamine-sulphonamide or -sulphone potentiating mixtures. Here there was a two- to threefold increase in the amount of drug needed to produce a similar result. No significant cross-resistance was observed to any of the standard antimalarials, including chloroquine, and it is therefore likely that the mode of action of the amidinourea is different from that of the standard antimalarials. CHIN et al. (1960a, b) and URBANSKI et al. (1964) concluded that nitroguanil showed no advantage in comparison with proguanil. RICHARD's results suggested that the amidinourea had little value as a causal prophylactic, but was able to clear the blood of asexual parasites as quickly as chloroquine in infected chicks.

**Table 2.** The antimalarial activity of 1-amidino-3-(3-chloro-4-cyanophenyl)urea compared with chloroquine, pyrimethamine and nitroguanil against normal laboratory strains of plasmodia. Seven oral doses of drug in 4 days

| Compound | *P. gallinaceum* $ED_{50}$ (mg base/kg) |
|---|---|
| 1-amidino-3-(3-chloro-4-cyano phenyl)urea | $7.1 \pm 1.6$ |
| Nitroguanil | $60 \pm 22$ |
| Chloroquine | $0.5 \pm 0.018$ |
| Pyrimethamine | $0.03 \pm 0.007$ |

$ED_{50}$, the level of drug which will reduce the parasitaemia to 50% of that of the untreated controls

**Table 3.** The antimalarial activity of 1-amidino-3-(3-chloro-4-cyanophenyl)urea, compared with chloroquine and nitroguanil against normal and drug-resistant strains of *P. gallinaceum*. Seven oral doses of drug, in milligrams base per kilogram in 4 days

| | *P. gallinaceum* Normal isolate (×1) | *P. gallinaceum* isolates with induced drug resistance (degree of resistance to individual drugs) | | | | | |
|---|---|---|---|---|---|---|---|
| | | Pyrimethamine (×3,000) | Cycloguanil[a] (×40) | Dapsone (×4) | Sulfadoxine (×40) | Dapsone + pyrimethamine (×20) | Sulfadoxine + pyrimethamine (×20) |
| $ED_{50}$ | | | | | | | |
| Chloroquine | 0.5 | 0.5 | 0.5 | 0.5 | 0.5 | 0.7 | 0.65 |
| Nitroguanil | 60 | 100 | 100 | 65 | 65 | 100 | 100 |
| 1-amidino-3-(3-chloro-4-cyanophenyl)urea | 7.1 | 10 | 10 | 7.5 | 7.5 | 15 | 20 |
| $ED_{99}$ | | | | | | | |
| Chloroquine | 2 | 4 | 4 | 2 | 4 | 4 | 4 |
| Nitroguanil | 100 | >100 | >100 | >100 | >100 | >100 | >100 |
| 1-amidino-3-(3-chloro-4-cyanophenyl)urea | 15 | 20 | 20 | 25 | 30 | 30 | 30 |

[a] The triazine metabolite of proguanil: 4,6-diamino-1-*p*-chlorophenyl-1,2-dihydro-2,2-dimethyl-5-triazine

## VII. Quinolinemethanols

In 1938 AINLEY and KING described the first of the series, 6-methoxy-α-(2-piperidyl)-4-quinoline methanols, which was active against *P. relictum* in canaries. A variety of analogues were prepared without any obvious therapeutic advantage. In 1946 BUCHMAN et al. made the 6,8-dichloro-2-phenyl-α-(2-piperidyl)-4-quinolinemethanol, this compound proving active against blood stages of *P. gallinaceum* in chicks and *P. vivax* in man. It had no sporontocidal activity and demonstrated a severe phototoxicity in man (PULLMAN et al. 1948). The phototoxic side effects almost caused the series to be abandoned and further development of the 4-quinolinemethanols was thought to be worthwhile only if new analogues could retain and improve the antimalarial activity, while being free of the photosensitising side effects. Following extensive chemistry a number of novel drugs were made that met these requirements including the compound mefloquine, α-(2-piperidyl)-2,8-bis (trifluromethyl)-4-quinolinemethanol. The vast majority of the studies on this compound were made in rodent and simian models. There was, however, one report from Lucknow where KAZIM (1978) examined the schizontocidal effect of mefloquine against *P. gallinaceum* in chicks. Using a rather cumbersome method of infection, young chicks were infected with 25 million parasitised red blood cells intramuscularly, and dosed orally from the day of infection for 8 days. The controls died on day 9 (mean value). Mefloquine at 11.7 mg/kg suppressed a patent parasitaemia until day 10, when parasites were demonstrated in the blood. This, the author claims, was due to persisting exoerythrocytic stages seen at autopsy, the average survival time being 16.3 days. Drug levels of 1.3 mg/kg and 0.43 mg/kg were ineffective.

# D. Conclusion

The number of workers now using avian malaria models has now become very few. This was due primarily to the introduction of the rodent models as most investigators appeared to be of the opinion that a mammalian model has more relevance to human infections than an avian system. The latter, however, served an important role in malaria chemotherapy, especially during two World Wars. The avian malaria models will now, if used at all, probably be of use mainly to immunologists, biochemists, and those interested in morphology and taxonomy.

# References

Aikawa M, Beaudoin RL (1968) Primaquine induced changes in the morphology of the exoerythrocytic stages of malaria. Science 160:1233–1234

Aikawa M, Beaudoin RL (1969) Morphological effects of 8-amino-quinolines on the exoerythrocytic stages of *Plasmodium fallax*. Milit Med 134:986–999

Ainley AD, King H (1938) Antiplasmodial action and chemical constitution. Part II. Some simple synthetic analogues of quinine and cinchonine. Proc R Soc Lond Ser B 128:60–92

Ardias A (1948) La solfonoterapia della malaria. Arch Ital Sci Med Colon Parasitol 29:115–133

Baranger P, Filer MK (1953) De l'action protectrice de colliers dans la malaria aviaire. Essai d'ethrographie experimentale. Acta Trop 10:69–72
Bekhli AF, Kozibeva NP, Moshkovski SLD, Rabinovich SA, Maksakovskaya EV, Gladkikh VF, Lebdeva MN, Nichko ND, Soprunova NI (1977) Synthesis of manufactured benzo(g) quinolines XIII. New manufactured benzo(g) quinolines showing antimalarial activity. Med Parazitol Parazit Bolezni 46:71–72
Bishop A, Birket B, Gilchrist BM (1947) The response of blood-inoculated and sporozoite-induced infections of *Plasmodium relictum* to drugs. Parasitology 38:163–172
Buchman ER, Sargent H, Meyers TC, Howton DR (1946) Potential antimalarials (chloro-2-phenylquinolyl-4)-α-piperidylcarbinols. J Am Chem Soc 68:2710–2714
Buttle GAH, Stephenson D, Smith S, Dewing T, Foster GE (1937) The treatment of streptococcal infections in mice with 4:4′ diaminodiaphenylsulphone. Lancet I:1331–1334
Chin YCH, Wy YY, Serafin B, Urbanski T, Venulet J, Jakimowska K (1960 a) Antimalarial properties of some derivatives of phenylamidineurea. Bull Acad Pol Sci d3 8:109–112
Chin YCH, Wy YY, Serafin B, Urbanski T, Venulet J (1960 b) Antimalarial properties of some guanidine derivatives. Nature 186:170–171
Coatney GR, Cooper WC (1944) The prophylactic effect of sulphadiazine and sulphaguanidine against mosquito-borne *Plasmodium gallinaceum* infection in the domestic fowl. (Preliminary report.) Public Health Rep 59:1455-1458
Coatney GR, Roudabush RL (1949) A catalogue of the species of the genus *Plasmodium* and index of their hosts. In: Boyd's malariology, vol I. Saunders, Philadelphia
Coatney GR, Cooper WC, Eddy NB, Greenberg J (1953) Survey of antimalarial agents. Chemotherapy of *Plasmodium gallinaceum* infections: toxicity; correlation of structure and action. Public Health Monogr 9:322
Coggeshall LT, Maier J, Best CA (1941) The effectiveness of two new types of chemotherapeutic agents in malaria (promin and sulphadiazine). JAMA 117:1077–1081
Coggeshall LT, Porter RJ, Laird RL (1944) Prophylactic and curative effects of certain sulphonamide compounds on exoerythrocytic stages in *Plasmodium gallinaceum* malaria. Proc Soc Exp Biol Med 57:286–292
Colebrook L, Buttle GAH, OMeara RAQ (1936) The mode of action of *p*-aminobenzenesulphonamide and prontosil in haemolytic streptococcal infections. Lancet II: 1223–1326
Curd FHS, Davey DG, Richardson DN (1949) Synthetic antimalarials Part XLII. The preparation of guanylureas and biurets corresponding to "paludrine" and related diguanides. J Chem Soc 3:1732–1738
Danilewsky B (1885) Zur Parasitologie des Blutes. Biol Zentralb 5:529–537
Davey DG (1946) The use of avian malaria for the discovery of drugs effective in the treatment and prevention of human malaria I. Drugs for clinical treatment and clinical prophylaxis. Ann Trop Med Parasitol 40:453–471
Diaz de Léon A (1937) Treatment of malaria with sulphonamide compounds. Public Health Rep 52:1460–1462
Diaz de Léon A (1938) Sulphonamides in the treatment of malaria. Medicina (Mexico City) 18:89–90
Diaz de Léon A (1940) Malaria and its treatment with intravenous sulphonamides. Medicina (Mexico City) 20:551–558
Findlay GM (1951) Recent advances in chemotherapy, 3rd edn, Vol 2. Churchill, London, pp 1–597
Fink E, Dann O (1967) Eine Weiterentwicklung des Roehl-Test zur Prüfung von Malariamitteln an *Plasmodium cathemerium* beim Kanarienvogel durch intravenöse Verabreichung. Z Tropenmed Parasitol 18:466–474
Garnham PCC (1966) Malaria parasites and other haemosporidia. Blackwell Scientific, Oxford
Goodwin LG, Rollo IM (1955) The chemotherapy of malaria, piroplasmosis, trypanosomiasis, and leishmaniasis. In: Hutner SH, Lwoff A (eds) Biochemistry and physiology of protozoa, vol 2. Academic, New York, pp 225–276
Grassi B, Feletti R (1890) Parassiti malarici negli uccelli. Nota preliminare. Boll Mens Accad Gioenia Sci Nat Catania Fasc 13:3–6

Greenberg J (1949) The potentiation of the antimalarial activity of chlorguanide by *p*-aminobenzoic acid competitors. J Pharmacol Exp Ther 97:238–242
Greenberg J (1953) Reversal of activity of chlorguanide against *Plasmodium gallinaceum* by free or conjugated *p*-aminobenzoic acid. Exp Parasitol 2:271–279
Greenberg J, Richeson EM (1951) Effect of 2,4-diamino-5 (*p*-chlorophenoxy) -6-methylpyrimidine and 2,4-diamino-6,7-diaphenylpteridine on chlorguanidine-resistant strain of *Plasmodium gallinaceum*. Proc Soc Exp Biol Med 77:174–176
Guttman P, Ehrlich P (1891) Über die Wirkung des Methylenblau bei Malaria. Berl Klin Wochenschr 28:953–956
Haas BH, Willcox A, Laird RL, Ewing FM, Coleman N (1948) Response of exoerythrocytic forms to alterations in the life cycle of *Plasmodium gallinaceum*. J Parasitol 34:306–320
Hanson RO, Tatum AL (1951) Drug, host, and parasite relationships in the treatment of avian malaria (*Plasmodium cathemerium* in canaries). J Infect Dis 90:105–109
Hawking F (1953) Milk diet, *p*-aminobenzoic acid and malaria (*Plasmodium berghei*). Br Med J 1:1201–1202
Hegner R, Manwell R (1927) The effects of plasmochin on bird malaria. Am J Trop Med 7:279–285
Hill J (1963) Chemotherapy of malaria. Part 2. The antimalarial drugs. In: Schnitzer RJ, Hawking F (eds) Experimental chemotherapy, vol 1. Academic, New York, pp 513–601
Jaswant Singh, Narayandas MG, Ray AP (1953) Assay of antimalarial against the sporogony cycle of *Plasmodium gallinaceum*. Part 1. Indian J Malariol 7:33–39
Kazim M (1978) Schizonticidal activity of mefloquine in *Plasmodium gallinaceum* infection in chicks. Indian J Parasitol 2:121–183
Kikuth W (1932) Zur Weiterentwicklung synthetisch dargestellter Malariamittel. Über die chemotherapeutische Wirkung des Atebrin. Dtsch Med Wochenschr 58:530–531
Kopanaris P (1911) Die Wirkung von Chinin, Salvarsan und Atoxyl auf die Proteosoma (*Plasmodium praecox*) Infektion des Kanarienvogels. Arch Schiffs Trop Hyg 15:586–596
Labbé A (1893) Sur les parasites endoglobulaires du sang de l'allouette. C R Soc Biol (Paris) 45:739–741
Laveran A (1880) Nature parasitaire des accidents de l'impaludisme; déscription d'un nouveau parasite trouvé dans le sang des malades atteintes de fièvre palustre. Baillière, Paris, pp 104
Leiker DL (1956) Note on sulphone activity in malaria infection. Lepr Rev 27:66–69
Long PH (1950) Correspondence. Early experiences with DDS in man. Int J Lepr 18:247
Lourie EM (1934a) Studies on chemotherapy in bird malaria. II. Observations bearing on the mode of action of quinine. Ann Trop Med Parasitol 28:255–277
Lourie EM (1934b) Studies on chemotherapy in bird malaria. III. Difference in response to quinine treatment between strains of *Plasmodium relictum* of widely separated geographical origins. Ann Trop Med Parasitol 28:513–523
MacCullum W (1898) On the haematozoan infections of birds. J Exp Med 3:117–136
Maier J, Riley E (1942) Inhibition of antimalarial action of sulphonamides by *p*-aminobenzoic acid. Proc Soc Exp Biol Med 50:152–154
Manwell R (1930a) The varying effects of quinine and plasmochin therapy on the different avian malarias. J Parasitol 17:110
Manwell R (1930b) Further studies on the effect of quinine and plasmochin on the different avian malarias. Am J Trop Med 10:379–405
Manwell R (1934) Quinine and plasmochin therapy in infections with *Plasmodium circumflexum*. Am J Trop Med 14:45–59
Manwell R, Haring A (1938) Plasmochin and atebrin therapy in *Plasmodium vaughani* infections. Riv Parasitol 2:207–218
Marshall EK Jr, Litchfield JT Jr, White HJ (1942) Sulphonamide therapy of malaria in ducks. J Pharmacol Exp Ther 75:89–104
Moshkovskij SD, Rabinovich SA, Maksakovskaya EV (1978) Chemotherapeutic study of

a new antimalarial drug Dabequine. Fourth international congress of parasitology, 19–26 August 1978, Warsaw. Short communications, Section D, p 103. Available from Organizing Committee, ICOPA IV, Warsaw, Poland
Narayandas MG, Ray AP (1954) Assay of antimalarials against the sporogony cycle of *P. gallinaceum*. Indian J Malariol 8:137–141
Opie E (1898) On the hematozoa of birds. J Exp Med 3:79–101
Peters W (1970) Chemotherapy and drug resistance in malaria. Academic, London
Pullman TN, Eichelberger L, Alving AS, Jones R Jr, Craige B Jr, Whorton CM (1948) The use of SN-10275 in the prophylaxis and treatment of sporozoite-induced vivax malaria (Chesson strain). J Clin Invest [Suppl] 27:12–16
Ramakrishnan SP, Basu PC, Singh H, Singh N (1962) Studies on the toxicity and action of diaminodiphenylsulphone (DDS) in avian and simian malaria. Bull WHO 27:213–221
Ramakrishnan SP, Basu PC, Singh H, Wattal BL (1963) A study of the joint action of diaminodiphenylsulphone (DDS) and pyrimethamine in the sporogony cycle of *Plasmodium gallinaceum* potentiation of the sporontocidal activity of pyrimethamine by DDS. Indian J Malariol 17:141–148
Richards WHG (1966) Antimalarial activity of sulphonamides and a sulphone, singly and in combination with pyrimethamine against drug-resistant and normal strains of laboratory plasmodia. Nature 212:1494–1495
Roehl W (1926) Die Wirkung des Plasmochins auf die Vogelmalaria. Arch Schiffs Trop Hyg 30:311–318
Rollo IM (1955) The mode of action of sulphonamides, proguanil, and pyrimethamine on *Plasmodium gallinaceum*. Br J Pharmacol 10:208–214
Ross R (1898) Report on the cultivation of *Proteosoma*, Labbé, in grey mosquitoes. Indian Med Gaz 33:401–448
Sergent ED, Sergent ET (1921) Avantages de la quinisation préventère demonstrés et précisés éxpérimentellement (Paludisme des oiseaux). Ann Inst Pasteur (Paris) 35:125–141
Steck EA (1972) Chemotherapy of malaria. Chemotherapy of protozoan diseases, vol III. U.S. Government Printing Offices, Washington DC
Taylor DJ, Josephson ES, Greenberg J, Coatney GR (1952) The in vitro activity of certain antimalarials against erythrocytic forms of *Plasmodium gallinaceum*. Am J Trop Med Hyg 1:132–139
Terzian LA (1947) A method of screening antimalarial compounds in the mosquito host. Science 106:449–450
Terzian LA (1950) The sulphonamides as factors in increasing susceptibility to parasitic invasion. J Infect Dis 87:285–290
Terzian LA, Stahler N, Weathersby AB (1949) The action of antimalarial drugs in mosquitoes infected with *Plasmodium gallinaceum* J Infect Dis 84:47–55
Terzian LA, Stahler N, Ward PA (1951) The effect of antibiotics and metabolites on the immunity of mosquitoes to malarial infection. J Infect Dis 90:116–130
Thompson PE, Reinertson JW, Bayles A, Moore AM (1953) The curative action of antimalarial drugs against *Plasmodium lophurae* in chicks. J Infect Dis 92:40–51
Tréfouël J, Tréfouël J, Nitti F, Bovet D (1935) Activité du *p*-aminophénylsulfamide sur les infections streptococciques expérimentales de la souris et du lapin. C R Soc Biol (Paris) 120:756–758
Urbanski T, Serafin B, Clyde DF, Jakimowska K, Witkiewicz M, Nantka-Namiriski P, Venulet J, Schultz GO, Splwinski J, Potaczek T (1964) Nitro compounds. In: Proceedings of the international symposium held at the Polish academy of sciences, Warszawa, 18–20 September, 1963. Pergamon, Oxford, pp 463–468
Walker HA, Richardson AP (1948) Potentiation of the curative action of 8-aminoquinolines and naphthoquinones in avian malaria. J Nat Malar Soc 7:4–11
Walker HA, Stauber LA, Richardson AP (1948) Curative action of pamaquine naphthoate, quinacrine, hydrochloride, and quinine bisulphate in *Plasmodium cathemerium* infections of the duck. J Infect Dis 82:187–192

Wampler F (1930) A preliminary report on the early effects of plasmochin on *P. cathemerium*. Arch Protistenkd 69:1–6

Wasielewski TKWN von (1904) Vogelplasmodiose. In: Studien und Mikrophotogramme zur Kenntnis der pathogenen Protozoen. T.A. Barth, Leipzig, Heft 2, S. 64–134

Wiselogle FY (ed) (1946) A survey of antimalarial drugs, 1941–1945, vol 1. Ann Arbor, Michigan

Woods DD (1940) The relation of *p*-aminobenzoic acid to the mechanism of the action of sulphanilamide. Br J Exp Pathol 21:74–90

CHAPTER 8

# Rodent Malaria Models

A. L. AGER, JR.

## A. Introduction

The first isolation of rodent malaria was reported by VINCKE and LIPS (1948). This isolate, obtained from the tree rat *Thamnomys surdaster*, was discovered at Keyberg in the former Belgian Congo and named *Plasmodium berghei.*

Four chemotherapy studies using this new isolate passed into laboratory mice and rats were reported within the next 2 years by GOODWIN (1949), SCHNEIDER et al. (1949), HILL (1950), and THURSTON (1950). By 1978 946 papers had appeared in the literature (PETERS and HOWELLS 1978) on chemotherapy research using rodent malaria. In the two subsequent years over 150 additional papers were published.

The numerous species and subspecies of rodent malarias that have been isolated are divided into two main series, the *berghei* group and the *vinckei* group. The group used for the majority of chemotherapy research is the *berghei* group, containing *P. berghei* (KBG-173) isolated by VINCKE and LIPS (1948), *P. yoelii* 17X (LANDAU and KILLICK-KENDRICK 1966) and *P. y. nigeriensis* N67 (KILLICK-KENDRICK 1973) and other subspecies. The *vinckei* group contains *P. vinckei* and *P. chabaudi*, which also have several subspecies. Excellent reviews of taxonomy and detailed descriptions of the various types of rodent malaria have been published by CARTER and DIGGS (1977) and KILLICK-KENDRICK (1978). Other aspects are reviewed in KILLICK-KENDRICK and PETERS (1978).

Rodent malaria was first successfully transmitted through mosquitoes by YOELI et al. (1964) using *Anopheles quadrimaculatus.* This procedure was modified by VANDERBERG and YOELI (1965) and finally standardised by VANDERBERG and YOELI (1966). *Anopheles stephensi* is the most effective mosquito to transmit rodent malaria cyclically (YOELI et al. 1966). Various reviews on mosquito transmission of rodent malaria have been reported by WÉRY (1968), LANDAU and BOULARD (1978), LANDAU et al. (1979), VANDERBERG and GWADZ (1980), FOSTER (1980), and CARTER and GWADZ (1980).

Chemotherapy studies using rodent malaria are diversified and the proper standardisation of a test system involves the close scrutiny of a large number of variables. Rodent strains vary tremendously in their susceptibility to malaria (GREENBERG et al. 1953; GREENBERG and KENDRICK 1958; MOST et al. 1966; BAFORT 1971). Parasites themselves vary in their course of infection and degree of virulence (HARDGREAVES et al. 1975; EUGI and ALLISON 1979; KNOWLES and WALLIKER 1980). Concomitant infections can alter the course of parasite growth. Mice harbouring *Eperythrozoon coccoides* usually have a reduced parasitaemia with *P. berg-*

*hei* (PETERS 1965a; THOMPSON and BAYLES 1966; GOTHE and KREIER 1977; COX 1978). Rats infected with *Haemobartonella muris* have increased parasitaemia of *P. berghei*, enhanced virulence being observed (HSU and GEIMAN 1952). The level of *p*-aminobenzoic acid (PABA) in the rodents' diet can influence the suppressive activity of certain sulphonamides (JACOBS 1964; RICHARDS 1970; PETERS and RAMKARAN 1980). The type of red blood cells available for certain parasite lines markedly influences the parasitaemia (OTT 1968; HANSON and THOMPSON 1972; BÜNGENER 1979a, b).

Overall, the rodent malaria models for chemotherapy studies have proven to be extremely valuable in assessing the activity of established and potentially new antimalarial compounds. General reviews containing specifically rodent malaria chemotherapy sections include PETERS (1970, 1974, 1980), PETERS and HOWELLS (1978), HILL (1966a, b), THOMPSON and WERBEL (1972), STECK (1972), ELSLAGER (1974), AVIADO (1969), and ROZMAN and CANFIELD (1979). The rodent malaria models perform as a primary and secondary screen before monkey malaria screens. The correlation of data on compounds tested in rodent malaria systems with monkey malaria systems is, in most instances, in agreement (SCHMIDT 1973; SCHMIDT et al. 1977, 1978). There is a certain degree of fluctuation in effective dose levels between rodent and primate models. However, only three compounds or groups of chemicals have not shown the degree of activity in rodents that they have in primates. The first two examples (RC-12 and certain 5-phenoxy-8-aminoquinolines) have tissue schizontocidal activity in the rhesus monkey infected with *P. cynomolgi* but are devoid of such activity in rodents. The other discrepancy involves the blood schizontocidal activity of proguanil, which is active in primates but inactive in rodents. Interestingly though it is an active causal prophylactic in rodents. Since there is only one exoerythrocytic cycle in rodent malaria the system resembles somewhat *P. falciparum*. This complicates testing for causal prophylactic compounds as well as radical curative agents.

## B. Blood Schizontocides

### I. Single-Dose Regimens

#### 1. Rane's Test

This system is based on the use of mice, inoculated intraperitoneally with asexual blood parasites, and treated 3 days later with one subcutaneous injection of the test compound. Antimalarial activity is assessed by comparing survival times of treated mice to infected, non-treated controls (OSDENE et al. 1967). All mice are ICR/HA Swiss type, bred in the Rane Laboratory. Test male and female animals weigh from 18 to 20 g and are all approximately the same age. Each mouse receives about $6 \times 10^5$ parasitised erythrocytes drawn from donor mice infected 4 days earlier with *P. berghei*. The parasites are maintained by passing them every 4 days in separate groups of donors inoculated with 0.2 ml of a 1:435 dilution of heparinised heart blood, harbouring a parasitaemia of approximately 50%. Three days postinfection, when a 5%–15% parasitaemia has developed, treatment begins with a single dose of test compound given subcutaneously. Test compounds are dissolved or suspended in peanut oil by mixing with a glass mortar and pestle. Mice are kept at 24 °C until treated, then moved to a room at 29 °C for the duration of the experiment. Deaths that occur before the 6th day, when infected, untreated controls begin to die, are regarded as toxic deaths. Each compound is administered initially in three graded doses diluted fourfold into groups of five mice per dose level. The highest dose is 640, 320 or 160 mg/kg, depending on the amount of compound available for testing. The per cent free base of each compound is not calculated since all compounds are tested blindly. Active compounds are subsequently tested at six dose levels, diluted twofold from the highest dose. Successive six-level tests are performed at respectively lower doses if necessary until the lower limit of activity is reached. Active compounds are tested orally at similar doses administered subcutaneously. Each oral compound is ground with a mortar and pestle in 0.5% hydroxyethylcellulose 0.1% Tween-80. A compound toxic at each of the three levels initially tested is retested at six dose levels diluted twofold from the lowest toxic dose.

Drug activity is based upon survival times and the minimum effective dose (MED), which is defined as the minimum dose increasing the survival time of infected treated mice by 100% over the survival time of infected non-treated controls. Mice alive 60 days after infection are considered cured. Pyrimethamine administered to ten mice at one level (120 mg/kg) serves as the positive control. A therapeutic index is obtained based upon a maximum tolerated dose (highest dose up to 640 mg/kg which has no more than one toxic death) and the MED.

This test system began in 1961, since when over 250000 compounds have been tested, with approximately 8000 exhibiting some antimalarial activity. Data on some antimalarial compounds are shown in Table 2. All compounds currently used in humans infected with malaria are active in this rodent test system. Proguanil shows slight blood schizontocidal activity; however, it is also only marginally active in other rodent systems because of the rodent's inability to metabolise proguanil to its active metabolite, cycloguanil.

### 2. Fink and Kretschmar's Test

A single-dose test system described by FINK and KRETSCHMAR (1970) assessed antimalarial activity by determining the prolongation of survival of mice by 20% ($ÜD_{20}$). NMRI albino mice were inoculated intraperitoneally with $10^7$ red blood cells parasitised with *P. vinckei vinckei*, followed within a few hours by a single intraperitoneal injection of test compound at various dose levels. Infected untreated control mice die within 5–6 days. The percent prolongation data for each dose were plotted on probit-activity log-dose paper and the $ÜD_{20}$ was directly extrapolated from the graph. The $ÜD_{20}$ was considered to be a reliable MED. This test was developed as a simple test to save time (no blood films required), and to use a smaller amount of test compound. $ED_{50}$s and $ED_{90}$s can be determined from this test if blood films are made and percent reductions in parasitaemia are determined. A comparison of $ED_{50}$s, $ED_{90}$s, and $ÜD_{20}$s is shown for several standard antimalarials in Table 1.

**Table 1.** Suppressive action of standard antimalarials on *P. vinckei* in NMRI mice injected intraperitoneally on day 0 of infection with $10^7$ PE/mouse. Data from FINK and KRETSCHMAR (1970)

| Substance | Reduction of parasitaemia on day 2 post infection compared with controls | | Prolongation of survival time compared with controls |
|---|---|---|---|
| | $ED_{50}$ (mg/kg) | $ED_{90}$ (mg/kg) | $ÜD_{20}$ (mg/kg) |
| Chloroquine[a] | 1.5 | 4.5 | 2.7 |
| Primaquine[a] | 0.35 | 2.5 | 2.0 |
| Quinine[b] | 17.0 | 40.0 | 40.0 |
| Mepacrine[b] | 4.9 | 6.3 | 6.0 |
| Pyrimethamine | 0.11 | 0.68 | 0.45 |
| Cycloguanil[b] | 1.0 | 10.0 | 6.0 |
| Sulphadiazine | 0.06 | 0.6 | 0.17 |

[a] As diphosphate calculated as per cent free base
[b] As hydrochloride calculated as per cent free base

## II. Multiple-Dose Regimens

### 1. Early Test Procedures

The first chemotherapy studies using *P. berghei* were reported by GOODWIN (1949) and SCHNEIDER et al. (1949). Both workers utilised similar procedures which included infecting mice intraperitoneally on day 0 (D0) followed by treatment subcutaneously (SCHNEIDER et al. 1949) or orally (GOODWIN 1949) on D0, D+1, and D+2. Antimalarial activity was assessed on D+6 by taking blood films and determining patency. The lowest active dose allowed 75% of the test mice to be non-patent on D+6 and was called the MED. THURSTON (1950) infected mice intraperitoneally and gave them test compound by gavage for four consecutive days commencing on D0. Blood films were taken on D+4 and D+6. Activity, in terms of the MED, was the lowest dose level allowing a 1% parasitaemia to develop. THURSTON (1953) modified this test by reducing the parasite inoculum from $5–15 \times 10^6$ to $10^6$ parasitised erythrocytes. The MED was changed to the lowest dose level, reducing the parasitaemia on D+4 to 2% of the 1%–5% parasitaemia level of the control group. HILL (1950) administered compounds orally once a day for 3 days then, on D+4, twice in the day. Activity was measured in terms of the lowest dose reducing parasitaemia to 0.25%. RAMAKRISHNAN et al. (1951) administered compounds twice daily orally on D0, D+1, and D+2. The effective dose was the lowest level which cleared parasites for 3 days after the last day of treatment. The MED was replaced by the $SD_{50}$ value (dose level suppressing the parasitaemia by 50%) as used by two earlier research workers, JACOBS et al. (1963) and AVIADO (1967). The suppression of parasitaemia for each drug dose was calculated by the formula:

$$\frac{\text{average \% parasitaemia in controls (sham-treated)} - \text{average \% parasitaemia in treated mice}}{\text{average \% parasitaemia in controls (sham-treated)}} \times 100.$$

The dose of compound and its average per cent suppression of parasitaemia were plotted on logarithmic-probability paper. Regression lines were drawn and $SD_{50}$ values were read from the plot. PETERS (1965a) measured activity in terms of an $ED_{50}$. This $ED_{50}$ is derived by plotting the erythrocyte infection rates (the percentage of erythrocytes containing parasites in the treated group compared with the sham-control group) on a probit scale and the doses of test compound on the log scale. Regression lines are drawn and $ED_{50}$ values read. The $ED_{50}$, $ED_{90}$, $SD_{50}$ and $SD_{90}$ have been the most common values used to estimate drug activity in reports since the early 1960s.

A test system was reported by WARHURST and FOLWELL (1968) to eliminate the influence of any host immunity upon the assessment of antimalarial activity. The test is called a 2% test and basically measures the time taken by the treated mice to achieve a 2% parasitaemia compared with appropriate controls. For a full explanation of the mathematics involved in determining activity the orginal paper should be read. This test is too complicated to be used in an initial screening system.

## 2. Four-Day Test

The 4-day suppressive test has been widely used since it can be performed within a 1-week period. The test consists of the inoculation of parasitised erythrocytes on Monday, the 1st day of the experiment (D0), followed by an injection of the test compound, which is repeatedly administered on D+1, D+2, and D+3. On D+4 (Friday) blood films are taken and antimalarial activity is assessed either by calculating parasitaemias or by scoring parasite numbers on a predetermined scale (i.e. 0–5).

PETERS (1970) described a basic procedure using this 4-day test. Randomly bred, Swiss, albino, male mice weighing $20 \pm 2$ g are used. Parasites (*P. berghei* KBG-173) are collected either by cardiac puncture or from axillary blood vessels in a heparinised syringe from a donor mouse harbouring a 20% parasitaemia. Blood is diluted with TC medium 199 to a final concentration of $10^7$ infected erythrocytes per 0.2 ml infecting suspension. Each mouse is inoculated intravenously, producing a more uniform infection rate than an intraperitoneal administration of parasites.

Test compounds are prepared at initial doses of 3, 10, and 30 mg/kg in saline if soluble or in a suspension of 0.5% carboxymethylcellulose and 0.2% Tween-80 if insoluble. Some compounds are ultrasonicated to reduce the particle size or are ground in a mortar with pestle. Initially, test compounds are administered subcutaneously, then if activity is demonstrated they are administered orally. The compounds are administered once a day starting on D0, and continued on D+1, D+2, and D+3. Blood films are made from tail blood on D+4 and stained with Giemsa. The erythrocyte infection rates (EIR) are determined and plotted versus the corresponding dose levels on probit-log paper and $ED_{50}$s and $ED_{90}$s are read from regression lines (Table 2). Maximum tolerated doses (MTD) and an end point of activity can be attained by varying the doses of the compounds. The $ED_{50}$s and $ED_{90}$s are expressed as dose of compound received in 1 day as milligrams per

**Table 2.** A comparison of suppressive activity of PETERS et al. (1975 b), THOMPSON et al. (1969), and RANE (STRUBE 1975)

| Compound name or WR No. salt form | *P. berghei* (KBG-173) 4-day suppressive test $ED_{90}$ (mg/kg, s.c.) | *P. berghei* (KBG-173) 6-day suppressive test $SD_{90}$ (mg/kg, s.c.) | *P. berghei* MED (mg/kg, s.c.) | $CD_{50}$ (mg/kg, s.c.) |
|---|---|---|---|---|
| 4-Aminoquinoline | | | | |
| Chloroquine $2H_3PO_4$ | 3.3 | 3.0 | 80 | > 160 |
| Acridine | | | | |
| Mepacrine methane sulphonate | 5.5 | | 20 | > 640 |
| Quinine type | | | | |
| Quinine 2HCl | 87 | 90 | 640 | > 640 |
| Sulphonamides | | | | |
| Sulphadiazine | 0.3 | 0.3 | 160 | > 640 |
| Sulfadoxine | 1.6 | NT[a] | 10 | 80 |
| Sulphone | | | | |
| Dapsone | 0.4 | 2 | 320 | > 640 |
| Pyrimidines | | | | |
| Pyrimethamine | 0.44 i.p. | 0.4 | 20 | 80 |
| Trimethoprim | 190 | > 200 | > 640 | > 640 |
| Triazines | | | | |
| Cycloguanil HCl | 11.0 | 10.0 | | |
| Cycloguanil pamoate | | | 160 | > 640 |
| Clociguanil | 0.35 | 5 | | |
| Quinoline methanols | | | | |
| WR 30090 HCl | 2.7 p.o. | 1.5 | 5 | 40 |
| WR 142490 HCl | 8.5 | 4.5 | 10 | 20 |
| Phenanthrenemethanols | | | | |
| WR 33063 HCl | 18.5 | 14 | 160 | > 640 |
| WR 122455 HCl | 10.0 | 4.5 | 20 | 40 |
| Naphthoquinones | | | | |
| Menoctone | 1.5 | 10.5 | 40 | 320 |
| WR 6012 | | 14 | 40 | 320 |
| Antibiotic | | | | |
| Minocycline | 25.5 i.p. | 100 | 160 | 640 |

[a] Not tested

kilogram per day. This test system has been used extensively by RICHARDS (1966), PETERS et al. (1965 b), RAETHER and FINK (1979) and MERKLI et al. (1980).

## 3. Drug-Diet Methods

In several test systems, compounds have been administered with animal food, e.g. DARROW et al. (1952), BOX et al. (1954) and GARZA and BOX (1961). One specific test system was used by THOMPSON et al. (1969) to screen several hundred compounds. Female CF-1 mice were divided into groups of seven and treated by drug-

**Table 3.** Suppressive effects of CI-679 acetate[a] by drug-diet treatment against *P. berghei* in mice

| Drug in diet (%) | Drug intake (mg/kg/day) | No. mice patent total mice | Suppression of parasitaemia (mean %) |
|---|---|---|---|
| 0.0032 | 4.0 | 0/10 | 100 |
| 0.0008 | 1.0 | 0/10 | 100 |
| 0.0002 | 0.33 | 3/10 | 99 |
| 0.00005 | 0.07 | 10/10 | 28 |
| Controls | | 10/10 | 56[b] |

[a] After THOMPSON et al. (1970). CI-679 acetate is triaminoquinazoline
[b] Mean percentage of cells parasitised

diet for 6 days, starting 1 day prior to an intraperitoneal inoculation of $2.5 \times 10^6$ parasites (*P. berghei* KBG-173). A group of seven to ten mice were included as untreated controls (negative control group). Quinine sulphate used as a positive control at a diet level of 0.05% gave a 90% suppression of parasitaemia. Blood films and final group weights were taken on D + 5. Microscopic examination of Giemsa-stained blood films was made to determine the percentage of cells parasitised. Actual drug doses were calculated from determining the drug intake (milligrams per kilogram per day), by comparing the per cent weight change of animals D − 1 to D + 5, and the amount of diet consumed/mouse per day.

Drug tolerance was reflected by the mean per cent weight change and the proportion of mice surviving treatment. A range of drug-diet concentrations was used in each experiment. If mice had eaten sufficient medicated ration (at least 1.5 g/mouse per day), and if there was no significant reduction of parasitaemia at the highest concentration, the test compound was considered of no further interest. A food intake of 1 g/mouse per day did not permit normal development of parasitaemia. In such instances, it was not possible to distinguish between the effects of the compound and inanition. Additional testing of the compound at diet levels permitting consumption of at least 1.5 g/mouse per day was required for determination of specific effect.

The results of testing a triaminoquinazoline are shown in Table 3.

Four major limitations to a drug screen utilising test compounds administered in mouse feed are: (a) irregular dose-response curves due primarily to inadequate intake of food containing the test compounds; (b) excessive time required to prepare the medicated diet; (c) the determination of the amount of drug consumed throughout the duration of the experiment; and (d) if the test compound is bitter or unpalatable in any way to the mouse it will not feed, leading to a non-specific suppression of the parasitaemia.

## 4. Six-Day Test

Because of the limitations of the drug-diet delivery system and the desire to test compounds against established infections, a modification of the 4-day test was reported by PETERS (1965 b) and THOMPSON et al. (1969). In a basic 6-day suppressive test described by THOMPSON et al. (1969), and used subsequently in testing hundreds of compounds, mice are infected on a Friday (D0) and compounds are administered twice daily on D+3, D+4, and D+5. Blood films are taken on D+6 and parasitaemias are determined by examination of erythrocytes by the following procedure:

100 erythrocytes if parasitaemia is 10%–100%
200 erythrocytes if parasitaemia is 5%–10%
Ten fields (2,000 erythrocytes) until ten parasites found, 0.5%–5%
11–100 fields (2,200–20,000 erythrocytes) until a parasite found 0.01%–0.45%
100 fields or 20,000 erythrocytes examined without a parasite before mouse is considered 0%

An inoculum of $2.5 \times 10^6$ parasitised erythrocytes of *P. berghei* (KBG-173) is injected intraperitoneally. Test compounds are administered either orally or subcutaneously suspended in 0.5% hydroxyethylcellulose-0.1% Tween-80. Oral compounds are administered through a #18 gauge needle which has an enlarged smooth tip. Quinine is administered as a positive control compound and the activity of each test compound is compared with quinine, yielding a "quinine index". Most compounds are administered at 64, 16, 4 and 1 mg/kg per day. Doses required for a given degree of effect, such as 90% suppression or $SD_{90}$, are estimated graphically from plots made on log-probit paper. A comparison of $SD_{90}$ values obtained in this 6-day suppressive test with several other test systems is shown in Table 2.

## C. Tissue Schizontocides

### I. Most's Test

MOST et al. (1967) described a screening system to determine if certain test compounds administered to rodents challenged with sporozoites had antimalarial activity based upon visualisation of exoerythrocytic stages in the liver. They utilised an inbred strain of albino mice (A/J Bar Harborn), rats and hamsters infected with *P. berghei* (NK strain) sporozoites, collected by dissection or trituration from *A. stephensi.* Two routes of sporozoite inoculation were used, the intraperitoneal route with $2.5 \times 10^4$ sporozoites and the intravenous route with $10^4$ to $1.5 \times 10^4$ sporozoites. Additional animals in the control and treatment groups received $2 \times 10^5$ to $2.5 \times 10^5$ sporozoites and the livers from some of these animals were examined for exoerythrocytic stages. Test compounds were administered subcutaneously (except quinine, which was given orally) the day before infection (D−1) and the day of infection (D0). Antimalarial activity was assessed by examining the blood for parasites for a 60-day period by splenectomising selected mice exhibiting no parasitaemia, and by searching liver sections for exoerythrocytic schizonts in mice which were blood film negative.

Primaquine in a total dose of 50 mg/kg was considered to be a causal prophylactic drug when administered on D−1 and D0 as judged by lack of patency, lack of parasitaemia in splenectomised rats and mice, and lack of exoerythrocytic forms in the examined liver sections. Pyrimethamine (300 mg/kg total dose) was also judged to be a causal prophylactic drug when given on D – 1 and D0 to mice receiving sporozoites via the intraperitoneal and intravenous routes. All mice were blood film negative before and after splenectomy and no exoerythrocytic forms were found.

Chloroquine (100 mg/kg total dose) and dapsone (300 mg/kg total dose), both administered subcutaneously, and quinine (400 mg/kg total dose) administered orally on D – 1 and D0 were found to be non-causal prophylactic drugs.

Since no distinction was made between drug activity against the exoerythrocytic stages and activity against emerging intraerythrocytic stages, additional experiments were performed to determine the actual stage affected by the drugs. Mice were inoculated with $10^4$ sporozoites intravenously and drugs were administered commencing on the 3rd day of patency and continued for four consecutive days to determine if a cure could be attained. Other groups similarly infected were treated for ten consecutive days commencing on the 3rd day after patency. Two addi-

**Table 4.** Possible outcomes in a drug trial experiment with inactive and active causally prophylactic drugs. After Most and Montuori (1975)

| Drug (mg/kg total dose) | | Rat smears[a] | | | Sub-transfused mouse[b] | EE[c] | Splenectomy[a] | Effect of drug |
|---|---|---|---|---|---|---|---|---|
| | | D+6 | D+10 | D+15 | | | | |
| Control | | 7/7 | | | | 2/2 | | |
| Non-causal prophylactic compounds | | | | | | | | |
| Quinine | 400 | 7/7 | | | | 2/2 | | Inactive |
| Chloroquine | 100 | 0/7 | 7/7 | | | 2/2 | | Suppressive (prolongation at interval to patency) |
| Sulfadoxine | 340 | 0/7 | 7/7 | | | 2/2 | | |
| WR 202831[d] | 640 | 0/7 | 0/7 | 7/7 | | | | Prolonged suppression and therapeutic |
| WR 205439[d] | 640 | 0/7 | 0/7 | 7/7 | | | | |
| WR 212576[d] | 640 | 0/7 | 0/7 | 0/7 | 0/5 | 2±/2 | 2/2 | Prolonged suppression, therapeutic and curative? |
| DDS[d] | 400 | 0/7 | 0/7 | 0/7 | 0/5 | 2±/2 | 2/2 | |
| Pyrimethamine | 400 | 0/7 | 0/7 | 0/7 | 0/5 | 2±/2 | 2/2 | |
| Causal prophylactic compounds | | | | | | | | |
| Primaquine[d] | 50 | 0/7 | 0/7 | 0/7 | 0/5 | 0/2 | 0/2 | Causal prophylactic activity |
| WR 209521 | 640 | 0/7 | 0/7 | 0/7 | 0/5 | 0/2 | 0/2 | |

[a] No. of rats patent over total
[b] No. of mice patent over total
[c] No. of rats positive for exoerythrocytic stages. These rats received $2.5 \times 10^5$ sporozoites while all other rats received $1 \times 10^4$ sporozoites
[d] WR 202831 is a 7-methoxyquinoline; WR 205439 is a 4-aminoquinoline; WR 212576 is a naphthyliridine-4-amino compound; DDS is dapsone; WR 209521 is an 8-aminoquinoline (structure in Table 6)

**Table 5.** A comparison of causal prophylactic data for miscellaneous chemicals from MOST[a] (unpublished work) and DAVIDSON et al.[b] (1981)

| WR No. or type of compound | Structure | *P. berghei* rats Active dose or range (mg/kg)[c] | *P. y. yoelii* ICR/HA mice $ED_{50}$ (mg/kg)[c] | |
|---|---|---|---|---|
| | | s.c. | s.c. | Oral |
| 6012[b] | 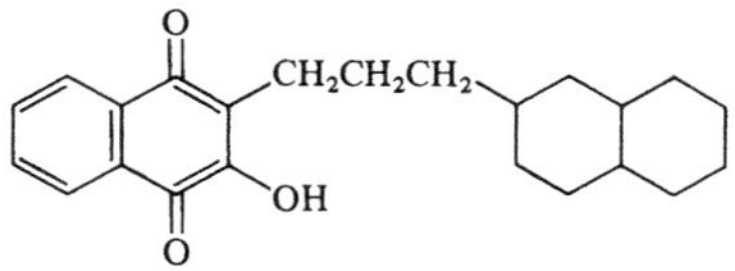 | 640 | 40 | 40 |
| 179305[b] | 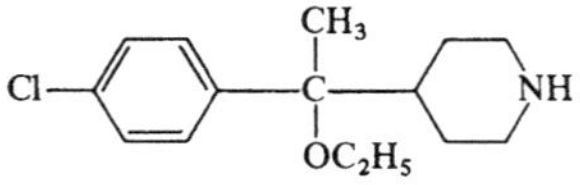 'trans' •HOCOCH=CHCOOH | 140 | 40 | 40 |
| 190729[b] | 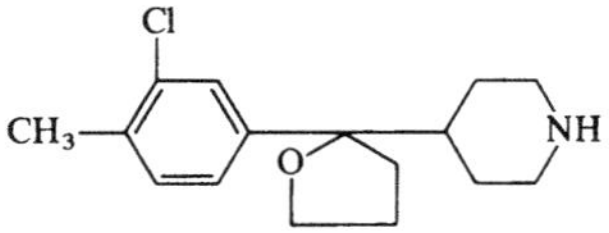 •HCl | 320 | 160 | 160 |
| 194905[b] | 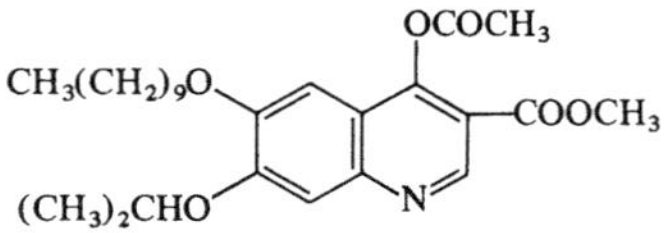 | 320 | 0.63 | 0.63 |
| 226626[b] | 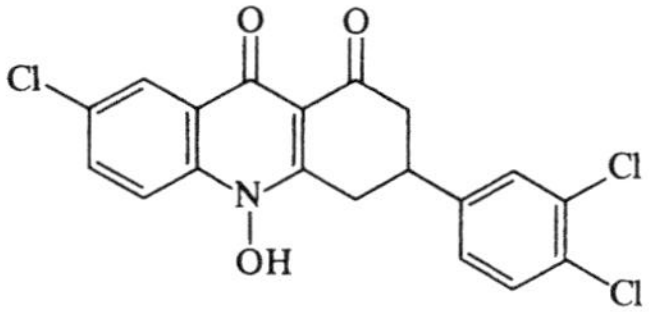 | 320[e] | 10 | 10 |

| | | | | |
|---|---|---|---|---|
| 40070 | 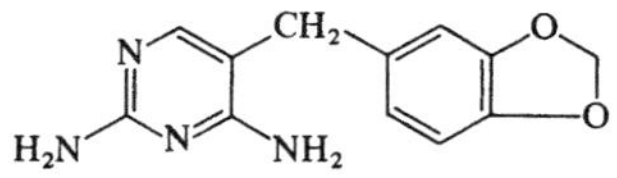 | 640 | 160 | 160 |
| 61112[b] | 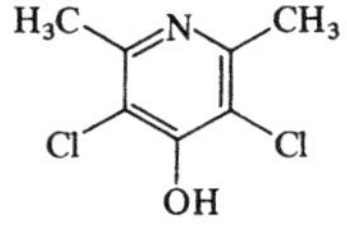 | 320 | 160 | 160 |
| 181953 | 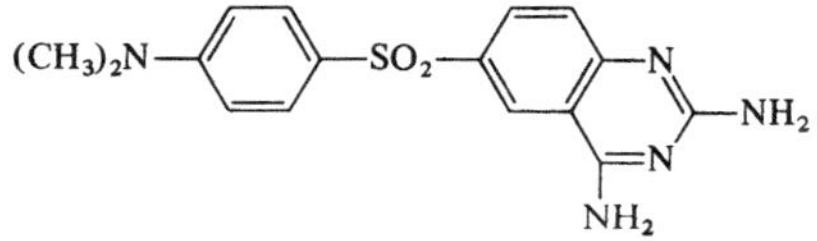 | 80–320 | 2.5 | 2.5 |
| 6798 Diformyl dapsone | 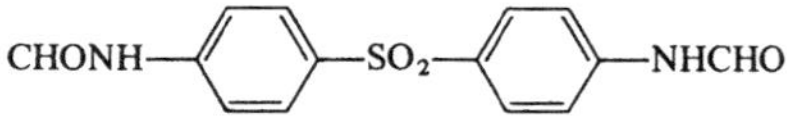 | 640 | 40 | 160 inactive |
| 6527 Tetracycline | 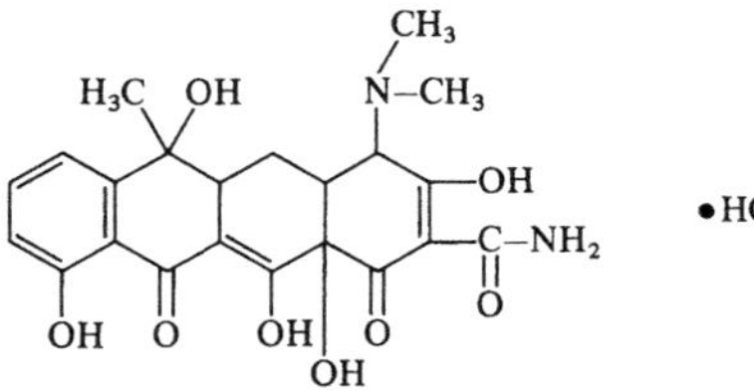 | 320 | 160 | 640 |

[a] Dr. HARRY MOST kindly gave permission to WRAIR to release his unpublished data
[b] Compounds published in DAVIDSON et al. (1981) while remaining compound data were supplied by Ager (unpublished)
[c] Total dose administered b.d. on D-1 and DO
[d] The lowest test dose permitting at least 50% of mice to survive the otherwise lethal inoculum of sporozoites
[e] Total dose administered once on DO

**Table 6.** A comparison of causal prophylactic data for 8-aminoquinolines from MOST[a] (unpublished work) and DAVIDSON et al. (1981)[b]

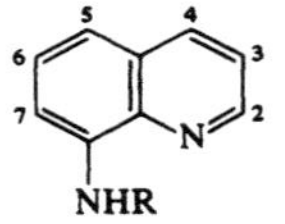

| Compound name or WR No. salt | Substituents in quinoline ring: 2 | 3 | 4 | 5 | 6 | R | *P. berghei* rats active dose or range (mg/kg)[c] s.c. | *P. yoelii yoelii* 17X ICR/HA mice $ED^{d}_{50}$ (mg/kg)[e] s.c. | Oral |
|---|---|---|---|---|---|---|---|---|---|
| Primaquine 2976[b] $H_3PO_4$ | | | | | $-OCH_3$ | $-CH(CH_2)_3NH_2$ with $CH_3$ on CH | 50 | 50 | 50 |
| 2-Methylprimaquine 182234[b] 2HCl | $-CH_3$ | | | | $-OCH_3$ | $-CH(CH_2)_3NH_2$ with $CH_3$ on CH | 160 | 40 | 40 |
| 4-Methylprimaquine 181023[b] $2H_3PO_4$ | | | $-CH_3$ | | $-OCH_3$ | $-CH(CH_2)_3NH_2$ with $CH_3$ on CH | 1–40 | 50 | 25 |
| 161085 $\cdot 2H_2O$ 2 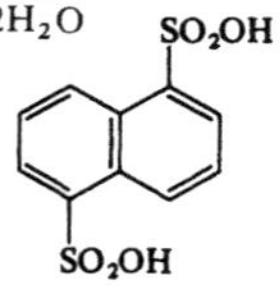 | | | | | $-OCH_3$ | $-CH(CH_3)CH_2CH_2CH_2NH-$ 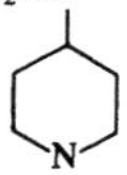 | 640 | 160 | 160 |
| 192515 3 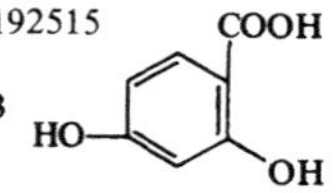 | $-CH_3$ | | $-CH_3$ | | $-OCH_3$ | $-CH(CH_3)CH_2CH_2CH_2CH_2NH_2$ | 80–320 | 80 | 80 |
| 193130 2 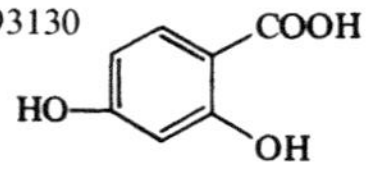 $\cdot H_2O$ | $-CH_3$ | | $-CH_3$ | | $-OCH_3$ | 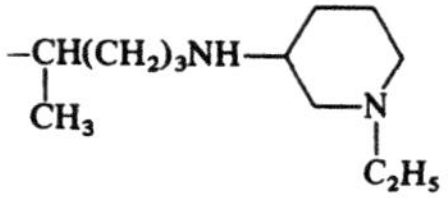 | 640 | 160 | 40 |
| 209521 $2H_3PO_4$ | | 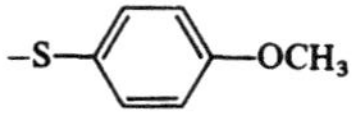 | | | $-OCH_3$ | $-CHCH_2CH_2CH_2NH$ with $CH_3$ on CH | 160–640 | 640 | 160 |

| | | | | | | | | |
|---|---|---|---|---|---|---|---|---|
| 225448[b] HOCOCH$_2$CH$_2$COOH | | —CH$_3$ | 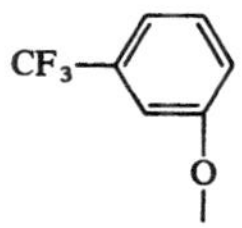 | —OCH$_3$ | —CH(CH$_3$)CH$_2$CH$_2$CH$_2$NH$_2$ | 2.5–40 | 40 | 40 |
| 227681 6HCl · H$_2$O | | —CH$_3$ | | —OCH$_3$ | 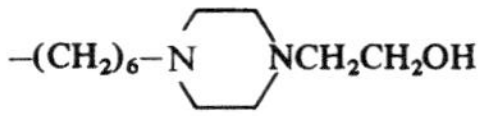 | 20 | 80 | >80 |
| 231033 HOCOCH$_2$CH$_2$COOH | | —CH$_3$ | 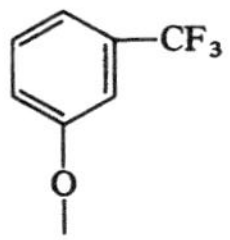 | —OCH$_3$ | —(CH$_2$)$_3$CH(CH$_3$)NH$_2$ | 2.5–20 | 20 | 10 |
| 231350 H$_3$PO$_4$ | | —CH$_3$ | | 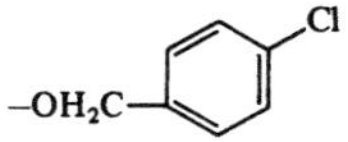 | —CH(CH$_3$)(CH$_2$)$_3$NH$_2$ | 40–80 | 160 inactive | 160 |
| 231030 HOCOCH$_2$CH$_2$COOH ·2H$_2$O | | —CH$_3$ | 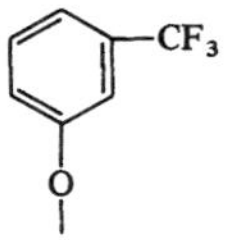 | —OCH$_3$ | —(CH$_2$)$_4$CH(CH$_3$)NH$_2$ | 2.5–20 | 40 | 10 |
| 228710 HOCOCH$_2$CH$_2$COOH | | —CH$_3$ | —OCH$_3$ | —OCH$_3$ | —CH(CH$_3$)CH$_2$(CH$_2$)$_3$NH$_2$ | 32 | 5 | 5 |
| 228456 H$_3$PO$_4$ | —CH$_3$ | —CH$_3$ | —OCH$_3$ | —OCH$_3$ | —(CH$_2$)$_3$CH(CH$_3$)NH$_2$ | 1–32 | 20 | 20 |
| 228457 H$_3$PO$_4$ | —CH$_3$ | | —OCH$_3$ | —OCH$_3$ | —(CH$_2$)$_3$CH(CH$_3$)NH$_2$ | 20 | 50 | ND[f] |
| 218335 2H$_3$PO$_4$ | | —CH$_3$ | | —OCH$_3$ | —(CH$_2$)$_3$CH(NH$_2$)CH$_2$CH$_3$ | 2.5–40 | 40 | 40 |
| 127854 2HCl | | —CH$_3$ | | —OCH$_3$ | —(CH$_2$)$_5$NHCH(CH$_3$)$_2$ | 2.5–20 | 160 | ND[f] |
| 226984 HCl | | —CH$_3$ | | —OCH$_3$ | 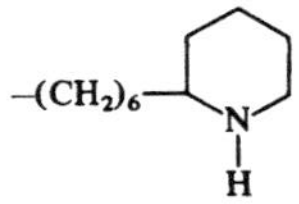 | 2.5–10 | 40 | 40 |
| 221527 CH$_3$SO$_3$H | | —CH$_3$ | —OCH$_3$ | —OCH$_3$ | —(CH$_2$)$_3$CH(NH$_2$)CH$_3$ | 2.5–10 | 10 | 10 |

**Table 6** (continued)

| Compound name or WR No. salt | 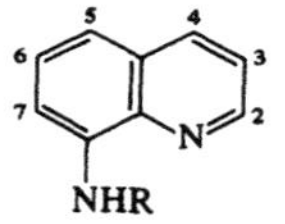 Substituents in quinoline ring 2 | 3 | 4 | 5 | R 6 | R | *P. berghei* rats active dose or range (mg/kg)[c] s.c. | *P. yoelii yoelii* 17X ICR/HA mice $ED_{50}^{d}$ (mg/kg)[e] s.c. | Oral |
|---|---|---|---|---|---|---|---|---|---|
| 22693 | | | —$CH_3$ | | —$OCH_3$ | 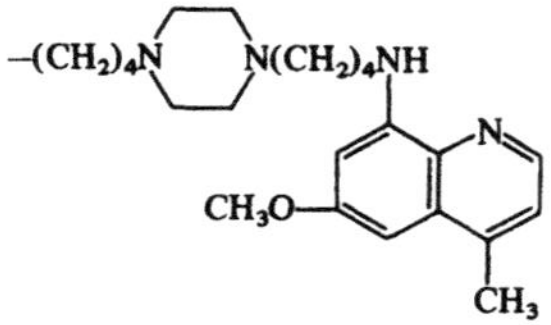 | 160 | 160 inactive | ND[f] |
| 211814 $4H_3PO_4 \cdot 3H_2O$ | | —$CH_3$ | | | —$OCH_3$ | —$CH(CH_3)CH_2CH_2CH_2NH_2$ | 10–80 | 40 | 40 |
| 183538 $2H_3PO_4 \cdot H_2O$ | 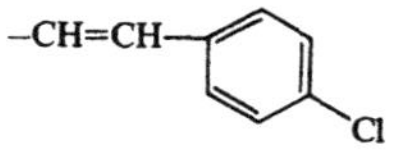 | | | | —$OCH_3$ | —$CH(CH_3)(CH_2)_3NH_2$ | 40 | 160 | 160 |

[a] Dr. Harry Most kindly gave permission to WRAIR to release his unpublished data
[b] Compounds published in Davidson et al. (1981) while remaining compound data were supplied by Agar (unpublished work)
[c] Total dose administered b.d. on D-1 and DO
[d] The lowest test dose permitting at least 50% of mice to survive the otherwise lethal inoculum of sporozoites
[e] Total dose administered once on DO
[f] Not determined

tional groups of mice were infected with erythrocytic parasites and treated for either four or ten consecutive days after patency was achieved. The authors concluded from these experiments that radical cures of patent, sporozoite-induced infections (treated for ten days with chloroquine, pyrimethamine and DDS) were due to activity directed against the asexual stages in the blood, rather than against the exoerythrocytic stages. For routine testing the distinction between causal prophylactic drugs and long-lived suppressive drugs (action only on erythrocytic stages) was still not resolved.

A modified experimental design was described by MOST and MONTUORI (1975) which simplified the previous procedures and attempted to separate blood schizontocidal from causal prophylactic drugs. Three additional parameters were measured with this test: (a) the suppression of parasitaemia, (b) the therapeutic index and (c) the curative activity of test compounds.

In each test six 19-day-old female rats (Sprague-Dawley) were injected intravenously with sporozoites. Four of these rats received $10^4$ sporozoites and two received $2.5 \times 10^5$, which were used 43–45 h later for liver biopsies. Sporozoites were harvested from dissected salivary glands, or concentrated from infected, crushed females using a density gradient concentration procedure. Test compounds were administered twice daily subcutaneously on D – 1 and D0. A total dose of 640 mg/kg was used initially unless toxicity was apparent, and a minimum causal prophylactic dose was achieved with all compounds. Blood smears were taken on D+6, D+10, and D+15 for determination of patency. Any rats inoculated with $10^4$ sporozoites, treated, and determined to be blood film negative were killed and bled. This blood was pooled and 0.2-ml aliquots were injected intraperitoneally into each of five female mice (6- to 8-week-old CF-1, and A/J strains). Blood films were taken 6 and 10 days after subinoculation and examined for parasites. If these mice were blood film negative, the liver biopsy material from the two rats inoculated with $2.5 \times 10^5$ sporozoites was examined for exoerythrocytic stages, and these rats were subsequently splenectomised. A drug was classified as causal prophylactic if: (a) treated rats were non-patent for 15–20 days, (b) subtransfused blood from these rats did not elicit a parasitaemia in mice, (c) livers of rats were negative by visual examination for exoerythrocytic stages 43–46 h after sporozoite inoculation, and (d) splenectomised rats did not develop parasitaemia.

Two 8-aminoquinolines, primaquine (50 mg/kg total dose) and WR 209521 (640 mg/kg total dose), were the only true causal prophylactic drugs mentioned of the several hundred compounds tested (Table 4). Certain compounds non-causal prophylactic in action, suppressed patency for prolonged periods of time. However, when splenectomy was performed, parasites were detected as were exoerythrocytic stages in the livers (Table 4). A comparison of causal prophylactic data for miscellaneous compounds from MOST (unpublished work) and DAVIDSON et al. (1981) are presented in Table 5. A similar comparison for 8-aminoquinolines is shown in Table 6.

Three main disadvantages of this test procedure are: (a) the large number of sporozoites required to produce enough exoerythrocytic schizonts for detection in the liver, (b) the time required to prepare liver sections for microscopic examination to detect exoerythrocytic schizonts and (c) the time needed to remove spleens and examine the peripheral blood for parasites.

## II. Berberian's Test

BERBERIAN et al. (1968) compared the causal prophylactic action of menoctone with that of primaquine in a sporozoite-induced test. Mice (A/J strain from Jackson Laboratories) were injected intravenously with $2.4 \times 10^4$ sporozoites (*P. berghei* NK 65). Compounds were suspended in 10% gelatine for oral administration or dissolved in sesame oil for parenteral injections. Causal prophylactic activity was determined by (a) examining blood films for four consecutive weeks on D+7, D+14, D+21, and D+28 after sporozoite inoculation and (b) subinoculation of blood from mice surviving 8 weeks after sporozoite injection. A dose level of test compound protecting 50% of the mice ($PD_{50}$) for 28 days postinfection was determined by plotting the data on log-probit paper.

Several drug regimens were used to show that menoctone was more active than primaquine. When chloroquine or quinine were administered in conjunction with menoctone the $PD_{50}$ value for menoctone was reduced.

Inability to distinguish causal prophylactic compounds from blood schizontocidal compounds is the major limitation of this test system. An added liability is the excessive time needed to blood film surviving mice on four different occasions and, in addition, the recipient mice of the subinoculated groups must also be examined.

## III. Vincke's Test

VINCKE (1970) reported a test to detect pre-erythrocytic antimalarial activity in young albino rats and Gif/TB albino mice infected with the ANKA strain of *P. berghei* obtained from *A. stephensi*. Sporozoites were harvested between days 15 and 25 and administered intravenously to test rodents. Two drugs (pyrimethamine isethionate and sulfadoxine) were used, each administered on the day before sporozoite inoculation (D−1) and the day sporozoites were administered (D0). Blood films were taken daily from D+4 to D+15. Mice exhibiting no parasitaemia on D+15 were then splenectomised and their blood was monitored for parasites 7 and 14 days later. Additional infected and treated mice were killed 46 h after sporozoite inoculation. Their livers were examined for exoerythrocytic stages and their blood was subinoculated into clean mice. Livers were examined microscopically with at least 100 serial sections being carefully searched before the rodent was classified as being negative. Blood films were examined in subinoculated mice to detect any parasitaemia.

VINCKE (1970) reported that both pyrimethamine and sulfadoxine administered alone as well as in combination produced a highly toxic effect against the exoerythrocytic forms.

This system does not distinguish adequately between residual blood schizontocidal activity and true tissue schizontocidal activity. It is also a very laborious system, requiring extended time periods to examine microscopically liver sections for exoerythrocytic forms.

## IV. Gregory and Peters' Test

GREGORY and PETERS (1970) developed a test system to distinguish true causal prophylactic compounds from those exhibiting residual blood schizontocidal activity. This system was later modified by PETERS et al. (1975a).

**Table 7.** The evaluation of causal prophylactic activity to show the method of calculation[a]

| Compound | Dose as base (mg/kg) | Group patency | | | Group mean pre-2% period | | | Activity[b] | | Comment |
|---|---|---|---|---|---|---|---|---|---|---|
| | | $C^0$, $T^0$ | XC | $C^x$, $T^x$ | $p^f$, $p^h$ | $p^b$ | $p^c$, $p^e$ | Residual (i) | On EE stages (ii) | |
| Control | | 3/3 | 3/3 | 3/3 | 5.12 | 4.39 | 4.15 | | | |
| T 1237 | 300 | 3/3 | | 3/3 | 4.80 | | 3.96 | −0.21 | −0.11 | Inactive |
| Control | | 4/5 | 3/3 | 5/5 | 6.01 | 4.75 | 4.46 | | | |
| T 1237 | 600 | 2/3 | | 3/3 | 5.89 | | 4.14 | −0.36 | +0.24 | Inactive |
| T 1237 | 1,000 | 3/3 | | 3/3 | 5.80 | | 3.87 | −0.64 | +0.43 | Inactive |
| Conclusion: Inactive, non-toxic at 1000 mg/kg | | | | | | | | | | |
| Control | | 4/5 | 3/3 | 3/3 | 5.26 | 3.58 | 4.23 | | | |
| WR 5990 | 10 | 2/3 | | 3/3 | 5.24 | | 3.98 | −0.17 | +0.15 | Inactive |
| WR 5990 | 30 | 0/3 | | 0/3 | | | | | | $LD_{100}$ |
| Conclusion: Inactive at maximum tolerated dose of 30 mg/kg | | | | | | | | | | |
| Control | | 3/3 | 3/3 | 3/3 | 5.65 | 4.33 | 4.35 | | | |
| Metachloridine | 10 | 2/3 | | 3/3 | 8.67 | | 4.41 | +0.06 | +2.96 | Slighty active |
| Metachloridine | 30 | 1/3 | | 3/3 | 11.26 | | 4.45 | +0.10 | +5.51 | Active |
| Metachloridine | 100 | 0/3 | | 3/3 | 14.00 | | 4.74 | +0.39 | +7.96 | Fully active |
| Conclusion: Fully active, MFAD 30–100 mg/kg, no residual activity | | | | | | | | | | |
| Control | | 4/4 | 3/3 | 3/3 | 5.82 | 4.49 | 4.15 | | | |
| ICI 56780 | 0.3 | 2/3 | | 3/3 | 11.26 | | 3.84 | −0.36 | +5.80 | Active |
| ICI 56780 | 1.0 | 1/3 | | 3/3 | 11.19 | | 4.54 | +0.45 | +4.98 | Active |
| ICI 56780 | 3.0 | 0/3 | | 3/3 | 14.0 | | 8.56 | +5.11 | +3.07 | Fully active? |
| Conclusion: Fully active, MFAD 1–3 mg/kg, marked residual activity at 3 mg/kg | | | | | | | | | | |

[a] All treatments on DO, 2 h after inoculation (Peters et al. 1975a)

[b] (i) Calculated from the formula $\frac{(p^b-a)(p^e-a)}{(p^c-a)}-(p^b-a)$, where $a=2.0$; (ii) calculated from the formula $(p^h-p^f-(i)$. (Note that i may be a negative value)

[c] C, control, T, treated mice inoculated with sporozoites ($C^0$, $T^0$), trophozoites (XC) or both ($C^x$, $T^x$). p, number of days required to reach a 2% parasitaemia level in group $C^0$ ($p^f$), $T^0$ ($p^h$), $C^x$ ($p^c$), $T^x$ ($p^e$), or XC ($p^b$)

**Table 8.** A comparison of causal prophylactic data for 8-aminoquinolines obtained from PETERS et al. (1975a) and DAVIDSON et al. (1981)[a]

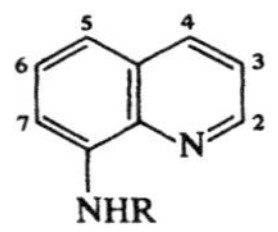

| Compound name or WR No. salt | Substituents in quinoline ring: 2 | 3 | 4 | 5 | 6 | R | *P. yoelii nigeriensis* N67 (CFW mice) MFAD (mg/kg s.c. x1) | *P. yoelii yoelii* 17X ICR/HA mice $ED_{50}$ (mg/kg): s.c. | oral |
|---|---|---|---|---|---|---|---|---|---|
| Primaquine[a] $2H_3PO_4$ | | | | | $-OCH_3$ | $-CH(CH_2)_3NH_2$<br>\|<br>$CH_3$ | 30–60 | 50 | 50 |
| 5990 $2H_3PO_4$ | | | | $-OCH_3$ | $-OCH_3$ | $-CH(CH_2)_3NH_2$<br>\|<br>$CH_3$ | Inactive at MTD | I | I |
| 182234[a] 2HCl | $-CH_3$ | | | | $-OCH_3$ | $-CH(CH_2)_3NH_2$<br>\|<br>$CH_3$ | 3–10 | 160 | 40 |
| 181023[a] $2H_3PO_4$ | | | $-CH_3$ | | $-OCH_3$ | $-CH(CH_2)_3NH_2$<br>\|<br>$CH_3$ | 30–100 | 50 | 25 |
| 210550 $2HNO_3$ | | $-CH_3$ | $-CH_3$ | | $-OCH_3$ | $-CH(CH_2)_3NH_2$<br>\|<br>$CH_3$ | 30–100 | >160 Inactive | 160 |
| 208442 2HBr | | | $-C_2H_5$ | | $-OCH_3$ | $-CH(CH_2)_3NH_2$<br>\|<br>$CH_3$ | 30–100 | 160 | 160 |
| 210551 $2HNO_3$ | | $-CH_3$ | $-CH_3$ | | $-OCH_3$ | $-CH(CH_2)_3NHCH(CH_3)_2$<br>\|<br>$CH_3$ | >MTD (100) | >160 Inactive | 160 |
| 211815 $2H_3PO_4 \cdot \frac{1}{2}H_2O$ | | $-CH_3$ | | | $-OCH_3$ | $-CH(CH_2)_3NHCH(CH_3)_2$<br>\|<br>$CH_3$ | > 30 (RA) | >160 Inactive | >160 Inactive |
| 183489 $HNO_3$ | | | | 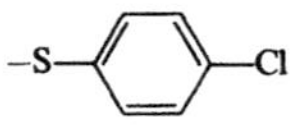 | $-OCH_3$ | $-CH(CH_2)_3NH_2$<br>\|<br>$CH_3$ | >750 | >640 Inactive | >640 Inactive |

| | | | | | | | | |
|---|---|---|---|---|---|---|---|---|
| 182232[a] hydrate | | | 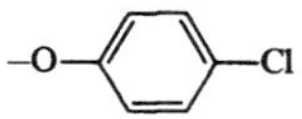 | —$OCH_3$ | —$CH(CH_2)_3NH_2$ with $CH_3$ | > 300 | > 640 Inactive | > 160 Inactive |
| 211532[a] fumarate | —$CH_3$ | | 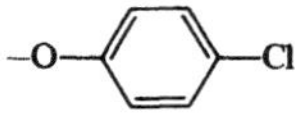 | —$OCH_3$ | —$CH(CH_2)_3NH_2$ with $CH_3$ | > 300 (RA) | > 160 Inactive | > 160 Inactive |
| 205439 maleate | 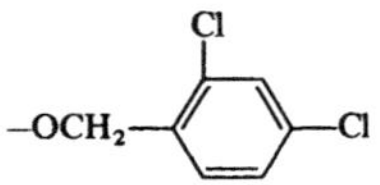 *cis* | | | —$OCH_3$ | —$CH(CH_2)_3NH_2$ with $CH_3$ | 1–3 | 160 | 160 |
| 106147 2HCl | 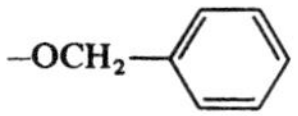 | | | —$OCH_3$ | —$CH(CH_2)_3NH_2$ with $CH_3$ | 10–30 | 160 | 160 |
| 206027 2HCl | | —$CH_3$ | | —$OCH_3$ | —$(CH_2)_3NH_2$ | MTD (100) | > 640 Inactive | NT |
| 161085 2 naphthalene disulphonate $2H_2O$ | | | | —$OCH_3$ | 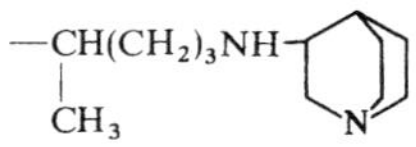 | 30 inactive | 160 | 160 |
| 189294 | | | | —$OCH_3$ | 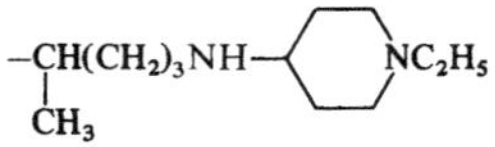 | 30–100 | 160 | NT |
| 188303 | | | 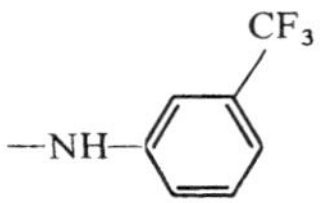 | —$OCH_3$ | 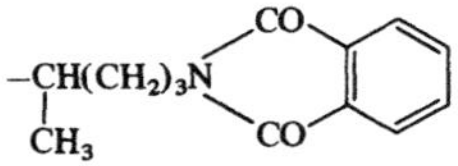 | 1,000 inactive | > 160 Inactive | NT |
| 182230 | | —$CH_3$ | | —$OCH_3$ | 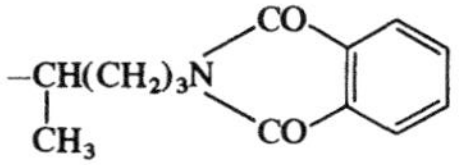 | > 1,000 | > 640 Inactive | > 160 Inactive |
| 181721 | | | 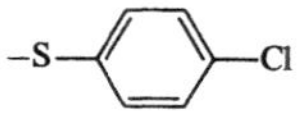 | —$OCH_3$ | 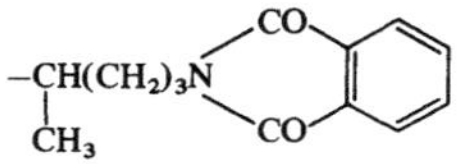 | 1,000 inactive | > 160 Inactive | NT |

**Table 8** (continued)

| Compound name or WR No. salt | Substituents in quinoline ring 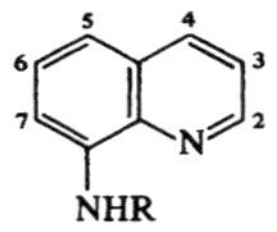 2 | 3 | 4 | 5 | 6 | R | *P. yoelii nigeriensis* N67 (CFW mice) MFAD (mg/kg s.c. x1) | *P. yoelii yoelii* 17X ICR/HA mice $ED_{50}$ (mg/kg) s.c. | oral |
|---|---|---|---|---|---|---|---|---|---|
| 181517 HCl | $—CH_3$ | | | | $-OCH_3$ | 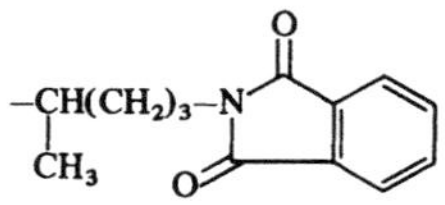 | 30–100 | 160 | > 160 Inactive |
| 7312 HCl | | | | | $—OCH_3$ | $-CH_2-C(OH)(CH_3)N[CH_2CH_2CH(CH_3)_2]_2$ | 1,000 inactive | > 640 Inactive | > 160 Inactive |
| 179443 | | | $—CH_3$ | | $—OCH_3$ | —H | 300 inactive | > 160 Inactive | > 160 Inactive |
| 49577 2HBr | | | | —OH | —OH | $—(CH_2)_5NHCH(CH_3)_2$ | > MTD (30) | > 160 Inactive | NT |
| 202437 sesqui β resorcylate | | | $—CH_3$ | | $—OCH_3$ | 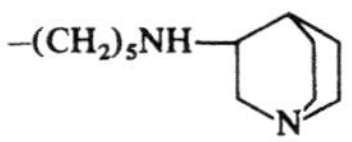 | 10–30 | 80 | 80 |
| 203607 2 β resorcylate | | | $—CH_3$ | | $—OCH_3$ | 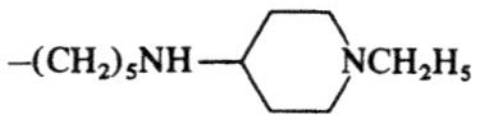 | 30–100 | 160 | 160 |
| 203608 2 β resorcylate | | | $—CH_3$ | | $—OCH_3$ | 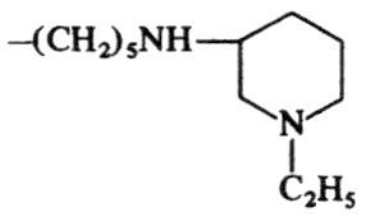 | 1–3 | 160 | 160 |

| | | | | | | | |
|---|---|---|---|---|---|---|---|
| 196469 Maleate | | —O— 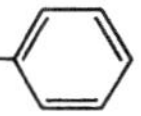 | —$OCH_3$ | —$(CH_2)_5NH$— 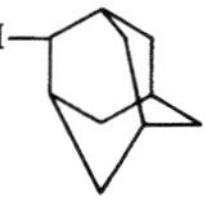 | 30 inactive 100 ± (RA) | > 160 Inactive | > 160 Inactive |
| 6025 | | —Cl | —$OCH_3$ | —$CH_2)_6N(C_2H_5)_2$ | 300 inactive | > 640 Inactive | > 640 Inactive |
| 6026 2HCl | —$CH_3$ | | —$OCH_3$ | —$(CH_2)_6N(C_2H_5)_2$ | 100 inactive | 80 | 40 |
| 29634 2HBr | | | —$OCH_3$ | —$(CH_2)_9N(C_2H_5)_2$ | 30–100 | | |

[a] Compounds reported by DAVIDSON et al. (1981); all other compounds were tested by AGER (unpublished work)

In each test there are two groups receiving the test compound and two control groups. All four groups are injected intravenously on D0 with an inoculum of sporozoites. Three hours after sporozoite inoculation two groups ($C^{\circ}$,$T^{\circ}$ and $C^{x}$,$T^{x}$) receive a single, subcutaneous injection of test compound (30 mg/kg). Forty-eight hours after administration of sporozoites two groups ($C^{x}$,$T^{x}$, XC) receive an intraperitoneal injection of $10^7$ parasitised erythrocytes. One remaining control group (C) receives nothing but the initial sporozoite injection. Blood films are made daily from D+3 to D+14 and parasitaemia levels are calculated. The determination of causal prophylactic activity is made via numerous mathematical computations explained completely in the original article of GREGORY and PETERS (1970). A compound is considered to be a causal prophylactic if no parasites are found in group $C^{\circ}$,$T^{\circ}$ from D+3 to D+14 while a parasitaemia develops in groups $C^{x}$,$T^{x}$ and XC.

This test system uses randomly bred, male, Swiss white mice (CFW line) inoculated with sporozoites of *Plasmodium yoelii nigeriensis* N 67. The parasitised erythrocytes used in groups $C^{x}$,$T^{x}$ and XC are also *P. yoelii nigeriensis*. The sporozoites are grown in *A. stephensi* and collected between days 11 and 14 after an infected blood meal. Whole infected mosquitoes are anaesthetised with carbon dioxide or ether, and the wings and legs are removed before grinding in a Teflon tube containing a small amount of 50% (V/V) calf serum and Grace's insect TC medium, or Ringer's solution. This suspension is placed in a refrigerated centrifuge and spun slowly to remove large pieces of mosquito exoskeletons and internal organs. The sporozoites are not quantitated but each mouse receives the equivalent of sporozoites found in two mosquitoes injected intravenously in 0.2-ml aliquots. Data are presented in Table 7 to show the method of calculation for this test. Comparative data for standard antimalarials are shown in Table 8.

## V. Hill's Test

HILL's test system (1975) modified and extended the causal prophylactic screen of GREGORY and PETERS (1970). For a compound to be considered truly causal prophylactic in nature it must pass through four different phases, the last of which meticulously tests for residual effects upon blood stage parasites.

In this system mice (Charles River strain) were inoculated with *P. yoelii nigeriensis* (N 67 strain) sporozoites from *A. stephensi* (Edinburgh strain). Sporozoites were harvested 8–11 days after the infected blood meal. Whole mosquitoes were ground in a Tenbroech grinder with Tyrode's Ringer glucose solution. Each mouse received approximately $10^4$–$10^5$ sporozoites intravenously in a total volume of 0.2 ml. Sporozoites were not always quantitated, but rather an infecting inoculum of 13 female mosquitoes per millilitre was utilised.

The basic test procedure for detecting causal prophylactic activity (phase I) involved administering test compounds 3 h after a sporozoite inoculation. During the ensuing 14-day period, blood films were taken until a 2% parasitaemia was achieved. If parasitaemia was not detected for 14 days the compound was considered to be fully protective for mice. It was then tested for residual activity directed against blood-stage parasites (phase II) by administering a single dose of test compound 48 h before $10^4$ trophozoites were injected intravenously. If the time interval

**Table 9.** Activity against the tissue stages of *P. berghei*: doses with little or no residual effects (HILL 1975)

| Compound | Dose (mg/kg) | Route | Phase I Proportion of mice developing parasitaemia from sporozoites | Phase II Residual drug effect on trophozoites (Mean pre-2% period in days of treated control) |
|---|---|---|---|---|
| Sulfadoxine | 250 | p.o. | 10/16[a] | 2(5.7/3.5) |
| Cycloguanil | 100 | p.o. | 0/4 | 0(5.11/4.56) |
| | 4 | p.o. | 0/6 [b] | |
| | 1 | p.o. | 3/5 [b] | |
| | 4 | s.c. | 0/4 [b] | 0(3.2/3.05) |
| | 1 | s.c. | 0/4 [b] | |
| | 0.5 | s.c. | 1/4 [b] | |
| | 0.125 | s.c. | 4/4 [b] | |
| Clindamycin | 1,000 | p.o | 0/4 | 0(5.46/4.56) |
| | 80 | p.o. | 0/4 [b] | |
| | 20 | p.o. | 4/4 [b] | |
| Doxycycline | 500 | p.o. | 0/4 | 0(5.05/3.65) |
| | 250 | p.o. | 1/4 [b] | |
| | 62.5 | p.o. | 3/4 [b] | |
| Spiramycin | 1,000 | p.o. | 0/14[c] | 0(5.9/4.56) |
| | 250 | p.o. | 4/4 | |
| Tetracycline | 2,000 | p.o. | 0/6 [b] | 0(3.8/3.05) |
| | 1,000 | p.o. | 2/4 [b] | |

[a] Combined results of four experiments
[b] A direct comparison
[c] Combined results of two experiments

to reach 2% parasitaemia was similar to that of the control group then it was considered that no residual activity had occurred. A dose delaying parasitaemia for more than 7 days, compared with infected, untreated controls, was not used. The results of six compounds tested in phases I and II are shown in Table 9. Compounds suspected of prolonged residual activity were tested (phase III) by giving sporozoites followed by drug 3 h later. After an additional 48 h had elapsed, 0.2 ml blood was removed from each mouse and injected intraperitoneally into a clean mouse (blood samples were never pooled). Blood films from recipient mice were examined for a 14-day period or until patency developed. Residual activity was noted if less than 50% of the recipients developed parasitaemia. A compound had no residual activity if 75% or more recipient mice developed patent infections. The results of five compounds tested in phase III are presented in Table 10.

An additional procedure (phase IV) was implemented to clarify whether or not a compound had a residual effect on the erythrocytic stages during the 48-h period of drug exposure in vivo. If no residual effect occurred then these parasites should remain infective. To determine if the erythrocytic parasites were still viable mice were injected intravenously with $10^4$ trophozoites 48 h after the compound had

**Table 10.** Activity against the tissue stages of *P. berghei*: doses with prolonged residual activity (HILL 1975)

| Compound | Dose (mg/kg) | Route | Phase III Proportion of mice developing parasitaemia | |
|---|---|---|---|---|
| | | | Recipients | Controls |
| Mepacrine hydrochloride | 250 | p.o. | 7/8 | 5/6 |
| Acedapsone | 1,000 | s.c. | 2/10 | 5/5 |
| Mepacrine hydrochloride | 250 | p.o. | 10/10 | |
| Acedapsone | 1,000 | s.c. | 1/10 | |
| Control donors | – | – | 10/10 | – |
| Acedapsone | 1,000 | s.c. | 0/10 | |
| | 250 | s.c. | 0/6 | 4/4[a] |
| Control donors | – | – | 5/6 | |
| Acedapsone | 100 | s.c. | 3/7 | |
| | 12.5 | s.c. | 5/7 | 4/4 |
| Control donors | – | – | 7/7 | |
| Cycloguanil pamoate | 100 | s.c. | 0/6 | 6/6 |
| Mepacrine hydrochloride | 250 | p.o. | 5/5 | |
| Sulfadoxine | 1,000 | p.o. | 0/10 | 4/4 |
| Control donors | – | – | 10/10 | |
| 12278 R.P. | 500[b] | p.o. | 7/8 | 4/4 |
| Control donors | – | – | 8/8 | |

[a] One mouse was negative on the 4th day although positive by the 7th day
[b] Maximum tolerated dose

been given. After an additional 3–4 h 0.2 ml of blood was removed and injected into clean recipient mice. Blood films were taken and a comparison of the time interval to reach 2% parasitaemia was made with that of control mice. If the time intervals were similar no permanent damage had been done to the parasites and thus no residual activity was present. Three compounds were tested in phase IV and the pre 2%-periods (days) were as follows.

| Compound | Dose (mg/kg) | Days |
|---|---|---|
| Acedapsone | 1,000 s.c. | 4.07 |
| Cycloguanil pamoate | 1,000 s.c. | 4.3 |
| Sulfadoxine | 1,000 p.o. | 4.19 |
| Control | – | 4.5 |

## VI. Fink's Test

FINK (1972) described a causal prophylactic test (slightly modified by FINK 1974) in which activity was measured in terms of a mean causal prophylactic dose ($CPD_{50}$). Randomly bred NMRI mice were inoculated intravenously with $10^4$

**Table 11.** A comparison of causal prophylactic data obtained by FINK (1974), PETERS et al. (1975a) and DAVIDSON et al. (1981)[a]. (All doses in mg/kg base or salt as indicated, administered once on DO, 2–4 h after sporozoite inoculation.)

| Compound | *P. yoelii yoelii* 17X (NMRI mice) $CPD_{50}$ (i)[b] (95% limits) | *P. yoelii nigeriensis* N67 (CFW mice) MFAD (ii)[c] | *P. yoelii yoelii* 17X (ICR/HA mice) $ED_{50}$ (iii)[d] |
|---|---|---|---|
| Chloroquine | Inactive at MTD | Inactive at MTD | Inactive at MTD |
| Quinine | Inactive at MTD | Inactive at MTD | Inactive at MTD |
| Mepacrine | Inactive at MTD | Inactive at MTD | Inactive at MTD |
| Primaquine | 6.6 (4.5–9.0) | 30–60 | 50 |
| Dapsone | 20 (13–32) | 3–10 | 40 |
| Sulphadiazine | 30 (15–60) | 30–60 | 160 |
| Sulfadoxine | 84 (60–118) | 3–10 | 40 |
| Proguanil | 1.6 (1.0–2.5) | 3–10 | 10 |
| Cycloguanil | 0.3 (0.2–0.4) | 1–2 | 5 |
| Pyrimethamine | 0.1 (0.07–0.14) | 0.3–1.0 | 1.25 |
| RC 12 | Inactive at MTD (200) | Slight activity at 300 | Inactive at 160 |
| Ni 147/36[e] | 4.0 (2.4–6.8) | 1–3 | NT[g] |
| Ba 138/111[e] | 23 (16–23) | 10–30 | NT[g] |
| Clindamycin | NT[g] | 10–30 | 40 |
| U-24779 A[f] | 2.0 (1.4–2.8) | 0.3–1 | NT[g] |

[a] Compounds published in DAVIDSON et al. (1981) while remaining compound data were supplied by AGER (unpublished)
[b] As base, i.p.
[c] As salt except pyrimethamine, dapsone and sulphonamides. s.c. except pyrimethamine, which is i.p.
[d] As salt except for pyrimethamine, dapsone and sulphonamides. All compound administered s.c.
[e] 6-aminoquinolines FINK (1974)
[f] U-24729 is *N*-demethyl-4′-pentyl-clindamycin
[g] Not tested

sporozoites of *P. yoelii yoelii* (17X strain) followed 2–3 h later by a single, intraperitoneal injection of test compound. Parasitaemias were followed until D+10 and if no parasites were observed the mouse was considered cured. Splenectomies were performed on some of these "cured" mice, to see if parasitaemia would ensue, but all were found to be negative. Livers were examined histologically for exoerythrocytic stages, but this proved too cumbersome a task and required excessive amounts of test compounds. To ensure that compounds were not giving false-positive results due to residual blood schizontocidal activity, blood-induced infections were started 48 h after administration of test compound to a group of mice. Mice remaining negative were considered to have been cured by residual blood schizontocidal action, whereas mice exhibiting parasitaemia were considered to have been given a compound with true causal prophylactic activity. Data on standard antimalarial compounds are shown in Table 11.

The line of *P. yoelii yoelii* (17X strain) used was avirulent in the NMRI mice since a parasitaemia greater than 10% was rarely observed and the infection was not normally fatal.

## VII. King's Test

KING et al. (1972), using *P. berghei* sporozoites in HA/ICR female mice, reported testing over 700 compounds for causal prophylactic activity. Fourteen days after an infective blood meal the mosquitoes were stunned by being placed in a freezer for 3 min, removed and then ground in a glass mortar with 10% inactivated rabbit serum in saline. This suspension was centrifuged for 5 min at 1,000 rpm. Each mouse was inoculated intraperitoneally with a 0.2-ml aliquot containing the sporozoites equivalent to three mosquitoes. Test compounds were administered subcutaneously at dose levels of 160, 40, and 10 mg/kg on D − 1, D0 and D + 1. Control mice, infected but not treated, did not die but attained a maximum parasitaemia on D + 14 followed by recovery. Blood films were taken from treated mice on days 6, 10, 14, 21, and 28 postinfection and parasitaemias were calculated. A compound was judged active if patency was not attained through 28 days.

To differentiate between causal prophylactic and residual blood schizontocidal activity mice were infected and treated with the lowest active dose in the initial test. Seventy-two hours later the mice were bled and their livers removed. Blood samples were pooled and subinoculated into clean recipient mice, using the same procedure for the liver samples. The rationale for this subinoculation of blood and liver homogenates resides in the understanding that true causal prophylactic compounds will kill all exoerythrocytic stages, resulting in an absence of merozoites in the pooled blood and liver samples. Thus the recipient mice will not develop parasitaemia while the mice receiving subinoculations from mice treated with active blood schizontocidal compounds will become patent.

Four compounds were reported to be causal prophylactics (cycloguanil pamoate, dapsone, pyrimethamine, and primaquine) while cholorquine and mepacrine were shown to be active only as blood schizontocidal agents.

The major flaw in this system concerns delaying the subinoculations for 72 h after sporozoite infection. Since the test compound is administered on D − 1, D0, and D + 1 it could easily be retained by the mouse until blood stage parasites develop. Any residual blood schizontocidal compound would have at least 30 h in which to kill the merozoites emerging from the exoerythrocytic stages, as well as subsequently developed blood parasites.

## VIII. Rane and Kinnamon's Test

RANE and KINNAMON (1979) described a procedure for assessing prophylactic antimalarial activity in mice inoculated with sporozoites 4 h after the experimental test compounds were injected. Activity was monitored by survival for a 30-day period. *P. yoelii yoelii* (17X strain) sporozoites were grown in *A. stephensi* mosquitoes. All compounds were suspended in peanut oil. Primaquine (100 mg/kg or 50 mg/kg) utilised as a positive control allowed mice to survive for a 30-day period. Infected, untreated control mice survived for approximately 9.7 days (range 6–13 days).

Thirty-five compounds were tested and the results were compared with a mouse system (GREGORY and PETERS 1970; PETERS et al. 1975a) and a monkey system (SCHMIDT et al. 1966; WHO 1971). Four compounds gave a false positive result in comparison to the mouse screen of GREGORY and PETERS (1970) and PETERS et al. (1975a). Six compounds were false positive when compared with the monkey screen of SCHMIDT et al. (1966) and WHO (1971). These false-positive results were due to their having persistent blood schizontocidal activity, while being devoid of tissue schizontocidal action.

This procedure has since been standardised by DAVIDSON et al. (1981) and utilised in testing over 4,000 compounds. Sporozoites are collected from female mosquitoes ground with a mortar and pestle in a 1 : 1 mixture of mouse plasma and saline. The suspension is filtered and sporozoites are quantitated so that each mouse receives approximately $2.5 \times 10^5$ in a 0.2-ml aliquot.

All experimental compounds are suspended in 0.5% hydroxyethylcellulose-0.1% Tween-80 and ground with a mortar and pestle. The initial dilutions used were 160, 40, and 10 mg/kg administered subcutaneously and, if active, lower dilutions were tested until an end point was reached. Active compounds were also tested orally. No correction for salt was made since most compounds were tested blindly. For each test, three control groups were used. The first group was injected only with sporozoites and served as a negative control group. These mice commenced dying 7 days later and were usually all dead within 1 week (majority dead on days 8 and 9). Another control group received 125 mg/kg of 4-methylprimaquine and served as a positive control. The third control group received 100 mg/kg chloroquine and served as an additional negative control. A test compound was considered active if at least two of five mice (at the highest non-toxic dose) survived a 30-day period.

The results of tests on some miscellaneous compounds are depicted in Table 5 while the antimalarial activity of some 8-aminoquinolines is shown in Table 6. The major limitation of this test is that it does not separate residual blood schizontocidal activity from true causal prophylactic action. It is a good primary screen and active compounds need to be checked in a secondary screen such as that of PETERS et al. (1975a) or HILL (1975). Only the pyrocatechol RC-12, and a series of compounds (5-phenoxy-8-aminoquinolines) were not active in rodent causal prophylactic systems but exhibited secondary tissue schizontocidal activity against *Plasmodium cynomolgi* in rhesus monkeys DAVIDSON et al. (1981).

## D. Residual Blood Schizontocides

### I. Schneider's Test

The ideal antimalarial compound is one which would retain its suppressive activity for 6 months or longer. Several systems to screen compounds for long-lasting (residual, or repository) activity have been reported, e.g. by SCHNEIDER et al. (1965) and BENAZET (1967).

SCHNEIDER et al. (1965) administered one oral dose of test compound to three groups of mice which were infected 7, 14, and 28 days respectively after treatment. Blood films were taken daily for 3 weeks in all mice starting on the 3rd day after inoculation of blood parasites. Mice, parasite free on D+7 and D+21, were bled and 0.2 ml of whole blood was injected into two clean recipient mice. Blood films of these recipients were examined two to three times a week for 2 weeks. Mice were judged cured if parasitaemia did not appear in these recipient mice. Several bis-4-aminoquinolines were shown to possess repository activity. BENAZET (1967) modified this procedure by infecting mice intraperitoneally, then administering test compounds on D0, D+1, D+2, and D+3. Blood films were taken on D+4 through D+21. Activity was measured in terms of a dose ($ED_{50}$) that kept 50% of the mice clear of parasites for 3 weeks.

## II. Thompson's Test

One test system, used by THOMPSON et al. (1963) to test cycloguanil pamoate, and THOMPSON et al. (1965) to test 4′, 4-diacetylaminodiphenylsulphone (DADDS) involved administering the test compound at one or more levels, suspended in a special vehicle, to several groups of mice, then challenging intraperitoneally with trophozoites a different group at monthly intervals. Blood films were made 7 and 14 days after challenge with trophozoites and parasitaemias were determined. All mice, (usually female to avoid fighting) were challenged only once to avoid any variables due to immunity. A dose level of the test compound was considered protective if challenged mice were parasitaemia negative at 7 and 14 days after inoculation of parasites.

Two different vehicles were used to suspend the test compound. The first was a lipid vehicle composed of 40% benzyl benzoate and 60% castor oil, while the second vehicle was aqueous and comprised 1.5% pectin with 0.1% Tween-60 in water. Test compounds were usually given in 5-ml amounts subcutaneously in the axillary region as a single injection. The results of one experiment using DADDS are shown in Table 12. Cycloguanil pamoate was the best repository compound found by THOMPSON et al. (1963) and it retained activity in the mouse system for 9 weeks at 660 mg/kg injected subcutaneously. ELSLAGER (1969) reviewed repository antimalarial drugs and gave data on a series of promising pyrimethamine salts. The experimental procedures used in this review are primarily that of THOMPSON et al. (1963). Several criteria were used in judging a repository compound. (a) It must be active enough to allow the release of an effective drug concentration over extended periods in a single dose regimen. (b) It must be absorbed slowly from the injection site or other localised depot. (c) The compound should be selectively toxic to the parasite and not the host cells or tissues. (d) The compound or its metabolic byproducts should not produce a cumulative effect within the body but, rather, should be excreted at a uniform rate. (e) An active respository compound should be able to eliminate all the asexual blood parasites from a challenge infection of asexual blood stages.

To test for curative effects of a compound three procedures are recommended (THOMPSON et al. 1970 and GARZA and BOX 1961). First, mice must be blood film negative for several weeks after challenge with asexual blood stages. Secondly, blood (about 0.2 ml) should be removed (via the ocular route) from challenged mice and subinoculated into clean recipient mice (do not pool samples). Blood films made on these recipients should remain parasite free. The third procedure involves taking the original mice soon after blood has been removed for subinocu-

**Table 12.** Repository effects of DADDS in mice against subsequent challenge with *P. berghei*. (THOMPSON et al. 1965)

| Dose (mg/kg) | Vehicle[a] | Weeks after dose 1 | 2 | 4 | 6 | 7 | 8 | 10 | 12 | 13 | 14 |
|---|---|---|---|---|---|---|---|---|---|---|---|
| Treated: Positive/total and (mean % suppression of parasitaemia) | | | | | | | | | | | |
| 400 | 1 | 0/10(100) | 0/5 (100) | 0/10(100) | 1/15(99) | 0/9(100) | 0/9 (100) | 2/10 (94) | 1/10 (94) | 3/5(63) | 0/10(100) |
| 200 | 1 | 3/10 (99) | 2/10 (99) | 1/10 (99) | 1/10(91) | | 2/10 (99) | 0/5 (100) | | | |
| 100 | 1 | 4/10 (98) | 10/10 (91) | 10/10 (96) | 5/5 (98) | | | | | | |
| 50 | 1 | 4/5 (46) | | | | | | | | | |
| 50 | 2 | 5/5 (7) | | | | | | | | | |
| Controls: Positive/total and (mean % cells parasitised) | | | | | | | | | | | |
| 0 | 1 | 12/12(39) | 2/2(64) | 7/7(48) | 9/9(41) | 5/5(44) | 8/8(46) | 6/6(62) | 5/5(39) | 5/5(49) | 3/3(48) |
| 0 | 2 | 5/5 (28) | | | | | | | | | |

[a] 1, 40% benzylbenzoate and 60% castor oil; 2, 1.5% pectin, 0.1% Tween 60 and water

**Table 13.** Cure of *P. berghei* in mice by different regimens of oral treatment with a fixed total oral dose of CI-679 acetate [a]

| Treatment (mg/kg and regimen) | No. of mice remaining negative after treatment | Data on surviving mice | | | | No. mice judged cured |
|---|---|---|---|---|---|---|
| | | Mouse No. | Blood film results | Sub-inoculation results | Rechallenge results (% cells infected) | |
| 100×1 | 0 | 3 | + | + | 0.2 | 0 |
| | | 9 | + | + | 0.3 | |
| 50×2×1 | 4 | 1 | − | − | 30.0 | 4 |
| | | 3 | − | − | [b] | |
| | | 4 | − | − | 31.0 | |
| | | 6 | − | − | [b] | |
| 25×2×2 | 4 | 1 | − | − | [b] | 4 |
| | | 3 | + | + | 0 | |
| | | 4 | + | + | 0.01 | |
| | | 6 | − | − | 18.0 | |
| | | 8 | − | − | 22.5 | |
| | | 10 | − | − | [b] | |
| 12.5×2×4 | 10 | 1 | − | − | 13.0 | 10 |
| | | 2 | − | − | 22.0 | |
| | | 3 | − | − | [b] | |
| | | 4 | − | − | 11.0 | |
| | | 5 | − | − | 19.0 | |
| | | 6 | − | [c] | 30.0 | |
| | | 7 | − | [c] | 15.0 | |
| | | 8 | − | [c] | 12.0 | |
| | | 9 | − | [c] | 27.5 | |
| | | 10 | − | [c] | 12.0 | |
| Rechallenge controls | | 1 | | | 41.5 | |
| | | 2 | | | 61.0 | |
| | | 3 | | | 52.5 | |
| | | 4 | | | 54.0 | |
| | | 5 | | | 49.5 | |
| | | 6 | | | 42.0 | |
| | | 7 | | | 43.0 | |
| | | 8 | | | 66.0 | |
| | | 9 | | | 79.0 | |
| | | 10 | | | 42.5 | |

[a] Groups of ten mice
[b] Not determined due to death from bleeding for subinoculation
[c] Not done

lation, and rechallenging them with asexual blood parasites. If they are cured there should be no immunity and they should be susceptible to reinfection. Therefore upon rechallenge, these original mice should develop parasitaemia if they had been cured. Experimental data using these procedures on a triaminoquinazoline (CI-679) were reported by THOMPSON et al. (1970) and are shown in Table 13.

## III. Sustained Release Implant Test

The practical advantages of sustained release antimalarials for field use that led THOMPSON et al. (1963) to develop cycloguanil pamoate were, unfortunately, not realised with their product for a variety of reasons. Nevertheless the basic principle was still attractive (see Part II, Chap. 7) and other approaches remained. HOWELLS and JUDGE (1981) attempted to prolong the activity of several compounds either by packing them into very small silicone rubber tubes, or incorporating them into a silicone rubber mix prior to vulcanisation. The silicone rubber (polydimethylsiloxane) tubes or pellets were implanted subcutaneously into groups of mice which were challenged after various intervals with $10^7$ erythrocytes infected with *P. berghei* N strain. These workers were unable to prolong significantly the blood schizontocidal effects of primaquine, chloroquine, cycloguanil, sulphadiazine, the dihydrotriazines WR 99209 or 99210, menoctone or mefloquine by implanting them in silicone rubber tubes. However, pyrimethamine base remained active for 3 months in tubular implants and for 5–6 months when incorporated into the polymethylsiloxane matrix.

The availability of biodegradable polymers led JUDGE et al. (1981) to study the duration of activity of several compounds when incorporated into a dihydropyran-based polymer. The detailed technique by which cycloguanil hydrochloride, pyrimethamine base and sulphadiazine were incorporated into the polymer to yield small pellets suitable for subcutaneous implantation into mice should be read in the original paper. It is important to note that the first two compounds interfered with the polymerisation process, which subsequently required modification. The polymers containing 10% cycloguanil HCl, 10%, 20% or 30% pyrimethamine, or 10%, 20% or 30% sulphadiazine were prepared as thin films from which round discs 7 mm in diameter were cut with a cork borer or were cryogenically milled,

**Table 14.** The protective action of 20% dihydropyran polymer implants against *P. berghei* N strain challenge in mice. (Adapted from JUDGE et al. 1981)[a]

| Group | Mean implant weight (mg) | Days challenged postimplantation | Day implant removed/reinfected | No. of mice infected[b] |
|---|---|---|---|---|
| Pyrimethamine | | | | |
| 1 | 47 | D+0, 84, 179, 252 | D+279/294 | 0/3 |
| 2 | 49 | D+28, 112, 206 | D+279/294 | 2/3 |
| 3 | 48 | D+56, 140, 224 | D+279/294 | 2/2 |
| Sulphadiazine | | | | |
| 1 | 42 | D+7, 84, 192 | D+275/289 | 4/4 |
| 2 | 44 | D+28, 126, 220 | D+275/289 | 1/2 |
| 3 | 43 | D+56, 165, 248 | D+275/289 | 3/3 |

[a] Polymers prepared by coprecipitation technique
[b] Blood films remained negative up to 294 days in the pyrimethamine and 289 days in the sulphadiazine groups. Rechallenge after removal of the implants was followed by parasitaemia in four out of eight of the pyrimethamine- and eight out of nine of the sulphadiazine-treated animals

then compressed into small, implantable pellets of about the same diameter. Both types or preparation were well tolerated. A preliminary study using a mixture of powdered polymer containing both pyrimethamine and sulphadiazine showed that suspended powders were of little value in prolonging the action of these drugs.

Mice with cycloguanil HCl disc implants were only protected for up to 14 days against challenge with *P. berghei* N strain. When pyrimethamine pellets were prepared by a coprecipitation technique they protected mice against multiple challenge with this parasite for at least 279 days. That this effect was not due to an immunising effect of repeated challenge was proven when the same animals became parasitaemic within 14 days of surgically excising the residual pellets. Similarly, sulphadiazine pellets produced by the same process protected mice for at least 275 days. The total amount of each drug was approximately 8–10 mg/mouse as a 20% implant weighing about 45 mg each (Table 14).

## E. Residual Tissue Schizontocides

A test system to evaluate compounds for residual antimalarial activity in mice inoculated with sporozoites was developed by SCHOFIELD et al. (1981) and has been operating for 1 year at the Rane Laboratory, Miami, Florida (unpublished). This system tests for either residual causal prophylactic or residual blood schizontocidal activity in mice injected with sporozoites. The experimental test design is divided into three phases. In the first phase compounds are tested for residual activity for a 3-day period when administered both orally and subcutaneously to the same mice. In the second phase all compounds exhibiting residual activity for 3 days are tested for 7, 14 or 21 days duration when administered both orally and subcutaneously to each mouse. In the third and final phase, compounds lasting 21 days are administered orally to one group of mice and subcutaneously to another, and challenged with parasites 21 days later. The following account incorporates several minor changes in technique as used in our own laboratory.

Phase I: In this phase mice are treated orally and subcutaneously with 80 mg/kg of the test compound on DO. This means each mouse receives a total dosage of 160 mg/kg. As all compounds are tested blindly, no per cent free base figures are calculated. Three days later (D+3) the mice are inoculated intraperitoneally with approximately $2.5 \times 10^5$ sporozoites of *P. yoelii yoelii* 17X. Blood films are taken on D+9 and the parasitaemias calculated. Mortality data are collected for all mice until D+16. Any mice alive on D+16 have blood films taken and parasitaemias determined.

Each experiment includes one control group (negative control) which receives 0.2 ml of 0.5% hydroxyethylcellulose-0.1% Tween-80 orally and subcutaneously. A positive control group also included in each experiment receives cycloguanil pamoate at 80 mg/kg orally and subcutaneously.

The parasitaemia of mice on D+9 and D+16 is estimated from Giemsa-stained blood films and scored 0 through + + + + +. The following system is used in scoring parasitaemias (using a microscope with a $\times$ 100 objective and $\times$ 10 eyepiece).

| | |
|---|---|
| 0 | = negative (no parasites in ten fields) |
| + | = very scanty ($\leqq$ five parasitised cells in ten fields) |
| ++ | = scanty ($\leqq$ five parasitised cells in one field) |
| +++ | = moderate ($\leqq$ 20% parasitaemia) |
| ++++ | = heavy ($\leqq$ 50% parasitaemia) |
| +++++ | = very heavy (> 50% parasitaemia) |

Phase II: Each compound is administered both orally (80 mg/kg) and subcutaneously (80 mg/kg) to mice in three groups. The first group of mice receives the compound on DO, the second group on D+7 and the third group on D+14. Each mouse receives a total of 160 mg/kg of the test compound.

The control groups are treated also on DO, D+7, and D+14, one with only HEC-Tween-80 (termed the negative control group) and the second with 80 mg/kg of WR 228258 (an amodiaquine analogue) both orally and subcutaneously (termed the positive control group).

On D+21 all mice are inoculated intraperitoneally with $2.5 \times 10^5$ sporozoites. Blood films are taken on D+27 and D+34 and parasitaemias scored 0 through +++++ as described in phase I. Each day mortalities are recorded.

Phase III: Two groups of mice are required for the testing of each compound. One group receives 80 mg/kg of the compound orally while the other group receives 80 mg/kg of the compound subcutaneously on DO. Four control groups are used for each day challenged: (a) one negative control group receives only HEC-Tween-80 orally, (b) the second negative control group receives only HEC-Tween-80 subcutaneously and (c, d) the third and fourth controls are positive controls, one receiving 80 mg/kg of WR 228258 subcutaneously and the other 80 mg/kg of WR 228258 orally.

On D+21 all mice are inoculated with $2.5 \times 10^5$ sporozoites intraperitoneally. Blood films are taken on D+27 and D+34 and parasitaemias are scored 0 through +++++ as described in phase I. Mortalities of all mice are recorded daily until D+34.

The negative control mice receiving only HEC-Tween-80 before the inoculation of sporozoites normally commence dying 7 days after sporozoite injection. By day 14, after receiving sporozoites, the majority of mice in this group will be dead and any remaining will exhibit very heavy parasitaemia ($\simeq$50% parasitaemia).

The positive control group (receiving cycloguanil pamoate) from phase I is blood film negative on D+9 and D+16. In phase II the positive control (receiving WR 228258) is usually completely suppressive for blood films taken on D+27 and D+34. For phase III WR 228258 is active at 80 mg/kg subcutaneously (blood films negative on D+27 and D+34). However, it does not retain oral residual activity for 21 days.

The following compounds were inactive in phase I: chloroquine phosphate, quinine sulphate, mepacrine hydrochloride, dapsone, sulphadiazine, tetracycline and primaquine phosphate. Several compounds exhibiting residual activity are shown in Table 15. This test system does not differentiate between residual causal prophylactic and residual blood schizontocidal activity. These two residual activities should be separated using the method of PETERS et al. (1975a) or HILL (1975).

**Table 15.** Compounds exhibiting residual activity against sporozoite-induced infections

| Compound WR No. | Structure | Days sporozoite inoculation after administration of test compound | | | No. mice out of 5 patents days after sporozoite inoculation | |
|---|---|---|---|---|---|---|
| | | Phase I | Phase II | Phase III | 6 | 13 |
| 5473 | 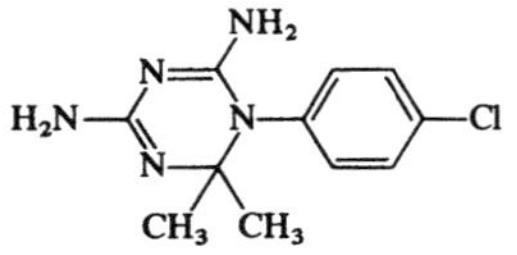 Pamoate salt | 3 | | 0 | 0 | 0 |
| | | | 7 | 1 | 1 | 1 |
| | | | 14 | 3 | 3 | 3 |
| | | | 21 | 5 | 5 | 5 |
| 181023 | 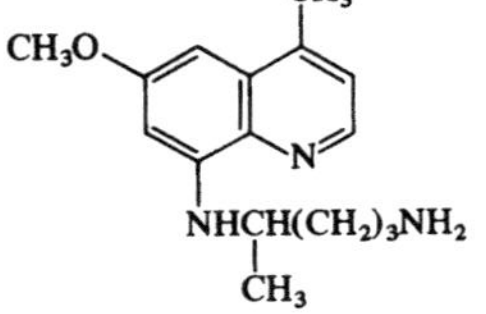 $\bullet 2H_3PO_4$ | 3 | | | 0 | 0 |
| | | | 7 | | 5 | 5 |
| | | | 14 | | 5 | 5 |
| | | | 21 | | 5 | 5 |
| 244160 | 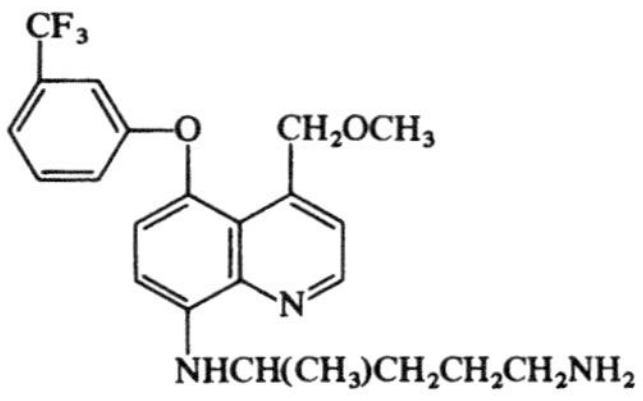 $\bullet 2H_3PO_4$ $\bullet C_2H_5OH$ $\bullet H_2O$ | 3 | | | 0 | 0 |
| | | | 7 | | 0 | 0 |
| | | | 14 | | 0 | 0 |
| | | | 21 | | 4 | 4 |

| | | | | | | |
|---|---|---|---|---|---|---|
| 171699 | 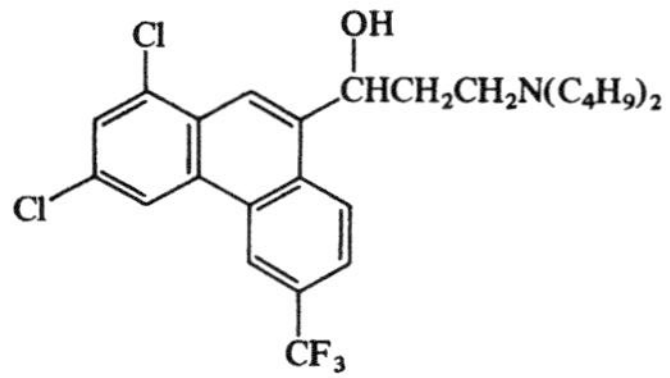 | 3 | 7 | | 0 | 0 |
| | | | 14 | | 0 | 0 |
| | | | 21 | | 0 | 1 |
| | | | | | 5 | 5 |
| 235693 | 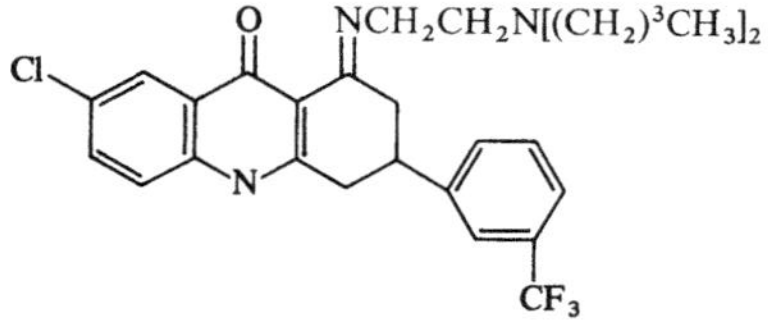 | 3 | | | 0 | 0 |
| | | 3 | 7 | | 0 | 2 |
| | | | 14 | | 3 | 3 |
| | | | 21 | | 5 | 5 |
| 159680 | 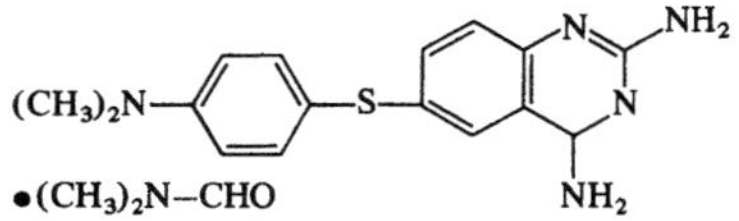 | 3 | | | 0 | 0 |
| | | | 7 | | 0 | 0 |
| | | | 14 | | 0 | 0 |
| | | | 21 | | 0 | 0 |
| | | | | 21 s.c. | 0 | 0 |
| | | | | 21 p.o. | 5 | 5 |
| 228258 | 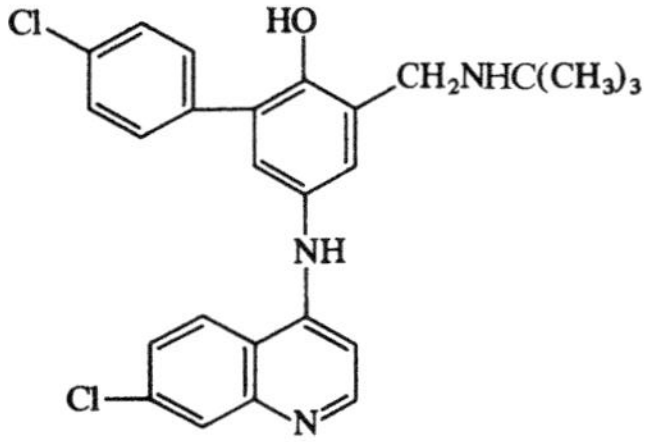 | 3 | | | 0 | 0 |
| | | | 7 | | 0 | 0 |
| | | | 14 | | 0 | 0 |
| | | | 21 | | 0 | 0 |
| | | | | 21 s.c. | 0 | 0 |
| | | | | 21 p.o. | 5 | 5 |

## References

Aviado D (1967) Pathologic physiology and chemotherapy of *Plasmodium berghei* I. Suppression of parasitemia by sulfones and sulfonamides in mice. Exp Parasitol 20:88–97

Aviado D (1969) Chemotherapy of *Plasmodium berghei*. Exp Parasitol 25:399–482

Bafort J (1971) The biology of rodent malaria with particular reference to *Plasmodium vinckei vinckei*. Ann Soc Belge Med Trop 51:1–204

Benazet F (1967) Activité d'un nouvel antimalarique, le 16.126 R.P. sur le paludisme expérimental des animaux de laboratoire. Bull Soc Pathol Exot 60:221–228

Berberian DA, Slighter RG, Freele HW (1968) Causal prophylactic effect of menoctone (a new hydroxynaphthoquinone) against sporozoite-induced *Plasmodium berghei* infection in mice. J Parasitol 54:1181–1189

Box E, Gingrich W, Celaya B (1954) Standardization of a curative test with *Plasmodium berghei* in white mice. J Infect Dis 94:78–83

Büngener W (1979a) Malariaplasmodien in der Maus Befall von reifen und unreifen Erythrozyten durch *Plasmodium berghei*, *Plasmodium yoelii* und *Plasmodium chabaudi*. Tropenmed Parasitol 29:198–205

Büngener W (1979b) Weitere Beobachtungen über den Verlauf der *Plasmodium berghei*-Infektion in der Maus. Tropenmed Parasitol 30:24–34

Carter R, Diggs C (1977) Plasmodia of rodents. In: Kreier J (ed) Parasitic protozoa, vol III. Academic, New York, pp 359–449

Carter R, Gwadz R (1980) Infectiousness and gamete immunization in malaria. In: Kreier J (ed) Malaria, vol III. Academic, New York, pp 263–293

Cox F (1978) Concomitant infections. In: Killick-Kendrick R, Peters W (eds) Rodent malaria. Academic, New York, pp 309–337

Darrow E, Gingrith W, Prine J (1952) The effect of antibiotics on experimental malaria (*Plasmodium cathemerium* and *Plasmodium berghei*). Am J Trop Med Hyg 1:927–931

Davidson D, Ager A, Brown J, Chapple F, Whitmire R, Rossan R (1981) Recent developments of tissue schizonticidal antimalarial drugs. Bull WHO 59:463–479

Elslager E (1969) Progress in malaria chemotherapy Part I. Repository antimalarial drugs. In: Jucker E (ed) Progress in drug research, vol XIII. Birkhäuser, Basel, pp 171–216

Elslager E (1974) New perspectives on chemotherapy of malaria, filariasis, and leprosy. In: Jucker E (ed) Progress in drug research, vol XVIII. Birkhäuser, Basel, pp 99–172

Eugi E, Allison A (1979) Malaria infections in different strains of mice and their correlation with natural killer activity. Bull WHO 57:231–238

Fink E (1972) Kausalprophylaktische Wirkung von Standard-Malariamitteln bei der Nagetiermalaria (*Plasmodium berghei yoelii*). Z Tropenmed Parasitol 23:35–47

Fink E (1974) Assessment of causal prophylactic activity in *Plasmodium berghei yoelii* and its value for the development of new antimalarial drugs. Bull WHO 50:213–222

Fink E, Kretschmar W (1970) Chemotherapeutische Wirkung von Standard-Malariamitteln in einem vereinfachten Prüfverfahren in der *Plasmodium vinckei*-Infektion der NMRI-Maus. Z Tropenmed Parasitol 21:167–181

Foster W (1980) Colonization and maintenance of mosquitoes in the laboratory. In: Kreier J (ed) Malaria, vol II. Academic, New York, pp 103–144

Garza BL, Box ED (1961) Evaluation of test of cure procedures in mice treated for *Plasmodium berghei* infections. Am J Trop Med Hyg 10:804–811

Goodwin L (1949) Response of *Plasmodium berghei* to antimalarial drugs. Nature 164:1133

Gothe R, Kreier J (1977) *Aegyptianella*, *Eperythrozoon*, and *Haemobartonella*. In: Kreier J (ed) Parasitic protozoa, vol IV. Academic, New York, pp 263–287

Greenberg J, Kendrick L (1958) Parasitemia and survival in mice infected with *Plasmodium berghei*. Hybrids between Swiss (high parasitemia) and Str (low parasitemia) in mice. J Parasitol 44:492–498

Greenberg J, Nadal E, Coatney G (1953) The influence of strain, sex, and age of mice on infection with *Plasmodium berghei*. J Infect Dis 93:96–100

Gregory KG, Peters W (1970) The chemotherapy of rodent malaria, IX Causal prophylaxis, part I: A method for demonstrating drug action on exoerythrocytic stages. Ann Trop Med Parasitol 64:15–24

Hanson WL, Thompson PE (1972) The relation of polychromatophilia to parasitemia and mortality in CF1 mice with drug-resistant and parent lines of *Plasmodium berghei*. Proc Helmintol Soc Wash 39:309–317

Hardgreaves BJ, Yoeli M, Nussenzweig RS (1975) Immunological studies in rodent malaria. I. Protective immunity induced in mice by mild strains of *Plasmodium berghei yoelii* against a virulent and fatal line of this plasmodium. Ann Trop Med Parasitol 69:289–299

Hill J (1950) The schizonticidal effect of some antimalarials against *Plasmodium berghei*. Ann Trop Parasitol 44:291–297

Hill J (1966a) Chemotherapy of malaria. Part 2: The antimalarial drugs. In: Schnitzer R, Hawking F (eds) Experimental chemotherapy, vol I. Academic, New York, pp 513–601

Hill J (1966b) Chemotherapy of malaria. Part 2: the antimalarial drugs. (Supplement to vol 1.) In: Schnitzer R, Hawking F (eds) Experimental chemotherapy, vol IV. Academic, New York, pp 448–462

Hill J (1975) The activity of antibiotics and long-acting compounds against the tissue stages of *Plasmodium berghei*. Ann Trop Med Parasitol 69:421–427

Howells R, Judge R (1981) Sustained-release implants in the chemotherapy of experimental rodent malaria I. A comparison of the effects of some antimalarials in polydimethylsiloxane matrices. Ann Trop Med Parasitol 75:495–510

Hsu D, Geiman Q (1952) Synergistic effect of *Haemobartonella muris* on *Plasmodium berghei* in white rats. Am J Trop Med Hyg 1:747–760

Jacobs RL (1964) Role of *p*-aminobenzoic acid in *Plasmodium berghei*. Infection in the mouse. Exp Parasitol 15:213–225

Jacobs RL, Alling DW, Cantrell WF (1963) An evaluation of antimalarial combinations against *Plasmodium berghei* in the mouse. J Parasitol 49:920–925

Judge B, Howells R, Graham N, McNeill M (1981) Sustained-release implants in the chemotherapy of experimental rodent malaria II. The effects of sulphadiazine, pyrimethamine, and cycloguanil in biodegradable polymer matrices. Ann Trop Med Parasitol 75:511–519

Killick-Kendrick R (1973) Parasitic protozoa of the blood of rodents. The life cycle and zoogeography of *Plasmodium berghei nigeriensis* subsp. nov. Ann Trop Med Parasitol 67:261–277

Killick-Kendrick R (1978) Taxonomy, zoogeography, and evolution. In: Killick-Kendrick R, Peters W (eds) Rodent malaria. Academic, New York, pp 1–48

King ME, Shefner AM, Schneider MD (1972) Utilization of a sporozoite induced rodent malaria system for assessment of drug activity. Proc Helminthol Soc Wash 39:288–291

Knowles G, Walliker D (1980) Variable expression of virulence in the rodent malaria parasite *Plasmodium yoelii yoelii*. Parasitology 81:211–219

Landau I, Boulard Y (1978) Life cycles and morphology. In: Killick-Kendrick R, Peters W (eds) Rodent malaria. Academic, New York, pp 53–82

Landau I, Killick-Kendrick R (1966) Note préliminaire sur le cycle évolutif des deux *Plasmodium* du rongeur *Thamnomys rutilans* en République Centrafricaine. C R Acad Sci [D](Paris) 268:873–875

Landau I, Miltgen F, Boulard Y, Chabaud A, Baccam D (1979) Etudes sur les gamétocytes des *Plasmodium* du groupe "vivax": morphologie, évolution prise par les *Anophelles* et infectivité des microgametocytes de *Plasmodium yoelii*. Ann Parasitol Hum Comp 54:145–161

Merkli B, Richle R, Peters W (1980) The inhibitory effect of a drug combination on the development of mefloquine resistance in *Plasmodium berghei*. Ann Trop Med Parasitol 74:1–9

Most H, Montuori W (1975) Rodent systems (*Plasmodium berghei-Anopheles stephensi*) for screening compounds for potential causal prophylaxis. Am J Trop Med Hyg 24:179–182

Most H, Nussenzweig R, Vanderberg J, Herman R, Yoeli M (1966) Susceptibility of genetically standardized (JAX) mouse strains to sporozoite- and blood-induced *Plasmodium berghei* infections. Milit Med 131:915–918

Most H, Herman R, Schoenfeld C (1967) Chemotherapy of sporozoite and blood-induced *Plasmodium berghei* infections with selected antimalarial agents. Am J Trop Med Hyg 16:572–575

Osdene TS, Russell PB, Rane L (1967) 2,4,7-Triamino-6-ortho-substituted arylpteridines. A new series of potent antimalarial agents. J Med Chem 10:431–434

Ott KJ (1968) Influence of reticulocytosis on the course of infection of *Plasmodium chabaudi* and *P. berghei*. J Protozool 15:365–369

Peters W (1965a) Competitive relationship between *Eperythrozoon coccoides* and *Plasmodium berghei* in the mouse. Exp Parasitol 16:158–166

Peters W (1965b) Drug resistance in *Plasmodium berghei* I. Chloroquine resistance. Exp Parasitol 17:80–89

Peters W (1970) Techniques for the study of drug response in experimental malaria. Chemotherapy and drug resistance in malaria. Academic, New York, pp 64–136

Peters W (1974) Recent advances in antimalarial chemotherapy and drug resistance. Adv Parasitol 13:69–114

Peters W (1980) Chemotherapy of malaria. In: Kreier J (ed) Malaria, vol I. Academic, New York, pp 145–283

Peters W, Howells R (1978) Chemotherapy. In: Killick-Kendrick R, Peters W (eds) Rodent malaria. Academic, New York, pp 345–384

Peters W, Ramkaran AE (1980) The chemotherapy of rodent malaria, XXXII. The influence of *p*-aminobenzoic acid on the transmission of *Plasmodium yoelii* and *P. berghei* by *Anopheles stephensi*. Ann Trop Med Parasitol 74:275–282

Peters W, Davies EE, Robinson BL (1975a) The chemotherapy of rodent malaria, XXIII. Causal prophylaxis, part II: Practical experience with *Plasmodium yoelii nigeriensis* in drug screening. Ann Trop Med Parasitol 69:311–328

Peters W, Portus JH, Robinson BL (1975b) The chemotherapy of rodent malaria, XXII. The value of drug-resistant strains of *P. berhei* in screening for blood schizontocidal activity. Ann Trop Med Parasitol 69:155–171

Raether W, Fink E (1979) Antimalarial activity of Floxacrine (HOE 991) I. Studies on blood schizonticidal action of Floxacrine against *Plasmodium berghei, P. vinckei*, and *P. cynomolgi*. Ann Trop Med Parasitol 73:505–526

Ramakrishnan S, Prakash S, Krishnaswami A (1951) Studies on *Plasmodium berghei* III. Latency relapse and immunity in albino rats with blood-induced infections. Indian J Malariol 5:447–454

Rane DS, Kinnamon KE (1979) The development of a "high volume tissue schizonticidal drug screen" based upon mortality of mice inoculated with sporozoites of *Plasmodium berghei*. Am J Trop Med Hyg 28:937–947

Richards WHG (1966) Antimalarial activity of sulfonamides and a sulfone, singly and in combination with pyrimethamine, against drug resistant and normal strains of laboratory plasmodia. Nature 212:1494–1495

Richards WHG (1970) The combining action of pyrimidines and sulphonamides or sulphones in the chemotherapy of malaria and other protozoal infections. Adv Pharmacol Chemother 8:121–147

Rozman R, Canfield C (1979) New experimental antimalarial drugs. Adv Pharmacol Chemother 17:1–43

Schmidt L, Rossan R, Fradkin R, Woods J, Schulemann W, Kratz L (1966) Studies on the antimalarial activity of 1,2-dimethoxy-4-(bisdiethyl-aminoethyl)-amino-5-bromobenzene. Bull WHO 34:783–788

Schmidt LH (1973) Infections with *Plasmodium falciparum* and *Plasmodium vivax* in the owl monkey – model systems for basic biological and chemotherapeutic studies. Trans R Soc Trop Med Hyg 67:446–474

Schmidt LH, Alexander S, Allen L, Rasco J (1977) Comparison of the curative antimalarial activities and toxicities of primaquine and its *d* and *l* isomers. Antimicrob Agents Chemother 12:51–60

Schmidt LH, Crosby R, Rasco J, Vaughan D (1978) Antimalarial activities of various 4-quinolinemethanols with special attention to WR 142490 (Mefloquine). Antimicrob Agents Chemother 13:1011–1030

Schneider J, Decourt PH, Montézin G (1949) Sur l'utilisation d'un nouveau plasmodium (*Pl. berghei*) pour l'étude et la recherche de médicaments antipaludiques. Bull Soc Pathol Exot 42:449–452

Schneider J, Bouvry M, Quellec J (1965) *Plasmodium berghei* et chimiothérapie. Ann Soc Belge Med Trop 45:435–449

Schofield P, Howells RE, Peters W (1981) A technique for the selection of long-acting antimalarial compounds using a rodent malaria model. Ann Trop Med Parasitol 75:521–531

Steck E (1972) The chemotherapy of protozoan diseases, vol III. U.S. Government Printing Office, Washington DC

Strube R (1975) The search for new antimalarial drugs. J Trop Med Hyg 78:171–185

Thompson PE, Bayles A (1966) Eradication of *Eperythrozoon coccoides* with oxophenarsine in normal and drug-resistant lines of *Plasmodium berghei* in mice. J Parasitol 52:674–678

Thompson PE, Werbel L (1972) Evaluation of antimalarial activity. Antimalarial agents chemistry and pharmacology. Academic, New York, pp 47–60

Thompson PE, Olszewski BJ, Elslager EF, Worth DF (1963) Laboratory studies on 4,6-diamino-1-(*p*-chlorophenyl)-1,2-dihydro-2,2-dimethyl-*s*-triazine pamoate CI-501 as a repository antimalarial drug. Am J Trop Med Hyg 12:481–493

Thompson PE, Olszewski BJ, Waitz J (1965) Laboratory studies on the repository antimalarial activity of 4,4′-diacetylaminodiphenylsulphone, alone and mixed with cycloguanil pamoate (CI-501). Am J Trop Med Hyg 19:12–26

Thompson PE, Bayles A, Olszewski B (1969) PAM 1392 [2,4-diamino-6(3,4-dichlorobenzylamino)-quinazoline] as a chemotherapeutic agent: *Plasmodium berghei, P. cynomolgi, P. knowlesi,* and *Trypanosoma cruzi.* Exp Parasitol 25:32–49

Thompson PE, Bayles A, Olszewski B (1970) Antimalarial activity of 2,4-diamino-6[(3,4-dichlorobenzyl)-nitrol-amino] quinazoline (CI-679 base) and CI-679 acetate. Am J Trop Med Hyg 19:12–26

Thurston J (1950) The action of antimalarial drugs in mice infected with *Plasmodium berghei.* Br J Pharmacol Chemother 5:409–416

Thurston J (1953) The chemotherapy of *Plasmodium berghei* I. Resistance to drugs. Parasitology 43:246–252

Vanderberg J, Gwadz R (1980) The transmission by mosquitoes of plasmodia in the laboratory. In: Kreier J (ed) Malaria, vol II. Academic, New York, pp 154–218

Vanderberg J, Yoeli M (1965) Some physiological and metabolic problems related to maintenance of the *P. berghei* cycle in *Anopheles quadrimaculatus.* Ann Soc Belg Med Trop 45:419–426

Vanderberg J, Yoeli M (1966) Effects of temperature on sporogonic development of *Plasmodium berghei.* J Parasitol 52:559–564

Vincke IH (1970) The effects of pyrimethamine and sulphormethoxine on the preerythrocytic and sporogonous cycle of *Plasmodium berghei berghei.* Ann Soc Belge Med Trop 50:339–358

Vincke I, Lips M (1948) Un nouveau *Plasmodium* d'un rongeur sauvage du Congo, *Plasmodium berghei* n.sp. Ann Soc Belge Méd Trop 28:97–104

Warhurst D, Folwell R (1968) Measurement of the growth rate of the erythrocytic stages of *Plasmodium berghei* and comparisons of the potency of inocula after various treatments. Ann Trop Med Parasitol 62:349–360

Wéry M (1968) Studies on the sporogony of rodent malaria parasites. Ann Soc Belge Med Trop 48:1–137

WHO (1971) Report of procedures for screening potential antimalarial compounds held 26–29 October 1971. WHO/MAL 72:763

Yoeli M, Most H, Boné G (1964) *Plasmodium berghei:* cyclical transmission by experimentally infected *Anopheles quadrimaculatus*. Science 144:1580–1581

Yoeli M, Upmanis R, Vanderberg J, Most H (1966) Life cycle and patterns of development of *Plasmodium berghei* in normal and experimental hosts. Milit Med 131:900–914

CHAPTER 9

# Malaria Models in Simian Hosts

R. N. ROSSAN

## A. Introduction

Recognition by MOORE and LANIER (1961) and YOUNG and MOORE (1961) of *Plasmodium falciparum* strains resistant to chloroquine, coupled with the disease among United States service personnel caused by such resistant strains, required the finding of a small, readily obtainable animal susceptible to human plasmodia for the evaluation of candidate antimalarial drugs. At Gorgas Memorial Laboratory YOUNG et al. (1966) demonstrated that the Panamanian *Aotus trivirgatus* (owl monkey) would support development of *Plasmodium vivax* obtained from a human patient. A year later, GEIMAN and MEAGHER (1967) reported the successful adaptation of an East African strain of *P. falciparum* in *A. trivirgatus* of Colombian origin. The Colombian *A. trivirgatus* model, infected with strains of *P. falciparum* of diverse susceptibilities and/or resistance to chloroquine, pyrimethamine, and quinine, afforded the basis for intensive investigations. SCHMIDT (1969) recognised the value of the owl monkey model for evaluating new antimalarials.

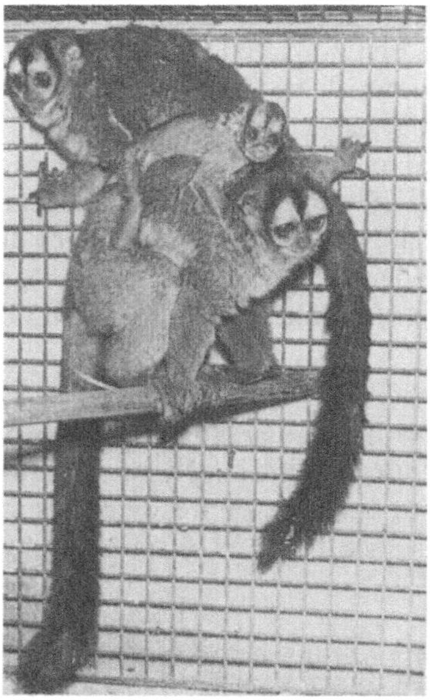

**Fig. 1.** The owl monkey or douroucouli (*Aotus trivirgatus*)

The spectrum of susceptibility of New World monkeys to human plasmodia has been the subject of various review articles by YOUNG (1970) and YOUNG et al. (1975, 1976). As will be discussed subsequently, only *A. trivirgatus* and, to a lesser extent, the squirrel monkey (*Saimiri sciureus*) have served as experimental hosts in drug evaluation studies. Prior to the establishment of the New World monkey model, the rhesus monkey, *Macaca mulatta,* infected with *P. cynomolgi* was most extensively used for chemotherapy trials. The literature through 1969, associated with such studies was reviewed by PETERS (1970) and only later studies will be discussed here. Details of techniques and of the course of infection in some simian hosts are provided in PETERS (1980).

## B. Use in Blood Schizontocide Studies

### I. Simian Plasmodia

#### 1. *Plasmodium cynomolgi*

For more than 30 years, trophozoite- and sporozoite-induced *P. cynomolgi* infection in the rhesus monkey (*Macaca mulatta*) has served as a model for evaluating potential antimalarial agents for use against *P. vivax* in man. While the utility of the simian malaria system has been overshadowed by the development of the *P. vivax – A. trivirgatus* model, some reports were published during the past 11 years using *P. cynomolgi.*

a) Quinazolines

Infections of the B strain of *P. cynomolgi* were used to evaluate 2,4-diamino-6-(3,4-dichlorobenzylamino) quinazoline (PAM 1392) by THOMPSON et al. (1969). Doses of 100.0 mg/kg for 5 days, or 50.0 mg/kg for 10 days cured such infections.

A second quinazoline, 2,4-diamino-6-[(3,4-dichloro-benzyl)nitrosamino] quinazoline (CI 679) was first evaluated by THOMPSON et al. (1970). The base form of the drug cured infections of the B strain of *P. cynomolgi* when administered orally twice daily for 5 days at a dose of 2.5 mg/kg. A single intramuscular dose of 10.0 mg/kg also proved to be curative. The acetate form of CI 679, at a total oral dose of 50.0 mg/kg cured infections in 14 of 15 rhesus monkeys. This curative capacity was observed at a single 50.0 mg/kg dose or at a dose as low as 3.125 mg/kg, twice daily, for 8 days. When administered in a repository form, both the base and acetate of CI 679 protected monkeys for at least 105 days against repeated trophozoite challenge.

SCHMIDT and ROSSAN (1979) further evaluated CI 679 against pyrimethamine sensitive (Ro) and pyrimethamine-resistant (Ro/PM) strains of *P. cynomolgi.* The total amount of drug required to cure infections of the Ro/PM strain was ten times the amount needed to cure the Ro strain, indicating cross-resistance with the pyrimethamine strain. Resistance to CI 679 became evident rapidly in both strains.

b) Antibiotics

The schizontocidal activity of three chlorinated lincomycin analogues against the B strain of *P. cynomolgi* was assessed by POWERS (1969). These analogues cured infections, but at doses of 50.0 and 100.0 mg/kg administered for 5 days and required 3–6 days for parasite clearance.

One of these agents, *N*-demethyl-4-pentyl-7-chlorolincomycin (U 24729A), was evaluated in a 7-day course of treatment by SCHMIDT et al. (1970) also against the B strain. Doses of U 24729A at 10.0 and 40.0 mg/kg cured infections, but the slow schizontocidal activity was again noted.

c) Pyrimidines

Trimethoprim, 2,4-diamino-5-(3′,-4′,5′-trimethoxybenzyl)-pyrimidine, was used by SCHMIDT et al. (1969) against two strains of *P. cynomolgi* – Ro (pyrimethamine susceptible) and Ro/PM (pyrimethamine resistant). Doses of 100.0 mg/kg cured infections of the Ro strain; two of three infections were cured at a dose of 50.0 mg/kg. In contrast, doses of up to 100.0 mg/kg had little or no activity against infections of the pyrimethamine-resistant strain. These data indicate a cross-resistance between the two folic acid antagonists –pyrimethamine and trimethoprim.

In the *P. cynomolgi*–rhesus system, SCHMIDT et al. (1977b) examined the synergism of pyrimethamine and sulphadiazine. Against a pyrimethamine-sensitive strain (Ro), the curative activity of pyrimethamine was increased 16–32 times by the concomitant administration of sulphadiazine at 1%–2% of the dose which would produce a 50% cure rate when administered alone. The activity of pyrimethamine against a pyrimethamine-resistant strain (Ro/PM) was increased at least 30 times when the compound was given in combination with 1.56 mg/kg of sulphadiazine (a non-curative dose).

d) Dihydroacridinedione

The evaluation of floxacrine (HOE 991) against the B strain of *P. cynomolgi* was published by RAETHER and FINK (1979). Cure was achieved by oral administration at doses of 15.0 and 20.0 mg/kg for 7 days, or intramuscular administration of doses of 1.25–7.5 mg/kg again for 7 days. However, drug resistance was readily induced. The prophylactic/radical curative capacity of this compound is discussed in the appropriate section of this review.

e) 9-Phenanthrenemethanol and Quinoline Methanol

DAVIDSON et al. (1976) have described their use of the *P. cynomolgi* – rhesus monkey model for evaluating antimalarial drugs. Data were presented for standard compounds and two experimental compounds. WR 33063, a phenanthrenemethanol, had a slightly suppressive activity at a dose of 100.0 mg/kg administered for 7 days. A quinolinemethanol, WR 30090, cured trophozoite-induced infections, but at high doses, 100.0 and 316 mg/kg for 7 days.

## 2. *Plasmodium knowlesi*

The *P. knowlesi* – rhesus system has been used to a lesser extent than the *P. cynomolgi* model for chemotherapy studies.

a) Pyrimidines

Trimethoprim, in addition to its evaluation against *P. cynomolgi* by SCHMIDT et al. (1969), was tested against *P. knowlesi* by ROTHE et al. (1969). The latter group showed that when trimethoprim was administered alone, doses of 50.0 mg/kg and lower only suppressed parasitaemias. The high sensitivity of *P. knowlesi* to sulphonamides was confirmed in that sulphalene (2-sulphanilamido-3-methoxypyrazine) cured infections in doses ranging from 50.0 to 0.5 mg/kg for 7 days. In combination, trimethoprim at a dose of 25.0 mg/kg with sulphalene at a dose of 0.5 mg/kg was curative, demonstrating a synergistic activity.

b) Quinazolines

THOMPSON et al. (1969) also used *P. knowlesi* to evaluate the quinazoline, PAM 1392. A dose of 100.0 mg/kg for 5 days cured the infection in two of three rhesus monkeys.

c) Antibiotics

POWERS et al. (1976) examined the activity of clindamycin (U 21) and its *N*-demethyl-4-pentyl analogue (U 24) against trophozoite-induced infections of *P. knowlesi* in rhesus monkeys. A single 100.0 mg/kg dose of U 21 cleared parasitaemias, but did not cure the infection. When U 21 or U 24 were administered twice daily for 5 days at a dose of 50.0 mg/kg, infections were cured; a dose of 10.0 mg/kg administered in this regimen was also curative. In contrast, a single daily 10.0 mg/kg dose of chloroquine administered for 3 days cured these infections. While both forms of the antibiotic were curative, parasite clearance was slower than with chloroquine.

## II. Human Plasmodia

### 1. *Plasmodium falciparum* and *P. vivax*

The establishment of human plasmodia in *A. trivirgatus* afforded an unique opportunity to evaluate the activity of experimental drugs directly against the parasites in a laboratory animal. Studies on the establishment in *A. trivirgatus* of diverse strains of *P. falciparum* and *P. vivax*, the courses of untreated infections, and the responses of these strains to chloroquine, pyrimethamine, and quinine have been detailed by SCHMIDT (1973, 1978a, b, 1979d), and drug susceptibilities are summarised in Table 1.

a) Pyrimidines

SCHMIDT et al. (1977b) assessed the activity of combined treatment with pyrimethamine and sulphadiazine against two pyrimethamine-resistant *P. falciparum* strains, Malayan Camp-CH/Q and Vietnam Smith. Both strains are maximally resistant to 2.5 mg pyrimethamine/kg per day. Administration of this dose of pyrimethamine with 5.0 mg/kg of sulphadiazine cured five of seven infections of the Malayan Camp strain and one of five infections of the Vietnam Smith strain. In no case did the cure rate approach 100%. The authors argue that this failure is due to extremely high resistance of both strains to pyrimethamine, and project that failures of combined therapy in human cases may be the result of such resistance.

When both pyrimethamine and sulphadiazine were administered against infections of the pyrimethamine-resistant Vietnam Palo Alto strain of *P. vivax*, the ac-

**Table 1.** Antimalarial susceptibility/resistance of eight strains of *P. falciparum* and two strains of *P. vivax* in *Aotus trivirgatus*. Adapted from SCHMIDT (1978 b)

| Strain | Response to | | |
|---|---|---|---|
| | Chloroquine | Pyrimethamine | Quinine |
| *P. falciparum* | | | |
| Cambodian I | S | RIII | S |
| Malayan IV | RII | RIII | S |
| Malayan Camp-CH/Q | S(R-I) | RIII | S |
| Malayan Camp-Sadun | S | RIII | S |
| Uganda Palo Alto | S | RIII | S |
| Vietnam Monterrey | RIII | RII | RII |
| Vietnam Oak Knoll | RIII | S | RIII |
| Vietnam Smith | RIII | RIII | RIII |
| *P. vivax* | | | |
| New Guinea Chesson | S | S | RI(S) |
| Vietnam Palo Alto | S | RII | S |

S, cured; RI, parasite clearance, with recrudescence; RII, only suppression of parasitaemia; RIII, no effect on parasitaemia or no more than marginal suppression. (S) and (RI) signify occasional response in group predominantly RI or S

tivity of the former compound was increased 16 times and that of the latter 64 times.

b) Quinazolines

WR 158122 [2,4-diamino-6-(2-naphthyl)-sulphonylquinazoline] and WR 159412 [2,4-diamino-6-(5-trifluoromethylphenyl)-thioquinazoline] were assessed against *P. falciparum* infections by SCHMIDT (1973, 1978 c, 1979 b). Cures of the pyrimethamine-susceptible Vietnam Oak Knoll strain were obtained with a low dose, 0.025 mg/kg for 7 days. Primary infections of the pyrimethamine-resistant Malayan Camp-CH/Q strain were cured also, although the dose required was at least 16 times that required for the Oak Knoll strain. Infections of the multiresistant Vietnam Smith strain were not uniformly cured at doses five to ten times those that consistently cured infections of the Malayan Camp-CH/Q strain. Thus, the activity of WR 158122 and WR 159412 proved to be inversely related to the level of pyrimethamine resistance exhibited by these three strains.

Additionally, subcurative treatment with WR 158122 and WR 159412 of the Malayan Camp and Oak Knoll strains rapidly produced strains highly resistant to these quinazolines. For example, quinazoline-resistant Oak Knoll strains could not be cured with a dose 500 times greater than that which cured the normal strain.

Cross-resistance between WR 158122 and pyrimethamine also occurred in *P. vivax* infections (SCHMIDT 1979 a). The calculated $CD_{90}$ for cures of the pyrimethamine-resistant Vietnam Palo Alto strain was about 15 times greater than that required for the pyrimethamine-sensitive New Guinea Chesson strain. Repeated treatments with WR 158122 of infections of the Vietnam Palo Alto strain resulted in resistance to the compound.

SCHMIDT (1973, 1979b) then examined the activities of WR 158122 and WR 159412, both dihydrofolic acid reductase inhibitors, when administered in combination with a *p*-aminobenzoic acid inhibitor, sulphadiazine. Such combination therapy did prevent emergence of *P. falciparum* parasites resistant to WR 158122 and WR 159412 and the activities of both compounds were increased, so that small doses of WR 158122 cured infections of the highly pyrimethamine-resistant Vietnam Smith strain and the Vietnam Palo Alto strain of *P. vivax*.

In addition to WR 158122 and WR 159412, five other 2,4-diamino-6-substituted quinazolines were tested by SCHMIDT (1979a) against infections of the chloroquine-resistant Vietnam Oak Knoll and pyrimethamine-resistant Malayan Camp-CH/Q strains of *P. falciparum*. Overall, these five compounds possessed less curative activity than WR 158122 and WR 159412.

### c) 4-Aminoquinolines

A group of seven 4-aminoquinolines was evaluated by SCHMIDT et al. (1977c) for antimalarial activity against chloroquine-susceptible and chloroquine-resistant strains of *P. falciparum*. The compounds were chloroquine, amodiaquine, amopyroquine, dichloroquinazine (12278 RP), SN 8137, SN 9584, and SN 10274. All of the compounds possessed similar activity against chloroquine-sensitive strains. As would be anticipated, the activities of amodiaquine, amopyroquine, and dichlorquinazine were less against the chloroquine-resistant strains; however, these compounds did cure, at well-tolerated doses, infections by such strains. Since the cross-resistance between certain 4-aminoquinolines and chloroquine-resistant falciparum strains in the *Aotus* model was limited, SCHMIDT et al. (1977c) cogently argued for the continued, targeted development of 4-aminoquinolines which could prove to be effective against chloroquine-resistant strains.

### d) Aminoalcohols

*α) 4-Quinolinemethanols.* The antimalarial assessment of some twelve 4-quinolinemethanols against chloroquine-sensitive and chloroquine-resistant *P. falciparum* strains and the Vietnam Palo Alto and New Guinea Chesson strains of *P. vivax* was reported by SCHMIDT (1973) and SCHMIDT et al. (1978a). One of these compounds, WR 142490 [α-(2-piperidyl)-2,8-(bis-trifluoromethyl)-4-quinolinemethanol hydrochloride] (subsequently named mefloquine), proved to be the most active of the 4-quinolinemethanols. The $CD_{90}$s to cure the pyrimethamine-resistant Malayan Camp-CH/Q strain and the chloroquine-resistant Vietnam Oak Knoll strain were identical (in 7-day administration, the $CD_{90}$ was a total of 14.0 mg/kg). To cure infections of the multiresistant Vietnam Smith strain, the $CD_{90}$ was a total of 28.0 mg/kg. Moreover it was shown that the curative activity of mefloquine is a function of the total amount of drug administered, either as a single dose, or the same total amount administered over a period of 3 or 7 days.

Mefloquine was highly active against vivax infections. The $CD_{90}$s, in a 7-day regimen, against the Palo Alto and Chesson strains of *P. vivax* were total doses of 8.0 and 14.0 mg/kg, respectively.

The activities of two other 4-quinolinemethanols were detailed by SCHMIDT et al. (1978d): WR 184086 [α-(*Tert*-butylaminoethyl)-2,8-bis-(trifluoromethyl)-4-quinolinemethanol] and WR 226253 [α-(2-piperidyl)-2-trifluoromethyl-6,8-dichloro-4-quinolinemethanol]. The total curative dose of WR 184806 required for infections of the Vietnam Smith strain was two to three times that required for the Vietnam Oak Knoll strain. WR 184804 was about one-third as active as mefloquine against the Vietnam Smith strain. WR 226253 was five to ten times more active than WR 184806 against the Vietnam Smith strain. Moreover, WR 226253 was twice as active as mefloquine against infections with this multiresistant drug strain. The curative activities of both WR 184806 and WR 226253 were shown to be a function of the total dose administered, whether delivered as a single dose, or three or seven daily doses.

The antimalarial activity of the above 4-quinolinemethanols was greater against infections of the Vietnam Palo Alto *P. vivax* strain than against both *P. falciparum* strains.

*β) 9-Phenanthrenemethanols.* A total of 17 compounds in this chemical class was assessed by SCHMIDT (1978b) and SCHMIDT et al. (1978b) against *P. falciparum* infections. WR 122455 proved to be the most active compound, with a $CD_{90}$ of 25.0 mg base/kg administered for 7 days against chloroquine-resistant and chloroquine-sensitive strains, as well as pyrimethamine-sensitive and pyrimethamine-resistant strains. Moreover, in comparison with chloroquine, WR 122455 was two to four times more active against chloroquine-susceptible falciparum strains. Cures were effected with single, 3-day, or 7-day doses, efficacy being related to the total dose administered.

A second, active compound in this class was WR 171669 (now also called halofantrine). While it was equally active against a chloroquine-resistant (Vietnam Oak Knoll) and a chloroquine-sensitive strain (Malayan Camp-CH/Q), it was less active against these strains when compared with WR 122455.

*γ) 4-Pyridinemethanols.* SCHMIDT et al. (1978c) and SCHMIDT (1979d) assessed the activities of 2,6-substituted-4-pyridinemethanols against *P. falciparum* strains of diverse drug susceptibility and resistance. Of ten compounds evaluated, three (two were diastereoisomers) were two to three times more active than chloroquine against infections of a chloroquine-sensitive strain; at the same doses they were similarly effective against the multiresistant Vietnam Smith strain.

Further assessment of two compounds, WR 172435 and WR 180409, against the Smith strain of *P. falciparum* and the chloroquine-sensitive Vietnam Palo Alto strain of *P. vivax* indicated the following: (a) with oral administration of the same total dose, 3-day and 7-day treatment schedules were similarly effective and somewhat better than a single-dose administration; (b) the activity of WR 172435 was somewhat greater than that of WR 180409; (c) the phosphate salt of WR 180409 could be administered intravenously and proved to be effective; (d) more rapid control of parasitaemia was obtained with either compound than any standard or new antimalarial compound; and (e) the therapeutic indices of the two drugs were four to eight times that of chloroquine against chloroquine-susceptible strains, with similar indices against drug-resistant strains.

e) Miscellaneous

A dihydro-acridinedione, floxacrine [7-chloro-10-hydroxy-3-(4-trifluoromethyl-phenyl)-3,4- dihydroacridine-1,9(2H, 10H)-dione], was evaluated by SCHMIDT (1979c) against two *P. falciparum* strains, Smith and Oak Knoll, and the Palo Alto strain of *P. vivax*. While floxacrine was equally suppressive against the three strains, it was less effective as a curative agent. From 6 to 64 times the dose required for parasite clearance was required for cure. To cure infections of the two falciparum and one vivax strain, more than a tenfold increase in doses was necessary. Floxacrine resistance occurred rapidly while treating the *P. vivax* infections. The prophylactic and radical curative activity of floxacrine against *P. cynomolgi* infections is discussed in a subsequent section.

Activities of two *o*-cresol derivatives, WR 194965 [2-(*t*-butyl-aminomethyl)-4-*t*-butyl-6-(4-chlorophenyl)-phenol] and WR 204165 [3,6-bis-(*t*-butyl)-8-(4-chlorophenyl)-2*H*, 4*H*-1,3-benzo-oxazine] were assessed against the Vietnam Smith strain of *P. falciparum* by SCHMIDT and CROSBY (1978). This pilot evaluation showed that both compounds had similar $CD_{90}$s, total doses of 27.0 and 35.0, respectively, and that these values were similar to that of mefloquine (WR 142490). Further studies with WR 194965 against the Vietnam Smith strain of *P. falciparum* and Vietnam Palo Alto strain of *P. vivax* indicated that the antimalarial activity was similar whether the drug was administered in a single dose, or divided into three or seven daily doses. Parasitaemias were cleared rapidly. WR 194965 was about twice as active against infections of the Vietnam Palo Alto strain as against the Vietnam Smith strain.

SCHMIDT et al. (1977b), using the pyrimethamine-resistant Vietnam Palo Alto strain of *P. vivax*, showed that the curative activity of pyrimethamine was increased 16 times and sulphadiazine 64 times when these two compounds were administered in combination. The curative dose of pyrimethamine in the combined regimen proved to be equivalent to the dose in a single drug regimen against the pyrimethamine-sensitive New Guinea Chesson vivax strain.

Using the *P. falciparum* Camp strain, VOLLER et al. (1969) cured an infection with a single oral administration of sulfadoxine plus pyrimethamine, at doses of 20.0 mg/kg and 2.0 mg/kg, respectively. Intramuscular treatment of an infected monkey with 5.0–30.0 mg/kg doses, only cleared the parasitaemia, while the recrudescence was cured with a similar regimen.

The activity of two chlorinated lincomycin analogues against the chloroquine-resistant Vietnam Oak Knoll strain of *P. falciparum* was examined by POWERS and JACOBS (1972). Seven-day oral administration of U 24 (*N*-demethyl-4-pentyl clindamycin hydrochloride) proved to be curative at doses of 10.0 and 50.0 mg/kg. Clindamycin hydrochloride (U 21) was curative at 75.0 mg/kg. Parasite clearance was slow, and they suggested that lincomycin should be combined with chloroquine or quinine.

GLEW et al. (1978) reported on the experimental induction, by subcurative therapy, of RIII quinine resistance in the *P. falciparum* Panama II strain. This was the first such occurrence using a non-human primate model. The authors were concerned that, although RIII quinine resistance in the field is unusual, increased quinine resistance may appear in many areas.

# C. Use in Tissue Schizontocide Studies

## I. Simian Plasmodia

### 1. *Plasmodium cynomolgi* in *Macaca mulatta* (Rhesus Monkey)

#### a) Aminobenzene

RC 12 [1,2-dimethoxy-4-(bis-diethhylaminoethyl)-amino-5-bromo-benzene] was the subject of two reports. SCHMIDT et al. (1966) found that RC 12 acted as a prophylactic against *P. cynomolgi* when administered 1 day before sporozoite inoculation, on the day of inoculation, and for 7 days after. Radical cures were achieved when RC 12, in conjunction with chloroquine, was administered daily for 14 days.

In a series of experiments, SODEMAN et al. (1972) confirmed that RC 12 does possess causal prophylactic capability against *P. cynomolgi* in rhesus monkeys. Following a single weekly administration of a 25.0 mg/kg dose for 6 weeks, a group of rhesus was challenged with sporozoites and treatment continued for an additional 3 weeks. No patent infections developed in the treated animals. To test for radical curative activity, patent parasitaemias were cleared by quinine or chloroquine, and then groups of five rhesus each were treated with 25.0 mg/kg of RC 12, for 5, 6 or 7 days. No regimen proved able to eradicate completely the tissue stages, as relapses occurred in animals in each group.

#### b) Quinoline Ester

RYLEY and PETERS (1970) examined the causal prophylactic activity of a quinoline ester (ICI 56780) in the rhesus model. A total of ten daily doses at 20.0 mg/kg did protect monkeys from infection, no infections developed in primaquine-treated comparison subjects and patent parasitaemias developed in untreated controls.

#### c) 8-Aminoquinolines

While primaquine is the only drug currently available for the radical cure of *P. vivax* infections, it is sometimes toxic in individual people who have glucose-6-phosphate dehydrogenase (G6PD) deficiency. Primaquine is a racemic mixture. Recently SCHMIDT et al. (1977 a) were able to compare the radical curative activity of the *d* and *l* isomers with the racemate against *P. cynomolgi* infections in the rhesus monkey. All three forms were equivalent in their curative capacity when administered for 7 days with chloroquine. The therapeutic index of *d*-primaquine proved to be at least twice that of primaquine. Based upon their observations, the authors suggested that human trials with the *d* isomer should be carried out and projected that a 7-day dosage regimen might not cause haemolytic reactions in patients with G6PD deficiency.

In a report covering the period 1946–1975, SCHMIDT et al. (1977 d) dealt with the total dose concept for radical cure by various 8-aminoquinolines. They showed that 7-day and 14-day dosage regimens of pamaquine, pentaquine or isopentaquine (with quinine as a blood schizontocide) were equally effective in radically curing infections with the M strain of *P. cynomolgi*. Primaquine (with chloroquine) was as effective in a 7-day dosage regimen as in a 14-day regimen in curing infections of the B strain of *P. cynomolgi*. Primaquine or 4-methyl primaquine (with chloroquine) proved to be equally effective in single dose, 3-day and 7-day dosage regimens as curative agents for B strain infections. Thus, duration of treatment with 8-aminoquinolines is not the critical factor in achieving radical cure, the total dose administered being the essential element. This supports the concepts of seeking new radical curative agents, less toxic than primaquine, which will produce radical cure in 1- or 3-day dosage regimens.

d) 4-Quinolinemethanol

The blood schizontocidal properties of mefloquine were discussed in a previous section. Mefloquine does not possess the capacity to act as a prophylactic or radical curative agent against sporozoite-induced *P. cynomolgi* infections, as shown by Schmidt et al. (1978a). However, when mefloquine was used in conjunction with primaquine for radical cure, it proved to be as effective as chloroquine.

e) Dihydroacridinedione

The activity of floxacrine against trophozoite-induced infections of human plasmodia was indicated in a previous section. Evaluation of floxacrine by Schmidt (1979c) for prophylactic activity showed that, when administered after inoculation of *P. cynomolgi* sporozoites, it afforded complete protection in rhesus monkeys. Of particular interest is that floxacrine does not act as a radical curative agent. No previous compound has exhibited such divergent activity against tissue schizonts. As the compound produced a haemorrhagic syndrome in some treated monkeys, its potential usefulness as a prophylactic agent may be limited.

f) 2,4-Diamino-6-Substituted Quinazolines

The evaluation by Schmidt and Rossan (1979) of CI 679, 2,4-diamino-6- [(3,4-dichlorobenzyl)-nitrosoamino]-quinazoline, against pyrimethamine-sensitive (Ro) and pyrimethamine-resistant (Ro/PM) strains of *P. cynomolgi* showed that the compound possesses neither causal prophylactic nor radical curative activity against either strain. There was, however, a dose-related delay in the onset of patency in both strains, as well as extensions of relapse intervals in the radical curative activity component.

g) Antibiotics

Two reports were concerned with the effect of antibiotics on exoerythrocytic stages.

Schmidt et al. (1970) showed that both 7-chlorolincomycin (U 21251F) and *N*-demethyl-4-pentyl-7-chloro-lincomycin (U 24729A) delayed the onset of parasitaemia during causal prophylactic studies of *P. cynomolgi* (B strain) in rhesus monkeys. Similar delays ensued when the compounds were tested against the pyrimethamine-susceptible (Ro) and -resistant (Ro/PM) strains of *P. cynomolgi*. U 24729A effected a longer delay in the onset of patency than did U 21251F and examination of liver sections showed that the former's activity was directly against the developing pre-erythrocytic stages. Radical cures of *P. cynomolgi* infections were not achieved with U 21251F, but U 24729A administered at a dose of 10.0 mg/kg for 7 days cured one of eight infections, and at a dose of 40.0 mg/kg for 7 days cured two of three infections.

On day 3 and 4 following inoculation of *P. vivax* sporozoites into a chimpanzee, GARNHAM et al. (1971) administered oxytetracycline (Terramycin) because of secondary illness in the animal. No exoerythrocytic stages could be demonstrated in sections from a liver biopsy obtained on day 8 and patency was delayed 12 days. This observation prompted a further study, using sporozoites of *P. cynomolgi ceylonensis* in the rhesus monkey. An untreated control had normal exoerythrocytic schizonts in an 8-day liver biopsy, and a patent infection beginning the same day. A second rhesus, treated with oxytetracycline on days 3 and 4 postinoculation, had small and abnormal exoerythrocytic schizonts on days 8 and 11. The prepatent period was 12 days.

h) Cyclopentane

WR 14997 (1-aminocyclopentane-carboxylic acid) was shown by OMAR and COLLINS (1974) to have no prophylactic activity against *P. cynomolgi.*

i) 9-Phenanthrenemethanol

Assessment by SCHMIDT et al. (1978 b) of the tissue schizontocidal activities of WR 122455 showed that administration of the drug during the incubation period following inoculation of *P. cynomolgi* sporozoites had no effect on the developing preerythrocytic forms. Patent parasitaemias in the treated animals occurred on the same day as the untreated controls. While retreatment of the patent infections cleared the parasites, subsequent relapses indicated that WR 122455 has no activity against the secondary tissue schizonts.

### 2. *Plasmodium fieldi*

COLLINS and CONTACOS (1971) reported the first chemotherapeutic studies with this malaria species in rhesus monkeys. Sporozoite-induced infections of three *P. fieldi* strains were treated with curative blood schizontocidal doses of quinine (300 mg × 5 or 7 days) or chloroquine (50 mg × 3 days or 150 mg × 2 days). Relapses occurred in seven of seven monkeys, multiply treated, during 1 year's observation. In one rhesus, 15 such relapses were observed, following administration of 300 mg quinine for 7 days.

The authors concluded that this model would be suitable for additional chemotherapy studies.

## II. Human Plasmodia

A definitive non-human primate model for the testing of causal prophylactic and/ or radical curative agents has yet to be established, the issue being more critical for *P. vivax* than for *P. falciparum* as there are no persisting exoerythrocytic forms for the latter species. An ideal system would require the following:

1. Production, in a vertebrate host, of infectious gametocytes during relatively defined periods
2. An efficient vector, in which the salivary glands become heavily infected with sporozoites
3. A consistently reproducible prepatent period in monkey recipients and all sporozoite-inoculated, untreated animals should develop patent parasitaemias

No mosquito–New World monkey system has been found to satisfy all of these criteria, as the data summarised in Table 2 show. When sporozoites of *P. vivax* were inoculated in *A. trivirgatus*, the per cent of animals in which patent infections developed varied from 7 to 75, while the prepatent period ranged from 8 to 48 days. Fewer trials have been reported for *P. falciparum* transmission attempts, but COLLINS et al. (1977, 1979) were relatively successful in obtaining patent infections in *A. trivirgatus*, 74% and 86%, respectively, of those inoculated. Prepatent periods, however, ranged from 17 to 67 days. None of these models could be considered useful for examining the prophylactic potential of compounds, according to the third desiderata stated above. The *P. vivax* system might serve a limited use in evaluating radical curative efficacy. Such a system was developed for the squirrel monkey (*Saimiri sciureus*) infected with *P. vivax*.

DEANE et al. (1966) first reported the susceptibility of *S. sciureus* to *P. vivax* by the inoculation of infected human blood. YOUNG et al. (1971) and ROSSAN et al. (1972) showed that squirrel monkeys could be infected with blood containing an *Aotus*-adapted *P. vivax* strain and extended this observation by establishing sporozoite-induced infections. The model was then used by ROSSAN et al. (1975) to evaluate the activity of standard antimalarial compounds. Trophozoite-induced infections were cured by a single 20.0 mg base/kg dose of chloroquine, or by three daily doses of 10.0, 10.0, and 5.0 mg base/kg. The 3-day regimen of chloroquine, plus primaquine given for 14 days at a dose of 1.0 mg base/kg daily cured sporozoite-induced infections.

When sporozoite-induced infections in *S. sciureus* were treated with chloroquine at a single 10.0 mg base/kg dose or a total 25.0 mg base/kg dose administered in 3 days, relapses occurred in three of seven surviving monkeys and also in un-

**Table 2.** Summary of attempts to obtain sporozoite-induced infections of *P. vivax* and *P. falciparum* in *Aotus trivirgatus*

| Monkeys No. positive/ No. inoculated | Prepatent period (days range) | Reference |
|---|---|---|
| *P. vivax* | | |
| 3/44 | 18-26 | BAERG et al. (1969) |
| 21/207 | 8–42 | D. C. BAERG, R. N. ROSSAN, M. D. YOUNG (unpublished data) |
| 12/22 | 14–48 | COLLINS et al. (1973a) |
| 2/11 | 30–32 | COLLINS et al. (1980) |
| 3/4 | 12–42 | WARD et al. (1969) |
| *P. falciparum* | | |
| 1/1 | 36 | COLLINS and CONTACOS (1972) |
| 6/9 | 19–67 | COLLINS et al. (1973b) |
| 20/27 | 17–46 | COLLINS et al. (1977) |
| 6/7 | 17–19 | COLLINS et al. (1979) |
| 1/2 | 33 | HAYES and WARD (1977) |
| 1/2 | 18 | WARD and HAYES (1972) |

treated control animals. Infections relapsed in *A. trivirgatus* inoculated with vivax sporozoites and treated only with chloroquine in three daily doses of 10.0, 10.0, and 5.0 mg base/kg. These results were the first chemotherapeutic evidence for the persistence of exoerythrocytic stages of *P. vivax* in New World monkeys.

## D. Conclusion

During the past decade, the development of the *Aotus*–human *Plasmodium* model for the testing of experimental antimalarial drugs proved to be an invaluable asset in the field of chemotherapy. Evaluations of numerous drugs in at least eight chemical classes have been reported, resulting in a wide spectrum of efficacy against the blood stages of *P. falciparum* and *P. vivax*. The most promising new agent is mefloquine, a 4-quinolinemethanol, possessing significant activity against the multidrug-resistant Vietnam Smith strain of *P. falciparum*.

SCHMIDT et al. (1977c) showed that the cross-resistance between chloroquine and amodiaquine in resistant strains of *P. falciparum* was not absolute, thus arguing for the development of other, potentially effective, 4-aminoquinoline analogues.

No single outstanding new drug was evaluated against the trophozoite stages of *P. cynomolgi* in the rhesus monkey model. Of interest, however, is that an antibiotic, lincomycin, proved to have both blood schizontocidal and some causal prophylactic activity. In the latter instance, the activity was manifested by a delay in the onset of patent infections following inoculation of *P. cynomolgi* sporozoites.

The problems associated with primaquine as a radical curative agent may be obviated based upon studies by SCHMIDT et al. (1977a, d). The use of the *d* isomer of primaquine in a 7-day dosage regimen may cure naturally acquired infections of *P. vivax* and not produce a haemolytic crisis in glucose-6-phosphate dehydrogenase-deficient patients, since this isomer is less toxic than the normally used drug.

The search for effective new antimalarial drugs must continue as new geographical areas with drug-resistant *P. falciparum* strains are continually being identified.

*Dedication.* This chapter is dedicated to Dr. LEON H. SCHMIDT, who pioneered the development of non-human primate models, using simian and human plasmodia, for the assessment of experimental antimalarial drugs. His work has contributed significantly to the advancement in chemotherapy of human malarias.

## References

Baerg DC, Porter JA Jr, Young MD (1969) Sporozoite transmission of *Plasmodium vivax* to Panamanian primates. Am J Trop Med Hyg 18:346–350

Collins WE, Contacos PG (1971) Observations on the relapse activity of *Plasmodium fieldi* in the rhesus monkey. J Parasitol 57:29–32

Collins WE, Contacos PG (1972) Transmission of *Plasmodium falciparum* from monkey to monkey by the bite of infected *Anopheles freeborni* mosquitoes. Trans R Soc Trop Med Hyg 66:371–372

Collins WE, Contacos PG, Stanfill PS, Richardson BB (1973a) Studies on human malaria in *Aotus* monkeys. I. Sporozoite transmission of *Plasmodium vivax* from El Salvador. J Parasitol 59:606–608

Collins WE, Neva FA, Chaves-Carballo E, Stanfill PS, Richardson BB (1973 b) Studies on human malaria in *Aotus* monkeys. II. Establishment of a strain of *Plasmodium falciparum* from Panama. J Parasitol 59:609–612

Collins WE, Warren McW, Skinner JC, Chin W, Richardson BB (1977) Studies on the Santa Lucía (El Salvador) strain of *Plasmodium falciparum* in *Aotus trivirgatus* monkeys. J Parasitol 63:52–56

Collins WE, Warren McW, Skinner JC, Richardson BB, Chin W (1979) Studies on the West African I strain of *Plasmodium falciparum* in *Aotus trivirgatus* monkeys. J Parasitol 65:763–767

Collins WE, Warren McW, Contacos PG, Skinner JC, Richardson BB, Kearse TS (1980) The Chesson strain of *Plasmodium vivax* in *Aotus* monkeys and anopheline mosquitoes. J Parasitol 66:488–497

Davidson DE Jr, Johnsen DO, Tanticharoenyos P, Hickman RL, Kinnamon KE (1976) Evaluating new antimalarial drugs against trophozoite induced *Plasmodium cynomolgi* malaria in rhesus monkeys. Am J Trop Med Hyg 25:26–33

Deane LM, Ferreira Neto J, Silveira IPS (1966) Experimental infection of a splenectomized squirrel monkey, *Saimiri sciureus*, with *Plasmodium vivax*. Trans R Soc Trop Med Hyg 60:811–812

Garnham PCC, Warren McW, Killick-Kendrick R (1971) The action of "Terramycin" on the primary exoerythrocytic development of *Plasmodium vivax* and *Plasmodium cynomolgi ceylonensis*. J Trop Med Hyg 74:32–35

Geiman QM, Meagher MJ (1967) Susceptibility of a New World monkey to *Plasmodium falciparum* from man. Nature 215:437–439

Glew RH, Collins WE, Miller LH (1978) Selection of increased quinine resistance in *Plasmodium falciparum* in *Aotus* monkeys. Am J Trop Med Hyg 27:9–13

Hayes DE, Ward RA (1977) Sporozoite transmission of falciparum malaria (Burma-Thau strain) from man to *Aotus* monkey. Am J Trop Med Hyg 26:184–185

Moore DV, Lanier JE (1961) Observations on two *Plasmodium falciparum* infections with abnormal response to chloroquine. Am J Trop Med Hyg 10:5–9

Omar MS, Collins WE (1974) Studies on the antimalarial effects of RC-12 and WR 14997 on the development of *Plasmodium cynomolgi* in mosquitoes and rhesus monkeys. Am J Trop Med Hyg 23:339–349

Peters W (1970) Chemotherapy and drug resistance in malaria. Academic, New York

Peters W (1980) Chemotherapy of malaria. In: Kreier JP (ed) Malaria, vol I. Academic, New York, pp 145–283

Powers KG (1969) Activity of chlorinated lincomycin analogues against *Plasmodium cynomolgi* in rhesus monkeys. Am J Trop Med Hyg 18:485–490

Powers KG, Jacobs RL (1972) Activity of two chlorinated lincomycin analogues against chloroquine-resistant falciparum malaria in owl monkeys. Antimicrob Agents Chemother 1:49–53

Powers KG, Aikawa M, Nugent KM (1976) *Plasmodium knowlesi:* Morphology and course of infection in rhesus monkeys treated with clindamycin and its *N*-demethyl-4-pentyl analog. Exp Parasitol 40:13–24

Raether W, Fink E (1979) Antimalarial activity of Floxacrine (HOE 991). I. Studies on blood schizontocidal action of Floxacrine against *Plasmodium berghei, P. vinckei,* and *P. cynomolgi.* Ann Trop Med Parasitol 73:505–526

Rossan RN, Baerg DC, Young MD (1972) Characterization of *Plasmodium vivax* infections in *Saimiri sciureus* (squirrel monkeys). Proc Helminth Soc Wash 39:24–28

Rossan RN, Young MD, Baerg DC (1975) Chemotherapy of *Plasmodium vivax* in *Saimiri* and *Aotus* models. Am J Trop Med Hyg 24:168–173

Rothe WE, Jacobus DP, Walter WG (1969) Treatment of trophozoite-induced *Plasmodium knowlesi* infection in the rhesus monkey with trimethoprim and sulfalene. Am J Trop Med Hyg 18:491–494

Ryley JF, Peters W (1970) The antimalarial activity of some quinoline esters. Ann Trop Med Parasitol 64:209–222

Schmidt LH (1969) Chemotherapy of the drug-resistant malarias. Annu Rev Microbiol 23:427–454

Schmidt LH (1973) Infections with *Plasmodium falciparum* and *Plasmodium vivax* in the owl monkey-model systems for basic biological and chemotherapeutic studies. Trans R Soc Trop Med Hyg 67:446–474

Schmidt LH (1978a) *Plasmodium falciparum* and *Plasmodium vivax* infections in the owl monkey (*Aotus trivirgatus*). I. The courses of untreated infections. Am J Trop Med Hyg 27:671–702

Schmidt LH (1978b) *Plasmodium falciparum* and *Plasmodium vivax* infections in the owl monkey (*Aotus trivirgatus*) II. Responses to chloroquine, quinine, and pyrimethamine. Am J Trop Med Hyg 27:703–717

Schmidt LH (1978c) *Plasmodium falciparum* and *Plasmodium vivax* infections in the owl monkey (*Aotus trivirgatus*) III. Methods employed in the search for new blood schizonticidal drugs. Am J Trop Med Hyg 27:718–737

Schmidt LH (1979a) Studies on the 2,4-diamino-6-substituted quinazolines. II. Activity of selected derivatives against infections with various drug-susceptible and drug-resistant strains of *Plasmodium falciparum* and *Plasmodium vivax* in owl monkeys. Am J Trop Med Hyg 28:793–807

Schmidt LH (1979b) Studies on the 2,4-diamino-6-substituted quinazolines. III. The capacity of sulfadiazine to enhance the activities of WR 158122 and WR 159412 against infections with various drug-susceptible and drug-resistant strains of *Plasmodium falciparum* and *Plasmodium vivax* in owl monkeys. Am J Trop Med Hyg 28:808–818

Schmidt LH (1979c) Antimalarial properties of floxacrine, a dihydroacridinedione derivative. Antimicrob Agents Chemother 16:475–485

Schmidt LH (1979d) Experimental infections with human plasmodia in owl monkeys – their contribution to development of new broadly active blood schizonticidal drugs. Adv Pharmacol Ther 10:79–90

Schmidt LH, Crosby R (1978) Antimalarial activities of WR 194965, and α-amino-o-cresol derivative. Antimicrob Agents Chemother 14:672–679

Schmidt LH, Crosby R (1978) Antimalarial activities of WR 194965, an α-amino-o-cresol Antimalarial activities of 2,4-diamino-6-[(3,4-dichlorobenzyl)-nitroso-amino]-quinazoline (CI-679) as exhibited in rhesus monkeys infected with the Ro or Ro/PM strains of *Plasmodium cynomolgi*. Am J Trop Med Hyg 28:781–792

Schmidt LH, Rossan RN, Fradkin R, Woods J, Schulemann W, Kratz L (1966) Studies on the antimalarial activity of 1,2-dimethoxy-4-(bis-diethyl-aminoethyl)-amino-5-bromobenzene. Bull WHO 34:783–788

Schmidt LH, Harrison J, Ellison R, Worcester P (1969) Activities of trimethoprim against infections with pyrimethamine susceptible and resistant strains of *Plasmodium cynomolgi*. Proc Soc Exp Biol Med 131:294–297

Schmidt LH, Harrison J, Ellison R, Worcester P (1970) The activities of chlorinated lincomycin derivatives against infections with *Plasmodium cynomolgi* in *Macaca mulatta*. Am J Trop Med Hyg 19:1–11

Schmidt LH, Alexander S, Allen L, Rasco J (1977a) Comparison of the curative antimalarial activities and toxicities of primaquine and its *d* and *l* isomers. Antimicrob Agents Chemother 12:51–60

Schmidt LH, Harrison J, Rossan RN, Vaughan D, Crosby R (1977b) Quantitative aspects of pyrimethamine-sulfonamide synergism. Am J Trop Med Hyg 26:837–849

Schmidt LH, Vaughan D, Mueller D, Crosby R, Hamilton R (1977c) Activities of various 4-aminoquinolines against infections with chloroquine-resistant *Plasmodium falciparum*. Antimicrob Agents Chemother 11:826–843

Schmidt LH, Fradkin R, Vaughan D, Rasco J (1977d) Radical cure of infections with *Plasmodium cynomolgi:* a function of total 8-aminoquinoline dose. Am J Trop Med Hyg 26:1116–1128

Schmidt LH, Crosby R, Rasco J, Vaughan D (1978a) Antimalarial properties of various 4-quinolinemethanols with special attention to WR 142490 (mefloquine). Antimicrob Agents Chemother 13:1011–1030

Schmidt LH, Crosby R, Rasco J, Vaughan D (1978b) Antimalarial activities of various 9-phenanthrene-methanols with special attention to WR 122455 and WR 171669. Antimicrob Agents Chemother 14:292–314

Schmidt LH, Crosby R, Rasco J, Vaughan D (1978c) Antimalarial activities of 4-pyridinemethanols with special attention to WR 172435 and WR 180409. Antimicrob Agents Chemother 14:420–435

Schmidt LH, Crosby R, Rasco J, Vaughan D (1978d) The antimalarial activities of the 4-quinolinemethanols, WR 184806 and WR 226253. Antimicrob Agents Chemother 14:680–689

Sodeman TM, Contacos PG, Collins WE, Smith CS, Jumper JR (1972) Studies on the prophylactic and radical curative activity of RC-12 against *Plasmodium cynomolgi* in *Macaca mulatta*. Bull WHO 47:425–428

Thompson PE, Bayles A, Olszweski B (1969) PAM 1392 [2,4-diamino-6-(3,4-dichlorobenzylamino)-quinazoline] as a chemotherapeutic agent: *Plasmodium berghei, P. cynomolgi, P. knowlesi,* and *Trypanosoma cruzi*. Exp Parasitol 25:32–49

Thompson PE, Bayles A, Olszewski B (1970) Antimalarial activity of 2,4-diamino-6-[(3,4-dichlorobenzyl)-nitros-amino]-quinazoline (CI-679 base) and CI-679 acetate. Laboratory studies in mice and rhesus monkeys. Am J Trop Med Hyg 19:12–26

Voller A, Richards WHG, Hawkey CM, Ridley DS (1969) Human malaria (*Plasmodium falciparum*) in owl monkeys (*Aotus trivirgatus*). J Trop Med Hyg 72:153–160

Ward RA, Hayes DE (1972) Sporozoite transmission of falciparum malaria (Vietnam, Smith strain) from monkey to monkey. Trans R Soc Trop Med Hyg 66:670–671

Ward RA, Rutledge LC, Hickman RL (1969) Cyclical transmission of Chesson vivax malaria in subhuman primates. Nature 224:1126–1127

Young MD (1970) Natural and induced malarias in Western hemisphere monkeys. Lab Anim Care 20:361–367

Young MD, Moore DV (1961) Chloroquine resistance in *Plasmodium falciparum*. Am J Trop Med Hyg 10:317–320

Young MD, Porter JA Jr, Johnson CM (1966) *Plasmodium vivax* transmitted from man to monkey to man. Science 153:1006–1007

Young MD, Baerg DC, Rossan RN (1971) Sporozoite transmission and serial blood passage of *Plasmodium vivax* in squirrel monkeys (*Saimiri sciureus*). Trans R Soc Trop Med Hyg 65:835–836

Young MD, Baerg DC, Rossan RN (1975) Experimental hosts for human plasmodia. Exp Parasitol 38:136–152

Young MD, Baerg DC, Rossan RN (1976) Studies with induced malaria in *Aotus* monkeys. Lab Animal Sci 26:1131–1137

CHAPTER 10

# Surrogate Models for Antimalarials

S.-C. Chou, K. A. Conklin, M. R. Levy, and D. C. Warhurst

## A. Isolated Enzyme Systems

M. R. Levy and S.-C. Chou

### I. Introduction

In recent years studies concerned with the mode of action of antimalarial drugs such as chloroquine have shifted from those concerned primarily with the effects on a particular enzyme or enzyme system to studies concerned with the consequences of the ability of chloroquine to act as a lysosomotropic agent. As a result of this new emphasis, chloroquine has become a useful tool in analysing a variety of cellular processes such as receptor-mediated endocytosis, regulation of the numbers of various membrane-associated receptors, the secretion, uptake and delivery of lysosomal enzymes, and means by which cells degrade various classes of materials.

In the case of the malaria parasite, chloroquine accumulates in red cells, and especially in infected red cells, where the concentration of the drug may be as much as 1 000 times that of the plasma (Macomber et al. 1966; Fitch 1969). Using this information, together with the observation that chloroquine caused a clumping of haemoglobin infected red cells, Homewood et al. (1972a) suggested that chloroquine could act to raise the pH of the malarial cell food vacuole, thereby reducing haemoglobin breakdown. Subsequently, studies on the proteolytic system of the parasite were undertaken in the hope that inhibition of this system might serve to stop haemoglobin digestion and inhibit cell growth (Levy and Chou 1975).

Interest in possible action of chloroquine at the level of the lysosome was stimulated when De Duve et al. (1974) illustrated that this compound, as well as other weak bases, could accumulate within the organelle. These lysosomotropic substances become trapped within lysosomes in their protonated forms and may inhibit lysosomal function by raising the pH within the organelle enough that the hydrolases fail to act (Ohkuma and Poole 1978), by inhibiting various lysosomal hydrolases (Wibo and Poole 1974; Matsuzawa and Hostetler 1980), or by a combination of these processes.

Lysosomotropic agents, including chloroquine, have now been shown to prevent intracellular degradation in a number of situations that involve participation of lysosomes in the degradative processes. Such studies have also contributed to the concept of the existence of lysosomal and non-lysosomal pathways of degradation (Ballard 1977; Seglen et al. 1979).

More recently, chloroquine and other antimalarials have been used to help elucidate the events that occur in a variety of receptor-mediated processes. In some cases, the effects are probably due to the lysosomotropic actions of the drugs, but in other cases the sites of action may be elsewhere.

In studies on receptor-mediated endocytosis, chloroquine has yielded information on the uptake into the cell and the subsequent fate of a variety of hormones and other compounds, as well as the fate of receptors for some of these compounds. Similarly, chloroquine has been useful in studies dealing with the delivery of newly formed lysosomal enzymes to their appropriate destinations, as well as in studies dealing with the intracellular movements of the receptors for these enzymes. Thus recent evidence indicates that chloroquine interferes with cellular uptake of glycoproteins and also causes premature release of cellular acid hydrolases (Wiesmann et al. 1975; Sando et al. 1979; Fischer et al. 1980; Gonzalez-Noriega et al. 1980; Hasilik and Neufeld 1980a; Tietze et al. 1980). In either case, the effect may be due to an impairment of the normal intracellular flow of receptors that can bind to glycoproteins bearing specific recognition markers.

This section will focus primarily on the effects of chloroquine and related agents on the cellular uptake and fate of hormones and other ligands, and on the uptake and release of lysosomal enzymes. The latter discussion will include data to suggest a possible role of chloroquine on intracellular movement of receptors for the delivery and/or uptake of lysosomal enzymes. Finally, the effects of protease inhibitors on parasite proteases and on the ability of the parasite to synthesise macromolecules will also be discussed.

## II. Effects of Chloroquine on Receptor-Mediated Endocytosis

There have been numerous studies dealing with the effects of chloroquine on various aspects of the lysosomal system. Chloroquine and other lysosomotropic agents accumulate within lysosomes (De Duve et al. 1974), and may raise the pH of the organelle by as much as 1.5 pH units in cultured macrophages (Ohkuma and Poole 1978). Similar results were obtained when isolated rat liver lysosomes were incubated with chloroquine (Reijngoud and Tager 1976). In either case, chloroquine concentrations within the organelle may exceed 50 m*M*. A number of groups have shown that cells treated with chloroquine have an impaired capacity to degrade endocytosed materials and, in some situations, endogenous materials. Thus, Lie and Schofield (1973) reported that chloroquine inhibited in vivo degradation of mucopolysaccharides by cultured human fibroblasts and suggested that the antimalarial activity of chloroquine and related compounds could be due to an inhibition of normal lysosomal activity. Similarly, Wibo and Poole (1974) found that chloroquine inhibited protein degradation in cultured rat fibroblasts. The rate of degradation of proteins with long half-lives was inhibited by 25% while that of proteins with short half-lives was inhibited by 15%. It was suggested that the effect was due to an inhibition of cathepsin B, as high concentrations of chloroquine produced an apparent inhibition of this enzyme, when the protease was assayed using an artificial substrate.

Since these early observations, many groups have used chloroquine and other lysosomotropic amines to characterise the internalisation and subsequent fate of various compounds that are taken into the cell following binding to specific receptors. Such compounds include hormones, low-density lipoprotein, $\alpha_2$-macroglobulin, and others. Most of these studies have centred on the questions of whether the particular ligand in question is internalised and degraded within lysosomes and, if so, either of these steps is necessary for the biological action of the substance in question.

### 1. Lipoproteins

GOLDSTEIN, BROWN, and co-workers utilized chloroquine to study the fate of low-density lipoprotein (LDL) in cultured fibroblasts. LDL is normally internalised following binding to specific receptors that are located within coated pits. The internalised material is delivered to lysosomes where the protein portion is degraded and the cholesteryl ester is hydrolysed to release free cholesterol (GOLDSTEIN and BROWN 1977). The release of cholesterol within the cell leads to a suppression of cellular levels of 3-hydroxymethyl coenzyme A reductase, the rate-limiting step in cholesterol synthesis, to the activation of an enzyme that re-esterifies the cellular cholesterol, and to a decreased synthesis of LDL receptors. Thus the release of cholesterol from endocytosed LDL serves to stop cellular cholesterol synthesis, to limit further uptake of LDL and to promote storage of intracellular cholesterol.

Chloroquine (20 $\mu M$) prevented the degradation of [$^{125}$I]LDL by these cells (GOLDSTEIN et al. 1975), as well as the hydrolysis of the cholesteryl esters (BROWN et al. 1975) but did not affect binding of LDL to its receptor. Since cell extracts degrade [$^{125}$I]LDL at pH 4, but not at pH 6, it seems likely that the action of chloroquine results from an increase in the intralysosomal pH. Similarly, the acid lipase that normally hydrolyses the cholesteryl ester within the LDL is probably inhibited. The inhibition of LDL degradation by chloroquine led to an accumulation of cholesteryl esters within the lysosome. Consequently, the three regulatory events described above failed to occur.

In related studies, STEIN et al. (1977) showed that chloroquine had no effect on the clearance of either circulating LDL or very low density lipoprotein (VLDL), but inhibited the degradation of both. Thus, pretreatment of animals with chloroquine for 3 h increased the amount of $^{125}$I-labelled VLDL (labelled in either the protein or lipid moiety) recovered in the liver 30 min after injection. When VLDL-containing [$^{3}$H]cholesterol was administered, the percentage of label that appeared as free, rather than as esterified cholesterol, after 45 min was markedly reduced in the chloroquine-treated animals.

Degradation of LDL or VLDL by the postnuclear supernatant of rat liver occurred optimally at pH 4.4, and was inhibited by chloroquine, although the degradation of other lipoproteins was less sensitive to the drug. It was concluded that lysosomal acid hydrolases normally act to degrade these various lipoproteins.

Similar results were obtained by OSE et al. (1980) for $^{125}$I-high-density lipoprotein in isolated rat fibroblasts, where chloroquine inhibited degradation by 50%, as did leupeptin (an inhibitor of some lysosomal proteases) or $NH_4Cl$ (another lysosomotropic agent). Similarly, chloroquine (or colchicine) inhibited hydrolysis of chyle cholesteryl ester by liver cells (FLOREN et al. 1977). The effect could be observed on hydrolysis of material taken up either prior or subsequent to administration of the drug. Most of the cholesteryl ester was associated with the large granule fraction.

A recent study indicates that chloroquine inhibits phospholipases A and C from delipidated rat liver lysosomes (MATSUZAWA and HOSTETLER 1980). The $ID_{50}$ in either case was 0.3 m$M$, but maximal inhibition of phospholipase A was only 55%. Phospholipase A was inhibited at pH 5.4 but not at 4.4, while the reverse was true for phospholipase C. A form of phospholipase A that catalyses the transacetylation step in the synthesis of monoglycerophosphate was not inhibited. In fact, chronic treatment of rats with chloroquine, which causes phospholipid accumulation in lysosomes, led to an increase in this particular form of the enzyme.

### 2. Hormones

#### a) Epidermal Growth Factor

Results similar to those described for LDL and the other circulating lipoproteins have been observed with a number of hormones. Thus, epidermal growth factor (EGF) in fibroblasts is rapidly internalised by a receptor-mediated process and is degraded within lysosomes (CARPENTER and COHEN 1976). The degradation, as measured by the release of [$^{125}$I]monoiodotyrosine into the medium following administration of [$^{125}$I]EGF, is inhibited by chloroquine at concentrations as low as 0.01 m$M$. However, the endocytosed EGF may remain in multivesicular bodies, rather than being transferred to lysosomes. This is in contrast to results obtained with macrophages, where chloroquine seems to enhance lysosome-phagosome fusion (HART and YOUNG 1978).

KING et al. (1980 a) have used chloroquine and other lysosomotropic agents to study the internalisation and fate of receptors for EGF. In the presence of EGF, receptor-hormone complexes are internalised and native [$^{125}$I]EGF declines by 60% after 1 h, indicating that the hormone has been degraded. In the presence of chloroquine or methylamine, more than 80% of the hormone remains undegraded, even after 6 h. Lysates of cells incubated with methylamine showed a 2.8-fold increase in total binding capacity for EGF, indicating that degradation of the receptors was also prevented. Cells incubated with methylamine in the absence of EGF exhibited a time-dependent loss of surface-binding capacity, suggesting that surface receptors may be internalised even in the absence of EGF. The half-life for the loss in surface binding was about 6 h in the presence of methylamine, and about 30 min in the presence of the amine and EGF. More recent studies support the concept that EGF receptors are continually internalised and degraded, and that occupancy of the receptors by EGF apparently changes the rate of degradation (KING et al. 1980 b).

In contrast to the effects of chloroquine, mepacrine seems to prevent the internalisation of [$^{125}$I]EGF (HAIGLER et al. 1980). The $ID_{50}$ was about 0.4 m$M$, the effect was reversible and binding was minimally affected. It was suggested that the effect of mepacrine was due to an inhibition of phospholipase $A_2$ ($PLA_2$), and several other $PLA_2$ inhibitors also prevented internalisation.

#### b) Insulin

Chloroquine has also been used to study the possible role of lysosomes in the metabolism of insulin in rat adipocytes (MARSHALL and OLEFSKY 1979). Cells incubated with [$^{125}$I]insulin and chloroquine showed a severalfold increase in cell-associated radioactivity as compared with untreated controls. The radioactivity was intracellular and was almost all recoverable as intact insulin. The chloroquine effect seemed to require internalisation of insulin, and it was suggested that the drug prevents the normal degradation or conversion of insulin within lysosomes.

Recent data indicate that insulin, EGF and $\alpha_2$-macroglobulin may all be internalised in the same vesicle, following patching of hormone-receptor complexes. Chloroquine (10 m*M*) does not seem to prevent the patching (SCHLESSINGER et al. 1978).

c) Human Choriogonadotropin

ASCOLI and PUETT (1978 a, b) have studied the effects of chloroquine on the degradation of receptor-bound human choriogonadotropin (HCG) and on gonadotropin-stimulated steroidogenesis by Leydig tumor cells. Binding of [$^{125}$I]HCG to these cells is normally followed by degradation of most of the hormone and the release of [$^{125}$I]monoiodotyrosine into the medium. The degradation was inhibited by chloroquine and ammonium chloride, as well as by protease inhibitors and inhibitors of energy metabolism. Binding of the hormone to the cell was not affected. Leupeptin, an inhibitor of several lysosomal proteases, also inhibited degradation of the receptor-bound hormone (ASCOLI 1979).

d) Progesterone

Chloroquine also inhibited HCG-stimulated progesterone secretion, and this was subsequently shown to be due to an inhibition of steroidogenesis (ASCOLI and PUETT 1978 b; ASCOLI 1978). Several lines of evidence suggest that the effects of chloroquine on steroidogenesis are distinct from those on HCG degradation. Thus, the $ID_{50}$ for inhibition of HCG breakdown was 4 μ*M*, while that for inhibition of steroidogenesis was 50 μ*M*. Also, the effects on degradation were reversible following removal of chloroquine from the medium, while those on steroidogenesis were not. In addition, ammonium chloride, which inhibited HCG degradation, was without effect on steroidogenesis. Chloroquine, but not ammonium chloride, was also able to inhibit cholera toxin or cyclic AMP-induced steroidogenesis. Since a number of other compounds also inhibited this process, it is possible that the effect is non-specific and due to impairment of cellular metabolism.

In a somewhat related study, chloroquine and other lysosomotropic agents were used to investigate a possible role of lysosomes in progesterone secretion by ovarian cells exposed to luteinising hormone (LH) (STRAUSS et al. 1978).

Chloroquine produced a dose-dependent inhibition of progesterone secretion in LH-treated cell suspension, the inhibition ranging from 10% at 5 μ*M* to 60% at 200 μ*M*. Chloroquine (50 μ*M*) also reduced cAMP-stimulated progesterone secretion back to the basal level. It did not prevent the ability of ovarian mitochondria to convert cholesterol to steroids, nor did it inhibit the incorporation of amino acids into protein, glucose oxidation or lactic acid production by ovarian cell suspensions. It was suggested that a portion of luteal cell cholesterol must be processed before it can enter the steroidogenic pool. This could involve the conversion of cholesteryl esters to cholesterol, a process that can occur in lysosomes. Depletion of cholesteryl esters is associated with increased steroidogenesis in LH-stimulated corpora lutea.

e) Prolactin

Chloroquine has also been used to study the fate of receptors for prolactin (Djiane et al. 1980). Binding of prolactin to mammary cell explants normally leads to a marked decrease in both free and total receptors. Chloroquine prevents this decrease, or "down regulation," presumably by preventing breakdown of the receptors in lysosomes. As was the case for EGF receptors, chloroquine caused a marked increase in the number of receptors even in the absence of prolactin, suggesting that there is normally a rapid turnover of the receptors.

More recently, chloroquine and ammonium chloride were shown to be without effect on the prolactin-induced synthesis of casein on rabbit mammary gland (Houdebine and Djiane 1980).These findings suggest that degradation of prolactin is not required for its actions. Similar conclusions were made concerning human choriogonadotropic hormone breakdown and steroidogenesis (Ascoli and Puett 1978 b).

In summary, numerous studies using chloroquine on receptor-mediated endocytosis of hormones and lipoproteins indicate that, while the drug does not prevent endocytosis of the receptor-ligand combination, it does inhibit the degradation of the internalised ligand. In at least several cases, the degradation of the internalised receptor is also inhibited. Finally, the finding that receptor number increases in the presence of chloroquine, even in the absence of ligand, suggests that at least some receptors are continually internalised and degraded within the lysosomes. Comparative findings on receptors for lysosomal and other glycoproteins will be discussed in the next section.

## III. Effects of Chloroquine on Uptake and Transport of Lysosomal Enzymes

A rather large number of recent studies have dealt with the observations that chloroquine may effect the uptake of lysosomal enzymes by the cell and may also cause an enhanced release of cellular lysosomal hydrolases. These studies have not only led to the suggestion by several groups that chloroquine may influence the recycling of intracellular receptors for lysosomal glycoproteins, but have helped to elucidate the mechanism by which lysosomal enzymes may be delivered to their organelle.

Wiesmann et al. (1975), studying the effects of lysosomotropic amines on the levels of a lysosomal enzyme in fibroblasts, noted that low concentrations (less than 5 $\mu M$) of chloroquine inhibited uptake of extracellular aryl sulphatase A and $\beta$-glucuronidase and accelerated the efflux of the cellular enzymes, even after the drug had been removed from the medium. The extracellular accumulation of enzymes was attributed to an inhibition of the uptake of normally secreted enzyme, rather than to direct effect on secretion. However, this interpretation is not supported by more recent evidence (see below).

Sando et al. (1979), studying the uptake of $\alpha$-L-iduronidase by cultured skin fibroblasts, noted that uptake was inhibitedby chloroquine ($ID_{50} = 20\ \mu M$) and by several other lysosomotropic amines. Since the inhibition was non-competitive, the authors concluded that the effect was not on binding of the enzyme to receptors. Uptake is thought to be mediated by receptors that recognise mannose-6-phosphate recognition markers on the enzyme (KAPLAN et al. 1977). The effect also was not due to an increased efflux of endocytosed enzyme. However, since iduronidase-deficient fibroblasts were used in the study, no information could be given on release of the endogenous enzyme. Inhibition required simultaneous presence of enzyme and amine. Preincubation of cells with chloroquine, followed by incubation with the enzyme in the absence of the drug, did not decrease uptake, despite the fact that 80% of the drug was still cell associated. The authors suggest that the amines interfere with the delivery of receptor-bound enzymes to lysosomes. It is of interest that in the studies described earlier, chloroquine did not seem to inhibit delivery of LDL and various hormones to lysosomes.

WILLCOX and RATTRAY (1979) attempted to distinguish between effects of chloroquine on enzyme uptake and enzyme secretion. Using cultured fibroblasts, these workers noted that increasing concentrations of chloroquine, from 5 to 100 $\mu M$, led to increasing amounts of extracellular $\beta$-hexosaminidase, with a concomitant decrease in cellular enzyme. To determine if the extracellular accumulation was due to an inhibition of uptake, cells were incubated with mannose-6-phosphate, which inhibits uptake by competing with the recognition marker on the enzyme. Whereas 50 $\mu M$ chloroquine caused a three fold increase in extracellular enzyme, there was only a 13% increase in the presence of mannose-6-phosphate. It was concluded that chloroquine acts by stimulating secretion rather than by inhibiting uptake, and more recent data seem to support this interpretation.

WILLCOX and RATTRAY (1979) also studied the isozyme pattern of hexosaminidase from cells and medium of chloroquine-treated cells. Chloroquine caused a depletion of the A isozyme (the more acidic form) with a concomitant increase in the medium. The amount of secreted B isozyme increased as well. Recent studies indicate that chloroquine may cause release of acid hydrolases that have not yet been delivered to lysosomes (HASILIK and NEUFELD 1980a; GONZALEZ-NORIEGA et al. 1980).

Several recent reports have suggested that chloroquine may act at the level of receptors that normally transport lysosomal glycoproteins, either delivering newly formed enzymes to lysosomes, or carrying endocytosed enzymes to the organelle. Thus, TOLLESHAUG and BERG (1979) studied the effects of chloroquine on hepatic membrane receptors for asialo-glycoproteins. Rat hepatocytes preincubated with chloroquine for 30–60 min had a marked decrease in the ability to take up [$^{125}$I]asialoorosomucoid (which binds to receptors specific for galactose residues exposed following removal of sialic acid). There was also an 85% reduction in binding capacity. Chloroquine itself did not affect binding. It was suggested that chloroquine may act by interfering with receptor recycling, possibly by preventing fusion between endocytic vesicles and lysosomes.

In studies on the biosynthesis and processing of lysosomal enzymes, HASILIK and NEUFELD (1980a) showed that several lysosomal enzymes were synthesised as precursors having a higher molecular weight, and then were progressively cleaved to their final form. There were marked disturbances of processing and of enzyme distribution in fibroblasts treated with chloroquine or with ammonium chloride. In these cells, as well as in untreated fibroblasts from patients with I-cell disease, almost all newly synthesised β-hexosaminidase was extracellular. The distribution between cells and medium of α-glucosidase and cathepsin D were more nearly normal, but intracellular processing was again incomplete. Chloroquine did not affect the phosphorylation of these enzymes, despite the change in intra- and extracellular distribution (HASILIK and NEUFELD 1980b). Administered $^{32}P$ was found on mannose-6-phosphate derived from the enzymes. Interestingly, phosphorylation was undetectable in enzymes from I-cell fibroblasts. The presence of the mannose-phosphate group is thought to be important for the correct intracellular transport of lysosomal enzymes (SLY 1980). Since phosphorylation was not inhibited by chloroquine, the release of enzymes from chloroquine-treated cells was not due to the absence of the recognition marker.

SLY'S group (GONZALEZ-NORIEGA et al. 1980) has studied the effects of chloroquine and ammonium chloride on pinocytosis and secretion of lysosomal enzymes by cultured human fibroblasts. Their data are of particular interest because they offer an explanation for the flow of enzymes through the cell.

Chloroquine (25 $\mu M$) treatment greatly enhanced secretion of newly synthesised hydrolases. The secreted enzymes bore the mannose-6-phosphate recognition marker for uptake. This marker is probably also responsible for delivery of the enzymes to lysosomes. The chloroquine-treated cells also had a reduced ability to pinocytose exogenous lysosomal enzymes bearing the mannose-6-phosphate marker. The reduced ability seems to result from a depletion of binding sites from the cell surface. Binding ability returns to normal rapidly following removal of chloroquine from the medium. The restoration is not prevented by cycloheximide, indicating the availability of receptors within the cell. Chloroquine had no effect on enzymes that had been previously endocytosed and which were presumably present in secondary lysosomes. These enzymes remained intracellular during chloroquine treatment, while newly synthesised cellular enzyme was secreted.

The authors offer the following explanation for their observations. Increased secretion is thought to occur because chloroquine reduces the availability of free receptors for attachment of newly synthesised enzymes. Thus, the new enzymes remain unbound in the intracisternal space and are secreted. The receptors normally deliver their enzymes to the lysosomes and then recycle back to the endoplasmic reticulum or Golgi region to pick up more enzyme. In a subsequent study (FISCHER et al. 1980) the existence of receptors for the mannose-6-phosphate forms of the lysosomal enzymes in the endoplasmic reticulum and Golgi apparatus was shown. The decrease in receptors would also account for the decreased pinocytosis of enzymes by the mannose-6-phosphate recognition marker. Further support for this explanation comes from the observation that β-glucuronidase dissociates very slowly from cellular membranes at pH above 6. The elevation of the lysosomal pH by chloroquine might therefore reduce the availability of receptors by reducing dissociation of receptor-enzyme complexes. This explanation would account for the observation by several groups that chloroquine-treated cells have elevated rates of secretion of lysosomal enzymes, as well as an impaired ability to take these up from the medium.

STAHL and his co-workers (STAHL and SCHLESSINGER 1980; TIETZE et al. 1980) have tested the effects of chloroquine on receptor-mediated endocytosis by peritoneal macrophages. These cells are capable of endocytosing glycoproteins and lysosomal enzymes that bear mannose or *N*-acetyl-glucosamine recognition markers. Chloroquine inhibited the uptake and subsequent degradation of [$^{125}$I]mannose bovine serum albumin. Binding was not affected, nor was internalisation of previously bound protein. The inhibition was time dependent, consistent with the idea that internalisation of receptors on the cell surface was required for the effect on uptake. It was suggested that chloroquine causes an inhibition of receptor recycling, possibly due to the requirement of a pH gradient for receptor retrieval, such as pH-sensitive separation of ligand from receptor. Such a concept is similar to that proposed by SLY'S group.

KUSIAK et al. (1980) have also studied the effects of chloroquine and other lysosomotropic agents on receptor-mediated endocytosis and on phagocytosis by cultured rat peritoneal macrophages. Chloroquine inhibited the receptor-mediated uptake of hexosaminidase, as well as the phagocytosis of latex beads. The various lysosomotropic agents inhibited the former process more effectively than the latter, suggesting that adsorptive pinocytosis and phagocytosis function independently of one another.

RICHES and STANWORTH (1980) have tested the effects of lysosomotropic amines on release of lysosomal enzymes from cultured mouse peritoneal macrophages. Chloroquine caused a release of 70% of the cellular $\beta$-glucuronidase. Quinine had a similar effect. The basis for the release is not known, but several explanations were offered including an alteration of intralysosomal pH, an activation of the alternative pathway of the complement system (a property of many of the compounds tested) to yield C3b, an inducer of lysosomal enzyme release or an enhancement of phagosome-lysosome fusion.

This last effect has been shown to occur in cultured macrophages where chloroquine was able to overcome the inhibition of lysosome-phagosome fusion in cells that had taken up virulent *Mycobacterium tuberculosis* (HART and YOUNG 1978). This and some other pathogens are apparently able to inhibit this fusion. Chloroquine also suppressed the intracellular multiplication of the bacterium. In addition, polyanions can inhibit phagosome-lysosome fusion, and this inhibition can be overcome by chloroquine and mepacrine.

In summary, there have been numerous reports that chloroquine treatment leads to an extracellular accumulation of lysosomal hydrolases, due probably to an enhanced secretion, as well as to an impaired ability to take up enzmye. These results may be explained by an effect on receptors that normally deliver newly formed enzyme to the correct intracellular site and which may also serve in endocytosis of extracellular enzymes which bear the correct recognition marker.

## IV. Protease Inhibitors: Effects on Parasite Protease and on Parasite Biosynthetic Processes and Growth

Erythrocytic stages of the malaria parasite degrade host cell haemoglobin to obtain aminoacids for growth. Degradation of many parasite organelles also occurs after the organism has invaded the host cell. These observations have prompted studies concerning the degradative system of the parasite and especially of parasite proteases. Not only could inhibition of this system be responsible for the effects of known antimalarial drugs (HOMEWOOD et al. 1972b), but it also offers a target at which potential new antimalarials may be directed.

### 1. Antimalarials as Protease Inhibitors

COOK et al. (1961) reported the existence of an alkaline and an acid protease in *Plasmodium berghei* and in *P. knowlesi*. The alkaline protease was the more active, and degraded globin more rapidly than it did haemoglobin. The acid protease was quite unstable. Cell-free extracts of *P. gallinaceum* degraded globin at pH 6.5, while haemoglobin was degraded much more slowly (MOULDER and EVANS 1946).

LEVY and co-workers reported that infected red cells of several species had much higher levels of an acid protease than did uninfected red cells (LEVY and CHOU 1973, 1974; LEVY et al. 1974). The pH optimum of the partially purified enzyme was 2.5–3.5, depending upon the species. Infected cells also had acid DNase and acid RNase activities (LEVY et al. 1976). The latter could not be detected in uninfected red cells. The protease was not inhibited by chloroquine nor by the sulphhydryl reagents iodoacetamide or *p*-chloromercuribenzoate (PCMB). EDTA was also without effect, as were the chloromethyl ketone derivatives of phenylalanine (TPCK) and lysine (TLCK). Phenylmethane sulphonylfluoride (PMSF), an inhibitor of serine proteases, was without effect on the protease from *P. falciparum* or *P. knowlesi*, but did inhibit that from *P. berghei*.

The parasite acid protease, as well as that from uninfected red cells, was inhibited by several potent protease inhibitors produced by actinomycetes. Several of these were effective at extremely low concentrations. Thus using a partially purified preparation of enzyme from *P. berghei*, $ID_{50}$s of 0.00025 μg/ml for pepstatin, 0.0005 μg/ml for chymostatin, 0.070 μg/ml for antipain and 0.2 μg/ml for leupeptin were obtained (LEVY and CHOU 1974). Pepstatin is an inhibitor of carboxyl proteases and chymostatin inhibits chymotrypsin-like proteases (UMEZAWA and AOYAGI 1977). These inhibitors are thought to be rather specific, so it is unusual that each was able to inhibit the parasite protease. These compounds also inhibited the protease from *P. knowlesi* and *P. falciparum*, as well as the enzyme from ghosts of the host red cells (LEVY et al. 1974). Again pepstatin was the most effective, suggesting that the protease involved is a carboxyl protease. Interestingly, pepstatin completely inhibited the acid protease ghosts of uninfected rhesus monkey red cells at concentrations of less than 0.8 ng/ml. The unusual sensitivity to inhibitors, as well as similarities in other products, suggest that the red cell and the parasite proteases are either identical or closely resemble one another.

More recently, CHARET et al. (1980) have reported the presence of an aminopeptidase in two species of rodent parasite, *P. yoelii* and *P. chabaudi*. This enzyme could degrade several short peptides, as well as the nitroanalide derivatives of several amino acids. The enzyme was sensitive to several antimalarials, including chloroquine (1 mM), mepacrine (0.1 mM) and primaquine (1 mM). Quinine had little effect.

The distribution of enzymes between red cell ghosts and parasites has been studied (Levy, unpublished data). While acetylcholinesterase and acid phosphatase were approximately equally distributed between the two, 60%–80% of the acid protease, acid RNase and DNase activities were in the parasite fraction. Over 85%

of the administered [$^{14}$C]-chloroquine appeared in the parasite fraction as well. Chloroquine treatment did not affect either the distribution or the specific activity of acid phosphatase, RNase or protease. The protease appeared to be present in a lysosome-like particle as enzyme, in particulate fractions obtained from parasites, exhibited a 50%–60% latency, even under the acidic conditions required for the assay.

## 2. Inhibition of Macromolecular Synthesis

The effects of various protease inhibitors on macromolecular synthesis of *Plasmodium* have been studied (LEVY and CHOU 1975). When *P. berghei*-infected mouse red cells were incubated with pepstatin for 4 h, there was an inhibition of incorporation of [$^{14}$C]-isoleucine into parasite protein. However, these results were variable and, in some experiments, pepstatin was without effect. Incorporation of orotic acid into RNA was also inhibited. Chymostatin, which is also a potent inhibitor of the protease, had little effect, while PMSF essentially completely inhibited incorporation of label into protein. Leupeptin, while not as potent an inhibitor of the parasite acid protease as pepstatin, inhibited incorporation of precursor into both RNA and protein of the infected red cells (LEVY et al. 1976). It also prevented the release of free amino acids, indicating that it was acting to prevent haemoglobin breakdown. The presence of a mixture of 15 amino acids did not overcome the inhibition.

Leupeptin and PMSF were also able to inhibit RNA and protein synthesis in parasites in monkey red cells infected with either *P. falciparum* (*Aotus* monkeys) or *P. knowlesi* (rhesus monkeys). Pepstatin and chymostatin, which are extremely potent inhibitors of the parasite protease, were without effect.

Several inhibitors of the parasite protease were tested for effects on parasitaemia in cultured infected cells (LEVY et al. 1976). Red cells from rhesus monkeys that had been infected with *P. knowlesi,* when cultured for 24 h in vitro showed a three fold increase in parasitaemia. Pepstatin (0.1–10 µg/ml) inhibited this increase by 35%–55%, while leupeptin (100 µg/ml) actually caused a marked decrease in parasitaemia. It is not known if the inhibition is due to an inability of the parasites to degrade haemoglobin, or to an inhibition of penetration of parasites into uninfected red cells. Injection of several of the protease inhibitors into mice infected with *P. berghei* did not prevent the development of parasitaemia.

Chloroquine and mepacrine both inhibited incorporation of precursors into protein and RNA in *P. berghei*-infected red cells incubated for 4 h in vitro. Mepcrine was the most effective, as 12.5 µg/ml inhibited protein synthesis by over 90%. Ten times as much chloroquine was required to produce the same effect. Interestingly, protein synthesis in cells infected with a chloroquine-resistant strain of *P. berghei* was equally sensitive to the drug (LEVY, unpublished data). Many of the protease inhibitors tested affected RNA synthesis even more effectively than they did protein synthesis. This was the case for chloroquine as well. In some cases, incorporation of label into RNA essentially stopped after 2 h. That this effect was not secondary to an inhibition of protein synthesis per se is indicated by the fact that the concentration of cycloheximide that inhibited protein synthesis by 75% had little effect on RNA synthesis.

## V. Summary

It seems clear that the cellular effects of antimalarial drugs such as chloroquine are quite complex. While early studies tended to concentrate on effects of these agents on various enzymes, it seems apparent that chloroquine can influence various cellular processes such as delivery of enzymes and receptors to their appropriate intracellular sites, the processing and degradation of intra- and extracellular materials, and the recycling of membrane proteins. Such observations should help to direct studies on the modes of action of antimalarial drugs on the parasites.

# B. Protozoa Other than *Plasmodium*

K. A. CONKLIN and S-C. CHOU

## I. Introduction

Protozoa have been extensively used as pharmacological and toxicological tools. The applicability of these organisms for screening chemotherapeutic agents, for investigating the mechanism of action or toxicity of drugs and for other pharmacological and related usages has been reviewed and documented by many authors (HUTNER 1964; HUTNER et al. 1968; JIROVEC 1963; KAVANAGH 1963).

In malaria research, protozoan models have provided a means to study antimalarials when other systems were not readily available. Indeed, paramecia and amoebae were utilised to study the action of quinine (BINZ 1867a, b) even before the discovery of the parasites that cause malaria by LAVERAN in 1880. However, other more recent work has shown the utility of protozoan models to screen for antimalarial activity and to investigate mechanisms of action of antimalarial drugs. The rationale for the use of these model systems instead of *Plasmodium* spp. includes the greater ease in culturing many protozoa, the shorter generation time of some protozoa which makes possible more rapid screening and the greater safety compared with the use of plasmodia which may infect humans.

## II. Experimental Models

The use of protozoan models for investigating antimalarial drugs encompasses three areas: (a) the use of parasitic or non-parasitic protozoa to screen for antimalarial activity, which involves the use of parasitised animals or free-living organisms in culture medium; (b) use in investigating the mechanism of action of antimalarial drugs, which generally involves the use of free-living organisms and subcellular preparations from the organisms; and (c) the testing of drugs with known antimalarial activity for potential use in the treatment of parasitic diseases other than malaria. With respect to this latter use, we will present only those investigations utilizing the free parasites in culture, but will not consider clinical trials.

### 1. Historical Notes

The use of protozoa and other microorganisms to investigate the action of antimalarial drugs preceded by several years the identification of the malaria parasites and the establishment of these organisms as causative agents of intermittent fever. In his classical works, BINZ (1867 a, b) demonstrated that quinine, in low concentrations, inhibits the movement of many protozoa by blocking the activity of cilia and flagella, and by inhibiting pseudopod formation. He showed that quinine kills *Paramecium* and numerous other microorganisms and that the amount of time it takes for cell lysis is dependent upon the drug concentration used. In organisms killed by quinine, he also noted the formation of black granules in the cytoplasm as well as darkening of the nucleus. Finally, he noted effects on pseudopod formation in human white blood cells similar to those observed in *Amoeba*. Indeed, the use of these protozoan test systems may actually have paved the way for identifying plasmodia and their relationship to malaria, as BINZ (1867 a) stated that the findings (i.e. that quinine kills *Paramecium*) might have some bearing on the nature of intermittent fever. If we interpret this statement to suggest a protozoan aetiology for malaria, the subsequent discovery of the intracellular protozoan parasites of the genus *Plasmodium* by LAVERAN (1880) may have been guided by his comments.

### 2. *Haemoproteus orizivorae*

During the search for reproducible antimalarial test systems, FOURNEAU et al. (1931) introduced *Haemoproteus orizivorae* to malaria drug testing. In this parasite of the Java rice bird, schizogony occurs in the endothelial cells of capillaries. The merozoites are released into the circulation and either enter erythrocytes, in which they develop into gametocytes, or re-enter endothelial cells to carry out further schizogony. FOURNEAU initially used this system to test for gametocytocidal activity, and later KIKUTH (1932, 1935) utilised the model to test for both schizontocidal and gametocytocidal activity. As discussed by PETERS (1970), *Haemoproteus* lost favour probably due to the introduction of *Plasmodium gallinaceum* as a model system for malaria chemotherapy.

### 3. Trypanosomes

*Crithidia fasciculata,* a flagellated protozoan of the parasitic family Trypanosomatidae, has been widely used as a model system for studying drug action (GOTTLIEB et al. 1972). This organism can be grown in bulk in defined medium and therefore lends itself to in vitro drug testing. Although it has been utilised primarily to investigate trypanocidal drugs, *C. fasciculata* requires an exogenous source of folic acid (as do plasmodia) and was investigated by NATHAN and COWPERTHWAITE (1954) as a possible system for preliminary evaluation of antifolate antimalarials. They investigated the growth inhibiting ability of three substituted 2,4-diaminopyrimidines on *C. fasciculata* grown in defined media, and suggested that this test system was superior to bacterial systems for determining potential antimalarial activity. They also demonstrated that quinine and mepacrine antagonise neither folic nor folinic acid in this test system, thus confirming that these agents interfere with a pathway other than that involving folic acid. *C. fasciculata* has also been used to screen other substituted diaminopyridines for antiprotozoal activity by measuring growth inhibition (MARKEES et al. 1968). Mepacrine, a trypanocidal as well as antimalarial drug, has also been shown to inhibit respiration of intact *C. fascicu-*

*lata,* and to inhibit succinic dehydrogenase activity and respiration of a mitochondrial preparation from this organism (HILL and HUTNER 1968). The effects of mepacrine in these systems, however, is less than that of other trypanocides.

Finally, another lower trypanosomatid, *Leptomonas,* has also been used to study several antiprotozoal drugs including antimalarials (GOLDBERG et al. 1974). Investigating growth inhibition and inhibition of respiration of intact cells and a particulate fraction, they demonstrated the sensitivity of the system to trypanocides. This trypanosome, however, proved not to be a satisfactory test system for antimalarials as neither mepacrine nor primaquine inhibited growth of this organism.

## 4. Amoebae

Many pathogenic and non-pathogenic amoebae have been used to study antimalarial drugs. BINZ (1867 b), of course, was the first to use non-pathogenic strains to study the effects of quinine. Others, however, have more recently used several strains of non-pathogenic amoebae to study antimalarials. HAWKINS and HAINTON (1972) demonstrated that chloroquine, 30 μg/ml, reduces the growth rate of *Amoeba proteus,* and in concentrations of 50 μg/ml and above kills these organisms after 2–3 days' exposure. The growth rate of *A. discoides* is much less affected. They also noted that both strains become flattened in appearance. PRASAD (1972) also investigated the effects of three antimalarials, mepacrine, chloroquine, and amodiaquine, on several strains of non-pathogenic amoebae. He found the free-living organisms *Schizopyrenus russelli, Naegleria gruberi, Didasculus thorntoni,* and *Tetramitus rostratus* to be insensitive to chloroquine in concentrations as high as 1 000 μg/ml, and were nearly as insensitive to amodiaquine. Mepacrine, however, in concentrations of 250–500 μg/ml, is amoebicidal to the first two parasites whereas the latter two are sensitive to concentrations of this drug as low as 31 μg/ml. PRASAD (1972) also demonstrated that the non-pathogenic *Entamoeba moshkovskii* and *E. invadens* (which is pathogenic only to reptiles) are sensitive to 62 μg/ml of mepacrine, whereas 1 000 μg/ml of chloroquine is non-amoebicidal to these organisms. Amodiaquine, at a concentration of 250 μg/ml, was found to be amoebicidal only against *E. invadens.*

Certain strains of the free-living amoebae of the genera *Naegleria* and *Hartmannella,* which have been associated with meningoencephalitis in humans and animals, have also been shown to be sensitive to antimalarials. Mepacrine, chloroquine, and amodiaquine, in concentrations of 16–125 μg/ml, are amoebicidal to *N. aerobia, H. culbertsoni* and *H. rhysodes* (PRASAD 1972). These effects are similar to those observed with comparable concentrations of emetine, a known amoebicide. CARTER (1969) demonstrated that quinine, 3.2 μg/ml, also has an immobilising effect on a pathogenic *Naegleria* sp. CASEMORE (1970), however, demonstrated only morphological changes in six strains of *H. castellanii* by chloroquine, 100 μg/ml, and no effect on these amoebae by the antifolate antimalarial, pyrimethamine (at 100 μg/ml).

*Entameoba histolytica,* the causative organism of amoebic dysentery, has also been evaluated for its sensitivity to antimalarial drugs. GORDEEVA (1965) showed that chloroquine causes decreased motility, rounding, and the formation of pycnotic nuclei in this organism. Both chloroquine (CONAN 1948; NEAL 1978) and mepacrine (DUTTA and YADAVA 1972; PRASAD 1972) were found to be amoebicidal when used singly against *E. histolytica,* although their potency was much less than that of emetine. The effect of chloroquine used singly, however, is controversial as DUTTA and YADAVA (1972) and PRASAD (1972) did not observe amoebicidal activity at a drug concentration of 1 000 μg/ml. Chloroquine (50–200 μg/ml), however, does appear to be an effective amoebicide when tested (in vitro) in combination with other amoebicidal drugs (NEAL 1978; YADAVA and DUTTA 1973).

### 5. *Tetrahymena pyriformis*

One of the many important protozoan models for biological research has been one or other member of the genus *Tetrahymena.* These ciliate protozoa have shown great value as tools for nutritional, pharmacological, and toxicological research (CORLISS 1965; HILL 1972a; HUTNER et al. 1973). *Tetrahymena* has been used extensively to investigate the mechanism of action of antimalarials utilising intact cells, and subcellular organelles and cell-free systems prepared from this organism. Its popularity as a test system is probably accounted for by the ease of culturing this free-living protozoan, its short generation time and its non-pathogenicity.

#### a) Studies Using Intact Cells; Effects on Cell Division

*Tetrahymena pyriformis* can be grown in defined medium, undefined but axenic medium, or medium that contains bacteria as a food source (HILL 1972b). Generally, studies of drug effects on intact cells are carried out in undefined but axenic medium which supports rapid growth of this organism (generation time of approximately 3 h). Effects of antimalarial drugs on cell growth and division are normally determined with cultures of cells in rapid logarithmic growth phase. This organism, however, has the further advantage that its cell division can be synchronised, which allows for drug testing when all cells are in the same growth phase. The technique most commonly employed is that of heat synchronisation (SCHERBAUM and ZEUTHEN 1954), which involves alternating exposure of the cells to 34 °C and 29 °C (for most strains), each for 30 min. The procedure involves seven consecutive temperature cycles, and is followed by division of nearly all cells 80 min after the last heat treatment. Division of heat-synchronised cells (which are considerably larger than logarithmic phase cells) will also continue for several generations in completely inorganic medium. This may also provide a certain benefit over other free-living organisms for drug testing, as binding to protein components of growth medium may interfere with drug activity.

The first use of *T. pyriformis* (*T. geleii*) as a test system for antimalarial drugs was by GROUPE (1945). He demonstrated that mepacrine in a concentration of 100 μg/ml is lethal to all cells, whereas the drug at 50 μg/ml completely inhibits cell division. Some cells, however, are still motile after 24 h of exposure to the lower drug concentration.

CLANCY (1968) also found mepacrine and several other antimalarials (chloroquine, primaquine, proguanil, and quinine) to be lethal to *T. pyriformis* in logarithmic growth phase (Table 1). He tested serial dilutions of each of the drugs for their ability to inhibit motility of the organism grown both at room temperature for 48 h (48 h RT) and at 37 °C for 1 h followed by room temperature for 48 h (37 °C/RT).

**Table 1.** Lethal effect of antimalarial drugs on *Tetrahymena pyriformis* W. Adapted from CLANCY (1968)

| Drug | Average minimum lethal concentration (μg/ml) | |
|---|---|---|
| | 48-h RT [a] | 37 °C/RT [b] |
| Mepacrine | 17 | 3 |
| Chloroquine | 1,475 | 79 |
| Primaquine [c] | 150 | 83 |
| | 163 | 80 |
| | 113 | 88 |
| | 113 | 88 |
| Proguanil | 90 | 49 |
| Quinine | 220 | 104 |

[a] Drugs tested for 48 h at room temperature
[b] Drugs tested for 1 h at 37 °C followed by 48 h at room temperature
[c] The values for primaquine designate the average lethal concentrations for preparations of the drug from four different sources

**Table 2.** Effect of antimalarial drugs on cell division in heat-synchronised cultures of *Tetrahymena pyriformis* GL. Adapted from CONKLIN and CHOU (1972a)

| Drug | Concentration ($mol/l \times 10^4$) | Cell division (percent of control) [a] |
|---|---|---|
| Quinine | 1.3 | 52 |
| | 2.5 | 15 |
| | 5.0 | 0 |
| Chloroquine | 3.5 | 68 |
| | 7.0 | 21 |
| | 14.0 | 0 |
| Primaquine | 1.8 | 53 |
| | 2.7 | 11 |
| | 5.4 | 0 |
| Mepacrine | 0.12 | 57 |
| | 0.18 | 7 |
| | 0.36 | 0 |

[a] The drug was added at the end of the heat synchronisation procedure, and cell division (compared with the control) was determined at 120 min

Drugs from different sources were also tested. The values in Table 1 are the average drug concentrations which completely inhibited motility. Mepacrine was by far the most potent drug tested at both temperatures. At room temperature, quinine, primaquine, and proguanil had comparable lethal effects, but less than that of mepacrine. Chloroquine, at room temperature, was much less active than the other drugs, although in tests at 37 °C its potency was similar to that of quinine, primaquine, and proguanil. All drugs were more potent at the higher temperature.

Antimalarial drugs also inhibit division of heat-synchronised cultures of *T. pyriformis* (CHOU et al. 1968; CONKLIN et al. 1969; CONKLIN and CHOU 1972a) as shown in Table 2. The effects of quinine and primaquine are similar in that 100% inhibition of cell division was observed at concentrations of approximately $5 \times 10^{-4}$ *M*. Mepacrine is significantly more potent in that complete inhibition was observed at $3.6 \times 10^{-5}$ *M*. The effect of chloroquine is less than that of the other drugs, requiring a drug concentration of $1.4 \times 10^{-3}$ *M* to inhibit cell division completely. This difference betwen chloroquine and the other antimalarial drugs, however, is not as great as that observed by CLANCY (1968).

Finally, MARKEES et al. (1968) has also used inhibition of cell division of *T. pyriformis* as a measure of antiprotozoal activity of substituted diaminopyridines.

b) Studies Using Intact Cells; Effects on Macromolecular Synthesis

Heat-synchronised and logarithmic-phase *T. pyriformis* actively incorporates exogenous precursors into nucleic acids, protein, and lipids. Studies with antimalarials, however, have been performed primarily with heat-synchronised cells in an inorganic medium, using $^{3}H$- or $^{14}C$-labelled macromolecular precursors.

The antimalarial drugs inhibit uptake and incorporation of precursors into nucleic acids and protein by intact cells. CHOU and RAMANATHAN (1968) demonstrated that mepacrine, at concentrations which inhibit cell division, inhibits incorporation of precursors (thymidine, uracil or uridine, and amino acids, respectively) into DNA, RNA, and protein. Subsequent studies (CONKLIN et al. 1969; CONKLIN and CHOU 1970, 1972a) also showed the inhibitory effect of mepacrine on these processes, and demonstrated that quinine, chloroquine, and primaquine have similar effects. The latter studies (CONKLIN and CHOU 1970, 1972a), however, showed that the degree of inhibition of precursor incorporation (into nucleic acids and protein) by quinine, chloroquine, and primaquine is the same or similar to the degree of inhibition of precursor uptake into the cell (Table 3). The degrees of inhibition of amino acid uptake and incorporation by mepacrine are also similar. These results were different from those observed with mepacrine (for thymidine and uridine), and with drugs that directly inhibit DNA, RNA, and protein synthesis (nalidixic acid, actinomycin D, and cycloheximide, respectively). Exposure of *T. pyriformis* to these drugs results in much greater inhibition of precursor incorporation than of precursor uptake. These data showed that direct inhibition of macromolecular synthesis results in much less inhibition of precursor uptake than incorporation, and suggested that mepacrine directly inhibits DNA and RNA synthesis. The results also suggested that the effects of quinine, chloroquine, and primaquine on precursor incorporation into nucleic acids and protein, and the effect of mepacrine on amino acid incorporation, may be secondary to inhibition of precursor uptake. To test this hypothesis, the effects of these antimalarial drugs on precursor uptake was investigated in cells in which DNA, RNA or protein synthesis was blocked by specific inhibitors (nalidixic acid, actinomycin D, and cycloheximide, respectively) of these processes. The results (CONKLIN and CHOU 1972a) demonstrated that in the absence of macromolecular synthesis, quinine, chloroquine, and primaquine inhibit uptake of thymidine, uridine, and amino acids, and that mepacrine inhibits uptake of amino acids (Table 4). It was concluded from

**Table 3.** Inhibition of precursor uptake and incorporation in synchronised cultures of *Tetrahymena pyriformis* GL. Adapted from CONKLIN and CHOU (1970, 1972a)

| Drug [a] | Precursor [b] | Percent inhibition [c] | |
|---|---|---|---|
| | | Uptake | Incorporation |
| Quinine | Thymidine | 47.0 ± 1.8 | 46.5 ± 1.2 [d] |
| Chloroquine | | 20.0 ± 2.4 | 27.3 ± 5.3 [d] |
| Primaquine | | 61.6 ± 0.8 | 67.9 ± 2.6 |
| Mepacrine | | 3.0 ± 0.8 | 22.9 ± 2.1 |
| Nalidixic acid | | 33.2 ± 2.1 | 51.7 ± 4.2 |
| Quinine | Uridine | 63.7 ± 1.0 | 63.7 ± 1.4 [d] |
| Chloroquine | | 42.0 ± 1.2 | 53.3 ± 1.7 |
| Primaquine | | 82.5 ± 0.8 | 87.5 ± 0.4 |
| Mepacrine | | 24.3 ± 0.7 | 42.8 ± 1.0 |
| Actinomycin D | | 42.6 ± 0.7 | 85.4 ± 0.7 |
| Quinine | Amino acids | 68.6 ± 2.1 | 73.0 ± 2.0 [d] |
| Chloroquine | | 75.6 ± 2.6 | 76.0 ± 3.5 [d] |
| Primaquine | | 57.8 ± 1.6 | 57.7 ± 4.4 [d] |
| Mepacrine | | 27.8 ± 0.8 | 30.2 ± 1.0 [d] |
| Cycloheximide | | 48.9 ± 0.9 | 95.5 ± 0.7 |

[a] Drug concentrations: quinine, $2.5 \times 10^{-4} M$; chloroquine, $7.0 \times 10^{-4} M$; primaquine, $2.7 \times 10^{-4} M$; mepacrine, $1.8 \times 10^{-5} M$; nalidixic acid, $8.5 \times 10^{-4} M$; actinomycin D, $4.0 \times 10^{-5} M$; cycloheximide, $5.0 \times 10^{-6} M$

[b] Precursors were, $^{14}C$-labelled. The amino acid mixture (algal profile) was a uniformly labelled preparation

[c] Mean ± SE compared with control after 80 min of incubation

[d] $P$ for uptake versus incorporation $> 0.05$

**Table 4.** Inhibition of macromolecular precursor uptake in synchronised cultures of *Tetrahymena pyriformis* GL in which precursor incorporation is blocked.[a] Calculated from data of CONKLIN and CHOU (1972a)

| Drug [b] | Percent inhibition of precursor uptake [c] | | |
|---|---|---|---|
| | Thymidine | Uridine | Amino acids |
| Quinine | 61 | 42 | 49 |
| Chloroquine | 19 | 26 | 59 |
| Primaquine | 69 | 66 | 29 |
| Mepacrine | 0 | 1 | 32 |

[a] Precursor incorporation was blocked by addition of nalidixic acid (for thymidine) actinomycin D (for uridine) or cyclohexamide (for amino acids)

[b] Drug concentrations: quinine, $2.5 \times 10^{-4} M$; chloroquine, $7.0 \times 10^{-4} M$; primaquine, $2.7 \times 10^{-4} M$; mepacrine, $1.8 \times 10^{-5} M$

[c] Mean percent inhibition ± SE compared with control after 60 min incubation. Precursors were $^{14}C$-labelled. The amino acid mixture (algal profile) was a uniformly labelled preparation

these studies that inhibition of precursor incorporation by quinine, chloroquine, and primaquine, and inhibition of amino acid incorporation by mepacrine were due, at least in part, to inhibition of precursor uptake by the cell.

Other studies with intact cells also demonstrated that the above four antimalarial drugs inhibit the incorporation of acetate into lipids of *T. pyriformis* (CHOU and RAMANATHAN 1968; CONKLIN et al. 1969). These results were interpreted to show inhibition of the cellular energy generating systems, and thus another potential site of drug action. The inhibition of energetics could also account for the inhibition of precursor incorporation into nucleic acids and protein since an energy source is necessary for nucleoside phosphorylation and amino acid activation.

These studies of antimalarial action on intact cells do provide information as to potential sites of action. However, the information is limited in that it cannot identify the exact intracellular site of drug action. For example, several mechanisms could explain the inhibition by antimalarial drugs of precursor incorporation into nucleic acids of intact cells. These mechanisms include inhibition of (a) uptake of the nucleosides thymidine and uridine by the cell (as suggested by CONKLIN and CHOU 1972a), (b) phosphorylation of the nucleosides to the nucleoside triphosphates, (c) transport of the nucleoside triphosphates into the nucleus or (d) the DNA and RNA polymerase reactions. Also, as mentioned above, the phosphorylation reactions and possibly the transport mechanisms for the precursors are dependent upon an energy source, so that inhibition of cellular energetics would also block precursor incorporation. Similarly, inhibition of amino acid incorporation could be due to inhibition of amino acid transport or activation, or an effect on cellular energetics. Therefore, elucidation of the exact site of drug action requires the use of subcellular systems.

c) Studies Using Subcellular Organelles

Intact and functional nuclei (LEE and SCHERBAUM 1965; CONKLIN and CHOU 1972b) and mitochondria (CONKLIN and CHOU 1972c) from *T. pyriformis* have been isolated and characterised as to functional capabilities and requirements. These organelles provide an excellent means of evaluating the effects of antimalarial drugs on individual cellular processes.

Nuclei isolated from *T. pyriformis* have been used to investigate the effect of antimalarial drugs on nucleic acid synthesis (CONKLIN and CHOU 1972b; CONKLIN et al. 1973). Nucleoside triphosphates were used to assay DNA and RNA synthesis, thus allowing for determination of the direct effects of the drugs on the nucleic acid polymerase reactions (Table 5). The effects of quinine and primaquine are similar in this assay system in that drug concentrations which inhibit cell division and precursor incorporation in intact cells (Tables 2, 3) do not produce a marked inhibition of DNA or RNA synthesis. Chloroquine, however, is a potent inhibitor of DNA synthesis in isolated nuclei but, as with the two other antimalarials, it produced little inhibition of RNA synthesis. These results suggest that inhibition of DNA synthesis accounts, at least in part for the action of chloroquine, but not quinine or primaquine. Also, direct inhibition of RNA synthesis does not appear to play a significant role in the activity of any of these three drugs.

Mitochondrial preparations have also been used to investigate the mechanism of action of antimalarial drugs. EICHEL (1956), using a cell-free homogenate of *T.*

**Table 5.** Inhibition of DNA and RNA synthesis in nuclei isolated from *Tetrahymena pyriformis* GL. Adapted from CONKLIN et al. (1973)

| Drug | Concentration (mol/l × $10^4$) | Percent inhibition [a] | |
|---|---|---|---|
| | | DNA synthesis | RNA synthesis |
| Quinine | 2.5 | 14 | 2 |
| | 5.0 | 24 | 8 |
| Chloroquine | 7.0 | 60 | 4 |
| | 14.0 | 81 | 11 |
| Primaquine | 2.7 | 18 | 7 |
| | 5.4 | 26 | 14 |

[a] Percent inhibition (compared with control) of radioactivity incorporated from (methyl-[$^3$H]-thymidine 5′-triphosphate (DNA synthesis) or 5-[$^3$H]-uridine 5′-triphosphate (RNA synthesis)

*pyriformis*, demonstrated that mepacrine ($7.2 \times 10^{-3}$ *M*) and quinine ($2.0 \times 10^{-3}$ *M*) markedly inhibit succinic acid oxidation. The inhibition by mepacrine could also be overcome by adding flavin mononucleotide. CONKLIN et al. (1971) also investigated the effect of antimalarial drugs on energetics of *T. pyriformis* mitochondria which were isolated and partially purified. They demonstrated that primaquine and chloroquine, at concentrations which completely inhibit cell division, stimulate oxidation of succinate and inhibit oxidative phosphorylation. These results suggest that these drugs act as uncoupling agents, and that this activity requires the quinoline nucleus and the diamino-alkane side chain common to these two drugs since quinine (which contains only the quinoline nucleus) and mepacrine (which contains only the side chain) did not affect succinate oxidation or oxidative phosphorylation. Primaquine, chloroquine, and quinine also inhibit oxidation of fumarate, malate, β-hydroxybutyrate, and glutamate, which indicates a direct inhibition of the enzyme systems which oxidise these substrates. The pattern of inhibition was similar and may be due to the quinoline moiety common to these three drugs. Mepacrine, at a concentration higher than that which inhibits synchronised cell division, has no significant effect on oxidation of any of the substrates. The difference between the results of these authors and those of EICHEL (1956), for quinine and mepacrine, is probably accounted for by the lower drug concentrations used by CONKLIN et al. (1971).

### d) Studies Using Cell-Free Systems

The effects of antimalarial drugs on macromolecular synthesis in cell-free systems from *T. pyriformis* have also been studied. CONKLIN and CHOU (1970) demonstrated that quinine, chloroquine, primaquine, and mepacrine, in concentrations that block uptake and incorporation of amino acids in intact cells, do not inhibit protein synthesis in a cell-free preparation. These results support the conclusion (CONKLIN and CHOU 1972a) that the in vivo effect of these antimalarial drugs is due to inhibition of amino acid uptake by the cell, and not due to direct inhibition of protein synthesis.

**Table 6.** Inhibition of DNA and RNA synthesis of solubilised DNA and RNA polymerases from *Tetrahymena pyriformis* GL. Adapted from CONKLIN et al. (1973)

| Drug | Concentration (mol/l × $10^4$) | Percent inhibition [a] | |
|---|---|---|---|
| | | DNA synthesis | RNA synthesis |
| Quinine | 2.5 | 1 | 2 |
| | 5.0 | 0 | 9 |
| Primaquine | 2.7 | 0 | 22 |
| | 5.4 | 0 | 25 |
| Chloroquine | 7.0 | 34 | 56 |
| | 14.0 | 67 | 73 |

[a] Percent inhibition (compared with control) of radioactivity incorporated from methyl-[$^3$H]-thymidine 5′-triphosphate (DNA synthesis) or 5-[$^3$H]-uridine 5′-triphosphate (RNA synthesis)

Solubilised and partially purified DNA and RNA polymerases from *T. pyriformis* have also been used to elucidate further the effects of antimalarial drugs on nucleic acid synthesis. CONKLIN et al. (1973) demonstrated that quinine and primaquine, at concentrations which inhibit cell division and nucleic acid precursor incorporation in vivo, have relatively little effect on DNA or RNA synthesis by the solubilised polymerases (Table 6). They concluded that the effects of these two antimalarial drugs in *T. pyriformis* is not due to inhibition of nucleic acid synthesis, and that the drugs possess another mechanism for blocking nucleic acid precursor incorporation in intact cells (e.g. inhibition of precursor uptake as suggested by CONKLIN and CHOU 1972a). Chloroquine, however, was shown to inhibit markedly DNA and RNA synthesis by the polymerases (Table 6), indicating that inhibition of nucleic acid synthesis probably accounts, in part, for the effects of this drug on *T. pyriformis*. For DNA synthesis, this result is consistent with the results using isolated nuclei.

Finally, antimalarial effects on lipid synthesis have also been investigated in cell-free preparations from *T. pyriformis*. Chloroquine and primaquine, at concentrations which block cell division, inhibit incorporation of acetate into all classes of lipids (PAN et al. 1974). These authors suggested that the inhibition of lipid synthesis could lead to alteration of membrane formation or function, and thus contribute to the inhibition of cell division and macromolecular precursor uptake. The inhibition of lipid synthesis could also account for the inhibition of acetate incorporation in intact cells (CHOU and RAMANATHAN 1968; CONKLIN et al. 1969). Quinine and mepacrine, however, do not significantly inhibit lipid synthesis in this cell-free system.

## 6. Other Protozoa

*Paramecium,* although not extensively used for drug testing, was shown by BINZ (1867a) to be sensitive to quinine. NEAL (1963) has also demonstrated the sensitivity of *Chilomonas paramecium* to 8-aminoquinolines, showing the potential usefulness of this organism for antimalarial testing. Finally, *Eimeria brunetti* may be of value for investigating antimalarial drugs as BULLOCK (1968) noted comparable coccidiostat and antimalarial activity for naphthoquinones between this organism and various *Plasmodium* species.

## III. Conclusion

Protozoa have provided useful models to investigate antimalarial drugs. Although their current usefulness may be limited due to the availability of reproducible in vitro culture techniques for *Plasmodium* species, their role in the progress of malaria research has been invaluable. The work of BINZ (1867a, b), which may have provided insight to the causality of intermittent fever, and that of others who utilised protozoa to screen antimalarials, has demonstrated the value of these models to clinical malariology.

Knowledge of the mechanisms of action of antimalarial drugs has also been furthered by the use of protozoan model systems. The use of many test systems (*Paramecium,* amoebae, trypanosomes, and *Tetrahymena pyriformis*) demonstrated the growth-inhibiting effect of these antiprotozoal agents. However, insight to the cellular and subcellular sites of drug action has also been provided, and most extensively by the use of the free-living ciliate protozoan *T. pyriformis*. These studies, utilising intact cells, subcellular organelles and cell-free systems, have provided considerable information as to the sites of action of four antimalarial drugs, three of which have current therapeutic value (quinine, chloroquine, and primaquine) and one of which (mepacrine) is primarily of historical interest for malaria chemotherapy. The effects of these agents on *T. pyriformis* can be summarised as follows:

1. Quinine, which inhibits cell division and incorporation of macromolecular precursors in intact cells, does not inhibit markedly DNA, RNA or protein synthesis in subcellular preparations. Since this agent inhibits precursor uptake by intact cells and substrate oxidation in mitochondria, its primary sites of action may be at the cell membrane and on mitochondrial energetics.

2. The effects of primaquine are qualitatively similar to those of quinine, except it also inhibits in vitro lipid synthesis and acts as an uncoupler of oxidative phosphorylation. Therefore, the primary sites of action of primaquine may also be at the cell membrane (membrane formation and transport functions) and on mitochondrial energetics.

3. Chloroquine, with effects on intact cells similar to quinine and primaquine, also inhibits nucleic acid synthesis by isolated nuclei (DNA synthesis only) and by the solubilised DNA and RNA polymerases. As precursor uptake, mitochondrial energetics and in vitro lipid synthesis were also inhibited by chloroquine, this antimalarial may have multiple mechanisms of action including direct inhibition of nucleic acid synthesis, effects on membrane formation and precursor transport, and effects on cellular energy generating systems.

4. Finally, we will consider the site of action of mepacrine, a drug which is known to interact with isolated DNA (HAHN et al. 1966; KURNICK and RADCLIFFE 1962; LERMAN 1961) and to inhibit synthesis of nucleic acids in *Plasmodium* species (LANTZ and VAN DYKE 1971; SCHELLENBERG and COATNEY 1961; VAN DYKE et al. 1969, 1970; VAN DYKE and SZUSTKIEWICZ 1969). This drug inhibits cell division

and synthesis of DNA and RNA in nuclei isolated from *T. pyriformis*, but has little effect on the uptake of nucleic acid precursors, mitochondrial energetics or in vitro lipid synthesis. These results demonstrate two things: a) the site of action of this drug is on DNA, a finding which may be of little significance in the light of the plethora of existing scientific literature about mepacrine and other acridines; b) more importantly, however, they demonstrate that the drug effects on *T. pyriformis* are the same as those observed in *Plasmodium*, the target organism for the clinical use of mepacrine. These results therefore, support the use of this protozoan test system to obtain valid information concerning the mechanism of action of chemotherapeutic agents.

## C. Drug-Induced Clumping Test

D. C. WARHURST

### I. Introduction

Drug-induced pigment clumping and its inhibition form a model for the study of antimalarial action which has not been widely used, in spite of its many advantages. It cannot be said to be truly a "surrogate" system, since clumping has been found to occur in all species of malaria tested, and is considered in this chapter only for convenience.

Following treatment with mepacrine, a new synthetic 9-aminoacridine (Fig. 1), intraerythrocytic forms of *Plasmodium vivax* were noted by JAMES (1934) first to develop aggregated pigment, and then to lose pigment entirely. BOCK (1939) found in *P. vivax*, *P. malariae*, and *P. ovale* treated with mepacrine that the first effect was an aggregation of pigment into one or more large clumps, as found normally in mature schizonts. BOCK and OESTERLIN (1938, 1939) found that this pigment clumping was preceded by a marked concentration of mepacrine into the intraerythrocytic stages of *P. inui* and *P. knowlesi*, as early as 10 min after administration of the drug. TATE and VINCENT (1934) found that, like quinine (which does not cause pigment-clumping), mepacrine was ineffective against tissue stages of malaria, and this was further emphasised by TONKIN'S (1946) observations on exoerythrocytic stages of *P. gallinaceum* in duck spleen explants in vitro.

THOMPSON et al. (1948) were able to show in *P. gallinaceum* that chloroquine (Fig. 1), the 4-aminoquinoline successor to mepacrine, had markedly similar morphological effects, the earliest being a clumping together of pigment granules. THURSTON (1952) also noted the peculiar morphological effects of chloroquine on *P. berghei* and, with the increasing use of electron microscopy, the ultrastructural

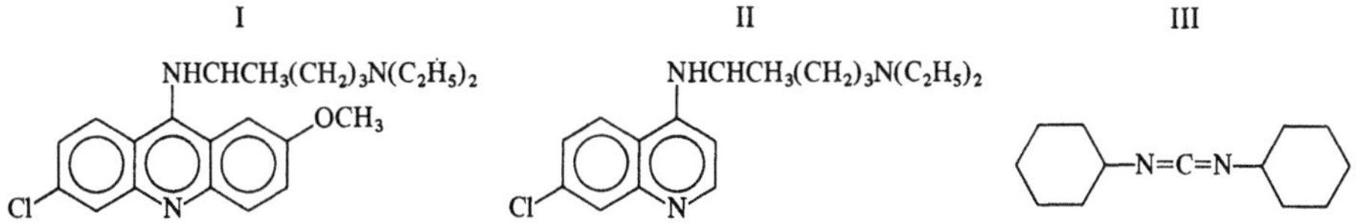


**Fig. 1.** Chemical structures. *I*, mepacrine; *II*, chloroquine; *III*, dicyclohexylcarbodiimide

details of the process began to be revealed (MACOMBER et al. 1967, *P. berghei;* WARHURST and HOCKLEY 1967, *P. berghei* and *P. cynomolgi*). The pigment granules in a growing intraerythrocytic malaria trophozoite such as *P. berghei* are localised in many small digestive vesicles, each one having been pinched off from a cytostomal vesicle containing ingested haemoglobin. The granules themselves, which are crystalline and electron-dense, are composed in part from the iron porphyrin haemin, a degradation product of haemoglobin (YAMADA and SHERMAN 1979). Within 80–120 min of the administration of chloroquine the pigment vesicles were found to be damaged and enclosed in a large vacuole which contained pigment crystals, haemoglobin, membranes, and ribosomal masses clearly derived from the cytoplasm. The similarity to autophagic vacuoles found in mammalian cells after various treatments (e.g. DE DUVE and WATTIAUX 1966) was clear. WARHURST and WILLIAMSON (1970) were able to show that ribosomal (17.4S and 24.2S) RNA of *P. knowlesi* became degraded after the formation of this autophagic vacuole, although no gross changes in RNA were detectable before its formation. WARHURST (1974) attempted to repeat these studies using *P. berghei* but found that, using the techniques then available, the extraction of undegraded ribosomal RNA was not possible.

WARHURST and ROBINSON (1971) tried to find cytotoxic agents of known mode of action which would cause pigment clumping in *P. berghei* in mice, in order to gain insights into the mode of action of chloroquine, but were unsuccessful. It was found, however, that chloroquine-induced clumping could be inhibited in vivo by a variety of agents, especially inhibitors of eukaryotic protein synthesis (WARHURST et al. 1971). In view of the difficulty of interpretation of actions of inhibitors in vivo, the pigment clumping technique was developed further in vitro (WARHURST and BAGGALEY 1972) and it then became possible to modify conditions more readily and to carry out more detailed analyses of antimalarial action (WARHURST et al. 1972a; WARHURST and THOMAS 1975; PETERS et al. 1975; PORTER and PETERS 1976) and of the process of autophagic vacuole formation itself (HOMEWOOD et al. 1972a, b; WARHURST et al. 1974; WARHURST and THOMAS 1978).

## II. Experimental Approach

### 1. Malaria and Mouse Strains

The test has been satisfactorily carried out using TO or TFW male, swiss albino mice, but there seems no reason why other strains should not be suitable. The infection with *P. berghei* N30 (K 173) or NK65 (PETERS 1970) is passaged weekly by inoculation of $10^6$ infected erythrocytes by the intraperitoneal (i.p.) or intravenous (i.v.) route. In the case of a mosquito-transmissible strain such as NK65 regular subpassaging should be carried out until gametocyte production is markedly diminished or lost. In preparation for experiments mice are inoculated on a Friday with a series of tenfold dilutions of infected blood in 50% calf serum/Ringer's solution (WARHURST and FOLWELL 1968) so that one or two animals with a suitable, rising parasitaemia will be available throughout the following week. Examination of tail bloodfilms unstained will indicate a suitable donor. Two to 10% of erythrocytes should contain pigmented parasites, and the majority should have "fine" pigment (Fig. 2).

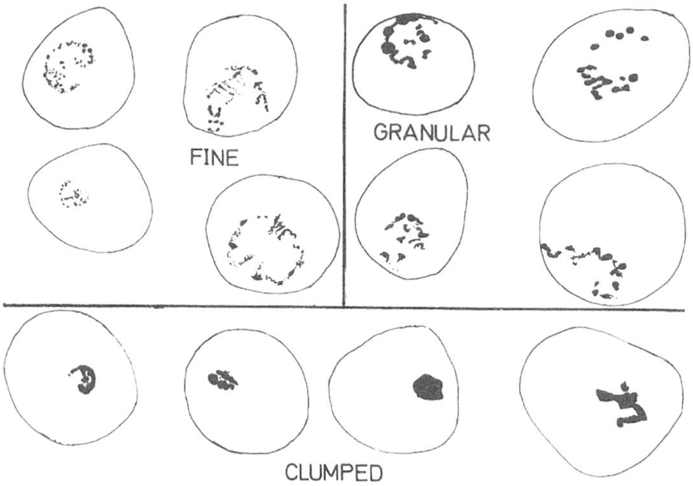


**Fig. 2.** Drawings of infected erythrocytes from unfixed, unstained, thin films of mouse blood after incubation in 199 medium. The distinction between "fine," "granular," and "clumped" pigment is illustrated (WARHURST et al. 1974)

## 2. Studies In Vivo

### a) Clumping Activity

A suitable dose of the drug is given i.p. or orally (p.o.). Thin blood films are taken from the tail before and for several hours after drug administration. The films need not be fixed and should not be stained. Consequently a good oil immersion objective and satisfactory lighting conditions are required for examination. Kohler illumination with the substage iris partially closed gives optimum results (some workers prefer to use a green filter). The erythrocytes in which pigmented parasites can be seen are graded into "fine," "granular," and "clumped" (Fig. 2).

### b) Inhibition of Clumping

The drug to be tested is injected at a suitable interval (15–30 min) before an injection of 30 mg/kg chloroquine. The chloroquine injection should be given subcutaneously (s.c.) and the test drug i.p. to prevent physical interactions between the two drugs. Thin blood films are prepared before the first and second drug doses, and at intervals for 2 h afterwards. Control infected animals injected with chloroquine alone are included in the study. The interval between administering the test drug and chloroquine can be varied as desired. The pigmented parasites are graded into fine, granular, and clumped as before, and the degree of inhibition of clumping assessed.

## 3. Studies In Vitro

### a) Culture Medium

Liquid 10 × concentrated 199 medium from Flow Laboratories or Gibco-Biocult, or dried medium from Wellcome Reagents, are suitable. After diluting or reconstituting the medium in distilled water, the requisite amounts of $NaHCO_3$ (0.148 g) and additional glucose (0.2 g) are added to each 100-ml quantity. Ten millilitres serum is then added (fetal or new-born calf serum from Flow Laboratories or Gibco-Biocult have proved suitable, but not "calf serum" or "bovine serum"). The medium is dispensed to form a shallow layer in the bottom of an Erlenmeyer flask, the flask stoppered or sealed with Parafilm, and brought to 37 °C. An alveolar air mixture (95% air: 5% $CO_2$) is then run in and the mixture is swirled, with the addition of more gas if necessary, until the phenol red indicator shows orange and the pH is 7.2–7.3. At this point the medium is distributed into tubes. Although glass test tubes (100 × 10 mm) with silicone-rubber stoppers have proved adequate, disposable, sterile, plastic, screw-capped 10-ml centrifuge tubes from Sterilin Ltd. are now preferred. From 3.8 to 3.9 ml medium is dispensed into each tube and the air space filled with 95% air: 5% $CO_2$ before replacing the stopper. Incubation then continues for 10 min, when the medium should be cherry-red, pH 7.4. When the tubes of culture medium have been prepared and equilibrated, the mouse selected is anaesthetised with chloroform and blood removed into a heparinised 1-ml syringe by cardiac or axillary puncture. Infected blood (0.05–0.02 ml) is then added to each tube, and a further 10 min are allowed to elapse before the addition of drugs begins.

### b) Preparation of Drugs

The solvent used for the drug should be added to control tubes in the highest concentration used in the experiment, to determine its effect on the parasites. Where possible drugs are dissolved in saline. In some cases dissolution is more easily achieved in distilled water. Addition of 0.1% NaOH or HCl is sometimes necessary. Other useful initial solvents are methanol and ethanol, and subsequent dilutions should be made in such cases in saline or distilled water. Addition of 0.1% Tween 80 is useful in this context. Stock solutions of drugs at concentrations more than $10^{-5}$ mol/litre can usually be stored adequately at −20 °C. It is important not to store aqueous dilutions of alcohol-soluble drugs, since irreversible precipitation will occur. Such dilutions should be used as soon as possible after preparation. For addition to suspensions of infected erythrocytes in culture medium drugs are made up at 40 × the desired concentration and added in 0.1-ml volumes. Where clumping alone is to be examined the initial volume of the medium is 3.9 ml (+0.02–0.05 ml blood) and there is one addition of 0.1 ml. Where inhibitory activity is being studied, 3.8 ml of medium is dispensed initially and two additions of 0.1 ml are made later.

### c) Detection and Measurement of Clumping Activity

α) *Screening*. After the addition of the drug to duplicate tubes at a final concentration of 1 μmol/litre, or 0.0005 mg/ml in the case of unknown drugs, incubation at 37 °C is continued in a roller-tube apparatus (about 12 rph) for 80 min. Controls with drug diluent and with 0.1 μmol/litre chloroquine are included. Then the tubes are centrifuged at 700 g for 5 min, supernatant is drained off and each pellet is resuspended in a drop of calf serum before preparing thin films. The original numbers of the films are covered using self-adhesive labels, and the slides are renumbered

**Table 7.** An experiment to detect pigment clumping activity

| | Tube No. | Fine | Granular | Clumped | % clumped (x) | – control (x–y) | As % of 88[a] |
|---|---|---|---|---|---|---|---|
| Control | 1 | 45 | 3 | 2 | 5 (y) | | |
| 0.1 ml solvent | 2 | 40 | 7 | 3 | | | |
| 0.1 μmol/litre | 3 | 1 | 6 | 43 | 86 | 81 | 92 |
| chloroquine | 4 | 0 | 10 | 40 | 80 | 75 | 85 |
| Drug A | 5 | 15 | 32 | 3 | 6 | 1 | 1 |
| 0.0005 mg/ml | 6 | 12 | 33 | 5 | 8.3 | 3.3 | 4 |
| Drug B | 7 | 0 | 4 | 46 | 92 | 87 | 99 |
| 0.0005 mg/ml | 8 | 1 | 8 | 41 | 82 | 77 | 88 |
| Drug C | 9 | 38 | 11 | 1 | 2 | – 3 | – 3 |
| 0.0005 mg/ml | 10 | 43 | 5 | 2 | 4 | – 1 | – 1 |

[a] 88 is the average maximum % "clumped" found by WARHURST and THOMAS (1975) for chloroquine. This figure may vary slightly depending on the individual interpretation of the worker counting the films

and examined "blind" under an oil immersion objective. On each slide 50 erythrocytes containing pigmented parasites are examined, and the numbers classified as fine, granular and clumped are noted. The results of a typical experiment may be as in Table 7.

The interpretation of this initial screening test is that drugs A and C show no sign of clumping induction at the concentration tested but drug B has a chloroquine-like effect.

*β) Dose Response*. The next step is to examine the crude dose-response relationship for the drugs tested. Routinely the drugs showing no clumping activity in the screening experiment are included in this study, to enable clumping activity at other drug concentrations to be detected. Self-inhibition at high concentrations by drugs which cause clumping at lower ones (e.g. chloroquine, Figs. 3, 4) is also detected in this test. A range of concentrations from 1 to 10 nmol/litre in tenfold steps is suitable. Drugs causing clumping are then further examined over a smaller range using twofold dilutions, to obtain an accurate estimate of the 50% clumping concentration which corresponds to the dissociation constant of the drug-receptor complex, $K_d$ or $K_m$ (WARHURST and THOMAS 1975). In examining large numbers of drugs for clumping activity it has been found useful to abbreviate the above procedure (WARHURST and GOULD 1982). After initial screening at 0.0005 mg/ml the dose-response experiment using serial tenfold dilutions, from 0.005 to 0.000005 mg/ml is carried out. In interpretation of the dose-response curve, the lowest concentration of drug producing between 70% and 100% clumping was taken as the reference point (P) for that drug. For example, in the case of chloroquine diphosphate, amodiaquine dihydrochloride, and mepacrine dihydrochloride, P was 0.00005 mg/ml (approxi-

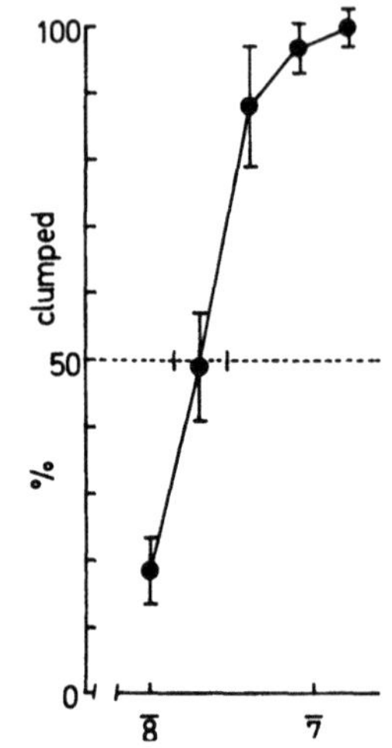


**Fig. 3.** Dose-response sigmoid relating percentage of parasites with clumped pigment (corrected) to log concentration of chloroquine. SD is indicated. The *interrupted line* crosses the *curve* at the 50% point and values + and − 2 SD are marked (five experiments, using duplicates)

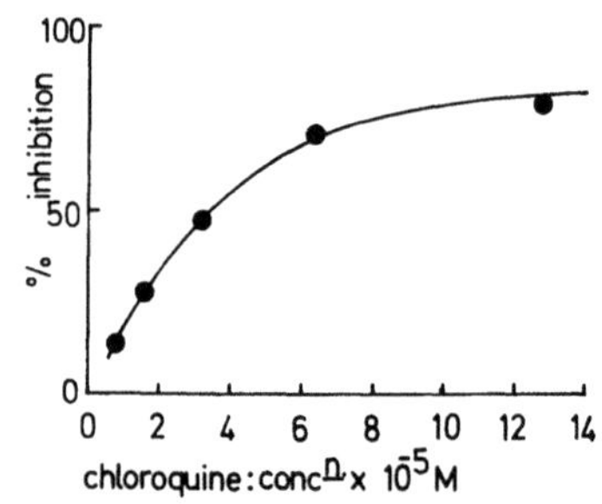


**Fig. 4.** Graph showing inhibition of clumping by chloroquine concentrations above 10 μmol/l

mately 0.1 μmol/litre). With reference to the standards chloroquine, amodiaquine, and mepacrine the "clumping index" (CI) for any drug was expressed as follows:

$$CI = \frac{0.00005}{P. drug}.$$

This method gives a CI of rather limited accuracy, which, however, can be used to compare series of structural variations on known drugs.

d) Detection and Measurement of Clumping Inhibition

Drugs to be tested are added in 0.1 ml saline at 40 × the desired concentration (0.005 mg/ml) to culture tubes containing 3.8 ml of equilibrated, infected blood with medium. Incubation at 37 °C on the roller tube apparatus continues for 15 min, then chloroquine at a final concentration of 0.1 μmol/litre is added. Incubation then proceeds for 80 min. Smears are prepared as usual. Comparison with controls with saline only, or saline and chloroquine detects inhibition. The "percentage inhibition" is calculated as follows:

$$\%_i = 100 - \left[\frac{\%\ \text{clumped with drug} + \text{chloroquine}}{\%\ \text{clumped with chloroquine alone}} \times 100\right].$$

(WARHURST et al. 1974)

In order to determine whether inhibition of clumping is competitive or non-competitive a classical pharmacological approach is used to determine how the dose-response curve of the agonist (chloroquine) is affected by the presence of the suspected antagonist. This involves carrying out at least four dose-response experiments for chloroquine in the presence of different concentrations of suspected antagonist. However, a simpler initial approach is to look at the dose-response curve of inhibitory effect of the drug in question against two or three different concentrations of chloroquine. If the per cent inhibition (%i) versus drug concentration curves shows the same 50% value, then non-competitive inhibition is assumed. Where inhibition is competitive a higher concentration of inhibitor will be needed in the presence of higher concentrations of chloroquine (1 and 0.1 μmol/litre) are suitable concentrations of chloroquine to use).

The results of a series of dose-response curves for chloroquine in the presence of different concentrations of inhibitory drug are treated as recommended by PATON (1970) using the equation:

$$DR - 1 = \frac{[i]^n}{K_i}$$

(GADDUM 1957).

(where DR is dose ratio, i.e. the ratio between the concentrations of agonist necessary to produce 50% clumping in the presence and absence of antagonist; $n$ is the number of molecules of antagonist competing with each molecule of agonist; [i] is the concentration of the antagonist; and $K_i$ is the dissociation constant of the antagonist-receptor complex).

The slope of the line obtained by plotting log (DR − 1) against log [i] is equal to $n$,

$$\log (DR - 1) = n \cdot \log [i] - \log K_i$$

and when $n = 1$

$$\log K_i = \log [i] - \log (DR - 1)$$

when $\log (DR - 1) = 0 \quad (DR - 1 = 1)$

$$\text{then } \log K_i = \log [i]$$

and this is the intercept on the abscissa

(PATON 1970).

It can be shown that when $n > 1$, then the $K_i$ value obtained is the geometric mean of $K_i$ values ('gm $K_i$') for $n$ molecules of antagonist, and the intercept on the abscissa represents mean log $K_i$

thus

$$DR-1=\frac{[i]^n}{gmK_i^n}$$

and

$$gmK_i=\left(\frac{[i]^n}{DR-1}\right)^{\frac{1}{n}}$$

which simplifies to

$$gmK_i=\frac{[i]}{(DR-1)^{\frac{1}{n}}}$$

In cases where $n$ is unknown, and is assumed to be 1 for the purpose of calculating a $K_i$ value, the magnitude of the error introduced depends on the true value of $n$ and on DR − 1, since as DR − 1 approaches 1 the error becomes infinitesimal (WARHURST and THOMAS 1975).

Examples of the application of this approach are given in Figs. 5–8).

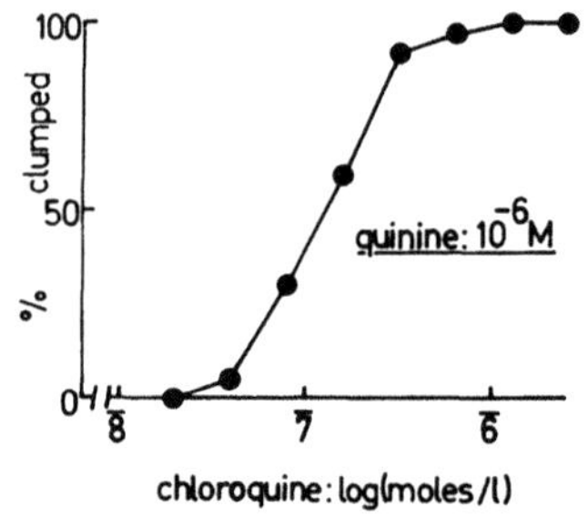


**Fig. 5.** Dose-response sigmoid in the presence of $10^{-6}$ mol/l quinine. Shape of curve is unaffected but the 50% point is moved along to the right

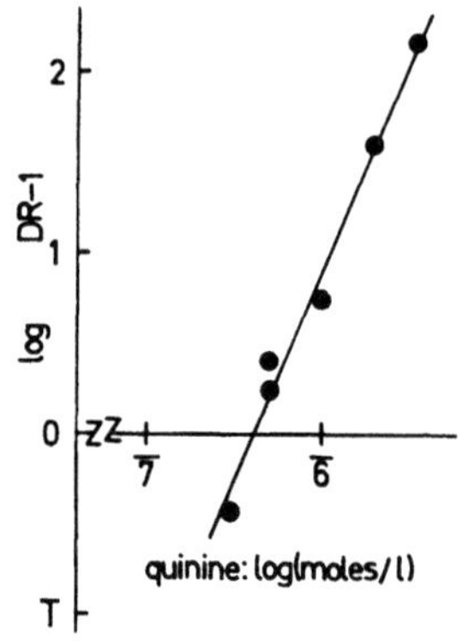


**Fig. 6.** Log(DR-1) plotted against log quinine concentration (slope = 2.3; intercept on abscissa is $\bar{7}.61$, corresponding to a $gmK_i$ of $4.1 \times 10^{-7}$ mol/l)

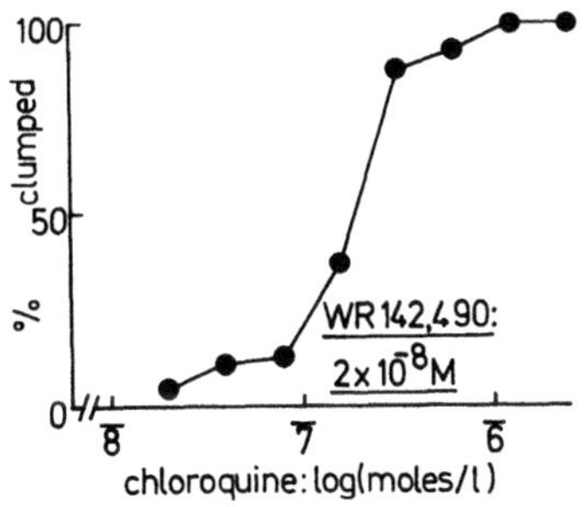


**Fig. 7.** Dose-response sigmoid in the presence of $2 \times 10^{-8}$ mol/l mefloquine (WR 142490). Shape of curve is unaffected but the 50% point is moved to the right

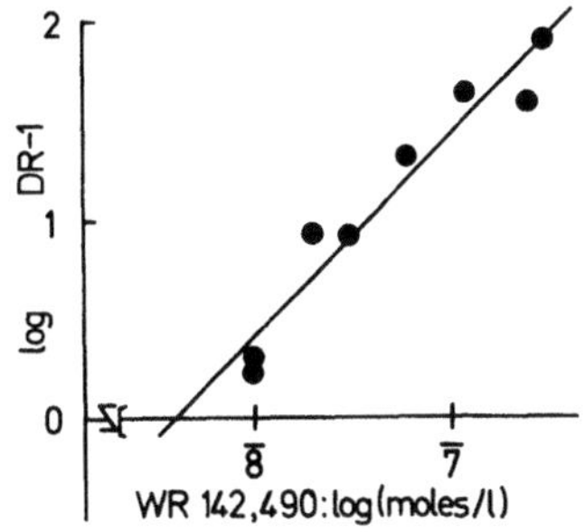


**Fig. 8.** Log(DR-1) plotted against log mefloquine (WR 142490) concentration (slope = 1.02; intercept on abscissa is $\bar{9}.6$, corresponding to a gm$K_i$ of $4 \times 10^{-9}$ mol/l

## III. Analysis of Autophagic Vacuole Formation

After a single intraperitoneal dose of 80 mg/kg chloroquine in the mouse, light microscope observation shows development of granular pigment within 20–30 min, followed by development of clumped pigment from 40 to 85 min. It is clear from the time course that finely pigmented parasites are the precursors of "granular," and "granular" are the precursors of "clumped" since, as the "granular" percentage rises, the "fine" percentage falls, and as the "clumped" percentage rises, the "granular" percentage falls. No alteration in parasitaemia occurs during this time (WARHURST and ROBINSON 1971). Although studies in vivo can be used to test drugs for clumping activity, it is recommended that the study of inhibition should be carried out in vitro, because of difficulties of interpretation owing to the need to take into account host distribution and absorption factors (see, for example, WARHURST et al. 1971).

The fate of parasites with clumped pigment has not been studied in vivo in any detail, although it is known that a decline in parasitaemia takes place over the 24 h following a chloroquine dose. Within 2–4 h after dosing the pigment clumps or autophagic vacuoles can be seen to have been expelled from the parasite and are located in the red-cell cytoplasm (THURSTON 1952).

The "fine" pigment grains of the normal *P. berghei* or *P. cynomolgi* parasite can be seen using electron microscopy to be localised within small vacuoles or "digestive vesicles," which are phagosome-like organelles where digestion of haemoglo-

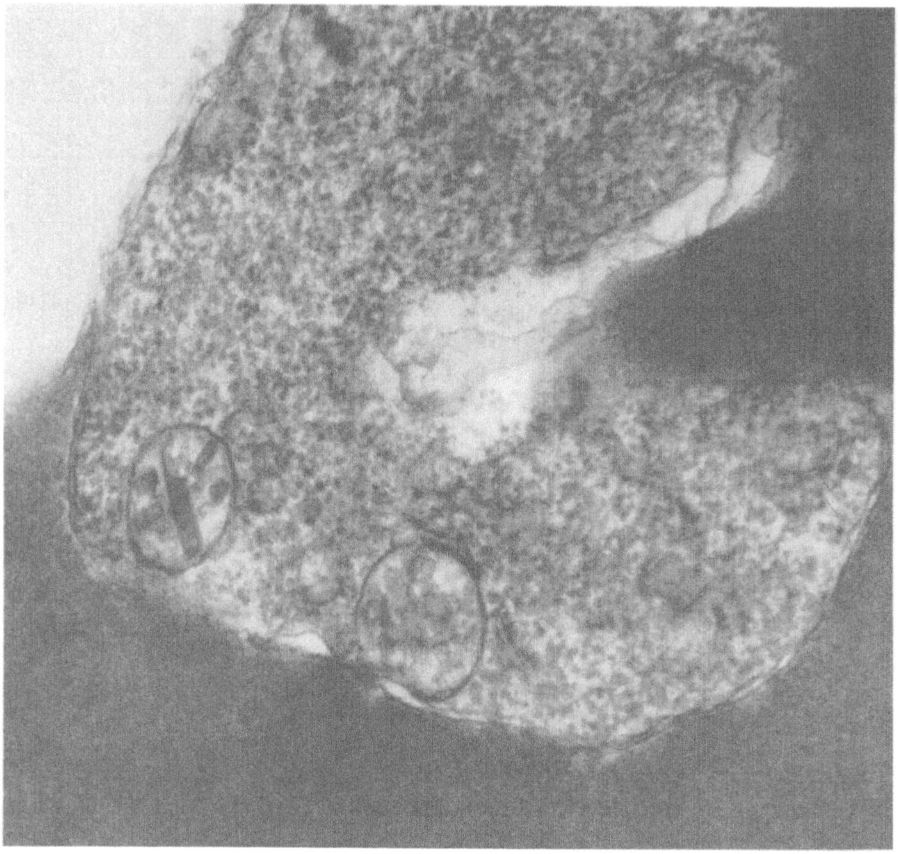

**Fig. 9.** *P. berghei* trophozoite after exposure to chloroquine in vivo for 20 min. The digestive vacuoles are enlarged and contain several pigment crystals, probably resulting from the fusion of adjacent vacuoles. "Granulation stage," ×30000

bin has taken place. Ultrastructurally the granulation stage of autophagic vacuole formation consists of swelling and fusion of adjacent digestive vesicles (Fig. 9). The clumping stage takes longer and appears to be a separate process, both by virtue of its sensitivity to inhibitors (see below), and because it involves the sequestration of fused digestive vesicles and cytoplasmic portions within what is, apparently, a newly synthesised membrane (Fig. 10). This process bears a strong similarity to autophagic vacuole formation in mammalian cells (DE DUVE 1963; NOVIKOFF and ESSNER 1962) or in other protozoa such as *Euglena* (BRANDES and BERTINI 1964). The presence of cytoplasmic ribosomes within the autophagic vacuole suggests that enzymatic breakdown of ribonucleoprotein must be taking place, and this is supported by the finding of WARHURST and WILLIAMSON (1970) that the eukaryotic-type ribosomal RNA of *P. knowlesi* (17.4S and 24.2S) became degraded after the formation of the chloroquine-induced autophagic vacuole.

Studies in vitro have successfully duplicated those in vivo (HOMEWOOD et al. 1971) and the time course, although shorter, shows the same characteristics (Fig.

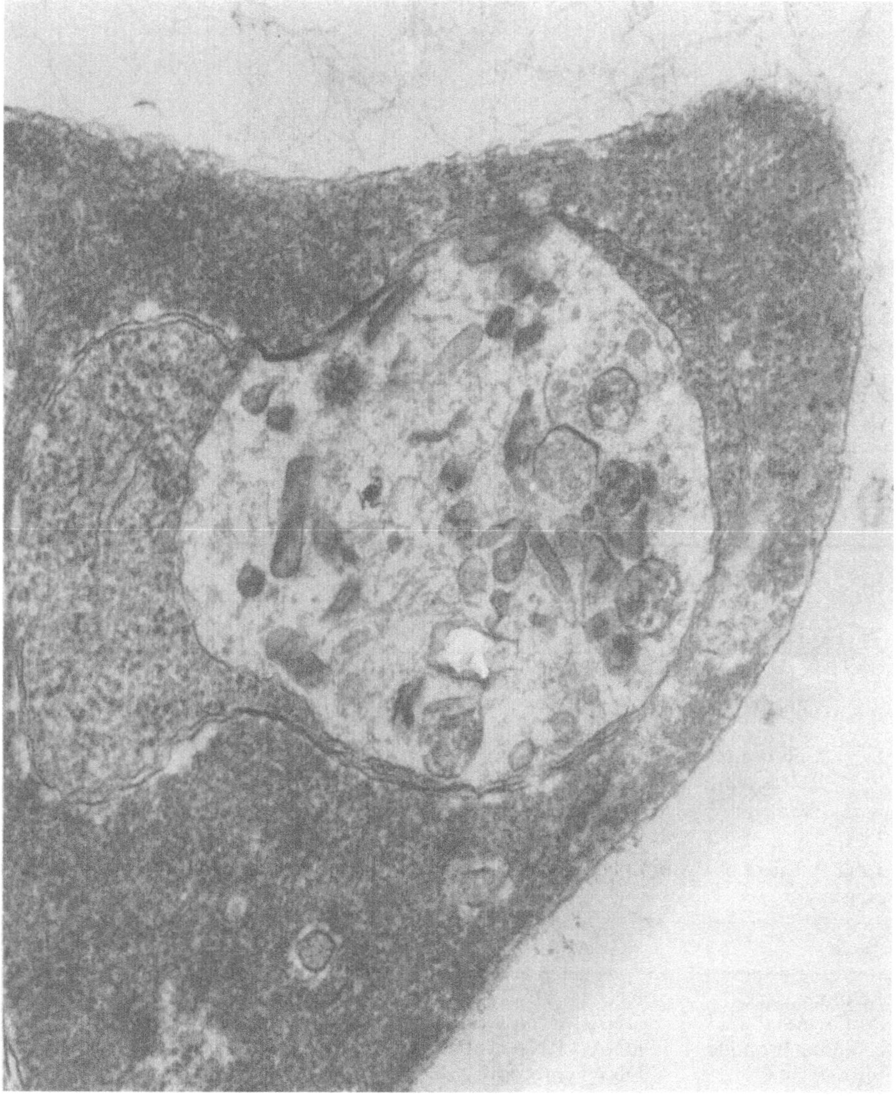

**Fig. 10.** *P. berghei* trophozoite after exposure to chloroquine in vivo for 60 min. The large autophagic vacuole (pigment clump) contains many free pigment crystals, cytoplasmic ribosomes and other debris (electron micrographs by courtesy of Dr. D. S. ELLIS). "Clumping stage," × 26000

11). Granulation occurred within 10 min, and clumping was complete by 70–80 min. The time course of granulation is comparable to that observed by POLET and BARR (1969) and FITCH (1969) for the primary phase of uptake of radiolabelled chloroquine into *P. knowlesi* and *P. berghei* respectively, and may be related to the effects of chloroquine concentrated on, or in, the digestive vacuoles (AIKAWA 1972).

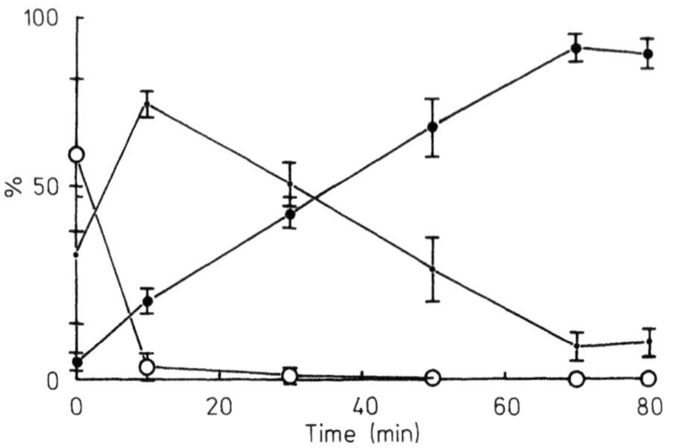


**Fig. 11.** Changes in pigment in *P. berghei* in vitro after addition of $10^{-6}$ mol/l chloroquine. *Ordinate,* percentage of erythrocytes showing fine (*open circle*), granular (*broken line*) or clumped (*full circle*) pigment after incubation for varying periods. *Abscissa,* time in minutes. (Two experiments, $n=4$. SD indicated). WARHURST et al. (1974)

**Table 8.** Effects of inhibitors of ribosomal protein synthesis on chloroquine-induced pigment clumping in vitro

| Agent | Action on | 50%i at | Non-competitive? |
|---|---|---|---|
| Cycloheximide | Eukaryotes | 30 μmol/l | Yes |
| Puromycin | Eukaryotes and prokaryotes | 3 μmol/l | Yes |
| Chloramphenicol | Prokaryotes | > 0.1 mmol/l | – |
| Tetracycline | | > 0.1 mmol/l | – |

**Table 9.** Effect of inhibitors of nuclei acid synthesis on chloroquine-induced pigment clumping in vitro

| Agent | Action on | 50%i at | Non-competitive? |
|---|---|---|---|
| Actinomycin D | RNA (+DNA) synthesis | 20 μmol/l | Yes |
| Proflavine | DNA+RNA synthesis | 8 μmol/l | Yes |
| Ethidium bromide | DNA+RNA synthesis | 60 μmol/l | ND |
| Mitomycin C | DNA synthesis | > 0.05 mg/ml | – |
| 6-Mercaptopurine | Purine interconversion | > 0.1 mmol/l | – |

ND, not done

Although the effects of cytotoxic drugs on clumping had been noted earlier (WARHURST et al. 1971) and inhibition by agents blocking nucleic acid and protein synthesis had been reported, a more detailed examination was possible in vitro. In particular the time course of inhibition could be carefully studied and the effects of abnormally high concentrations of drugs tested.

Evidence was found, using inhibitors, that autophagic vacuole formation following granulation was an active process, depending upon intact synthetic machinery in the parasite (see Tables 8,9) (WARHURST et al. 1974). These observations contradict the hypothesis of HAHN et al. (1966) that the primary target for chloroquine in malaria parasites is DNA-primed nucleic acid synthesis, although this is not ruled out as a secondary mode of action.

Time-course studies showed that the clumping stage was being affected by the active agents tabulated in Tables 8 and 9, since inhibition was noted even when the agents were added 30 min after chloroquine. The response to cycloheximide and the inactivity of chloramphenicol and tetracycline confirm that the malarial ribosomes are of eukaryotic type, as indicated by the earlier studies on ribosomes (COOK et al. 1971) and ribosomal RNA (WARHURST and WILLIAMSON 1970).

The findings of HOMEWOOD et al. (1971) that chloroquine at therapeutic concentrations (1 µmol/litre) in vitro had no effect on parasite nucleic acid synthesis for at least 1 h after addition, and that protein synthesis from isoleucine was similarly unaffected, support the idea that the autophagic vacuole is formed actively by the cell, and the results described earlier indicate that nucleic acid synthesis (probably RNA synthesis) and protein synthesis are involved in vacuole formation. HOMEWOOD and ATKINSON (1973) found that in the absence of serum in Eagle's medium without vitamins, clumping would still take place provided glucose [partially replaced by glycerol (55%) or lactate (25%)] was present together with the amino acids cystine and methionine. 2-deoxy D-glucose inhibited the process in the presence of glucose or glycerol. It was not found possible to replace glucose by pyruvate, ribose or stearic acid. The requirement for RNA and protein synthesis in autophagic vacuole formation probably relates to the need for synthesis of new membrane and possibly enzymes, which may involve synthesis of a messenger RNA and then ribosomal translation of the message into protein. The requirement for glucose or other energy source reflects two aspects. The first is the need for glucose for chloroquine uptake (FITCH et al. 1974) presumably related to the supply of ATP from glycolysis. The second is the probable need for ATP from glucose for the synthesis of nucleic acid and protein.

The interesting observation of FITCH et al. (1974) that 2,4-dinitrophenol at concentrations in the region of 1 mmol/litre would inhibit chloroquine uptake parallels the effect of this proton ionophore on chloroquine-induced autophagic vacuole formation (WARHURST and THOMAS 1978), where 50%i was found at 0.6 mmol/litre. In view of the almost complete dependence of erythrocytic stages of *P. berghei* on glycolysis as a source of energy (see, for example, HOMEWOOD 1977) the activity of this antimitochondrial drug, an uncoupler of electron transport from phosphorylation, was enigmatic, especially because, while reducing ATP levels it was shown to have no effect on glycolysis (FITCH et al. 1974). Studies on other antimitochondrial agents and inhibitors of membrane ion transport revealed that several agents were active inhibitors of chloroquine-induced autophagic vacuole formation. These fell into two groups (a) the proton ionophores such as monensin and 2,4-dinitrophenol where inhibition was non-competitive, and (b) the mitochondrial ATPase inhibitors such as oligomycin and venturicidin, where inhibition was found to be competitive. The cell membrane ($Na^{+}K^{+}$) ATPase inhibitor ouabain had no effect. It was also found that one inhibitor of mitochondrial ATPase, dicyclohexylcarbodiimide (Fig. 1c, DCCD), whilst not inhibiting autophagic vacuole formation, would, like chloroquine, induce the process, but with the relatively high $K_m$ value of 4.7 µmol/litre.

**Table 10.** Action of inhibitors of cell membrane and microsomal ($Na^+$, $K^+$) and mitochondrial ($Mg^{2+}$) ATPases compared with their effects on autophagic vacuole formation

| Inhibitor | Clumping (µmol/l) | | ATPase inhibition (µmol/l) | |
|---|---|---|---|---|
| | gmK | $K_m$ | $Na^+, K^+$ | $Mg^{2+}$ |
| Oligomycin B | 0.18 | – | 40 | 0.17 |
| Venturicidin | 0.41 | – | 5,000 | 0.31 |
| Ouabain | > 1,400 | – | 10 | No effect |
| DCCD | – | 4.7 | 1,000 | 2 |

For further details see WARHURST and THOMAS (1978)

The mitochondrial ATPase inhibitors have no structural similarity to chloroquine, unlike the antimalarials such as quinine which also inhibit autophagic vacuole formation competitively (see next section). Moreover, quinine did not inhibit the clumping effect of DCCD. In addition FITCH (personal communication) found that oligomycin did not inhibit uptake of [$^{14}$C]-chloroquine by *P. berghei*-infected erythrocytes. When the $K_i$ values for oligomycin and venturicidin and the $K_m$ for DCCD were measured, they compared closely with concentrations required for inhibition of mammalian mitochondrial ATPase (Table 10). It is known that chloroquine at concentrations between 10 and 100 µmol/litre inhibits respiration of mammalian mitochondria (GREILING and DORNER 1962) and it is probable that similar levels of chloroquine are to be found in the parasite cytoplasm after concentration by high-affinity sites (FITCH 1969), so that an effect of chloroquine on the malarial mitochondrion is not unlikely. It is, however, difficult to explain competition between oligomycin and chloroquine unless the mitochondrial site for chloroquine is overlapped by the, admittedly large, oligomycin site. DCCD also binds to the same component of mitochondrial ATPase (the $CF_0$ complex) as oligomycin and venturicidin (BEECHEY et al. 1967). It is thus apparent that the simple sequence of autophagic vacuole formation (WARHURST 1973) must be modified to include a mitochondrial component (see Fig. 12).

The ionophores active against autophagic vacuole formation are proton ionophores. No activity was noted using a calcium ionophore or a potassium ionophore such as valinomycin (WARHURST and THOMAS 1978; and WARHURST, in preparation). This points to the importance of hydrogen ion gradients in the uptake of drugs such as chloroquine and/or essential metabolites. Areas of probable proton excess in the parasite/host-cell complex include the red cell compartment and the digestive vesicles (HOMEWOOD et al. 1972a). A proton deficit might be expected in the mitochondrion. These gradients of pH are physiologically very significant, and if abolished will have major effects on metabolism (see HAROLD 1970, 1972, 1977). The modes of action of two highly active ionophores, monensin (50%i at 20 nmol/litre) and nigericin (50%i at 4 nmol/litre) are of interest. Monensin will dissolve in membranes and exchange $H^+$ for $Na^+$ (less readily $K^+$) without affecting the overall potential difference across the membrane. Thus if there is an excess of either $Na^+$ or $H^+$ on one side, and the other ion is available on the other side, an equili-

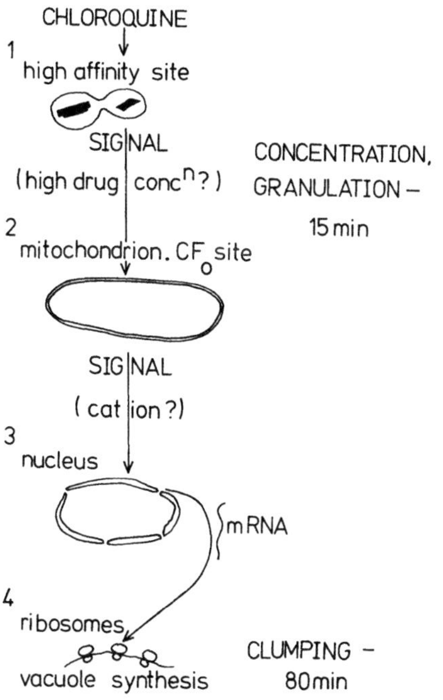


**Fig. 12.** Hypothetical course of events in chloroquine-induced pigment clumping (autophagic vacuole formation). *1*, site of competitive inhibition by quinine, mefloquine, etc.; *2*, site of action of DCCD. The chloroquine effect here is competitively inhibited by oligomycin and venturicidin; *3*, site of non-competitive inhibition by actinomycin D; *4*, site of non-competitive inhibition by cycloheximide

bration will occur, depending on concentration of $H^+$ and $Na^+$. Monensin is effective in normal high $Na^+$ media in abolishing hydrogen ion excess within membranes. Nigericin is similar to monensin but is specific for $K^+$. It is highly effective within cells, i.e. in areas of high $K^+$ concentration, in abolishing areas of $H^+$ excess (HAROLD 1977). The effectiveness of these ionophores in inhibition of chloroquine-induced autophagic vacuole formation, and the lack of effect of the purely $K^+$ ionophore valinomycin and the $Ca^{++}$ ionophore A 23187 indicates that hydrogen ion, rather than charge gradient, is of importance at some stage in the process. Monensin and nigericin both inhibit uptake of [$^{14}$C]-chloroquine by erythrocytic *P. berghei* (DIRIBE and WARHURST 1980) but the effect of nigericin is only manifested in the presence of a high $K^+$ concentration in the incubation medium. This is not needed for the nigericin effect on clumping, which is noticed, moreover, at a lower nigericin concentration. It would appear that the effect of nigericin on uptake is through its effect on the passage of chloroquine into the red cell, whilst the effect on clumping is achieved intracellularly.

It is interesting to note that in medium 199 in vitro exposure of *P. berghei* to chloroquine (10 µmol/litre) for 1 h led to very little decrease in infective potency (84% vs 100%) compared with undrugged controls (DAVIES 1973), although when a similar experiment was carried out in saline-glucose-reduced glutathione medium, potency was reduced to 10% (WARHURST and FOLWELL 1968). In the simple medium it is known that autophagic vacuole formation does not take place, although uptake of chloroquine proceeds as usual. It would therefore seem that the process of autophagic vacuole formation (and extrusion of the vacuole) may be delaying parasite death. Thus one possible mechanism of resistance to chloroquine might be an increase in the rate of autophagic vacuole formation. This possibility has not been investigated. Further evidence for the undiminished viability of *P. berghei* in erythrocytes in medium 199 1 h after chloroquine is provided by the observations of HOMEWOOD et al. (1971) on the undiminished incorporation of precursors into protein and nucleic acid during this period. Thus it appears that prolonged exposure to chloroquine is necessary for a lethal effect, whereas the morphological changes are stimulated by only a short exposure.

A surprising observation was that a marked inhibition of clumping was brought about by raising the temperature of incubation by 2°–3 °C (WARHURST 1973). This further supports the active nature of the clumping response.

## IV. Insights into Antimalarial Mode of Action

### 1. General Principles

Drugs which cause or inhibit autophagic vacuole formation are acting on the malaria parasite, and penetrating to their site of action within the time course of an experiment (80–95 min). The antimetabolite antimalarials sulphadiazine, sulfadoxine, pyrimethamine, and cycloguanil neither cause nor inhibit clumping (WARHURST et al. 1972b; WARHURST, unpublished). Apart from questions of permeability of the parasite-erythrocyte complex to the drugs in question, it is known that these agents affect the folate pathway (FERONE 1977), and inhibition of the formation of active derivatives of tetrahydrofolate manifests itself particularly in an inhibition of thymidylate synthesis for DNA. Since DNA synthesis does not seem to be involved in the course of autophagic vacuole formation, this may explain the inability of antimetabolite drugs to affect the process.

The 8-aminoquinolines are, in general, inactive in induction or inhibition of clumping. Exceptions are noted at high (0.005 mg/ml) concentrations of some 8-aminoquinolines which have a side chain containing two nitrogen atoms in addition to the 8-amino group (see PETERS et al. 1975 for examples, but note that the concentrations tested were 0.5 and 0.005 mg/ml not % as stated there). Although the quinolone WR 118176 inhibited clumping at 0.005 mg/ml, menoctone and some other tissue schizontocides were inactive. It would be of interest to examine the effects of metabolites of these and related drugs in the clumping system.

The blood schizontocides, that is those antimalarials which act solely on intra-erythrocytic malaria parasites, either cause or inhibit autophagic vacuole formation at relatively low concentrations (well below 0.005 mg/ml or 10 μmol/litre). Aryl methanol antimalarials such as the cinchona alkaloids, mefloquine and phenanthrenes, cause some swelling of digestive vesicles with apparent dissolution of pigment crystals, but no autophagic vacuole formation, at least in the first few hours (DAVIES et al. 1975; PETERS et al. 1977). These drugs will competitively inhibit both the uptake of [$^{14}$C]chloroquine (FITCH 1972) and the development of autophagic vacuoles after chloroquine (WARHURST et al. 1972a, b; WARHURST and THOMAS 1975). This evidence indicates that these drugs are concentrated by the same mechanisms as chloroquine; they interact with the same receptor site. There are differences between $K_i$ values for inhibition of [$^{14}$C]chloroquine uptake and $gmK_i$ values for clumping inhibition, the latter generally being lower, and more dependent on chemical structure (Table 11). These differences can be explained to some extent because autophagic vacuole formation is a more complex process than chloroquine uptake, and the $gmK_i$ values represent the combined effects of the drugs on several processes, including chloroquine uptake. It is also likely that high-affinity uptake sites are heterogeneous (WARHURST and THOMAS 1975).

It is noteworthy that the blood schizontocides which inhibit chloroquine-induced pigment clumping competitively have some activity against chloroquine-resistant strains of malaria, although the claim that drugs with an "$n$" value of $\sim 1$ are more often effective than those with a value of $> 1$ (WARHURST and THOMAS 1975) has not yet been properly investigated. Studies on clumping enable activity on chloroquine-resistant malaria to be predicted. This activity is probable if the antimalarial:

1. Has no effect in the clumping system
2. Causes non-competitive inhibition
3. Causes competitive inhibition

In 1. the drug is probably an antimetabolite or a tissue schizontocide. In 2. it may be an inhibitor of protein or nucleic acid (RNA) synthesis, or have effects on energy utilization. In 3. it may be a quinine-like drug or a drug acting via the parasite mitochondrion. Where a drug which causes autophagic vacuole formation is competitively inhibited by quinine, it is probably a drug of the chloroquine type and likely to have a reduced effect against chloroquine-resistant strains, but where a clumping inducer is not inhibited, or is inhibited non-competitively by quinine, activity against these strains can be expected.

## 2. Structure-Activity Relationships and Characteristics of the Receptor Site

On the basis of competitive inhibition of chloroquine-induced pigment clumping in vitro and antimalarial activities in vivo a model drug-receptor interaction was proposed by WARHURST and THOMAS (1975). The proposed receptor consisted of an electropositive group situated 6–8 Å away from an electronegative group, the two being separated by a planar lipophilic area. Ring-ring interactions were thought to occur between the planar area of the receptor and the quinoline rings of chloroquine and quinine. In chloroquine-like drugs the occurrence of a sterically restricted (hydrogen bonding or coordination?) link between the electropositive area of the receptor and aromatic nitrogen atom was suggested, because of the major deleterious effect of adjacent substitution on activity [see WARHURST and GOULD (1982) for further data on this point]. It was clear that such a restricted interaction was not taking place in quinine-like drugs, as substituents adjacent to the aromatic nitrogen had no marked deleterious effect, and in some cases enhanced activity. However, in contrast to chloroquine-like drugs (WARHURST and GOULD 1982) very strict steric restrictions apply to the side chain (quinuclidine nitrogen) of cinchona alkaloids. Epimerisation at C9 (giving epiquinine or epiquinidine) (Part II, Chap. 2) leads to loss of antimalarial activity (THOMPSON and WERBEL 1972). 9-epiquinine neither causes nor inhibits pigment clumping even at high concentrations (WARHURST and THOMAS 1975). In the model of 1975 this steric restriction of orientation in the side chain was thought to be related to the need for an internal hydrogen bond between the 9-hydroxyl group and the quinuclidine nitrogen, as suggested by CHENG (1971). However, recent studies by OLEKSYN and LEBIODA (1980) indicate that the hydrogen bond is formed in the 9-epimers but not in the antimalarial cinchona alkaloids! Emphasis is now being placed on interactions of blood schizontocides with ferriprotoporphyrin IX (haemin) since CHOU et al. (1980) have been able to show that this iron (III) porphyrin is an essential component of the blood-schizontocide receptor (Part II, Chap. 1). The structure of ferriprotoporphyrin IX corresponds closely to the hypothetical receptor proposed earlier. It has a central electropositive area, ferric iron bearing one excess positive charge, surrounded by a planar lipophilic ring system with potentially, negatively charged, carboxyl groups at a distance of 4.4–9.6 Å from the iron. Interactions of electronegative ligands with the electropositive iron atom are by axial coordination, i.e. the axis of the interaction is perpendicular to the plane of the porphyrin ring (BUCHLER 1975). Although it has been proposed that both chloroquine and quinine bind to ferriprotoporphyrin IX by means of a nitrogen-iron coordination link (WARHURST 1981 a), it has been possible to confirm this spectrophotometrically only in the case of quinine and other antimalarially active aryl methanols. Here, structure-activity relationships show that the side chain quinuclidine or piperidine nitrogen is involved. The absorption spectrum of the 1:1 complex in benzene shows a Soret peak, c. 410 nm, indicative of the iron atom in a high-spin pentacoordinate state, a new peak, c. 490 nm, indicating a transition of the $Fe^{+++}$ electrons (Table 11) and two charge-transfer peaks at c. 510 and 610 nm, indicative of ring/ring interactions (MAHLER and CORDES 1967) (Fig. 13). Epiquinine does not form a complex

**Table 11.** The relationship of various experimentally determined parameters in aryl methanol antimalarials

| Drug | DNA binding | Benzene-soluble complex with haemin giving 490-nm absorption peak[a] | $K_i$ (uptake)[b] (μM) | $gmK_i$ (clumping inhibition)[c] (μM) | Antimalarially active |
|---|---|---|---|---|---|
| Quinine | Yes[d] | Yes | 2 | 0.41 | Yes |
| 9-Epiquinine | Yes[e] | No | – | > 100 | No |
| Quinidine | – | Yes[e] | – | 0.10 | Yes |
| Cinchonine | – | Yes | – | 0.24 | Yes |
| Cinchonidine | – | Yes[e] | – | 0.67 | Yes |
| Mefloquine | No[f, g] | Yes | 2 | 0.004 | Yes |
| WR 177602 | – | Yes | – | 0.010 | Yes |
| WR 122455 | Yes[h] | Yes | 0.7 | 0.011 | Yes |
| WR 30090 | – | Yes[e] | 2 | 0.025 | Yes |
| RO 210960 | Yes[e] | Yes | – | 0.053 | Yes |

[a] WARHURST (1981 b)
[b] FITCH (1972)
[c] WARHURST and THOMAS (1975)
[d] HAHN et al. (1966)
[e] WARHURST (unpublished)
[f] PETERS et al. (1977)
[g] DAVIDSON et al. (1975)
[h] PORTER and PETERS (1976)

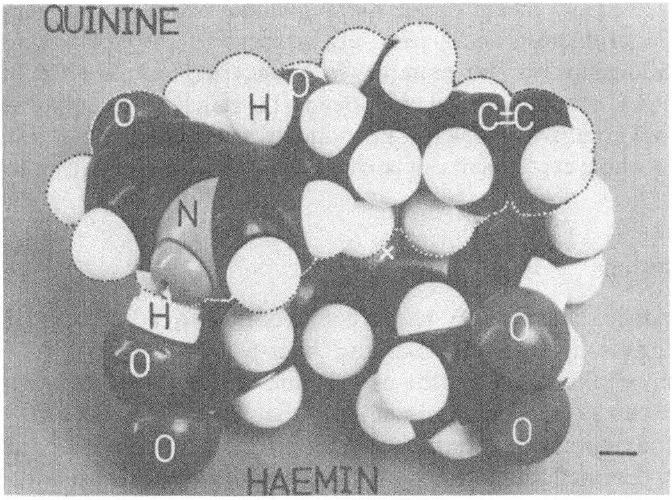


**Fig. 13.** Corey-Pauling-Koltun model of a possible quinine-haemin complex. The quinine molecule is outlined by a *dotted line*. *X* indicates the iron atom of haemin coordinating with the quinuclidine nitrogen atom of quinine. The *bar* represents 1 Å.

(WARHURST 1981b). Although chloroquine and mepacrine form water-soluble complexes with ferriprotoporphyrin IX at pH 7.4, which show charge transfer and Soret peaks, the electronic transition of $Fe^{+++}$ is not detectable (unpublished work), indicating that a coordination complex is not formed. It is possible that the 1:2 chloroquine-ferriprotoporphyrin IX complex described by CHOU et al. (1980) is made by interaction of one molecule of chloroquine with ferriprotoporphyrin IX oxo-dimer (COHEN 1969). These possibilities need further study, especially in the case of amodiaquine and its analogues where direct interactions with ferriprotoporphyrin IX are difficult to demonstrate, except at alkaline pH values.

Complexes of antimalarials and ferriprotoporphyrin IX may be developed during the formation of haemozoin pigment from haemoglobin in the digestive vacuole. It is possible that quinine-like drugs will complex directly with haemozoin, and this may explain its apparent dissolution following treatment. Unpublished observations in this laboratory indicate that chloroquine itself does not complex with crystalline haemozoin, confirming the report of MACOMBER et al. 1967. The drug/ferriprotoporphyrin IX complexes may have different effects on the parasite (clumping induction or clumping inhibition) related to their hydrophilic or lipophilic characteristics. It is known that ferriprotoporphyrin IX itself has membrane-damaging properties (TAPPEL and ZALKIN 1959). These may be enhanced (CHOU and FITCH 1980) or even diminished by complexation with antimalarial schizontocides.

## V. Drug-Screening Applications

Although primary screening in animal models and cultures of *P. falciparum* in vitro are of major importance, the use of drug-induced autophagic vacuole formation can be envisaged as a means of determining modes of action and relationships of drugs of special interest, and a relatively inexpensive way of studying structure-activity relationships (see, for example, WARHURST and GOULD 1982) In particular it avoids the use of radiolabelled compounds, the purchase, handling and disposal of which pose expensive problems. Economy of animals is another point in its favour, since a whole experiment can be carried out with the blood from one mouse.

## VI. Conclusions

The drug-induced clumping test has, in conjunction with radiolabelled drug studies and experiments in vivo advanced our knowledge of the mode of action of antimalarials significantly over the past decade. Although the technique has been criticised (HAHN 1974) conclusions on the probable unimportance of DNA as a site of high-affinity uptake of antimalarial schizontocides have been vindicated by the observation that mefloquine, a blood schizontocide par excellence with high activity in clumping inhibition, does not bind to DNA (DAVIDSON et al. 1975; PETERS et al. 1977) (Table 11). Now that continuous cultures of *P. falciparum* are available, it can be envisaged that these will provide major sources of new insights in the years to come, but studies on drug-induced autophagic vacuole formation will continue to give us useful information.

The clumping technique will detect and classify drugs which have a chloroquine-like or quinine-like mode of action. It will also detect agents which inhibit energy metabolism, protein synthesis or RNA synthesis, but it will not detect antimetabolites of the pyrimethamine-sulphonamide group, or other agents which have their main effects on DNA synthesis. The technique has been used to study structure activity relationships and to predict the topography of the blood-schizontocide receptor.

*Acknowledgment.* The author is grateful to colleagues in Liverpool and London for their collaboration, and to Professor W. PETERS for his constant encouragement. WHO, MRC, and the Research and Development Command of the US Army have given financial assistance to the author, who is now supported by the Public Health Laboratory Service.

## References

Aikawa M (1972) High resolution autoradiography of malarial parasites treated with $^3$H-chloroquine. Am J Pathol 67:277–284

Ascoli M (1978) Demonstration of a direct effect of inhibitors of the degradation of receptor-bound human chorionic gonadotropin on the steroidogenic pathway. J Biol Chem 253:7839–7843

Ascoli M (1979) Inhibition of the degradation of receptor-bound human choriogonadotropin by leupeptin. Biochim Biophys Acta 586:608–614

Ascoli M, Puett D (1978a) Degradation of receptor-bound human choriogonadotropin by murine Leydig tumor cells. J Biol Chem 253:4892–4899

Ascoli M, Puett D (1978b) Inhibition of the degradation of receptor-bound human choriogonadotropin by lysosomotropic agents, protease inhibitors, and metabolic inhibitors. J Biol Chem 253:7832–7838

Ballard FJ (1977) Intracellular protein degradation. Essays Biochem 13:1–37

Beechey RB, Roberton AM, Holloway CT, Knight IG (1967) The properties of dicyclohexylcarbodiimide as an inhibitor of oxidative phosphorylation. Biochemistry 6:3867–3879
Binz C (1867a) Über die Wirkung antiseptischer Stoffe auf Infusorien von Pflanzenjauche. Zentralb Med Wiss 5:305–308
Binz C (1867b) Über die Einwirkung des Chinin auf Protoplasma-Bewegungen. Arch Mikrosk Anat 3:383–389
Bock E (1939) Über morphologische Veränderungen menschlicher Malaria Parasiten durch Atebrineinwirkung. Arch Schiffs-Trop Hyg 43:209–214
Bock E, Oesterlin M (1938/1939) Über einige fluoreszenzmikroscopische Beobachtungen. Zentralbl Bakteriol (Naturwiss) 143:306–318
Brandes D, Bertini F (1964) Role of Golgi apparatus in the formation of cytolysomes. Exp Cell Res 35:194–217
Brown MS, Dana SE, Goldstein JL (1975) Receptor-dependent hydrolysis of cholesteryl esters contained in plasma low density lipoproteins. Proc Natl Acad Sci USA 72:2025–2029
Buchler JW (1975) Static coordination chemistry of metalloporphyrins. In: Smith KM (ed) Porphyrins and metalloporphyrins. Elsevier, Amsterdam, pp 157–231
Bullock FJ (1968) Antiprotozoal quinones. I. Synthesis of 2-hydroxy-3-alkyl-1,4-naphthoquinones as potential coccidostats. J Med Chem 11:419–424
Carpenter G, Cohen S (1976) $^{125}$I-labelled human epidermal growth factor. Binding, internalization, and degradation in human fibroblasts. J Cell Biol 71:159–171
Carter RF (1969) Sensitivity to amphotericin B of a *Naegleria sp.* isolated from a case of primary amoebic meningoencephalitis. J Clin Pathol 22:470–474
Casemore DP (1970) Sensitivity of *Hartmanella* (*Acanthamoeba*) to 5-fluorocytosine, hydroxystilbamidine, and other substances. J Clin Pathol 23:649–652
Charet P, Aissi E, Maurois P, Bouquelet S, Biguet J (1980) Aminopeptidase in rodent *Plasmodium*. Comp Biochem Physiol [B] 65:519–524
Cheng CC (1971) Structure and antimalarial activity of aminoalcohols and 2-(*p*-chlorophenyl)-2(4-piperidyl)-tetrahydrofuran. J Pharm Sci 60:1596–1598
Chou AC, Fitch CD (1980) Hemolysis of mouse erythrocytes by ferriprotoporphyrin IX and chloroquine. Chemotherapeutic implications. J Clin Invest 66:856–858
Chou SC, Ramanathan S (1968) Quinacrine: site of inhibition of synchronized cell division in *Tetrahymena*. Life Sci 7:1053–1062
Chou SC, Ramanathan S, Cutting WC (1968) Quinacrine: inhibition of synchronized cell division in *Tetrahymena*. Pharmacology 1:60–64
Chou AC, Chevli R, Fitch CD (1980) Ferriprotoporphyrin IX fulfils the criteria for identification as the chloroquine receptor of malaria parasites. Biochemistry 19:1543–1549
Clancy CF (1968) The lethal effect of certain antimalarial drugs on *Tetrahymena pyriformis*. Am J Trop Med Hyg 17:359–363
Cohen IA (1969) The dimeric nature of hemin hydroxides. J Am Chem Soc 91:1980–1983
Conan NJ (1948) Chloroquine in amebiasis. Am J Trop Med Hyg 28:107–110
Conklin KA, Chou SC (1970) Antimalarials: effects on in vivo and in vitro protein synthesis. Science 170:1213–1214
Conklin KA, Chou SC (1972a) The effects of antimalarial drugs on uptake and incorporation of macromolecular precursors by *Tetrahymena pyriformis*. J Pharmacol Exp Ther 180:158–166
Conklin KA, Chou SC (1972b) Studies on the mode of action of primaquine using *Tetrahymena pyriformis*. Proc Helminth Soc 39:261–264
Conklin KA, Chou SC (1972c) Isolation and characterization of *Tetrahymena pyriformis* GL mitochondria. Comp Biochem Physiol [B] 41:45–54
Conklin KA, Chou SC, Ramanathan S (1969) Quinine: Effect on *Tetrahymena pyriformis*. I. Inhibition of synchronized cell division and site of action. Pharmacology 2:247–256
Conklin KA, Chou SC, Heu P (1971) Quinine: Effect on *Tetrahymena pyriformis*. III. Energetics of isolated mitochondria in the presence of quinine and other antimalarial drugs. Biochem Pharmacol 20:1877–1882
Conklin KA, Heu P, Chou SC (1973) The effects of antimalarial drugs on nucleic acid synthesis in vitro in *Tetrahymena pyriformis*. Mol Pharmacol 9:304–310

Cook L, Grant PT, Kermack WO (1961) Proteolytic enzymes of the erythrocytic forms of rodent and simian species of malarial plasmodia. Exp Parasitol 11:372–379

Cook RC, Rock RC, Aikawa M, Fournier MJ (1971) Ribosomes of the malarial parasite *Plasmodium knowlesi* – I. Isolation, activity, and sedimentation velocity. Comp Biochem Physiol [B] 39:897–911

Corliss JO (1965) *Tetrahymena,* a ciliate genus of unusual importance in modern biological research. Acta Protozool 3:1–20

Davidson MW, Griggs BG, Boykin DW, Wilson WD (1975) Mefloquine, a clinically useful quinolinemethanol antimalarial which does not significantly bind to DNA. Nature 254:632–634

Davies EE (1973) Studies on the host-parasite relationship and chemotherapy of *Plasmodium berghei.* PhD Thesis, University of Liverpool

Davies EE, Warhurst DC, Peters W (1975) Action of quinine and WR 122455 (a 9-phenanthrenemethanol) on the fine structure of *Plasmodium berghei* in mouse blood. Ann Trop Med Parasitol 69:147–153

De Duve C (1963) The lysosome concept. In: de Reuck AVS, Cameron MP (eds) Lysosomes. Churchill, London, pp 1–31

De Duve C, Wattiaux R (1966) Functions of lysosomes. Annu Rev Physiol 28:435–492

De Duve C, De Barsy T, Poole B, Trouet A, Tulkens P, Van Hoof F (1974) Lysosomotropic agents. Biochem Pharmacol 23:2495–2531

Diribe CO, Warhurst DC (1980) Inhibitors of chloroquine uptake. Trans R Soc Trop Med Hyg 74:675–676

Djiane J, Kelly PA, Houdebine LM (1980) Effects of lysosomotropic agents, cytochalasin B, and colchicine on the "down regulation" of prolactin receptors in mammary gland explants. Mol Cell Endocrinol 18:87–98

Dutta GP, Yadava JNS (1972) Direct amoebicidal action of known antiamoebic drugs against axenically grown *Entamoeba histolytica.* Indian J Med Res 60:1156–1163

Eichel HJ (1956) Effects of atabrine and flavin mononucleotide on oxidation of succinic acid by *Tetrahymena* preparations. Biochim Biophys Acta 22:571–573

Ferone R (1977) Folate metabolism in malaria. Bull WHO 55:291–298

Fischer HD, Gonzalez-Noriega A, Sly WS, Morre DJ (1980) Phosphomannosyl enzyme receptors in rat liver. Subcellular distribution and role in intracellular transport of lysosomal enzymes. J Biol Chem 255:9608–9615

Fitch CD (1969) Chloroquine resistance in malaria: a deficiency of chloroquine binding. Proc Natl Acad Sci 64:1181–1187

Fitch CD (1972) Chloroquine resistance in malaria: Drug binding and cross resistance patterns. Proc Helminth Soc Wash 39:265–271

Fitch CD, Yunis NC, Chevli R, Gonzalez Y (1974) High affinity accumulation of chloroquine by mouse erythrocytes infected with *Plasmodium berghei.* J Clin Invest 54:23–33

Floren CH, Nordgren H, Nillson A (1977) Effects of chloroquine and colchicine on the degradation of chyle cholesteryl ester and phospholipids in vivo. Eur J Biochem 80:331–340

Fourneau, E, Tre'fouel J, Novet D, Benoit G (1931) Contribution à la chimiotherapie du paludisme, essais sur les calfats. Ann Inst Pasteur Paris 46:514–541

Gaddum JH (1957) Theories of drug antagonism. Pharmacol Rev 9:211–218

Goldberg B, Lumbros C, Bacchi J, Hutner SH (1974) Inhibition by several standard antiprotozoal drugs of growth and $O_2$ uptake of cells and particulate preparations of a *Leptomonas.* J Protozool 21:322–326

Goldstein JL, Brown MS (1977) The low-density lipoprotein pathway and its relation to atherosclerosis. Annu Rev Biochem 47:896–930

Goldstein JL, Brunschede GY, Brown MS (1975) Inhibition of the proteolytic degradation of low density lipoprotein in human fibroblasts by chloroquine, concanavalin A, and Triton WR 1339. J Biol Chem 250:7854–7862

Gonzalez-Noriega A, Grubb JH, Talhad V, Sly WS (1980) Chloroquine inhibits lysosomal enzyme pinocytosis and enhances lysosomal enzyme secretion by impairing receptor recycling. J Cell Biol 85:839–852

Gordeeva LM (1965) Morphologic changes in *Entamoeba histolytica* under the effect of some acridine derivatives and chloroquine in culture. Med Parazitol (Mosk) 34:713–719 (in Russian)
Gottlieb M, Zuhalsky M, Zuhalsky AC (1972) *Crithidia* as a model organism? J Parasitol 58:1008–1009
Greiling H, Dorner G (1962) Biochemische Untersuchungen zum Wirkungsmechanismus des Resochins. Z Rheumaforsch 21:316–324
Groupe V (1945) Effect of atabrine on *Tetrahymena geleii* (Protozoa, Ciliata). Proc Soc Exp Biol Med 60:321–323
Hahn FE (1974) Chloroquine (Resochin). In: Corcoran JW, Hahn FE (eds) Antibiotics, vol III. Springer, Berlin Heidelberg New York, pp 58–78
Hahn FE, O'Brien RL, Ciak J, Allison JL, Olenick JG (1966) Studies on modes of action of chloroquine, quinacrine, and quinine and on chloroquine resistance. Milit Med 131:1071–1089
Haigler HT, Willingham MC, Pastan I (1980) Inhibitors of $^{125}$I-epidermal growth factor internalization. Biochem Biophys Res Commun 94:630–637
Harold FM (1970) Antimicrobial agents and membrane function. Adv Microb Physiol 4:45–404
Harold FM (1972) Conservation and transformation of energy by bacterial membranes. Bacteriol Rev 36:172–230
Harold FM (1977) Ion currents and physiological functions in microorganisms. Annu Rev Microbiol 31:181–203
Hart PD'A, Young MR (1978) Manipulation of the phagosome-lysosome fusion response in cultured macrophages. Enhancement of fusion by chloroquine and other amines. Exp Cell Res 114:486–490
Hasilik A, Neufeld EF (1980a) Biosynthesis of lysosomal enzymes in fibroblasts. Synthesis as precursors of higher molecular weight. J Biol Chem 255:4936–4945
Hasilik A, Neufeld EF (1980b) Biosynthesis of lysosomal enzymes in fibroblasts. Phosphorylation of mannose residues. J Biol Chem 255:4946–4950
Hawkins SE, Hainton JM (1972) Sensitivity of amoebae to chloroquine or erythromycin. Microbios 5:57–63
Hill DL (1972a) The biochemistry and physiology of *Tetrahymena*. Academic, New York, pp 193–202
Hill DL (1972b) The biochemistry and physiology of *Tetrahymena*. Academic, New York, pp 15–18
Hill GC, Hutner SH (1968) Effect of trypanocidal drugs on terminal respiration of *Crithidia fasciculata*. Exp Parasitol 22:207–212
Homewood CA (1977) Carbohydrate metabolism of malarial parasites. Bull WHO [Suppl] 55:229–235
Homewood CA, Atkinson EM (1973) Chloroquine-induced pigment clumping in *P. berghei:* dependence on composition of the medium. Trans R Soc Trop Med Hyg 67:26–27
Homewood CA, Warhurst DC, Baggaley VC (1971) Incorporation of radioactive precursors into *Plasmodium berghei* in vitro. Trans R Soc Trop Med Hyg 65:10
Homewood CA, Warhurst DC, Peters W, Baggaley VC (1972a) Lysosomes, pH, and the antimalarial action of chloroquine. Nature 235:50–52
Homewood CA, Warhurst DC, Peters W, Baggaley VC (1972b) Electron transport in intraerythrocytic *Plasmodium berghei*. Proc Helminth Soc Wash 39:382–386
Houdebine LM, Djiane J (1980) Effects of lysosomotropic agents and of microfilament and microtubule-disrupting agents on the activation of casein-gene expression by prolactin in the mammary gland. Mol Cell Biol 17:1–15
Hutner SH (1964) Protozoa as toxicological tools. J Protozool 11:1–6
Hutner SH, Fromentin H, O'Connell KM (1968) Some biological leads to chemotherapy of blood protista, especially Trypanosomatidae. In: Weiman D, Ristic M (eds) Infectious blood diseases of man and animals, vol I. Academic, New York, pp 175–209
Hutner SH, Baker H, Frank O, Cox D (1973) *Tetrahymena* as a nutritional pharmacological tool. In: Elliott AM (ed) Biology of *Tetrahymena*. Hutchinson and Ross, Pennsylvania, pp 411–433

James SP (1934) The direct effect of atebrin on the parasites of benign tertian malaria. Trans R Soc Trop Med Hyg 28:3
Jirovec O (1963) Protozoa as models in biological research. In: Ludvik J, Lom J, Varra J (eds) Progress in protozoology. Academic, New York, pp 31–37
Kaplan A, Fischer HD, Achord D, Sly WS (1977) Phosphohexyl recognition is a general characteristic of pinocytosis of lysosomal glycosidases by human fibroblasts. J Clin Invest 60:1088–1093
Kavanagh F (1963) Analytical microbiology, vol I. Academic, New York
Kikuth W (1932) Chemotherapeutische Versuche mit neuen synthetischen Malariamitteln in ihrer Bedeutung für die Bekämpfung der Malaria. Zentralbl Bakteriol [Orig A] 127:172–178
Kikuth W (1935) Die experimentelle Chemotherapie der Malaria. Dtsch Med Wochenschr 15:573
King AC, Hernandez-Davis L, Cuatrecasas P (1980a) Lysosomotropic amines cause intracellular accumulation of receptors for epidermal growth factor. Proc Natl Acad Sci USA 77:3283–3287
King AC, Willis RA, Cuatrecasas P (1980b) Accumulation of epidermal growth factor within cells does not depend on receptor recycling. Biochem Biophys Res Commun 97:840–845
Kurnick NB, Radcliffe IE (1962) Reaction between DNA and quinacrine and other antimalarials. J Lab Clin Med 60:669–688
Kusiak JW, Quirk JM, Brady RO (1980) Factors that influence the uptake of $\beta$-hexosaminidase A by rat peritoneal macrophages. Biochem Biophys Res Commun 94:199–204
Lantz CH, Van Dyke K (1971) Studies concerning the mechanism of action of antimalarial drugs. II. Inhibition of the incorporation of adenosine-5′-monophosphate-$^3$H into nucleic acids of erythrocyte-free malarial parasites. Biochem Pharmacol 20:1157–1166
Laveran A (1880) Note sur un nouveau parasite trouvé dans le sang de plusieurs malades atteints de fièvre palustre. Bull Acad Med Natl (Paris) 9:1235–1236
Lee YC, Scherbaum OH (1965) Isolation of macronuclei from the ciliate *Tetrahymena pyriformis* GL. Nature 208:1350–1351
Lerman LS (1961) Structural consideration in the interaction of DNA and acridines. J Mol Biol 3:18–30
Levy MR, Chou SC (1973) Activity and some properties of an acid protease from normal and *Plasmodium berghei*-infected red cells. J Parasitol 59:1064–1070
Levy MR, Chou SC (1974) Some properties and susceptibility to inhibitors of partially purified acid proteases from *Plasmodium berghei* and from ghosts of mouse red cells. Biochim Biophys Acta 334:423–430
Levy MR, Chou SC (1975) Inhibition of macromolecular synthesis in the malarial parasite by inhibitors of proteolytic enzymes. Experientia 31:51–53
Levy MR, Siddiqui WA, Chou SC (1974) Acid protease activity in *Plasmodium falciparum* and *P. knowlesi* and ghosts of their respective red cells. Nature 247:546–549
Levy MR, Chou SC, Siddiqui WA (1976) Protease inhibitors and growth of the malarial parasite. Conference on acid proteases: structure, function, and biology, 1976. Oklahoma Medical Research Foundation, Oklahoma City
Lie SO, Schofield B (1973) Inactivation of lysosomal function in normal cultured human fibroblasts by chloroquine. Biochem Pharmacol 22:3109–3114
Macomber PB, O'Brien RL, Hahn FE (1966) Chloroquine: Physiological basis of drug resistance in *Plasmodium berghei*. Science 152:1374–1375
Macomber PB, Sprinz H. Tousimis AJ (1967) Morphological effects of chloroquine on *Plasmodium berghei* in mice. Nature 214:937–939
Mahler HR, Cordes EH (1967) Biological chemistry. Harper and Row, London
Markees DG, Dewey VC, Kidder GW (1968) The synthesis and biological activity of substituted 2,6-diaminopyridines. J Med Chem 11:126–129
Marshall S, Olefsky JM (1979) Effects of lysosomotropic agents on insulin interactions with adipocytes. Evidence for a lysosomal pathway for insulin processing and degradation. J Biol Chem 254:10153–10160

Matsuzawa Y, Hostetler KY (1980) Inhibition of lysosomal phospholipase A and phospolipase C by chloroquine and 4,4′-bis (diethylaminoethoxy) α,β-diethyl phenylethane. J Biol Chem 255:5190–5194
Moulder JW, Evans EA Jr (1946) The biochemistry of the malaria parasite VI. Studies of the nitrogen metabolism of the malaria parasite. J Biol Chem 164:145–157
Nathan HA, Cowperthwaite J (1954) Use of the trypanosomid flagellate, *Crithidia fasciculata,* for evaluating antimalarials. Proc Soc Exp Biol Med 85:117–119
Neal RA (1963) Protozoan tools in the study of antimalarial drugs. Proc 7th int cong trop med malaria, Rio de Janeiro, *5*,, 101–102. Available from: Gräfic Olimpica Editora, Luiz Franco, Rio de Janeiro
Neal RA (1978) Antiamoebic activity of drugs given singly and in combination against axenically grown *Entamoeba histolytica*. Arch Invest Med [Suppl] 9:387–392
Novikoff AB, Essner E (1962) Cytolysomes and mitochondrial degeneration. J Cell Biol 15:140–146
Ohkuma S, Poole B (1978) Fluorescence probe measurement of the intralysosomal pH by living cells and the perturbation of pH by various agents. Proc Natl Acad Sci USA 75:3327–3331
Oleksyn BJ, Lebioda LF (1980) Conformation-configuration relationship in cinchona alkaloids. Pol J Chem 54:755–762
Ose L, Røken I, Norum KR, Berg T (1980) The effect of ammonia, chloroquine, leupeptin, colchicine, and cytochalasin B on degradation of high density lipoproteins in isolated rat hepatocytes. Exp Cell Res 130:127–135
Pan HYM, Chou SC, Conklin KA (1974) Effects of antimalarial drugs and clofibrate on in vitro lipid synthesis in *Tetrahymena pyriformis* GL. Pharmacology 12:48–56
Paton WDM (1970) Receptors as defined by their pharmacological properties. In: Porter R, O'Connor M (eds) Molecular properties of drug receptors. Ciba Foundation Symposium. Churchill, London, pp 3–32
Peters W (1970) Chemotherapy and drug resistance in malaria. Academic, New York
Peters W, Portus JH, Robinson BL (1975) The chemotherapy of rodent malaria, XXII. The value of drug-resistant strains of *P. berghei* in screening for blood schizontocidal activity. Ann Trop Med Parasitol 69:155–171
Peters W, Howells RE, Portus J, Robinson BL, Thomas SC, Warhurst DC (1977) The chemotherapy of rodent malaria, XXVII. Studies on mefloquine (WR 142490). Ann Trop Med Parasitol 71:407–418
Polet H, Barr CF (1969) Uptake of chloroquine 3-$H^3$ by *Plasmodium knowlesi* in vitro. J Pharmacol Exp Ther 168:187–192
Porter M, Peters W (1976) The chemotherapy of rodent malaria, XXV. Antimalarial activity of WR 122455 (a 9-phenanthrene methanol) in vivo and in vitro. Ann Trop Med Parasitol 70:259–270
Prasad BNK (1972) In vitro effect of drugs against pathogenic and nonpathogenic free-living amoebae and on anaerobic amoebae. Indian J Exp Biol 10:43–45
Reijngoud DJ, Tager JM (1976) Chloroquine accumulation in isolated rat liver lysosomes. FEBS Lett 64:231–235
Riches DWH, Stanworth DR (1980) Primary amines induce selective release of lysosomal enzymes from macrophages. Biochem J 188:933–936
Sando GN, Titus-Dillon P, Hall CW, Neufeld EF (1979) Inhibition of receptor-mediated uptake of a lysosomal enzyme into fibroblasts by chloroquine, procaine, and ammonia. Exp Cell Res 119:359–364
Schellenberg KA, Coatney GR (1961) The influence of antimalarial drugs on nucleic acid synthesis in *Plasmodium gallinaceum* and *Plasmodium berghei*. Biochem Pharmacol 6:143–152
Scherbaum O, Zeuthen E (1954) Induction of synchronous cell division in mass cultures of *Tetrahymena pyriformis*. Exp Cell Res 6:221–227
Schlessinger J, Schecter Y, Willingham MC, Pastan I (1978) Direct visualization of binding, aggregation, and internalization of insulin and epidermal growth factor on living fibroblastic cells. Proc Natl Acad Sci USA 75:2659–2663

Seglen PO, Grinde B, Solheim AE (1979) Inhibition of the lysosomal pathway of protein degradation in isolated rat hepatocytes by ammonia, methylamine, chloroquine, and leupeptin. Eur J Biochem 95:215–225

Sly W (1980) Saccharide traffic signals in receptor-mediated endocytosis and transport of acid hydrolases. In: Svennerholm L, Mandel P, Dreyfus H, Urban PF (eds) Structure and function of the gangliosides. Plenum, New York

Stahl PD, Schlessinger PH (1980) Receptor-mediated pinocytosis of mannose/*N*-acetylglucosamine-terminated glycoproteins and lysosomal enzymes by macrophages. Trends Biochem Sci 5:194–196

Stein Y, Ebin V, Bar-On H, Stein O (1977) Chloroquine-induced interference with degradation of serum lipoproteins in rat liver, studied in vivo and in vitro. Biochim Biophys Acta 486:286–297

Strauss JF, Kirsch T, Flickinger GL (1978) Effects of lysosomotropic agents on progestin secretion by rat ovarian cells. J Steroid Biochem 9:71–78

Tappel AL, Zalkin H (1959) Lipid peroxidation in isolated mitochondria. Arch Biochem Biophys 80:326–332

Tate P, Vincent M (1934) The action of atebrin on bird malaria. Parasitology 34:523–530

Thompson PE, Werbel LM (1972) Antimalarial agents. Academic, New York

Thompson PE, Bayles A, Bush DL, Lilligren BL (1948) On the ability of *Plasmodium lophurae* to acquire resistance to chlorguanide, camoquin, and chloroquine. J Infect Dis 83:250–255

Thurston JP (1952) Biological investigations on animal parasites of interest in chemotherapy. PhD Thesis, University of London

Tietze C, Schlessinger P, Stahl P (1980) Chloroquine and ammonium ion inhibit receptor mediated endocytosis of mannose-glycoconjugates by macrophages: Apparent inhibition of receptor recycling. Biochem Biophys Res Commun 93:1–8

Tolleshaug H, Berg T (1979) Chloroquine reduces the number of asialoglycoprotein receptors in the hepatocyte plasma membrane. Biochem Pharmacol 28:2919–2922

Tonkin IM (1946) The testing of drugs against exoerythrocytic forms of *P. gallinaceum* in tissue culture. Br J Pharmacol 1:163–173

Umezawa H, Aoyagi T (1977) Activities of proteinase inhibitors of microbial origin. In: Barett AJ (ed) Proteinases in mammalian cells and tissues. North Holland, Amsterdam

Van Dyke K, Szustkiewicz C (1969) Apparent new modes of antimalarial action detected by inhibited incorporation of adenosine-8-$^3$H into nucleic acids of *Plasmodium berghei.* Milit Med 134:1000–1006

Van Dyke K, Szustkiewicz C, Lantz CH, Saxe LH (1969) Studies concerning the mechanism of action of antimalarial drugs – inhibition of the incorporation of adenosine-8-$^3$H into nucleic acids of *Plasmodium berghei.* Biochem Pharmacol 18:1417–1425

Van Dyke K, Lantz C, Szustkiewicz C (1970) Quinacrine: Mechanisms of anti-malarial action. Science 169:492–493

Warhurst DC (1973) Chemotherapeutic agents and malaria research. In: Chemotherapeutic agents in the study of parasites. Symp Br Soc Parasitol 11:1–28

Warhurst DC (1974) Malarial RNA. In: Bateman JB (ed) Basic research on malaria. Technical report ERO-5-74. European Research Office and Chelsea College, London, pp 196–200

Warhurst DC (1981 a) Mapping the blood-schizontocide receptor. Trans R Soc Trop Med Hyg 75:606

Warhurst DC (1981 b) The quinine-haemin interaction and its relationship to antimalarial activity. Biochem Pharmacol 30:3323–3327

Warhurst DC, Baggaley VC (1972) Autophagic vacuole formation in *P. berghei.* Trans R Soc Trop Med Hyg 66:5

Warhurst DC, Folwell RO (1968) Measurement of the growth rate of the erythrocytic stages of *P. berghei* and comparison of the potency of inocula after various treatments. Ann Trop Med Parasitol 62:349–360

Warhurst DC, Gould S (1982) The chemotherapy of rodent malaria, XXXIII. The activity of chloroquine and related blood schizontocides, and of some analogues in drug-induced pigment clumping. Ann Trop Med Parasitol 36:257–264

Warhurst DC, Hockley DJ (1967) Mode of action of chloroquine on *Plasmodium berghei* and *P. cynomolgi*. Nature 214:935–936
Warhurst DC, Robinson BL (1971) Cytotoxic agents and haemozoin pigment in malaria parasites (*Plasmodium berghei*). Life Sci 10:755–760
Warhurst DC, Thomas SC (1975) Pharmacology of the malaria parasite – a study of dose-response relationships in chloroquine-induced autophagic vacuole formation in *Plasmodium berghei*. Biochem Pharmacol 24:1047–1056
Warhurst DC, Thomas SC (1978) The chemotherapy of rodent malaria, XXXI. The effect of some metabolic inhibitors upon chloroquine-induced pigment clumping in *Plasmodium berghei*. Ann Trop Med Parasitol 72:204–211
Warhurst DC, Williamson J (1970) Ribonucleic acid from *Plasmodium knowlesi* before and after chloroquine treatment. Chem Biol Interact 2:89–106
Warhurst DC, Robinson BL, Howells RE, Peters W (1971) The effect of cytotoxic agents on autophagic vacuole formation in chloroquine-treated malaria parasites (*Plasmodium berghei*). Life Sci 10:761–771
Warhurst DC, Homewood CA, Baggaley VC (1972a) Observations *in vitro* on the mode of action of chloroquine and quinine in blood stages of *Plasmodium berghei*. J Protozool [Suppl] 19:53
Warhurst DC, Homewood CA, Peters W, Baggaley VC (1972b) Pigment changes in *Plasmodium berghei* as indicators of activity and mode of action of antimalarial drugs. Proc Helminth Soc Wash 39:271–278
Warhurst DC, Homewood CA, Baggaley VC (1974) The chemotherapy of rodent malaria, XX. Autophagic vacuole formation in *Plasmodium berghei in vitro*. Ann Trop Med Parasitol 68:265–281
Wibo M, Poole B (1974) Protein degradation in cultured cells. II. The uptake of chloroquine by rat fibroblasts and the inhibition of cellular protein degradation and cathepsin B1. J Cell Biol 63:430–440
Wiesmann UN, Didonato S, Herschkowitz NN (1975) Effects of chloroquine on cultured fibroblasts: Release of lysosomal hydrolases and inhibition of their uptake. Biochem Biophys Res Commun 66:1338–1343
Willcox P, Rattray S (1979) Secretion and uptake of *β-N*-acetylglucosaminidase by fibroblasts. Effect of chloroquine and mannose-6-phosphate. Biochim Biophys Acta 586:442–452
Yadava JNS, Dutta GP (1973) Combined action of antiamoebic drugs and antibiotics on axenically grown *Entamoeba histolytica*. Indian J Med Res 61:971–975
Yamada KA, Sherman IW (1979) *Plasmodium lophurae*. Composition and properties of hemozoin, the malaria pigment. Exp Parasitol 48:61–74

CHAPTER 11

# Interactions Between Chemotherapy and Immunity

G. A. T. TARGETT

## A. Introduction

It is perhaps not surprising that few planned studies on the interactions between chemotherapy of malaria and the immune status of infected individuals or animals have been carried out. Most antimalarial drugs have been developed in an empirical way, tested against acute-stage infection. Levels of specific resistance at the time of treatment, immunodepression as a result of infection or increased resistance to challenge as a result of chemotherapy have either been irrelevant or just not considered.

The past few years have seen major advances in our understanding of both immunological response to malarial infection and modes of action of antimalarial compounds. The details of these are given in other chapters of this book but, increasingly, it is being recognised that these two methods of control directed against the parasite can and do interact in both positive and negative ways, producing sometimes minor, sometimes profound, changes in levels of infection. Here I shall be considering (a) the effectiveness of drugs in relation to the immune status of the host; (b) malaria-linked immunopathogenic or immunopathological syndromes; (c) the immunodepressive effects of antimalarials; (d) the induction of immunity by chemotherapy; and (e) immunopotentiation and chemotherapy.

The modes of action of the commonly used antimalarials, so far as these are known, are discussed in detail elsewhere in the book (Part II, Chaps. 1–5, 9–15). The immune responses are also reviewed by MITCHELL (Chap. 4) but it is perhaps useful to begin by indicating briefly those aspects of the immune response in malaria that have, or might have, a particular relevance where chemotherapy is concerned.

## B. Immune Responses in Malaria

### I. Innate Resistance

Those mechanisms that have been elucidated in any detail at all relate only to the blood stages of infection. Virtually nothing is known about natural resistance as it affects sporozoites and exoerythrocytic development in the liver although the high, if not absolute, degree of species specificity of *Plasmodium* species indicates a genetic basis to susceptibility. Of the various innate determinants affecting either invasion of red cells or development within the erythrocyte (see review by TARGETT 1981 a), few can be linked with responses to chemotherapy. The intraerythrocytic factors suppress but rarely totally inhibit development of the parasite. Thus in individuals heterozygous (or indeed, homozygous) for haemoglobin S, development of *P. falciparum* is relatively normal under conditions of high oxygen tension, but greatly impaired at the lower oxygen tensions that might occur in the deeper circulation (PASVOL et al. 1978). ATP levels in red blood cells vary and low levels are thought to confer some resistance to *P. falciparum* (in black Americans), as a consequence, reducing the severity of the disease. Such individuals respond better to chemotherapy than those with normal ATP levels (POWELL et al. 1972), and the relatively lower levels of *P. falciparum* parasitaemias in Africans may be one reason why chloroquine resistance has appeared so much more slowly there than in Southeast Asia and South America (HALL and CANFIELD 1972).

## II. Acquired Immunity

It is important first to appreciate in broad terms the influence of acquired immune responses on the pattern of human disease. Where the disease is highly endemic, very young children are protected to a large extent, partly as a result of non-immunological factors (TARGETT 1982), and partly through maternally derived immunity. There follows a period of several years during which repeated infection produces high parasitaemias and correspondingly high rates of mortality (in *P. falciparum* infections) and morbidity. A lessening of the clinical aspects of the disease precedes the gradual acquisition of an antiparasitic immunity. Adults show strong immunity that keeps parasite levels very low, but this is maintained only if sporozoite challenge continues. In areas where transmission is irregular, an effective immunity may never be attained, the whole population rather than the children alone remaining susceptible to clinical malaria or, at best, semi-immune. This pattern is broadly true for both falciparum and vivax malaria. Development of immunity in simian, rodent and avian malaria infections used as laboratory models is, as we shall see later, usually different from that of the human disease. Commonly the hosts develop either a strong, acquired immune response following a single infection, or a fulminant infection which, untreated, is invariably fatal.

An important feature of the human disease is that resistance depends on continuous challenge and on the continued presence of parasites in the body. It is not a sterile immunity. *P. falciparum* infections die out within a year if there is no further exposure. *P. vivax* infections under similar circumstances last about 3 years because of the presence of dormant stages within the liver (KROTOSKI et al. 1980, and see Chap. 1). The waning of resistance is shown by the susceptibility to re-exposure in both cases and the development of relapse infections of *P. vivax*.

A point of obvious relevance to the present discussion is the stage or stages of the parasite life-cycle against which the immune responses are primarily directed.

Immune responses to sporozoites have not been clearly established. NARDIN et al. (1979) have recently demonstrated the presence of antisporozoite antibodies in individuals from a *P. falciparum* hyperendemic area. Since they occurred mainly in immune adults, it was suggested that they might effect a sterilising immunity.

Evidence of functional immune responses directed against exoerythrocytic stages of mammalian malaria parasites is also difficult to find. There is much to suggest that this phase of the life cycle is, in fact, unaffected by the immune response. However, VERHAVE (1975) exposed mice to sporozoites of *P. berghei* but provided drug cover to prevent the establishment of a blood infection. After two or three infections there was clear evidence of immunity – shown by reduction in the number of liver schizonts – though it was not clear whether this was directed against the sporozoites or the liver stages themselves. It may be that we shall have to revise our view that there is little or no effective immunity to pre-erythrocytic forms, and this clearly has some relevance when considering causal prophylactic and antirelapse drugs.

The antiparasitic immunity that develops is directed mainly against asexual stages in the blood, especially against schizonts and the extracellular merozoites. Growth of the parasite within the red cell brings about changes in the erythrocyte membrane through modification of host membrane components. It is this schizont stage in *P. falciparum* that becomes sequestered in the deep vasculature, probably as a result of a sequence of specific immunologically mediated changes (TARGETT 1981). Rupture of erythrocytes at schizogony is associated with release of considerable quantities of antigen, and antibody is developed which kills or blocks invasion by the extracellular merozoites (COHEN and BUTCHER 1971; MILLER et al. 1975). The released antigen may be detected circulating either as free antigen or complexed with antibody. In either form it can modulate the immune response to the parasite. Antigen and complexes are also deposited in various organs or tissues, contributing to the pathogenesis (e.g. anaemia) or initiating immunopathological changes (e.g. acute or chronic renal lesions) which respond variably to chemotherapy.

There are perhaps important links too between immune responses, gametocyte production, infectivity, and chemotherapy, since there is conflicting evidence on the infectivity of gametocytes in immune individuals.

## C. Immunodepression by Malaria Infections

Secondary immunodeficiency is a feature of malarial and, indeed, of many other infections. There are many clinical and experimental data on the nature of this depression (GREENWOOD 1974; WEDDERBURN 1974), which is relevant here since, as we shall see, chemotherapy can be linked with specific and non-specific immune effector mechanisms. MCGREGOR and BARR (1962) demonstrated a significantly lower antibody response to tetanus toxoid in malarious as opposed to chemoprophylactically protected children, and this was, in fact, the first demonstration of immunodepression associated with any parasite. Subsequent studies have shown that, in experimental malaria infections, depression of both antibody and cell-mediated immune responses can occur, the latter being demonstrable only when parasitaemias are high. It is generally true that, although immunodepression can be associated with low-grade chronic infections (WEDDENBURN and DRACOTT 1977), the degree of depression parallels the parasitaemia. Studies on patients have amply confirmed the original observation that antibody responses are depressed but have shown that cell-mediated responses in vivo (skin tests) or in vitro, and responses to mitogens, such as phytohaemagglutinin, are largely unimpaired (TERRY 1977).

A variety of mechanisms of immunodepression have been demonstrated. Impaired macrophage processing of antigen and its presentation to germinal centres

(WARREN and WEIDANZ 1976; BROWN et al. 1977) are probably a consequence of antigenic competition. Suppressor activity of macrophages (WYLER et al. 1979) and of T cells (JAYAWARDENA cited by PLAYFAIR 1980) have also been demonstrated. Mitogenic substances have been isolated from human and rodent malaria parasites (GREENWOOD and VICK 1975; FREEMAN and PARISH 1978) and are responsible for polyclonal activation, with the consequent reduced ability to respond to any antigenic challenge (TERRY 1977).

Although the severity of immunodepression is largely a consequence of the degree of parasitaemia, responses in chronic infections can remain impaired. WEDDERBURN and DRACOTT (1977) demonstrated reduced IgG responses associated with low-grade rodent malarias and, of particular interest, WILLIAMSON and GREENWOOD (1978) showed persistence of immunodepression after treatment of *P. falciparum* infections with chloroquine. Parasitaemic patients showed impaired immune responses to *Salmonella typhi* and to meningococcal vaccine. Treated patients rapidly recovered the ability to respond to *S. typhi*, probably because this was a secondary immune response, but there was prolonged depression of antibody production to the meningococcal vaccine, this being a primary response.

## D. Immune Dependence of Antimalarial Chemotherapy

There is much indirect evidence to link the effectiveness of chemotherapy with the immune status of the host. Treatment of the infected semi-immune individual is effective with lower dose schedules than those required for infected non-immunes (WHO 1973). Introduction of malaria control measures reduces the immunity of the population. Thereafter it is necessary to increase the dose of antimalarial to effect a clinical cure (AFRIDI and RAHIM 1962; PRINGLE and LANE 1966). Blood schizontocidal drugs such as quinine are more effective if treatment is given after the patient has experienced several paroxysms and is consequently developing some measure of acquired resistance (YORKE 1925). Experimentally, similar results have been obtained by treatment of *P. berghei* infections with chloroquine (GOLENSER et al. 1978). Quinine too was shown to be more effective against *P. gallinaceum* in intact rather than splenectomised or bursectomised chickens (TALIAFERRO 1948; TALIAFERRO and KELSEY 1948; TALIAFERRO and TALIAFERRO 1949), and against *P. knowlesi* in intact as opposed to splenectomised rhesus monkeys (NAUCK 1934). Chloroquine treatment of *P. knowlesi* has also been shown to be dependent on acquired immunity to be fully effective (DUTTA and SINGH 1978, cited by PETERS 1970).

We have recently investigated in some detail the effectiveness of three antimalarials, pyrimethamine, chloroquine, and quinine, against *P. chabaudi* and *P. yoelii* infections in intact CBA mice and in mice that were immunologically impaired (LWIN et al. 1984). In intact mice, *P. chabaudi* gives rise to a high but resolving parasitaemia followed by one or two small recrudescences, then immunological resolution of infection. The infection in T-cell-deprived mice is not fatal but it does not resolve (Fig. 1). *P. berghei*, on the other hand, is fatal in both intact and T-cell-deprived mice, though survival is significantly longer in the latter, i.e. when the "immune response" is impaired (Fig. 2). The therapeutic regimens of the three

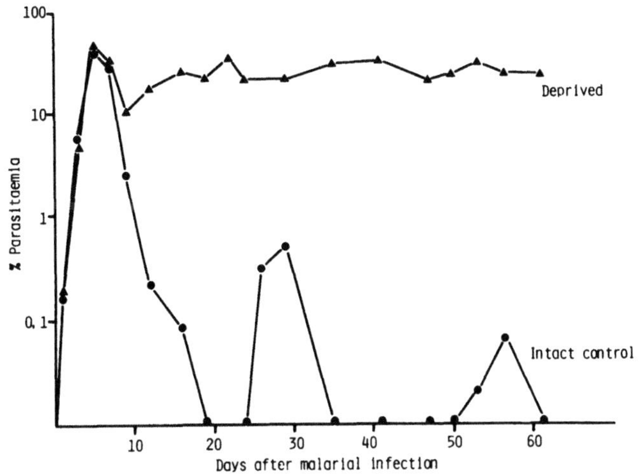


**Fig. 1.** *P. chabaudi:* mean parasitaemias in intact control (*circles*) and T-cell-deprived (*triangles*) CBA mice

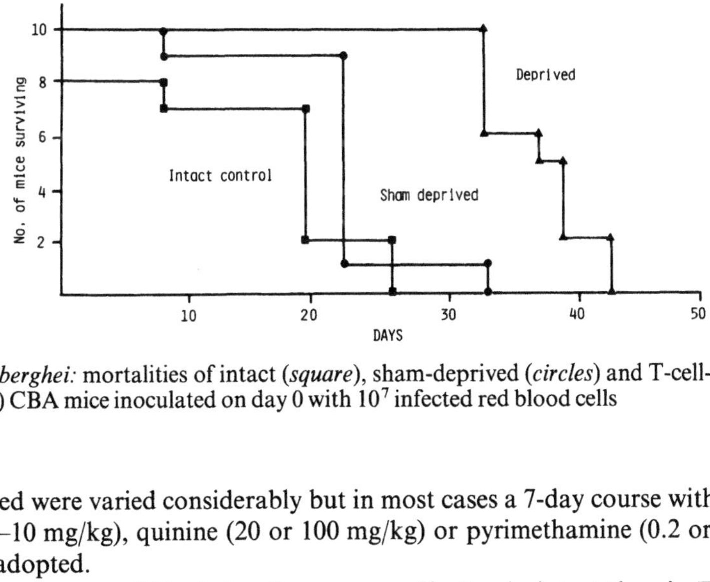


**Fig. 2.** *P. berghei:* mortalities of intact (*square*), sham-deprived (*circles*) and T-cell-deprived (*triangles*) CBA mice inoculated on day 0 with $10^7$ infected red blood cells

drugs used were varied considerably but in most cases a 7-day course with chloroquine (2–10 mg/kg), quinine (20 or 100 mg/kg) or pyrimethamine (0.2 or 2.0 mg/kg) was adopted.

Chemotherapy of *P. chabaudi* was more effective in intact than in T-cell-deprived mice (Lwin et al. 1979, and Figs. 3–5) but, in *P. berghei* infections, the reverse was generally true, a more effective response to chemotherapy being obtained in infected T-cell-deprived animals (Fig. 6). The effects were partly dose dependent. Where a large enough dose of drug was used, chemotherapy of *P. chabaudi* in T-cell-deprived mice could be as effective as treatment of infections in intact animals. Timing of drug treatment was also a contributing factor. Differences in responses of infections in T-cell-deprived and intact mice were more pronounced when treatment was begun later rather than very early in infection. Larger inocula of parasites (*P. chabaudi*) also meant that subsequent chemotherapy (e.g. with pyrimethamine,

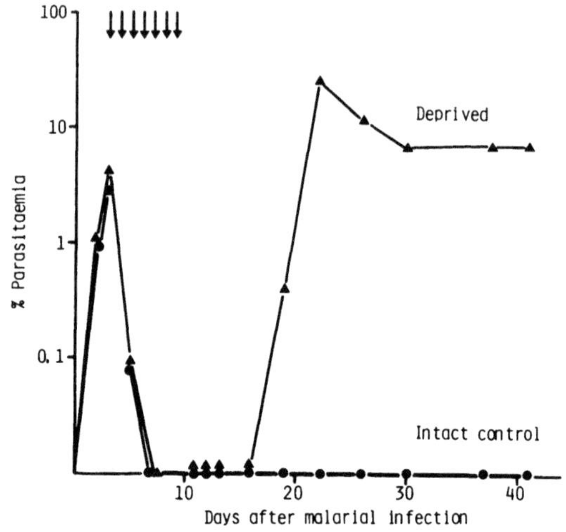


**Fig. 3.** *P. chabaudi:* mean parasitaemias in T-cell-deprived (*triangles*) and intact control (*circles*) CBA mice inoculated on day 0 with $10^7$ infected red blood cells and treated with chloroquine (*arrows*) 4 mg/kg (days 3–9) (LWIN 1978)

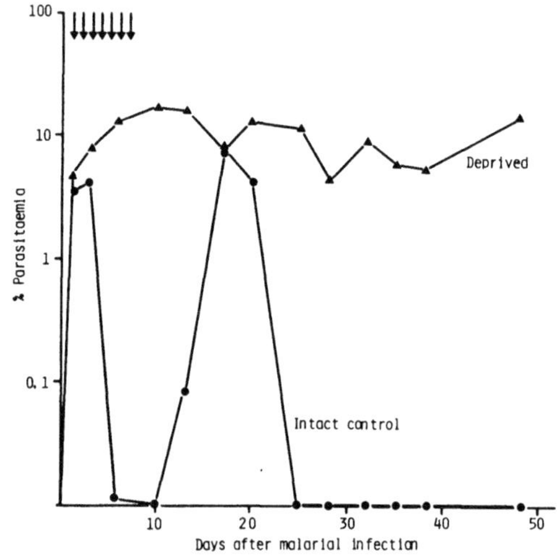


**Fig. 4.** *P. chabaudi:* mean parasitaemias in T-cell-deprived (*triangles*) and intact control (*circles*) CBA mice inoculated with $1.5 \times 10^8$ infected red blood cells on day 0 and treated with quinine (*arrows*) 100 mg/kg per day (days 1–7) (LWIN 1978)

2 mg/kg for 7 days) was likely to be less effective in immunologically impaired hosts.

Immunodepression produced by treatment with hydrocortisone acetate (200 mg/kg single dose or 30 mg/kg for 7 days) converted a normally resolving infection with *P. chabaudi* into one that was fatal. Again, when combined with chloroquine or quinine chemotherapy, there was evidence that the drug treatment was less effective in the immunodepressed host. Similar experiments with *P. berghei* were complicated by the depression of reticulocytosis induced by hydrocortisone, thus reducing the numbers of cells preferentially invaded by *P. berghei*.

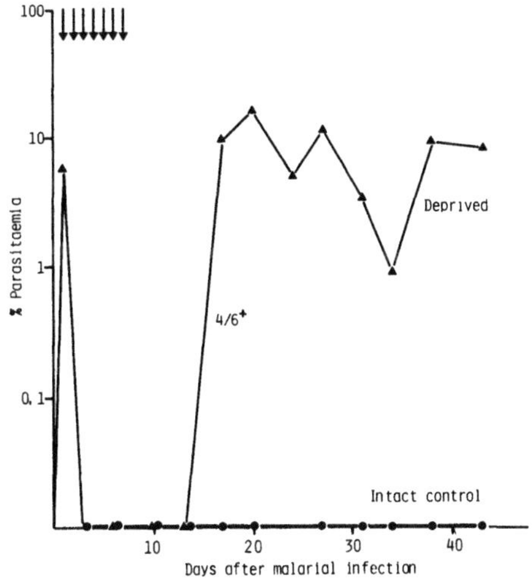


**Fig. 5.** *P. chabaudi:* mean parasitaemias in T-cell-deprived (*triangles*) and intact control (*circles*) CBA mice inoculated on day 0 with $1.5 \times 10^8$ infected red blood cells and treated with pyrimethamine (*arrows*) 2 mg/kg per day (days 1–7). Control mice were all cured of infection but in four out of six deprived mice infections recrudesced (LWIN 1978)

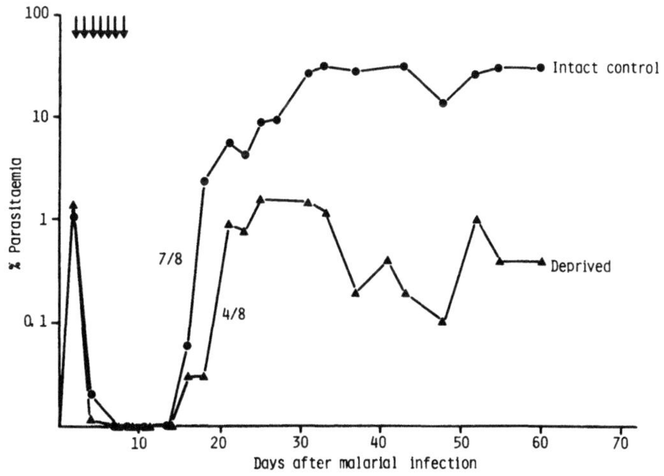


**Fig. 6.** *P. berghei:* mean parasitaemias in T-cell-deprived (*triangles*) and intact control (*circles*) CBA mice inoculated on day 0 with $10^7$ infected red blood cells and treated with chloroquine (*arrows*) 10 mg/kg per day (days 2–8). Seven out of eight control mice developed recrudescent infections and died (mean survival time $32 \pm 17.1$ days). Four out of eight treated T-cell-deprived mice recrudesced. One died (on day 62) while the three others became aparasitaemic (LWIN 1978)

It is not easy to identify the immunological mechanisms that determine these differences in response between the two parasites. We have seen that *P. berghei* infections are normally fatal, death occurring earlier in intact as opposed to T-cell-deprived hosts. *P. berghei* induces a profound immunodepression with production of T-suppressor cells (JAYAWARDENA, cited by PLAYFAIR 1980). Removal of these

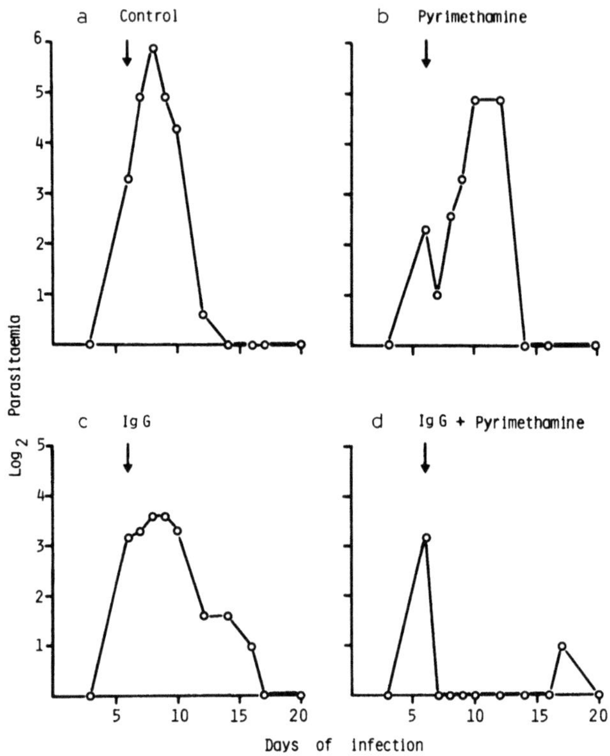


**Fig. 7 a–d.** *P. chabaudi:* the combined effect on infection of chemotherapy and passively transferred IgG (from mice hyperimmunised against *P. chabaudi*). Doses of drug and of antibody that were not curative when given alone were selected. **a** Control (*arrow*) 0.1 ml saline i.p. **b** 0.2 ml (1.0 mg/kg) pyrimethamine i.p. (*arrow*). **c** 0.2 (1.0 mg) IgG i.p. (*arrow*). **d** 0.2 ml pyrimethamine (1.0 mg/kg) + 1.0 mg IgG i.p. (*arrow*)

by T-cell deprivation might mean that where chemotherapy was not fully effective but greatly reduced the parasite load, impairment of suppressor mechanisms could allow a better immune respond than in intact mice. The greater effectiveness of chemotherapy of *P. chabaudi* infections in intact mice may be related to antibody production. This is impaired in T-deprived mice (JAYAWARDENA et al. 1977), especially IgG production. Experiments were also undertaken to determine whether drugs and passively transferred antibody (IgG) act additively or synergistically. IgG from mice hyperimmunised against *P. chabaudi* was administered to infected mice in doses that partially suppressed but did not eradicate parasitaemia. Combining this with subcurative chemotherapy (with chloroquine or pyrimethamine) was markedly more effective than either form of therapy used alone (Fig. 7) and, significantly as far as the present discussion is concerned, was demonstrable in deprived as well as in intact mice (LWIN et al. 1984). ROBERTS et al. (1977) also showed that recrudescence of *P. yoelii* infections in congenitally athymic (Nu/Nu) mice after treatment with clindamycin could be prevented by thymus grafting or by injection of hyperimmune serum.

One possibility resulting from relatively reduced effectiveness of chemotherapy in an immunodepressed host is selection for drug-resistant parasites. This is illustrated by studies on the interactions of chemotherapy and immune mechanisms in cancer. CARTER et al. (1973) showed that successful treatment of Gardner lymphosarcoma of mice with L-asparaginase was dependent on the host immune response. In immunologically intact animals, cutaneous grafts of the tumor disappeared completely following a single injection of L-asparaginase. The same treatment in T-cell-deprived mice caused the tumour to regress initially but a residue of surviving tumour cells gave rise to local and disseminated lymphosarcoma that was eventually fatal. The recurrent tumours were invariably asparaginase resistant; these would normally have been removed in the immunologically intact host by the immune response. In *P. chabaudi* malaria infections, although persistence or recrudescence of infection following chemotherapy was more likely in immunodepressed hosts, there was no evidence that this was due to selection for drug-resistant parasites. A difference might have been demonstrable if chemotherapy of infections in immunodeprived hosts had been repeated several times.

Immunosuppressant therapy with steroids is sometimes associated with management of nephrotic syndrome and treatment of cerebral malaria. The steroids reduce or prevent cerebral and pulmonary oedema, but very different views prevail on the value of this treatment as an adjunct to antimalarial chemotherapy. HALL (1977), in his review, concluded that steroid treatment of diffuse vascular disease such as that seen in severe *P. falciparum* malaria was probably not helpful. The experimental studies combining hydrocortisone and antimalarial therapy of *P. chabaudi* infection would tend to support this view as the antimalarials, especially quinine, were not as effective as when given alone.

Recently, THOMMEN-SCOTT (1981) has reported that cyclosporin A has a marked antimalarial activity in mice infected with *P. berghei* NK65 or *P. chabaudi*. This compound, a fungal metabolite, is used clinically and experimentally as an immunodepressant with selective antilymphocyte action, reversibly inhibiting transformation of stimulated T cells and suppressing both humoral and cell-mediated immunity. Significant antimalarial effects were obtained with five daily oral doses of 25 mg/kg. Further preliminary studies showed that the drug was effective against infections in congenitally athymic mice and against *P. falciparum* in vitro, implying that here the antimalarial activity was distinct from the modulating effect that the compound has on the immune system.

## E. Immunodepressive Effects of Antimalarial Drugs

Chemotherapy can influence the immune response in malaria basically in two ways. We shall be considering how the induction of antimalarial immunity is affected by suppression or cure of infection by chemotherapy. Here we are concerned with direct (i.e. non-specific) effects on the immune system by the antimalarials – their immunodepressive (or perhaps immunostimulatory) properties.

Chloroquine is known to be immunodepressive. In vitro studies show depressed lymphocyte responses to mitogens such as phytohaemagglutinin and to various antigens, due perhaps to the stabilising effect that chloroquine has on lysosomal membranes (HURVITZ and HIRSCHORN 1965). This property has been used in treatment of autoimmune collagen disease but prolonged therapy with high doses of the drug were necessary.

Quinine (THONG and FERRANTE 1978; GOLD et al. 1979) and primaquine (THONG et al. 1978) were also shown in vitro to have similar immunodepressive properties. Mefloquine had no effect on delayed-type hypersensitivity (DTH) responses but did suppress antibody production (THONG et al. 1979). The immunodepressive effects are, however, dose related and when THONG et al. (1981) tested the effects in vivo of chloroquine, quinine, and primaquine on antibody and DTH responses to sheep red blood cells they found that the clinically related doses, well below those used in vitro were not immunodepressive.

THONG and FERRANTE (1980) also tested pyrimethamine for its effect on the immune system in vivo. Here they reported immunopotentiation, both antibody and DTH responses to sheep erythrocytes being enhanced. Pyrimethamine also reversed immunodepression in tumour-bearing mice. The timing of drug and sheep-cell antigen administration was important, the most marked effect being when they were given simultaneously. However, the dose of pyrimethamine used (5 mg/kg or greater) was again much above that required for effective treatment of (mouse) malaria. In summary, marked non-specific changes in immune responsiveness as a result of malaria prophylaxis or therapy do not on the basis of available evidence seem to be likely.

## F. Chemotherapy and Induction of Immunity

The crucial question here is the extent to which antimalarial drugs modify the ability to mount an immune response to the malaria parasite. Drugs may be used prophylactically, curatively or as suppressives, and effects on levels of immunity may vary accordingly.

There seems to be very little doubt that effective causal prophylaxis precludes the development of any immunity since without subsequent drug cover the individual is fully susceptible to infection. Prophylaxis with blood schizontocides such as chloroquine does, however, allow normal development of the exoerythrocytic cycle. While there is no direct epidemiological evidence, it is conceivable that preventing asexual parasitaemia in this way could allow the development of a protective immunity to sporozoites and/or liver schizonts. VERHAVE (1975) showed that mice given chloroquine in drinking water to prevent any asexual parasitaemia when they were exposed to bites of *P. berghei*-infected mosquitoes soon showed a reduction in numbers of exoerythrocytic parasites, indicative of immunity to one or both of the early stages of infection. NARDIN et al. (1979) have shown that most adults in a *P. falciparum*-endemic area do have antisporozoite antibodies, but few of the children do so. Since the children are usually parasitaemic, the immunodepressive effects of infection might prevent the development of antisporozoite antibodies. The important implication would be that suppression of asexual parasitaemia could allow the development of a sterilising antisporozoite response. It would need to be 100% effective since, otherwise, once drug cover had been removed, the individual would be completely susceptible to blood-stage infection, immunity in malaria being highly stage specific.

Development of immunity to malaria in man is, as we have seen, a slow process, requiring repeated exposure to infection and waning quickly once that ceases. Consequently, curative therapy is inimical to development of resistance.

Experimental studies have generally shown that duration and/or levels of parasitaemia determine the level of resistance to subsequent challenge. Thus WAKI (1976) immunised mice by repeated infection with *P. berghei* and radical chemotherapy with sulphamonomethoxine (20 mg/kg per day for 4 days). Drug treatment began 3 days after inoculation of parasites. A single immunising dose conferred little resistance to subsequent homologous challenge, but four immunising infections gave a very effective immunity. LWIN (1978) was able to cure *P. chabaudi* infections with a 7-day course of chloroquine (10–40 mg/kg per day). A significant reduction in the level of challenge infection was achieved when chemotherapy began very early in infection (starting 1–6 days after the inoculation of parasites), but the strongest immunity was obtained when chemotherapy was delayed (Table 1).

Suppressive chemotherapy is frequently proposed as effective for the alleviation of clinical symptoms of infection without impairing the development of immunity. There is certainly considerable experimental evidence that resistance to normally virulent *Plasmodium* infections can be induced if the parasitaemia is held at a low-grade, chronic level for a sufficiently long time. Diets deficient in para-amino benzoic acid (PABA), such as milk, have been used to achieve immunity in this way (KRETSCHMAR 1965). Similar results have been achieved with PABA antagonists such as sulphonamide. ELING and JERUSALEM (1977) maintained *P. berghei*-infected mice on drinking water containing varying dose levels of sulphathiazole. Parasitaemias were suppressed to varying degrees, depending on the drug concentration. While it was possible to induce a strong immunity to challenge, drug concentrations used during the immunising period were crucial, too high a dose preventing the acquisition of antimalarial immunity. LWIN (1978) suppressed *P. chabaudi* parasitaemias to patent but low ($<0.4\%$) levels with chloroquine (2 mg/kg per day) given from days $-1$ to $+20$ of infection. Subsequent challenge did not produce infection patent by blood examination. Shorter periods of treatment, allowing varying degrees of recrudescence of the immunising infection, again

**Table 1.** The effect of curative chloroquine therapy (10 mg/kg per day × 7) at various stages of a *P. chabaudi* infection in mice on resistance to reinfection. Mice were challenged 68 days after the primary infection (LWIN 1978)

| Onset of treatment day | Mean peak parasitaemias (%) | |
|---|---|---|
| | Immunising infection | Challenge infection |
| 1 | 1.5 | 2.9 |
| 2 | 2.4 | 11.5 |
| 4 | 6.8 | 5.7 |
| 6 | 40.0 | 6.0 |
| 14 | 42.2 | 0.6 |
| Control | – | 36.0 |

showed that certain minimum levels of parasitaemia and periods of exposure to the parasite were necessary to induce effective resistance.

It is possible in rodent malaria infections to induce acquired resistance by eliminating the infection, i.e. producing a sterile immunity (WAKI 1976). An effective antimalarial immunity in man depends on the persistence of infection, and suppressive therapy would seem therefore to be most appropriate. There is still scope here for controlled investigations but there are also potential problems, not least being the possibility of selection of drug-resistant strains (PETERS 1970). A further complication is the possible effect on gametocytogenesis and hence on transmission. The evidence concerning development of antigamete or antigametocyte immunity is conflicting. Some epidemiological studies indicate clearly that, in highly endemic areas, the relatively non-immune children are the major source of infection, the semi-immune or immune adults, although they have circulating gametocytes, having presumably developed an acquired immunity that renders these non-infective (McCARTHY et al. 1978). Against this MUIRHEAD-THOMPSON (1954) and others have concluded that the gametocytes of such adults *are* an important source of infection. It is also unclear whether the development of acquired immunity to the asexual stages in any way triggers the production of gametocytes. COHEN and McGREGOR (1963), in their now classic passive transfer studies with children infected with *P. falciparum,* produced a dramatic reduction in asexual parasites by inoculation of immune IgG, but gametocyte numbers actually rose. Experimentally, TANDON and BHATTACHARYA (1970) enhanced *P. berghei* gametocytaemia markedly by treatment of mice with dexamethasone. This might appear to contrast with the passive transfer studies, since the steroid is immunodepressive. However, it also depresses reticulocytosis and this would serve to inhibit *P. berghei* infections. Clearly the interaction between chemotherapy, the acquisition of immunity and viable gamete production remains a very open question.

The importance of antigenic variation and of variant-specific responses in acquisition of immunity to malaria in man is still unknown but it is pertinent to remember that BROWN and his co-workers converted a normally fatal *P. knowlesi* infection in rhesus monkeys into a prolonged, low-grade infection by chemotherapy (with sulphadiazine and proguanil). The chronic infections were apparently maintained by continuous antigenic variations by the parasite, this inducing variant-specific, antibody-mediated, protective responses (BROWN and BROWN 1965; BROWN 1978).

## G. Immunopathological Changes in Malaria

The immunological basis of pathological changes occurring as a result of malaria infection and the consequences for chemotherapy demand consideration. These changes include the tropical splenomegaly syndrome (TSS), nephrotic syndrome and perhaps cerebral malaria.

### I. Tropical Splenomegaly Syndrome

TSS, a persistent splenomegaly in adults from highly endemic malarious regions, is linked with abnormal immunological responses to infection, particularly with *P.*

*malariae*. The syndrome is associated with high levels of malarial antibodies and high molecular weight IgM, but also circulating low molecular weight IgM (7S) and free light chains (FAKUNLE and GREENWOOD 1977), antiglobulins and heterophile antibodies. It is likely that TSS results from immunological malfunction, either abnormal responses to antigen-antibody complexes (WORLD HEALTH ORGANIZATION 1975) or a disorder of control of immunoglobulin production (FAKUNLE and GREENWOOD 1977). Prolonged treatment with antimalarials, e.g. primaquine and chloroquine (STUIVER et al. 1971), is necessary to effect a significant decrease in spleen size and an improvement in other symptoms.

### II. Renal Lesions

Acute glomerulonephritis is not uncommon with malaria infections, including *P. falciparum*. Deposition of immunoglobulins, mainly IgM, and complement has been shown (BHAMARAPRAVATI et al. 1973) but the condition responds readily to antimalarial therapy. In contrast, chronic nephropathies may develop as a result of *P. malariae* infection. Immunoglobulin (IgG and IgM) is found in granular deposits in capillary walls of glomeruli, often in association with complement and malarial antigen (HOUBA and LAMBERT 1974). The prognosis is generally poor because the nephropathy does not respond well to steroids and antimalarials (WORLD HEALTH ORGANIZATION 1977). This was shown to be particularly true in those patients with deposits of $IgG_2$ alone, an immunoglobulin that fixes complement poorly.

The reasons for the poor response to chemotherapy are unknown. Complexes are likely to be deposited through the formation of low-affinity antibodies (STEWARD 1977) and, although these initiate the damage, other auto-immune changes probably perpetrate the syndrome.

### III. Cerebral Malaria

Mention has been made already of chemotherapy associated with cerebral malaria, namely doubts concerning the use of combinations of steroids and antimalarials, such as quinine. The immunological basis of cerebral malaria is still debatable but it does seem likely that malarial antigen-antibody complexes through platelet and complement activation could give rise to the major features of cerebral malaria, namely increased vascular permeability, diffuse intravascular coagulation and the formation of microthrombi (ROITT et al. 1981). Steroids effectively depress the *early* stages of an immune response but have been shown to have no effect on *established* malarial infections (COX 1968). If the cerebral lesion is predominantly immunologically mediated, steroid therapy would therefore be expected neither to enhance nor potentiate the effects of an antimalarial drug.

## H. Immunopotentiation and Chemotherapy

HANSON (1981) has drawn attention to an area of possible interaction between chemotherapy and immunological resistance that deserves further investigation, namely the combination of antimalarial therapy with compounds that enhance immunity. A number of candidate substances are already being studied in relation to experimental malarias. CLARK, ALLISON and their co-workers (see ALLISON et al. 1979; CLARK 1979) have been investigating the development of non-specific resistance to rodent malaria and piroplasm infections by pretreatment with bacille Calmette-Guerin (BCG) *Corynebacterium parvum* and a variety of other agents. While it is not yet clear how the resistance obtained is mediated, it appears to be associated with activity of NK cells (EUGUI and ALLISON 1980), release of low molecular weight substances such as interferon, or tumour necrosis factor from macrophages (CLARK 1979) and, as a result, intraerythrocytic death of the parasites. The effects are variable with different species of *Plasmodium* but, even where the protective response is limited, combination with chemotherapy would be well worth testing. Similarly, muramyl dipeptide, one of a number of adjuvants being used in experimental vaccination programmes against *P. falciparum* malaria (SIDDIQUI et al. 1981) has also been shown to increase resistance to *Trypanosoma cruzi* if given alone prior to infection (KIERSZENBAUM and FERRARER 1979), perhaps in the same way as BCG.

A recent report on the combined use of chloroquine and glucan is strong support for this approach. Glucan is a known immunopotentiating agent, again when given alone or as an adjuvant (COOK et al. 1980). Against *P. berghei* malaria it is not very effective when used alone but BLIZNAKIV (1980, cited by HANSON 1981) has reported that glucan combined with chloroquine was much more active against *P. berghei* in mice than either compound used separately.

## J. Conclusions

The effectiveness of antimalarial drugs is undoubtedly affected by the immune status of the host, much higher doses being required to cure populations in epidemic situations following long periods of little or no exposure, or immunologically deprived infected animals. At the same time, there do seem to be good prospects for effective combination of chemotherapy and immunotherapy in a variety of ways.

The possible combination with immunopotentiating agents such as glucan has already been mentioned. These affect the immune responses non-specifically and their modes of action are still uncertain, but the results obtained by BLIZNAKIV (see above) should be a stimulus for concerted further effort. A totally unexplored area of interaction in protozoology as yet is targeting of drugs by means of antibodies. The experimental studies combining chemotherapy and passive immunisation with IgG referred to earlier were carried out with polyclonal immunoglobulin. Development of monoclonal antibodies now makes targeting a much more testable approach. Monoclonal antibodies to *P. falciparum* (PERRIN et al. 1981) and to rodent (FREEMAN et al. 1980; YOSHIDA et al. 1980) and avian (RENER et al. 1980) malaria parasites have already been produced. These include antibodies that react with surface determinants of sporozoites, merozoites or gametes, but of equal interest here would be those that react with the intraerythrocytic stages. It has been demonstrated that antimalarial antibodies can in fact enter infected red blood cells. A drug coupled to such an antibody might be highly specific in action and effective at low concentrations.

Finally, considerable effort is being directed towards the production of vaccines for malaria. The three main approaches are development of an antisporozoite vaccine to abort the infection at its source (COCHRANE et al. 1980), an antimerozoite vaccine to alleviate clinical disease (COHEN 1979), and an antigamete vaccine which blocks transmission (CARTER and GWADZ 1980). Reducing transmission is an essential part of any vaccination programme and one could envisage appropriate combinations of a vaccine to stop transmission and chemotherapy to suppress clinical malaria.

This is for the future, of course. Whatever form of vaccine is eventually developed is most unlikely on its own to control malaria. Combining chemotherapy and the immunological approach will be an essential element of any major control effort and it is crucial, therefore, to understand as fully as possible how chemotherapy relates to innate and acquired, specific, and non-specific immunological responses.

*Acknowledgements.* I am grateful to Dr. WILLIAM L. HANSON, who sent me a prepublication copy of his paper, and to Ms. JACKIE KING for typing the manuscript.

## References

Afridi MK, Rahim A (1962) Concluding observations on the interruption of malaria transmission with pyrimethamine (Daraprim). Rev Parasitol 23:249–266

Allison AC, Christensen J, Clark IA, Elford BC, Eugui EM (1979) The role of the spleen in protection against murine babesia infections. In: Role of the spleen in the immunology of parasitic diseases. Tropical Diseases Research Series No. 1. Schwabe, Basel, pp 151–182

Bhamarapravati N, Boonpucknavig S, Boonpucknavig S, Yaemboonruang C (1973) Glomerular changes in acute *Plasmodium falciparum* infection. An immunopathologic study. Arch Pathol 96:289–293

Brown IN, Watson SR, Slijivic VS (1977) Antibody response in vitro of spleen cells from *Plasmodium yoelii*-infected mice. Infect Immun 16:456–460

Brown KN (1978) Antigenic variation. In: Capron A, Lambert PH, Ogilvie B, Péry P (eds) Immunity in parasitic diseases. INSERM, Paris, pp 59–70

Brown KN, Brown IN (1965) Immunity to malaria: antigenic variation in chronic infections of *Plasmodium knowlesi*. Nature 208:1286–1288

Carter R, Gwadz RW (1980) Infectiousness and gamete immunization in malaria. In: Kreier JP (ed) Malaria, vol 3. Academic, New York, pp 263–297

Carter RL, Connors TA, Weston BJ, Davies AJS (1973) Treatment of a mouse lymphoma by L-asparaginase: success depends on the host's immune response. Int J Cancer 11:345–357

Clark IA (1979) Protection of mice against *Babesia microti* with cord factor, COAM, Zymosan, Glucan Salmonella, and Listeria. Parasite Immunol 1:179–196

Cochrane AH, Nussenzweig RS, Nardin EH (1980) Immunization against sporozoites. In: Kreier JP (ed) Malaria, vol 3. Academic, New York, pp 163–202

Cohen S (1979) Immunity to malaria. Proc R Soc Lond [Biol] 203:323–345

Cohen S, Butcher GA (1971) Serum antibody in acquired malarial immunity. Trans R Soc Trop Med Hyg 65:125–135

Cohen S, McGregor IA (1963) Gamma-globulin and acquired immunity to malaria. In: Garnham PCC, Pierce AE, Roitt I (eds) Immunity to protozoa. Blackwell, Oxford, pp 123–159

Cook JA, Holbrook TW, Parker BW (1980) Visceral leishmaniasis in mice: protective effect of glucan. J Reticuloendothel Soc 27:567–573

Cox FEG (1968) The effect of betamethasone on acquired immunity to *P. vinckei* in mice. Ann Trop Med Parasitol 62:295–300

Eling W, Jerusalem C (1977) Active immunization against the malaria parasite *Plasmodium berghei* in mice: sulfathiozole treatment of a *P. berghei* infection and development of immunity. Tropenmed Parasitol 28:158–174
Eugui EM, Allison AC (1980) Differences in susceptibility of various mouse strains to haemoprotozoan infections: possible correlation with natural killer activity. Parasite Immunol 2:277–292
Fakunle YM, Greenwood BM (1977) Low molecular weight (7S) IgM and free light chains in the sera of patients with the tropical splenomegaly syndrome. Clin Exp Immunol 28:153–156
Freeman RR, Parish CR (1978) Polyclonal B-cell activation during rodent malarial infections. Clin Exp Immunol 32:41–45
Freeman RR, Trejdosiewicz AJ, Cross GAM (1980) Protective monoclonal antibodies recognising stage-specific merozoite antigens of a rodent malaria parasite. Nature 284:366–368
Gold EF, Ophir R, Ben-Efraim S (1979) Inhibition of mixed lymphocyte reaction by quinine and lack of effect on plaque-forming cells and lymphoid-derived tumor cells. Int Arch Allergy Appl Immunol 58:447–453
Golenser J, Poels LG, Leeuwenberg ADEM, Verhave JP, Meuwissen JHET (1978) The influence of chloroquine on establishment of immunity against *P. berghei*. J Protozool 25:14B
Greenwood BM (1974) Immunosuppression in malaria and trypanosomiasis. In: Porter R, Knight J (eds) Parasites in the immunized host, mechanisms of survival. Elsevier, New York, pp 137–146
Greenwood BM, Vick RM (1975) Evidence for a malaria mitogen in human malaria. Nature 257:592–594
Hall AP (1977) Treatment of severe falciparum malaria. Trans R Soc Trop Med Hyg 71:367–378
Hall AP, Canfield CJ (1972) Resistant falciparum malaria in Vietnam: its rarity in negro soldiers. Proc Helminthol Soc Wash [Suppl] 39:66–70
Hanson WL (1981) Chemotherapy and the immune response in protozoal infections. J Protozool 28:27–30
Houba V, Lambert PH (1974) Immunological studies in tropical nephropathies. Adv Biosci 12:617–629
Hurvitz D, Hirschorn K (1965) Suppression of in vitro lymphocyte responses by chloroquine. N Engl J Med 273:23–26
Jayawardena AN, Targett GAT, Carter RL, Leuchars E, Davies AJS (1977) The immunological response of CBA mice to *P. yoelii* 1. General characteristics, the effects of T-cell deprivation and reconstitution with thymus grafts. Immunology 32:849–859
Kierszenbaum F, Ferrarer RW (1979) Enhancement of host resistance against *Trypanosoma cruzi* infections by the immunoregulatory agent muramyl dipeptide. Infect Immun 25:273–278
Kretschmar W (1965) The effects of stress and diet on resistance to *Plasmodium berghei* and malarial immunity in the mouse. Ann Soc Belge Med Trop 45:325–344
Krotoski WA, Krotoski DM, Garnham PCC, Bray RS, Killick-Kendrick R, Draper CC, Targett GAT, Guy MW (1980) Relapses in primate malaria: discovery of two populations of exoerythrocytic stages. Preliminary note. Br Med J 1:153–154
Lwin M (1978) Interaction of chemotherapy and the immune response in experimental malaria infections. PhD thesis of the University of London
Lwin M, Liston AJ, Doenhoff MJ, Targett GAT (1984) Interactions of chemotherapy and the immune responses on *Plasmodium chabaudi* and *P. berghei* malaria infections in mice. Ann Trop Med Parasitol (in press)
Lwin M, Targett GAT, Doenhoff MJ (1979) Chemotherapy of malaria (*P. chabaudi*) infections in immunosuppressed mice. Trans R Soc Trop Med Hyg 73:103
McCarthy VC, Clyde DF, Woodward WE (1978) *Plasmodium falciparum:* responses of a semi-immune individual to homologous and heterologous challenges, and non-infectivity of gametocytes in *Anopheles stephensi*. Am J Trop Med Hyg 27:6–8
McGregor IA, Barr M (1962) Antibody response to tetanus toxoid inoculation in malarious and non-malarious Gambian children. Trans R Soc Trop Med Hyg 56:364–367

Miller LH, Aikawa M, Dvorak JA (1975) Malaria (*Plasmodium knowlesi*) merozoites: immunity and the surface coat. J Immunol 114:1237–1242
Muirhead-Thomson RC (1954) Factors determining the true reservoir of infection of *Plasmodium falciparum* and *Wuchereria bancrofti* in a West African village. Trans R Soc Trop Med Hyg 48:208–225
Nardin EH, Nussenzweig RS, McGregor IA, Bryan JH (1979) Antibodies to sporozoites: their frequent occurrence in individuals living in an area of hyperendemic malaria. Science 206:597–599
Nauck EG (1934) Chemotherapeutische Versuche bei Affenmalaria (*P. knowlesi*). Arch Schiff Trop Hyg 38:313–326
Pasvol G, Weatherall DJ, Wilson RJM (1978) Cellular mechanism for the protective effect of haemoglobin S against *P. falciparum* malaria. Nature 274:701–703
Perrin LH, Ramirez E, Lambert PH, Miescher PA (1981) Inhibition of *P. falciparum* growth in human erythrocytes by monoclonal antibodies. Nature 289:301–303
Peters W (1970) Chemotherapy and drug resistance in malaria. Academic, London
Powell RD, McNamara JV, Rieckmann KH (1972) Clinical aspects of acquisition of immunity to falciparum malaria. Proc Helminthol Soc Wash [Suppl] 39:51–56
Playfair JHL (1980) Vaccines against malaria. In: Taylor AER, Muller R (eds) Vaccines against parasites. Blackwell, Oxford, pp 1–23
Pringle G, Lane FCT (1966) An apparent decline in the efficiency of small doses of chloroquine in suppressing malaria parasitaemias in semi-immune African schoolchildren. East Afr Med J 43:575–578
Rener J, Carter R, Rosenberg Y, Miller LH (1980) Anti-gamete monoclonal antibodies synergistically block transmission of malaria by preventing fertilization in the mosquito. Proc Natl Acad Sci USA 77:6797–6799
Roberts DW, Rank RG, Weidanz WP, Finerty JF (1977) Preventing recrudescent malaria in nude mice by thymic grafting or by treatment with hyperimmune serum. Infect Immun 16:821–826
Roitt IM, Male DK, Hay FC, Nineham LJ (1981) The biological role of immune complexes. Clin Immunol Allergol 14:169–176
Siddiqui WA, Kan S-C, Kramer K, Case S, Palmer K (1981) Use of a synthetic adjuvant in an effective vaccination of monkeys against malaria. Nature 289:64–66
Steward MW (1977) Affinity of the antibody-antigen reaction and its biological significance. In: Glynn LE, Steward MW (eds) Immunochemistry: an advanced textbook. Wiley, Chichester, pp 233–262
Stuiver PC, Ziegler JL, Wood JB, Morrow RH, Hutt MSR (1971) Clinical trial of malaria prophylaxis in tropical splenomegaly syndrome. Br Med J 1:426–429
Taliaferro WH (1948) The role of the spleen and the lymphoid-macrophage system in the quinine treatment of gallinaceum malaria. 1. Acquired immunity and phagocytosis. J Infect Dis 83:164–180
Taliaferro WH, Kelsey FE (1948) The role of the spleen and lymphoid-macrophage system in the quinine treatment of gallinaceum malaria. II. Quinine blood levels. J Infect Dis 83:181–199
Taliaferro WH, Taliaferro LG (1949) The role of the spleen and lymphoid-macrophage system in the quinine treatment of gallinaceum malaria. III. The action of quinine and of immunity on the parasite. J Infect Dis 84:187–220
Tandon N, Bhattacharya NC (1970) Gametogenesis of *Plasmodium berghei* in corticosteroid-treated albino mice. Bull WHO 43:344–347
Targett GAT (1981) Immunological and allergological aspects of malaria infection. Clin Immunol Allergol 14:301–309
Targett GAT (1982) Immunological aspects of malaria infections. In: Nahmias S, O'Reilly RJ (eds) Immunology of human infections, vol. II. Plenum, New York, pp 385–402
Terry RJ (1977) Immunodepression in parasite infections. In: Capron A, Lambert PH, Ogilvie B, Péry P (eds) Immunity in parasitic diseases. INSERM, Paris, pp 161–178
Thommen-Scott K (1981) Antimalarial activity of Cyclosporin A. Agents Actions 2:770–773
Thong YH, Ferrante A (1978) Inhibition of mitogen-induced lymphocyte proliferative responses by quinine. Am J Trop Med Hyg 23:354–356

Thong YH, Ferrante A, Rowan-Kelly B (1978) Primaquine inhibits mitogen-induced human lymphocyte proliferative responses. Trans R Soc Trop Med Hyg 72:537–539
Thong YH, Ferrante A (1980) Immunopotentiation by pyrimethamine in the mouse. Clin Exp Immunol 39:190–194
Thong YH, Ferrante A, Rowan-Kelly B, O'Keefe DE (1979) Effect of mefloquine on the immune response in mice. Trans R Soc Trop Med Hyg 73:388–390
Thong YH, Ferrante A, Secker LK (1981) Normal immunological responses in mice treated with chloroquine, quinine, and primaquine. Trans R Soc Trop Med Hyg 75:108–109
Verhave JP (1975) Immunization with sporozoites: an experimental study of *Plasmodium berghei* malaria. Thesis, Catholic University of Nijmegen
Waki S (1976) Protective immunity of *Plasmodium berghei* in mice induced by repeated infection and chemotherapy. Jpn J Parasitol 25:441–446
Warren HS, Weidanz WP (1976) Malaria immunodepression in vitro: adherent spleen cells are functionally defective as accessory cells in the response to horse erythrocytes. Eur J Immunol 6:816–819
Wedderburn N (1974) Immunodepression produced by malarial infection in mice. In: Porter R, Knight J (eds) Parasites in the immunized host: mechanisms of survival. Elsevier, New York, pp 123–135
Wedderburn N, Dracott BN (1977) The immune response to type III pneumococcal polysaccharide in mice with malaria. Clin Exp Immunol 28:130–137
World Health Organization (1973) Chemotherapy of malaria and resistance to antimalarials. WHO Tech Rep Ser No. 529
World Health Organization (1975) Developments in malaria immunology. WHO Tech Rep Ser No. 579
World Health Organization (1977) The role of immune complexes in disease. WHO Tech Rep Ser No. 606
Williamson WA, Greenwood BM (1978) Impairment of the immune response to vaccination after acute malaria. Lancet *I*:1328–1329
Wyler DJ, Oppenheim JJ, Koontz LC (1979) Influence of malaria infection on the elaboration of soluble mediators by adherent mononuclear cells. Infect Immun 24:151–159
Yorke W (1925) Further observations on malaria made during treatment of general paralysis. Trans R Soc Trop Med Hyg 19:108–122
Yoshida N, Nussenzweig RS, Potocnjak P, Nussenzweig V, Aikawa M (1980) Hybridoma produces protective antibodies directed against the sporozoite stage of malaria parasite. Science 207:71–73

# Preclinical and Clinical Trial Techniques

CHAPTER 12

# Preclinical Testing [1]

M. H. HEIFFER, D. E. DAVIDSON, JR., and D. W. KORTE, JR.

## A. Introduction

Since the establishment of the United States Army Antimalarial Drug Development Programme in 1963, there has been a continual evolution of the organisational structure, the philosophy, the approach and the methods used. This evolution reflects the rapid development of science and technology in these years, the gradual development of a multidisciplinary cadre of scientists and the evolution of ethical principles and statutory requirements. The philosophy, approaches and methods which will be discussed in this chapter are those which have been employed by the US Army Programme in the past, those which are presently being employed and those which will be incorporated in the future. As the science and technology of drug development continue to evolve, more rational and more efficient methods must be developed and applied to malaria research, to ensure the optimal use of the limited resources which have traditionally been allocated to this disease.

One may consider that preclinical testing includes all laboratory investigations performed on a candidate drug before it is introduced into man. While preclinical investigations are designed in part to satisfy the requirements set forth by various regulatory agencies, their real purpose should be to develop rational and safe protocols for human investigations. Information obtained in well-designed preclinical studies should exclude extreme toxicants, define target organ toxicity, predict initial dosage for phase I clinical pharmacology studies and form the basis from which human volunteers can more appropriately grant their informed consent to participate in phase I studies.

The major features of the antimalarial drug development process currently employed by the Programme are illustrated in Fig. 1 (CANFIELD and HEIFFER 1978). This process encompasses the entire development of a candidate drug, from its conception as a structural formula through chemical synthesis, physical-chemical characterisation, efficacy investigations, prep lab or pilot plant synthesis, chemical analysis and stability studies, development of analytical methods for biological fluids, preformulation and bioavailability studies, metabolic analysis and pharmacokinetic evaluation, pharmacodynamic characterisation, toxicological assessments, manufacture and analysis of dosage forms, and creation of a "notice of claimed investigational exemption for a new drug" (IND). The drug development

1 The authors dedicate this chapter to the late Dr. ROBERT S. ROZMAN, who devoted most of his later years to the development of antimalarial drugs

process culminates in phase I and phase II clinical pharmacology investigations and phase III clinical trials.

After carefully analysing efficacy data from in vivo and in vitro malaria test systems, a decision may be made to develop a medicinal chemical which clearly demonstrates superiority over existing drugs. In order to support all of the planned preclinical and clinical investigations it is necessary to synthesise kilogram quantities. Large-scale synthetic methods are developed through chemical research in either a pilot plant or a preparatory laboratory. A complete chemical analysis by an independent laboratory is performed on each bulk lot of drug. The analyst uses the most specific and sensitive methods that modern technology has made available. Accelerated stability studies are also performed on each unformulated lot. Although the analysis of pure antimalarial drug substances rarely poses problems, quantitative analysis of drug substances within biological fluids (e.g. blood) is significantly more difficult. Therefore, while the large-scale synthesis is being carried out, sensitive and specific analytical methods for accurately estimating small concentrations of parent drug in biological fluids are being developed. In addition, the physical-chemical properties of the drug are studied during this time, e.g. partition coefficients, dissociation constants, solubility, particle size, crystalline state, and protein-binding capacity. The candidate drug is also prepared in radiolabelled form to support pharmacokinetic and drug metabolism studies. When possible, pharmacokinetic estimates are quantitatively determined to ensure the early achievement of steady-state drug levels in subsequent subacute toxicological investigations. The design and extent of toxicological studies are determined by the intended clinical use of the drug, and by information previously obtained in studies of closely related drugs. In the initial stages, toxicological studies are conducted in sufficient depth and duration to support phase I clinical pharmacology and phase II studies in a small number of volunteers receiving a single dose of the candidate drug. In later stages of toxicological evaluation, studies are designed to support repeated administration, or use of the drug in either a large number of individuals or in a non-selected population.

Each investigation outlined in Fig. 1 culminates in a definitive report. These reports should be of such quality and contain sufficient detail to enable one to reconstruct unambiguously the actual experiment from reading these documents. Each report receives a careful and critical review by investigators from our staff, and no report is reviewed in isolation from previous reports on a particular drug. In the United States, an IND must be filed with the Food and Drug Administration before administering a new drug to human subjects. The major elements of the IND application are the proposed clinical protocol, detailed information on drug composition, a thorough description of manufacturing procedures and safety standards, results of all preclinical investigations including efficacy studies, qualifications (demonstrated by training and experience) of the proposed clinical investigators, and a series of documents including the appropriate informed consent agreements for human volunteers. The IND is written after all of the preclinical investigational reports have been reviewed, correlated, and evaluated, and after the proposed clinical protocols have been developed. At this point the decision to proceed with human investigations is reevaluated, after considering benefit to risk factors. The IND documents are sent for review to an independent advisory group

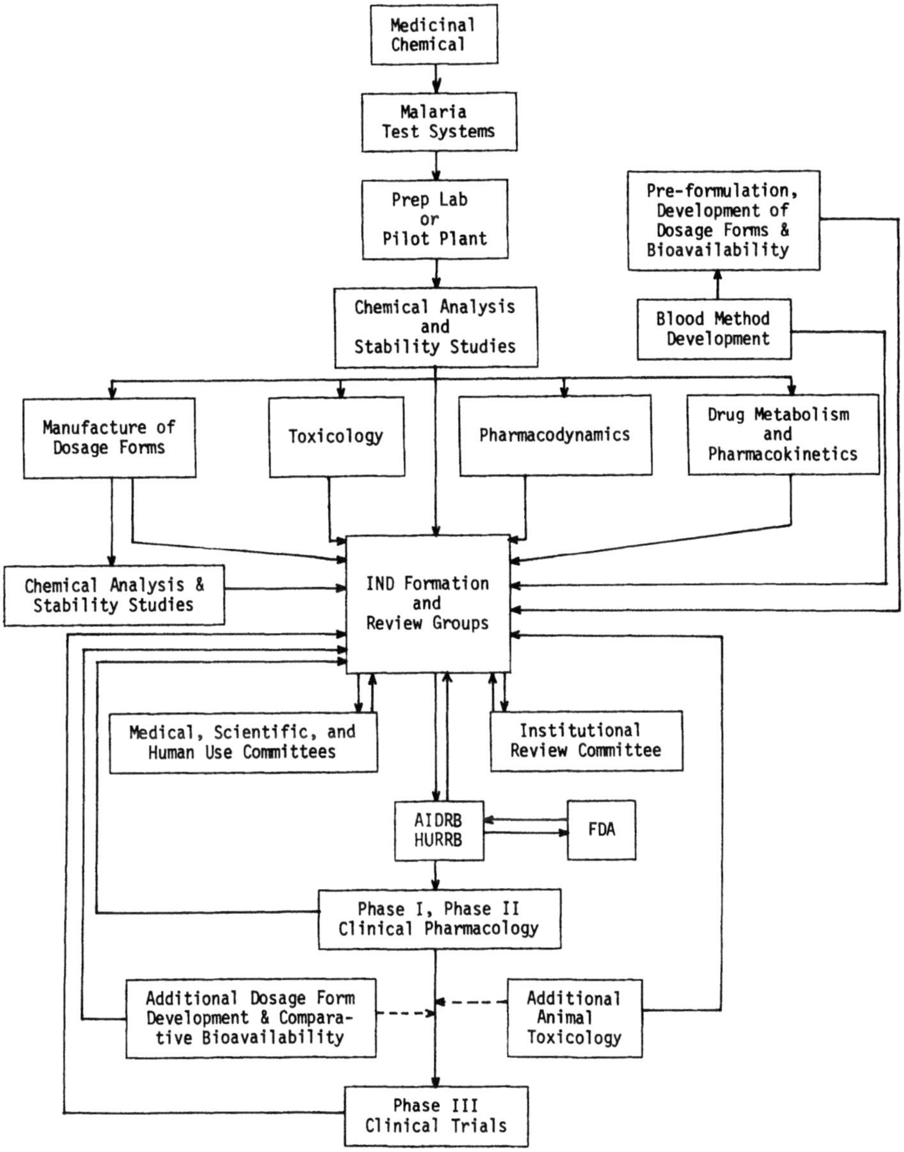


**Fig. 1.** Antimalarial drug development process. *AIDRB–HURRB,* Army Investigational Drug Review Board – Human Use Research Review Board; *FDA,* Food and Drug Administration

composed of highly qualified university and government scientists and leaders of the industrial community. The IND also receives a number of other independent medical, scientific, institutional, and human use reviews before it is sent to the US Food and Drug Administration (see Fig. 1). This review process and Food and Drug Administration regulations help to ensure that drug products are pure and stable; that specifications of drug substances and products are met; that claims pertaining to the drug are supported by scientifically valid data; that the drug is reasonably safe and efficacious; that all preclinical and clinical investigations follow the scientific method and good ethical practices; that the methods and results of all investigations are adequately documented; that all investigations are conducted by qualified personnel; that volunteers and patients are adequately and properly informed; and that peer review and institutional reviews are properly conducted.

The Army Programme is multidisciplinary and highly coordinated. Approximately 35% of the work is performed intramurally at the Walter Reed Army Institute of Research, and 65% is performed extramurally under contracts. The contract programme is viewed as an extension of the intramural programme, and is closely monitored and carefully coordinated. Emphasis is placed upon close integration of preclinical and clinical investigations. This ensures that clinical investigators have a thorough understanding of the potential hazards of a new drug before it is introduced into man, and provides continuous feedback of information to preclinical investigators which may be used to improve the design and relevance of preclinical studies. Usually each investigator performs three functions. He designs and conducts intramural research, monitors extramural research, and directs the development of one or more drugs to and through the IND stage. Once a medicinal chemical is selected for development, a member of the scientific staff is chosen to direct the process. This IND project director decides in meetings with contract monitors and other investigators what studies need to be performed, requests development of protocols, establishes schedules and deadlines and estimates costs. The IND project director then assures adherence to protocols and deadlines, reviews study reports, and directs the staff review process. This management technique promotes efficient and effective movement of a candidate drug through the preclinical stage of testing and assures that each IND project director develops a broad understanding of all aspects of drug development, and a thorough familiarity with the characteristics of the candidate drug.

In the sections of this chapter which follow, three major areas of preclinical testing will be described in further detail – preclinical efficacy testing (see also Chaps. 6–10), preclinical toxicology, and pharmacodynamic investigations. Other major components of preclinical development will be addressed elsewhere in the text.

## B. Efficacy Investigations

### I. Empirical Versus Rational Drug Synthesis

All drug development programmes utilise biological test systems in the search for new medicinally active substances. "Blind screening" and "lead-directed synthesis" are two approaches which have traditionally been used most effectively. Blind screening requires two ingredients, a very large number of medicinal chemicals and well-defined biological test systems capable of high throughput. Blind screening is the only practical method of discovering entirely new classes of drugs when biochemical rationale is lacking and when the nature of the drug receptors is unknown. Once an active compound of a new class is discovered through blind screening, improvement of activity and reduction of side effects can be approached through lead-directed synthesis. Testing of compounds synthesised as chemical analogues of active leads also requires well-defined biological test systems; and, to guide synthesis effectively, test results must be quantitative. For the future, a more rational approach to selection and design of new antimalarials may be possible. Advances in knowledge of the unique aspects of the metabolism of the plasmodial parasite and specific knowledge about drug receptors may permit greater application of rational drug development techniques. Unfortunately, the rational approach has had very limited applicability in the past because of the lack of detailed physical-chemical information concerning the receptors upon which antimalarial drugs act. In the past, information about receptors has been more helpful in explaining the mechanism of action of existing drugs than in designing new ones. The exception has been the development of drugs which are competitive inhibitors of the metabolism of *p*-aminobenzoic or folic acids. For the future, computer-assisted molecular modelling may come into greater use to assist in the prospective design of new drugs. To support molecular modelling, a better understanding of drug-receptor interactions must be obtained utilising X-ray diffraction, receptor mapping, electrostatic contour mapping, other physical and chemical tools and theoretical science (GRUND et al. 1980).

## II. Drug-Screening Models

A variety of avian, rodent, simian, and human plasmodial models have been used for the screening and evaluation of candidate antimalarial drugs. These malaria models have been established in a variety of laboratory animals, and short- and long-term plasmodial culture systems have been used extensively for chemotherapeutic studies. A number of books and reviews have been published which describe the characteristics of malaria model systems comprehensively (COATNEY et al. 1953, 1971; DAVEY 1963; JIANG 1978; KILLICK-KENDRICK and PETERS 1978; PETERS 1970; THOMPSON and WERBEL 1972; WISELOGLE 1946; WHO 1971, 1973; YOUNG et al. 1975). The discussion which follows is limited to a review of screening techniques and malaria models which have been selected for use in the US Army Antimalarial Drug Development Programme. The choice of malaria models has been dictated by programme objectives; by technical considerations such as sensitivity, reproducibility and breadth of response to known antimalarial compounds; and by practical considerations such as the required rate of testing, technical complexity, quantity of test compound needed and cost per test. Currently the availability and cost of subhuman primates is severely limiting, and this has dictated new testing strategy and stimulated efforts towards development of alternative models.

Each malaria model system has its individual characteristics, and no single model exists which can be said to be entirely predictive for man. Selection of candidate drugs for clinical trial in man and the design of clinical protocols are based upon consideration of data from a battery of test systems. Each species and strain of *Plasmodium* has its intrinsic spectrum of sensitivity to chemotherapeutic agents, and differences among species, and even among strains, may be considerable. Of perhaps even greater importance are differences among various laboratory animal hosts which influence the absorption, distribution, metabolism and elimination of test compounds. Host factors such as natural resistance and immune competence also influence the efficacy of test compounds in different models.

As in all organised drug development programmes, a hierarchial network of efficacy tests has been established to support efficiently and effectively the objectives of the Antimalarial Drug Programme (KINNAMON and ROTHE 1975). All compounds are assessed initially in one or more primary screening models. Ideally, primary "screens" have optimal sensitivity, a high degree of reproducibility, high throughput, require a minimum quantity of test compound and have a low cost per test. A compound which is considered "active" in a screening test by well-established criteria is considered for further evaluation in successively more critical tests. At the end of each successive stage of testing a decision is made to advance the compound to the next stage or to discontinue testing. These decisions are based upon review of all efficacy and tolerance data available at the decision point, and are influenced especially by comparison of the properties of the compound in question with those of its analogues. Secondary test systems and other advanced testing models are designed to verify and quantify the antimalarial activity of each candidate compound, to develop an understanding of its unique characteristics, to gain an appreciation of its limitations, to provide information to guide synthesis of analogues, and to provide information to guide development of a rational clinical protocol. Some pharmacological and toxicological information and clues to mode of action may be obtained in efficacy testing. However, definitive information in these areas generally requires special laboratory investigations outside of the province of routine testing. Relatively few compounds reach the final stages of efficacy testing. Between 1964 and 1980 the Programme screened over 275000 compounds at the primary level. More than 9000 had antimalarial activity, but only 30 were selected for advancement to phase I clinical investigation.

## C. Blood Schizontocidal Testing

### I. Primary Testing

The primary objective of developing new drugs for suppressive prophylaxis and treatment of drug-resistant falciparum malaria in man has been addressed by establishment of a hierarchial battery of blood schizontocidal tests. The mouse malaria model developed by RANE (OSDENE et al. 1967) has served as the principal primary screening test for blood schizontocidal activity since 1964. The rodent malaria parasite, *Plasmodium berghei*, has many practical advantages over the avian malarias which were used extensively prior to 1950 (COATNEY et al. 1953; WISELOGLE 1946). The genetic homogeneity of laboratory mice, their freedom from interfering bacterial and viral pathogens, their small body size, unlimited availability and ease of handling have permitted highly reproducible screening on a scale that would have been impracticable with avian models. The Rane test has a low cost per test because it uses mortality rather than parasitaemia as an end point, and because single rather than multiple test compound regimens are utilised. The sensitivity of this mouse model across a broad range of chemical classes has generated a large number of new leads for the Programme.

For a time, researchers utilised a trophozoite-induced *P. gallinaceum* mortality model in young chickens (OSDENE et al. 1967) as a supplementary primary blood schizontocidal screen, hoping to take advantage of the somewhat different spectrum of drug susceptibilities of this avian malaria. After 3–4 years of experience, this model was abandoned because many compounds active in the mouse model were inactive in the chick, and because it generated no significant leads which would not have been discovered by the mouse model. Short-term incubation of *P. berghei* was also used for primary screening in the early years of the Programme (CENEDELLA and SAXE 1967; CENEDELLA et al. 1970). In more recent years cultures of *P. falciparum* (DESJARDINS et al. 1979) have come into prominent use for selective primary screening.

## II. Secondary Testing

Compounds which are active in primary screens, and which appear to offer advantage over close analogues, may be selected for secondary blood schizontocidal testing. Initially, secondary testing generally utilises *P. berghei* in mice to confirm activity and to extend the data base on the compound. Quantitative determination of potency relative to standard antimalarials can be assessed using either mortality or parasitaemia parameters (THOMPSON et al. 1963). Information on optimal routes and regimens of administration, duration of suppressive prophylactic effect, and antagonism or synergism in combination with other drugs is obtained at this stage. A battery of drug-sensitive and drug-resistant lines of *P. berghei* have been developed by drug pressure techniques for initial determination of relative potency. Lines are available which are highly resistant to chloroquine, quinine, pyrimethamine, cycloguanil, dapsone, primaquine, mefloquine or primaquine, or to a number of experimental antimalarial drugs (PETERS 1965 a, b, 1966; PETERS et al. 1977; THOMPSON et al. 1965, 1967). Although many of these lines are far more resistant and more broadly cross-resistant than resistant human isolates of *P. falciparum* encountered to date, preliminary conservative estimates of the potential utility of experimental drugs against human resistant strains may be obtained in mice. The rodent malaria model may also be used to assess the liability of experimental drugs to induce resistance by continuous drug pressure or by "relapse" techniques (MERKLI and PETERS 1976; PETERS 1968, 1974).

In former years, the ability of test compounds to inhibit schizont maturation in short-term cultures of *P. falciparum* was used to assess the efficacy of experimental compounds across a battery of sensitive and resistant strains utilising techniques developed by RIECKMANN et al. (1968). This method predicted utility of drugs against resistant strains in man with a high degree of reliability. Following the development of long-term falciparum culture techniques by TRAGER and JENSEN (1976) and HAYNES et al. (1976), a more quantitative, semiautomated culture system was developed based upon incorporation of radiolabelled substrates (DESJARDINS et al. 1979). This enhanced capability has reduced dependence on *Aotus trivirgatus* monkeys and has increased the reliability of selection of clinical candidates.

Simian malaria models have been used for advanced-stage evolution of candidate blood schizontocidal drugs. Trophozoite-induced *P. knowlesi* in the rhesus monkey was used in the early years of the programme (ROTHE et al. 1969), but its spectrum of sensitivity is quite atypical. Mefloquine, for example, is ineffective in this model (unpublished data). Trophozoite-induced *P. cynomolgi* in the rhesus monkey has a spectrum of sensitivity which more nearly approximates drug-sensitive vivax and falciparum malaria in man (DAVIDSON et al. 1976; GENTHER et al. 1948), but use of this model for blood schizontocidal testing declined with the advent of the *Aotus* monkey model.

The development of drug-testing techniques utilising drug-sensitive and drug-resistant strains of *P. falciparum* in Colombian *Aotus trivirgatus* monkeys by SCHMIDT (1973, 1978 a, b, c) represented the first practical capability for preclinical evaluation of antimalarials against a human malaria parasite in vivo. The resistance of human isolates has remained remarkably stable after years of passage through *Aotus*. Although avian, rodent and simian malarias have proven to be extremely valuable in the development of antimalarials, only the *Aotus* models, in conjunction with falciparum culture techniques, have provided preclinical data which have had direct predictive value of efficacy against resistant human strains. In recent years, Panamanian *Aotus* monkeys have also been used successfully in preclinical antimalarial drug studies (YOUNG et al. 1975). Several strains of *P. vivax* have also been adapted to Colombian or Panamanian *Aotus* by trophozoite passage (ROSSAN et al. 1975; SCHMIDT 1973, 1978 a, b, c). This has permitted evaluation of candidate drugs as blood schizontocides against this human *Plasmodium* as well.

## D. Tissue Schizontocidal Testing

For the development of new drugs for causal prophylaxis of falciparum and vivax malaria and for radical cure of vivax malaria in man, a battery of tissue schizontocidal models has been utilised. Tissue schizontocidal testing is more complex and more costly than blood schizontocidal testing because of the need to maintain an insectary for production of infective sporozoites. Reproducibility of tissue schizontocidal models is more difficult to maintain because of limitations in methods currently available for harvesting, quantifying and assessing the infectivity of sporozoite inocula.

Avian, rodent, and simian malaria models may be used for causal prophylactic testing. The first causal prophylactic model used by the Programme was a sporozoite-induced *P. gallinaceum* model in young chickens (RANE and RANE 1972). Later, a primary causal prophylactic model in mice utilising *P. berghei* (RANE and KINNAMON 1979) was developed which was more reproducible and cost effective. This mouse model is still in use as a primary screen. A major limitation of *P. berghei* causal prophylactic models derives from the rapidity with which pre-erythrocytic schizogony is completed (less than 72 h). Candidate compounds with persistent blood schizontocidal activity frequently give false indications of causal prophylactic activity by causing abortion of infection as the erythrocytic infection is being established (GREGORY and PETERS 1970). A number of secondary *P. berghei* models have been developed to make the distinction between this so-called "residual" suppressive prophylactic effect and true causal prophylaxis. One model, developed by GREGORY and PETERS (1970), simultaneously assesses drug effects against sporozoite-induced parasitaemia and a delayed trophozoite-induced parasitaemia to make the distinction. Another model, developed by MOST and MONTUORI (1975), utilise direct microscopic examination of pre-erythrocytic tissue stages in the livers of infected rats.

Among laboratory malaria models currently available, sporozoite-induced *P. cynomolgi* malaria in rhesus monkeys most closely resembles human vivax malaria (SCHMIDT et al. 1963). It is the only laboratory model which permits assessment of activity against persistent tissue stages, and thus it is the only model available for assessment of candidate radical curative drugs (DAVIDSON et al. 1981). The rhesus model has also been used effectively for causal prophylactic studies (SCHMIDT et al. 1963). Vivax malaria has been successfully induced by sporozoites in several species of New World primates (YOUNG et al. 1975) but, to date, infection rates have not been sufficiently consistent to suggest utility in prophylactic testing.

There is a clear need for improved models and more reliable techniques for tissue schizontocidal drug testing. Culture techniques for exoerythrocytic stages would be particularly useful.

## E. Miscellaneous Models

Similarities between drug sensitivities of insect stages of malaria parasites and exoerythrocytic stages in the vertebrate host have been described by TERZIAN (1947) and TERZIAN et al. (1949). This concept has led to the development of sporontocidal models as an indirect approach towards development of tissue schizontocides. Avian, simian, and human sporontocidal models (GERBERG 1971) were developed and utilised as screens for a number of years prior to the development of high-volume, rodent causal prophylactic models.

The Programme has devoted considerable attention to compounds which inhibit the metabolism of folic acid as potential causal prophylactic and blood schizontocidal drugs. Although small amounts of plasmodial dihydrofolate reductase have been isolated and used to test a few candidate antifols (FERONE et al. 1969), the enzyme has not been available in sufficient quantity to support general screening. GENTHER and SMITH (1977) have utilised cultures of folate-dependent bacteria as an adjunct to in vivo antimalarial screening to guide development of antimalarial antifolates. In the future, it is hoped that dihydrofolate reductase as well as other plasmodial enzymes may be isolated from falciparum culture systems in quantity to support direct enzyme assays.

## F. Toxicological Investigations

### I. General

The purpose of preclinical toxicological investigation is to define the potential risk associated with proposed administration of a new drug, drug form or drug combination to human volunteers. Since it is impossible to eliminate all risk, the philosophy guiding toxicity testing in our programme has been one of conservatism and supererogation, tempered by budgetary realism. Our toxicological evaluation system is not a static, isolated entity, but rather a dynamic, interdisciplinary approach to the problem of risk assessment. Consequently, there has been a continual evolution of the approach to toxicological evaluation to include updating of study designs, incorporation of validated new testing procedures, and elimination of those studies or procedures that no longer represent an efficient utilisation of resources. In addition, toxicological evaluation of each drug is individualised based on structural characteristics; results from efficacy, metabolic, and pharmacokinetic studies; and feedback from clinical studies. Typically, the toxicological evaluation of a candidate antimalarial drug may be divided into three stages. In the first stage the phototoxic and mutagenic potential of the candidate new drug is assessed. These studies are performed concurrently with the advanced efficacy tests so that these data will be available at the critical decision point when an analogue is selected for development of an IND. The second stage of toxicological evaluation generally consists of acute and 28-day subacute testing, and provides a toxicological framework that supports development of the candidate drug through phase I into phase II clinical pharmacological investigations. Once the candidate drug has been shown to be efficacious in initial phase II studies, the drug, if selected for continued development, enters the third or extended study phase of toxicological evaluation. During this phase, reproductive/teratological studies, chronic toxicity/carcinogenic studies, reversal studies and appropriate special studies are performed as required. The remainder of this discussion will focus on those individual studies normally performed with a "typical" candidate antimalarial drug.

Antimalarial efficacy in a compound is customarily associated with a spectrum of pharmacological and toxicological activities. Consequently, a major goal of antimalarial drug development is to select those compounds which possess potent antimalarial activity relative to their other pharmacodynamic actions. Two toxicological properties that have been associated with antimalarial compounds are photosensitisation (ROTHE and JACOBUS 1968) and mutagenic activity (SCHÜPBACH 1979). Since these toxicological effects may be minimised, if not eliminated, by appropriate structural modifications (ROTHE and JACOBUS 1968; SCHÜPBACH 1979), it is imperative that the potential of a candidate drug to photosensitise or to induce genetic mutations be recognised early in its development. This is the rationale for the first or "early" phase of toxicological evaluation.

A screening procedure, developed at the Walter Reed Army Institute of Research (ROTHE and JACOBUS 1968), has been utilised to determine the phototoxic potential of candidate drugs. This procedure is based on the observation that albino mice develop minimal perceptible erythema after exposure to a standard dose of long-wave ultraviolet radiation for 72 h. Shorter periods of exposure will not produce erythema unless the mice are pretreated with a photosensitising agent. A candidate drug is considered a non-sensitiser if no erythema is observed at dosages of the drug that exceed the maximum tolerated dose. The second half of the early stage of toxicological evaluation is concerned with assaying the candidate drug for mutagenic potential. The system utilised is the *Salmonella*/mammalian microsome mutagenicity test, developed by AMES et al. (1975). The candidate drug is tested against histidine-dependent strains of *Salmonella typhimurium*, TA 1535, TA 1538, TA 98, and TA 100, alone or in the presence of a metabolic activation system (S-9 fraction obtained from livers of rats treated with Aroclor 1254). The number of revertants to histidine prototrophy is determined and compared with the spontaneous reversion rate in simultaneously exposed control plates. If the ratio of drug-induced revertants to spontaneous revertants is less than two, with or without metabolic activation, and if simultaneous positive control tests are indeed positive, the candidate drug is not considered to possess significant mutagenic potential.

The second stage of preclinical toxicological evaluation is initiated following selection of the candidate drug for continued development. The ultimate aim of this evaluation is to document the potential risk associated with administration of the candidate drug. In addition, these studies provide the foundation for extended toxicological evaluation. Tests included in this phase are single-dose, acute studies as well as multiple-dose, subacute studies.

## II. Acute Toxicity

The acute studies include $LD_{50}$ determinations in rats, mice, and either guinea pigs or rabbits, plus an approximate lethal dose determination in beagles. These studies are designed to determine a medial lethal dose and to establish the dose-response relationship of the lethal action of the drug in different species and by different routes of administration. Acute $LD_{50}$ experiments follow a standard protocol regardless of drug, animal species or route of administration. This rigidity of format maximises the usefulness of the $LD_{50}$ determinations since it facilitates direct comparison of the toxicities of structural analogues. In acute studies, animals are observed for at least 14 days after administration of drug and mortality data are then evaluated using probit analysis (FINNEY 1971). A single dose of the candidate drug is administered to different groups of animals by oral gavage and intraperitoneal injection or, occasionally, intravenous injection. Comparison of oral and parenteral $LD_{50}$'s may also provide an early approximation of the relative bioavailability of the drug.

The objective of the approximate lethal dose studies in beagles is to establish a lethality threshold or, at the minimum, a range of toxicity for the candidate drug when it is administered in a single oral dose. In addition, the data obtained from this study provide valuable insight into the pharmacological responses associated with accidental poisoning. The basic procedure is to dose two dogs, each at a different dosage level. The initial doses are selected based on previous experience with structurally similar drugs and the results of the $LD_{50}$ studies in other species. The dose levels selected for the second pair of dogs will be increased or decreased depending on the responses observed in the initial pair of dogs. Ideally, the dose(s) selected for the last pair of dogs would be used to confirm the approximation of the minimum lethal dose.

## III. Subacute Toxicity

The goal of subacute studies is to provide a detailed toxicological profile of the candidate drug in an attempt to anticipate human toxicity. This profile is then incorporated with other preclinical data into a phase I clinical pharmacology protocol designed to minimise any adverse drug reactions. Four objectives have been established to assist in attaining this goal. These objectives are to document drug-induced functional and morphological pathology, to establish a "no observable effect" dose, to define those clinical measurements that presage drug-induced tissue dysfunctions and to educe a mechanism for the toxic action(s) of the drug. Data acquisition in support of the study objectives is markedly dependent upon the animal species and the drug doses selected.

In subacute toxicological studies, the candidate drug is administered for 28 consecutive days. These studies provide information on the effect of repeated exposure to sublethal levels of the candidate drug and determine how these effects are related to dose. The design of multiple-dose studies permits one to monitor progressive dysfunction with increasing duration of drug exposure and to assess drug-induced morphological changes.

Historically, the rat and beagle have been the species most often chosen for the subacute studies. These two species are readily available and the toxicological data base that has been generated for them is large. Furthermore, the rat and beagle are extremely sensitive to the effects of most antimalarial drugs. For example, our testing experiences have indicated that the beagle is a more sensitive species than the rhesus monkey for subacute studies for all classes of aminoquinoline and aminocarbinol antimalarials, with the exception of the 8-aminoquinolines. Thus, during the subacute testing phase for 8-aminoquinolines, studies in the rhesus monkey have been performed in addition to studies in the beagle and the rat. Although the metabolism in these species has not always correlated with the metabolic profile derived from subsequent clinical studies, the inherent sensitivity of the rat and beagle to these classes of compounds justifies their use in the subacute toxicological evaluation.

Doses selected for multiple-dose studies should include a high dose that produces significant toxicity, a low dose that produces no observable toxic effects and an intermediate dose for dose-response estimates. The dosage regimens employed in the subacute studies are determined following a pharmacokinetic appraisal of the candidate drug in the appropriate species. Our philosophy is that the animals should be presented with a steady-state concentration of the drug during most of the period of drug exposure. Since many antimalarials have long half-lives, this has necessitated the incorporation of a loading dose into the dosage regimen of some candidate drugs. Selection of actual dose levels is derived from the acute studies as well as from information obtained in efficacy studies and previous subacute studies with structurally similar compounds.

Young animals (6- to 8-month-old beagles and 5- to 6-week-old rats) are utilised for these toxicity studies. These animals are pubescent at study initiation and during this period of rapid growth and development are more susceptible to the toxic manifestations of a candidate drug. The rate of weight gain has been found to be a sensitive index of drug toxicity in evaluating candidate antimalarials. In addition to body weight determinations, a variety of tests are conducted in each animal during the subacute studies to document drug-induced toxicity. These tests and observations include daily clinical signs, weekly food and water consumption, weekly urine and faecal analysis (beagle only), pre- and post-dosing ophthalmological examinations (beagle only), periodic haematological and clinical chemical tests, plus terminal organ weights and histopathological examination of all tissues.

A summary of the predominant acute and subacute toxicological observations for several classes of antimalarials currently in extended clinical testing is presented in Table 1. The $LD_{50}$ values listed in the table are for the most toxic member of each class. These values reflect the relative potency of the entire class in both the acute and subacute toxicity studies. The most striking phenomena observed with repeated administration of the candidate antimalarial compounds are the histo-

**Table 1.** Predominant toxicological observations for the major classes of antimalarial compounds evaluated in the US Army Drug Development Programme

| Class | Compounds tested | Oral $LD_{50}$ male rats[a] (mg/kg) | Clinical pathology/target organs from subacute toxicity studies[b] | |
|---|---|---|---|---|
| | | | Rat | Dog |
| Folate metabolism inhibitors | 4 | 926 | ↓ Weight gain<br>↓ WBC<br>Lymphoid tissue<br>GI tract | ↓ Weight gain<br>↓ WBC, ↓ reticulocytes<br>↑ BUN<br>Lymphoid tissue<br>Bone marrow<br>GI tract, kidney |
| Pyridine-carbinols | 2 | 518 | ↓ Weight gain<br>↑ WBC, ↑ SGOT, ↑ SGPT<br>↑ alk. phos., ↑ BUN<br>Lymphoid tissue<br>GI tract<br>Skel. muscle | ↓ Weight gain<br>Emesis, ↑ SGPT<br>Lymphoid tissue<br>Bone marrow |
| Quinoline-carbinols | 3 | 745 | ↓ Weight gain<br>↓ WBC, ↑ SGOT<br>↑ SGPT, ↑ BUN<br>GI tract, kidney<br>Liver | ↓ Weight gain<br>Emesis, ↑ SGOT<br>↑ SGPT, ↑ alk. phos.<br>↓ Reticulocytes<br>Lymphoid tissue<br>Bone marrow<br>GI tract, liver<br>Kidney |
| Phenan-threne-carbinols | 3 | $\gg 1000$ | Alopecia, ↑ WBC<br>↓ Weight gain<br>↓ Reticulocytes<br>↑ SGOT, ↑ SGPT<br>Lymphoid tissue<br>Bone marrow<br>Skel. muscle | Emesis, ↑ WBC<br>↓ Weight gain<br>↓ Reticulocytes<br>↑ SGPT, ↑ BUN<br>Lymphoid tissue<br>Bone marrow<br>GI tract, kidney |
| 8-Amino-quinolines | 3 | 177 | Rough hair coat<br>↓ Weight gain<br>↑ Reticulocytes<br>↑ WBC, ↑ Hct<br>↓ Platelets<br>↑ SGOT, ↑ SGPT<br>Heart, Skel. muscle<br>Liver, kidney | Cyanosis, ↑ SGOT<br>↓ Weight gain<br>↑ MetHb<br>↑ Reticulocytes<br>↓ Platelets<br>↑ Haptoglobins<br>Heart, liver<br>Lymphoid tissue |

[a] $LD_{50}$ value given is for the most toxic compound in each class
[b] Observations are those that were present in a majority of compounds in each class
↓, decrease; ↑, increase; *WBC*, total leucocyte count; *BUN*, blood urea nitrogen; *GI tract*, Gastrointestinal tract; *SGOT*, serum glutamic oxaloacetic transaminase; *SGPT*, serum glutamic pyruvic transaminase; *alk. phos.*, alkaline phosphatase; *Hct*, haematocrit; *metHb*, methamoglobin

pathological changes observed in the lymphoid tissue and bone marrow. These dose-dependent changes include vacuolar degeneration of reticuloendothelial cells of the thymus, lymph nodes or spleen; lymphoid depletion of the tonsil, thymus, and lymph nodes; and an elevated myeloid-to-erythroid ratio in the bone marrow. Histopathological alterations of the liver, kidney, skeletal muscle, and gastrointestinal tract are commonly associated with higher doses of the candidate antimalarials. Increases in leucocyte count, decreases in the number of reticulocytes and elevated serum concentrations of SGOT, SGPT, and BUN are frequently observed following antimalarial drug administration and are reflective of underlying histopathological changes.

The exception to this toxicity profile is the class containing the 8-aminoquinoline compounds. These compounds are considerably more toxic than the other classes described and possess a different profile. Degenerative changes in the heart, skeletal muscle and liver are the most significant histopathological alterations reported for the 8-aminoquinolines. Characteristic haematological changes occur with repeated administration of these compounds and include methaemoglobin formation, with an increased number of reticulocytes and a decreased platelet count. These haematological changes dominate the toxicity profile of the 8-aminoquinolines; consequently, a recent objective of the programme has been to investigate different assay systems for determining the relative methaemoglobin-forming potential of the most promising drugs of this class prior to their selection for preclinical toxicological evaluation.

During the past 15 years more than 50 compounds have been tested through the second preclinical stage of toxicological evaluation. This has produced an extensive data base against which the relative safety of a candidate drug may be compared. At the completion of this second stage, data derived from toxicological evaluation, pharmacological studies and efficacy testing are synthesised into a risk/benefit analysis which establishes the rationale for introduction of the candidate drug to man.

## IV. Chronic Toxicity

The third or extended phase of toxicological evaluation begins after analysis of phase II clinical pharmacological studies clearly indicates promising therapeutic potential of the candidate drug. Information about the metabolic and pharmacokinetic characteristics of the candidate drug in several species, including man, at this stage of development makes it possible to individualise the design of these advanced stages of toxicological investigation. This stage of evaluation generally includes carcinogenic, chronic toxicity, and reproductive/teratological studies. Often reversal studies or other special studies are necessary to define more completely the toxicity of the candidate drug.

The scope of chronic toxicity testing is dependent in part on the proposed clinical use of the candidate drug. A drug proposed for single-dose therapy may only require 3–6 months of toxicological testing while a proposed prophylactic agent may require studies of 2 years' duration or longer. The design of long-term toxicity studies is similar to that of subacute studies previously described except that dose levels must be adjusted appropriately based on the results of the subacute toxicity studies, pharmacokinetic and metabolic studies, and the proposed therapeutic dosing regimen. In addition, the number of animals is increased and the intervals for sampling of blood for haematological and clinical chemical determinations are lengthened.

Routinely, the chronic toxicity study in mice and rats is combined with carcinogenic studies as this combination provides for a more efficient and economical use of laboratory resources and personnel. During this 2-year study, the drug is incorporated into the feed to provide a constant daily dose rate per kilogram body weight. A minimum of 50 animals per sex is assigned to at least three drug dose levels to ensure an adequate sample size in surviving groups at study termination. Currently, studies are initiated in pubescent animals rather than in utero as in a two-generation study. The current procedure was designed to assess the carcinogenicity of drugs being developed for a rather restricted target population, young adult males; however, future carcinogenic studies may require a multigenerational approach, as the target population will have a broader base.

A major aspect of the extended phase of toxicological evaluation is assessing the action of a candidate drug on the reproductive performance of test animals. These studies are routinely performed in three segments. Segment 1 is an investigation of a drug's effect on general reproductive performance and fertility, segment 2 is a determination of the teratogenic potential of a drug, and segment 3 is an evaluation of the prenatal and postnatal toxicities of a drug. Although dose selection is critical for all toxicological studies, it is especially critical for reproductive studies because of the added complexity of parent-offspring interactions. Dose selection is further complicated by the long half-lives of many candidate antimalarials, which cause a significant lag period before steady-state conditions are attained. The interpretation of results from segment 2 and 3 studies is especially difficult under these circumstances because these studies require relatively short-term dosing regimens. Consequently, we have incorporated loading doses into these studies which ensure early attainment of steady-state conditions throughout the period of drug exposure. Currently, three dose levels of the candidate antimalarial are utilised in each segment in an attempt to ensure that a maximally tolerated dose and a no-effect dose are administered.

Often questions are raised during the toxicological evaluation of a candidate drug which cannot be answered with the standard battery of tests. A frequently asked question is whether or not a lesion is reversible. This question may be answered by performing a reversal study in which an antidote is incorporated or in which the candidate drug is withdrawn during the later stages of the study. The observation of adverse effects on fertility by a candidate drug during segment 1 reproductive testing in the male may necessitate performing a dominant lethal study to pinpoint the stage of spermatogenesis most sensitive to the drug's actions. For those drugs being developed for intravenous administration, studies of their potential to induce venous toxicity are performed. These studies are modifications of the procedures utilised by the National Cancer Institute for antineoplastic drugs. In this procedure the lateral marginal ear vein of the rabbit is used to assess vasotoxicity. Other studies designed to answer specific questions concerning an individual drug's toxicity include blood compatibility studies, neurological studies in monkeys and special electron microscope studies. It must be emphasised that the toxicological evaluation of a candidate drug is not a rigid screening of a compound, but rather it is a systematic, individualised assessment of the toxicological potential of a new drug which is performed to gain a thorough knowledge concerning the relative risk of administering the candidate antimalarial to man. This permits the design of safer, more efficient clinical protocols.

## G. Pharmacodynamic Investigations

Antimalarial drugs possess a broad spectrum of pharmacodynamic actions in addition to their antimalarial activity. Historically, the cinchona alkaloids were known to produce significant effects on cardiac rhythm (BIGGER and HOFFMAN 1980). The relationship of antimalarial efficacy and antiarrhythmic activity has been retained with the synthetic antimalarials such as primaquine (BASS et al. 1972), chloroquine, and amodiaquine (ARORA et al. 1956). In addition to their effects on cardiac rhythm, antimalarial drugs have been shown to depress cardiac muscle in vitro (MARSHALL and OJEWOLE 1978). Many antimalarial drugs interact with the autonomic nervous system. Quinine has significant atropine-like activity (DIPALMA 1971) as well as appreciable alpha adrenergic blocking activity (MECCA et al. 1980). In addition, the 8-aminoquinolines have been reported to attenuate central sympathetic reflexes (MOE et al. 1949) and to exert a $\beta$-adrenergic blocking action (BASS et al. 1972). Some antimalarials may have significant effects on respiration. For example, quinine has recently been shown to produce marked effects on respiratory rate, minute volume, and dynamic airways resistance (CALDWELL and NASH 1978). These cardiovascular, autonomic, and respiratory effects become increasingly important when antimalarials are administered intravenously as in the emergency treatment of cerebral malaria.

A major goal of drug development is to provide a selective advantage for the therapeutic action of a drug versus its other pharmacodynamic effects. The more efficacious, synthetic analogues of quinine i.e. chloroquine and amodiaquine) possess three times the potency of quinidine in reverting auricular fibrillation (ARORA et al. 1956). However, experimental studies with mefloquine, a quinolinemethanol which is extremely efficacious in the treatment of chloroquine-resistant strains of *Plasmodium falciparum*, suggest that mefloquine possesses only 20% of the antiarrhythmic potency of quinidine (HEMWALL and DIPALMA 1979). Consequently, continued development of this class of compounds may produce a drug which could be formulated into a relatively safe, yet highly effective intravenous preparation.

Fortunately, the effects of antimalarials on the cardiovascular, respiratory and autonomic nervous system are generally benign when these drugs are administered orally. The primary purpose of early pharmacodynamic screening of a candidate antimalarial is to characterise its effects on the cardiovascular, respiratory and autonomic nervous systems. These studies are expanded considerably for those compounds selected for development as intravenous formulations. Any unusual or unexpected findings observed in screening will necessitate additional studies to describe the mechanism of action or to determine whether the effects may be reversed or attenuated by standard clinical procedures.

Pharmacodynamic screening is divided into three phases, each of which utilises 10- to 15-kg beagles, anaesthetised with sodium pentobarbital, as the experimental model. The first phase is the dose-response portion of the screen in which standardised cardiorespiratory measurements are obtained during administration of a series of progressively increasing, bolus intravenous doses of the candidate drug. The second phase consists of a slow, intravenous infusion of the drug over a 45- to 60-min period during which electrocardiographic intervals and arterial blood gas values are determined periodically in addition to the standard cardiorespiratory measurements. This second phase is conducted in an attempt to simulate, experimentally, what would occur clinically under conditions most favourable for rapid absorption of an orally administered drug. The third, or drug-interaction, phase of the screen is conducted to provide preliminary information on whether the candidate drug modifies the cardiorespiratory responses to a series of cardioactive compounds, e.g. noradrenaline, isoproterenol, serotonin, histamine, angiotensin, and acetylcholine.

The results from the dose-response phase of the pharmacodynamic screen for representative quinolinemethanols, 8-aminoquinolines and other antimalarial compounds are summarised in Table 2. Inspection of these results suggests that the most frequently observed response to a bolus intravenous injection of a candidate drug is a transient decrease in mean arterial pressure. This hypotensive response is usually accompanied by an increase in respiratory rate which may be considered reflexive because of its temporal relationship to the hypotensive response. The chronotropic response is more heterogeneous, with the majority of drugs producing less than a 10% change from baseline at this dose. A slow, intravenous infusion produces a characteristic cardiorespiratory profile that is different from the effects

**Table 2.** Cardiorespiratory responses of anaesthetised dogs to a 5s bolus intravenous injection (10 mg/kg) of representative antimalarials [a]

| Antimalarial | Heart rate | Mean arterial pressure | Respiratory rate |
|---|---|---|---|
| Quinolinecarbinols | | | |
| Mefloquine [b] | −20 | −41 | 428 [d] |
| WR 177602 | −36 | −47 | 91 |
| WR 184806 [c] | nc | −15 | 20 |
| 8-Aminoquinolines | | | |
| Primaquine [b] | nc | −15 | 16 |
| WR 6026 | nc | −43 | 28 |
| WR 181023 | nc | −11 | 25 |
| WR 225448 | nc | −14 | 50 |
| Others | | | |
| WR 172435 (pyridinecarbinol) | 14 | −20 | nc |
| WR 180409 [b] (pyridinecarbinol) | −33 | −61 | 464 [d] |
| WR 194965 (phenylphenol) | 32 | −49 | 200 [d] |
| WR 228258 (4-aminoquinoline) | nc | −61 | 63 |

[a] Percentage change from baseline; < 10% considered as no change (nc)
[b] Response reported is for a 3-mg/kg dose; 10 mg/kg was lethal in this model
[c] Response reported is for an 8-mg/kg dose
[d] Respiratory response was short, usually less than 1 min in duration

**Table 3.** Cardiorespiratory responses to slow intravenous infusions of representative antimalarials in the anaesthetised dog

| Drug | Infusion rate (mg/kg/min) | Total dose (mg/kg) | Percent change from baseline at completion of infusion [a] | | | Duration of drug response following infusion (h) |
|---|---|---|---|---|---|---|
| | | | Heart rate | Mean arterial pressure | Respiratory rate | |
| Mefloquine | 0.58 | 35 | −26 | nc | nc | >2 |
| WR 177602 | 0.58 | 35 | nc | nc | nc | 0 |
| WR 228258 | 0.46 | 20.7 | −35 | −15 | 100 | 0.6 |
| Primaquine | 0.59 | 17.6 | nc | nc | −18 | 1 |
| WR 225448 | 0.42 | 12.7 | nc | nc | 23 | 1 |
| WR 6026 | 0.48 | 21.6 | −17 | nc | −23 | 1.5 |
| WR 172435 | 0.50 | 30 | −14 | nc | nc | >2 |
| WR 180409 | 0.25 | 15 | −12 | nc | nc | >1 |
| WR 194965 | 0.50 | 30 | −31 | nc | −32 | >2 |

[a] Change from baseline must equal or exceed 10% to be reported. Responses of less than 10% were considered to be 'no change' (nc)

[b] Two-hour observation period following completion of infusion for all drugs except WR 180409, which had a 1-h observation period

of bolus injections (Table 3). Slow infusion attenuates the hypotensive response observed following bolus injection and reveals a negative chronotropic action for most compounds. An interesting aspect of this analysis is the observation that WR 177602, the *threo* isomer of mefloquine, produces less than a 10% change in cardiorespiratory indices when administered as a slow intravenous infusion. WR 177602 would be a logical candidate for continued development as an intravenous preparation.

Following pharmacodynamic screening, a more intensive cardiovascular and respiratory assessment of the candidate antimalarial drug is performed prior to extensive clinical investigation or development as an intravenous preparation. This advanced pharmacodynamic evaluation includes measurement of the following cardiovascular indices: arterial and left ventricular pressure, left ventricular dP/dt, peripheral leads of the electrocardiogram, heart rate, pulmonary artery and wedge pressures, cardiac output, and pulmonary vascular resistance. Respiratory evaluations include tidal volume, dynamic airways resistance and compliance, as well as measurements of arterial and venous $pO_2$, $pCO_2$, pH values, and venous haematocrit. The candidate drug is infused into a pentobarbital-anaesthetised dog at one of three infusion rates over a 20-min period and responses are monitored prior to, during and for 120 min following the infusion. Thus, these investigations provide a detailed prediction of the cardiovascular and respiratory effects which may be experienced by volunteers exposed to doses of the candidate drug that range from non-toxic or minimally toxic to moderately or severely toxic. Studies of mefloquine methanesulphonate, an intravenous preparation, indicated that administration at a dosage rate of 1 mg/kg per minute had little or no effect on monitored cardiorespiratory indices while higher doses produced a temporary decrease in tidal volume and dynamic airways resistance with an increased respiratory rate, while elevating pulmonary artery and wedge pressure and depressing arterial pressure (CALDWELL and NASH 1977). These cardiorespiratory responses were qualitatively similar but less severe than the responses reported for equimolar doses of quinine hydrochloride in the same experimental model (CALDWELL and NASH 1978).

During the preclinical testing of a compound, unusual or unexpected results may be encountered which require additional investigation. These studies should define in more detail the pharmacological activity of a candidate drug and therefore aid in interpreting toxicological findings or provide a rationale for the management of potential side effects or adverse responses in man. For example, WR 194965, when administered subacutely to beagles at lethal doses, produced a characteristic pattern of toxic signs but no observable changes in haematology, clinical chemistry, and histopathology (LEE et al. 1977). The nature and duration of the toxic signs, which included emesis, salivation, diarrhoea, tremors, convulsions, lethargy, and weakness, suggested that the lethal action of this compound was due in part to a profound but temporary augmentation of parasympathetic activity. Pharmacodynamic screening also suggested that WR 194965 enhanced parasympathetic tone. A more detailed investigation of the cardiovascular actions revealed that atropine pretreatment or bilateral vagotomy significantly attenuated the negative chronotropism produced by this drug (KORTE et al. 1978), thereby supporting the hypothesis that enhancement of parasympathetic tone is a major component of the pharmacological response following administration of WR 194965.

Candidate antimalarial drugs possess the potential for considerable pharmacodynamic activity especially on the cardiovascular, autonomic, and respiratory systems. Consequently, it is imperative that the preclinical assessment of a candidate drug should include pharmacodynamic studies. These studies provide the basis for the rational synthesis of compounds which will enhance the selective advantage of the candidate antimalarial versus its other pharmacological actions, and may also suggest a novel therapeutic indication.

## H. Concluding Remarks

To establish effective control of malaria, one must completely interrupt the life cycle of the parasite. One approach is the continuous development of drugs which prevent or cure this disease. In order to accomplish this goal, one must have an effective drug development process. This chapter describes the approach to preclinical development which has evolved in the US Army Antimalarial Drug Development Programme. The approach is not presented as a model for those agencies or institutions who may wish to pursue antimalarial or other drug development objectives, but rather it portrays how one organisation has maximised the resources available to it. We believe, however, that both the close integration and coordination of all phases of preclinical investigation and the integration of preclinical and clinical studies are essential to any programme if resources are to be applied efficiently and effectively, and if maximum safety during clinical investigation and ultimate clinical use of a drug is to be assured.

Another approach to drug development is rational synthesis, which is not used at present due to a lack of specific knowledge about the biochemical action of drugs and information about the interaction of drugs with receptors at the molecular level. With this information, a more rational approach could be made which would facilitate the drug development process by reducing both the time to identify a new lead and the cost of the process.

There is genuine need for the establishment of additional multidisciplinary drug development teams in other countries dedicated to the search for more effective drugs to prevent or treat malaria and other major infectious diseases. To complement this endovour, a continuous training programme to ensure a continuity of capable professional and technical personnel is needed. If the various governments throughout the world follow historical precedent, there will be a strong tendency to dismantle the resources dedicated to the search for new antimalarials with the appearance in the near future of one or two drugs on the market. One has a tendency to forget that it requires approximately 9–10 years to market a drug after its initial synthesis, but that parasite resistance, to that drug may emerge considerably earlier.

## References


Ames BN, McCann J, Yamasaki E (1975) Methods for detecting carcinogens and mutagens with the *Salmonella*/mammalian-microsome mutagenicity test. Mutat Res 31:347–363

Arora RB, Madan BR, Patnak RK (1956) Antiarrhythmics: Part VIII: Chloroquine, amodiaquine, procaine amide, and quinidine in experimental auricular arrhythmias simulating clinical disorders. Indian J Med Res 44:453–462

Bass SW, Ramirez MA, Aviado DM (1972) Cardiopulmonary effects of antimalarial drugs. VI. Adenosine, quinacrine, and primaquine. Toxicol Appl Pharmacol 21:464–481

Bigger JT Jr, Hoffman BF (1980) Antiarrhythmic drugs. In: Gilman AG, Goodman LS, Gilman A (eds) The pharmacological basis of therapeutics. McMillan, New York, p 768

Caldwell RW, Nash CB (1977) Pulmonary and cardiovascular effects of mefloquine methanesulfonate. Toxicol Appl Pharmacol 40:437–448

Caldwell RW, Nash CB (1978) Cardiopulmonary effects of IV quinine HCl(Q). Fed Proc 37:689

Canfield CJ, Heiffer MH (1978) The US Army drug development program. In: Adolphe M (ed) Advances in pharmacology and therapeutics, vol 10, Chemotherapy. Oxford, New York, pp 99–108

Cenedella RJ, Saxe LH (1967) Automated mass screening of compounds for antimalarial activity. Automation in analytical chemistry. Technicon symposium. Technicon Corporation, New York, pp 281–285

Cenedella RJ, Saxe LH, Van Dyke K (1970) An automated method of mass drug testing applied to screening for antimalarial activity. Chemotherapy 15:158–176

Coatney GR, Cooper LC, Eddy NB, Greenberg J (1953) Survey of antimalarial agents. Chemotherapy of *Plasmodium gallinaceum* infections: Toxicity; correlation of structure and action. Public health monograph number 9, US Government Printing Office, Washington, DC

Coatney GR, Collins WE, Warren M, Contacos PG (1971) The primate malarias. US Department of Health, Education and Welfare Publication, US Government Printing Office, Washington, DC

Davey DG (1963) Chemotherapy of malaria. Biological basis of testing methods. In: Schnitzer RJ, Hawkin F (eds) Experimental Chemotherapy. Academic, New York, p 487

Davidson DE, Johnson DO, Tanticharoenyos P, Hickman RL, Kinnamon KE (1976) Evaluating new antimalarial drugs against trophozoite-induced *Plasmodium cynomolgi* malaria in rhesus monkeys. Am J Trop Med Hyg 25:26–33

Davidson DE, Ager AL, Brown JL, Chapple FE, Whitmire RE, Rossan RN (1981) New tissue schizonticidal antimalarial drugs. Bull WHO 59:463–479

Desjardins RE, Canfield CJ, Haynes JD, Chulay JD (1979) Quantitative assessment of antimalarial activity in vitro by a semiautomated microdilution technique. Antimicrob Agents Chemother 16:710–718

DiPalma JR (1971) Chemotherapy of protozoan infections 1: Malaria. In: DiPalma JR (ed) Drill's Pharmacology in Medicine, McGraw-Hill, New York, p 1783

Ferone R, Burchall JJ, Hitchings GH (1969) *Plasmodium berghei* dihydrofolate reductase. Isolation, properties, and inhibition by antifolates. Mol Pharmacol 5:49–59

Finney DJ (1971) Probit Analysis. Cambridge University Press, Cambridge

Genther CS, Smith CC (1977) Antifolate studies. Activities of 40 potential antimalarial compounds against sensitive and chlorguanide triazine resistant strains of folate-requiring bacteria and *Escherichia coli*. J Med Chem 20:237–243

Genther CS, Squires W, Fradkin R, Schmidt LH (1948) Malaria chemotherapy: 1. The response of trophozoite-induced infections with *Plasmodium cynomolgi* to various antimalarial drugs. Fed Proc 7:221

Gerberg EJ (1971) Evaluation of antimalarial compounds in mosquito test systems. Trans R Soc Trop Med Hyg 65:358–363

Gregory KG, Peters W (1970) The chemotherapy of rodent malaria. IX. Causal prophylaxis, I: A method for demonstrating drug action on exo-erythrocytic stages. Ann Trop Med Parasitol 65:15–24

Grund P, Andose JD, Rhodes JB, Smith GM (1980) Three-dimensional molecular modeling and drug design. Science 208:1425–1431

Haynes JD, Diggs CL, Hines FA, Desjardins RE (1976) Culture of human malaria parasites *Plasmodium falciparum*. Nature 263:767–769

Hemwall E, DiPalma JR (1979) Cardiovascular and antiarrhythmic effects of mefloquine. Pharmacologist 21:200

Jiang JB (1978) Plasmodium: Experimental animals for human malaria and research needs. A review. Exp Parasitol 46:339–352

Killick-Kendrick R, Peters W (1978) Rodent malaria. Academic, New York

Kinnamon KE, Rothe WE (1975) Biological screening in the US Army antimalarial drug development program. Am J Trop Med Hyg 24:174–178

Korte DW Jr, Herman A, Neidig MH Jr, Heiffer MH (1978) Cardiovascular activity of the candidate antimalarial drug (1-*t*-butyl)-2-(*t*-butylaminomethyl)-6-(4-chlorophenyl)-phenol phosphate (WR 194965·$H_3PO_4$) in the dog. Pharmacologist 20:253

Lee CC, Kowalski JJ, Kintner LD, Hong CB, Girven JD, Ellis ER (1977) Subacute oral toxicity of 4-(*t*-butyl)-2-(*t*-butylaminomethyl)-6-(4-chlorophenyl)phenol phosphate, WR 194965·$H_3PO_4$, in dogs. Supplement to interim report No. 113, Midwest Research Institute, Kansas City, MO. USAMRDC Contract DAMD 17-74-C-4036

Marshall RJ, Ojewole JA (1978) Comparative effects of some antimalarial drugs on isolated cardiac muscle of the guinea pig. Toxicol Appl Pharmacol 46:757–768

Mecca TE, Elam JT, Nash CB, Caldwell RW (1980) *alpha*-Adrenergic blocking properties of quinine HCl. Eur J Pharmacol 63:159–166

Merkli B, Peters W (1976) A comparison of two different methods for the selection of primaquine resistance in *Plasmodium berghei berghei*. Ann Trop Med Parasitol 70:473–474

Moe GK, Peralta B, Seevers MH (1949) Central impairment of sympathetic reflexes by 8-aminoquinolines. J Pharmacol Exp Ther 95:407–414

Most H, Montuori WA (1975) Rodent systems (*Plasmodium berghei-Anopheles stephensi*) for screening compounds for potential causal prophylaxis. Am J Trop Med Hyg 24:179–182

Osdene TS, Russell PB, Rane L (1967) 2,4,7-Triamino-6-ortho-substituted arylpteridines. A new series of potent antimalarial agents. J Med Chem 10:431–434

Peters W (1965a) Drug resistance in *Plasmodium berghei* Vincke and Lips, 1948. I. Chloroquine resistance. Exp Parasitol 17:80–89

Peters W (1965b) Drug resistance in *Plasmodium berghei* Vincke and Lips, 1948. II. Triazine resistance. Exp Parasitol 17:90–96

Peters W (1966) Drug responses of mepacrine- and primaquine-resistant strains of *Plasmodium berghei* Vincke and Lips, 1948. Ann Trop Med Parasitol 60:25–30

Peters W (1968) The chemotherapy of rodent malaria, V. Dynamics of drug resistance, Part I: Methods for studying the acquisition and loss of resistance to chloroquine by *Plasmodium berghei*. Ann Trop Med Parasitol 62:277–287

Peters W (1970) Chemotherapy and drug resistance in malaria. Academic, New York

Peters W (1974) Prevention of drug resistance in rodent malaria by the use of drug mixtures. Bull WHO 51:379–383

Peters W, Portus J, Robinson BL (1977) The chemotherapy of rodent malaria, XXVIII. The development of resistance to mefloquine (WR 142490). Ann Trop Med Parasitol 71:419–427

Rane DS, Kinnamon KE (1979) The development of a "high volume tissue schizonticidal drug screen" based upon mortality of mice inoculated with sporozoites of *Plasmodium berghei*. Am J Trop Med Hyg 23:937–947

Rane L, Rane DS (1972) A screening procedure, based on mortality, with sporozoite-induced *Plasmodium gallinaceum* malaria in chicks. Proc Helminthol Soc Wash 39:283–287

Rieckmann KH, McNamara JV, Frischer H, Stuckert TA, Carson PE, Powell RD (1968) Effects of chloroquine, quinine, and cycloguanil upon the maturation of asexual erythrocytic forms of two strains of *Plasmodium falciparum in vitro*. Am J Trop Med Hyg 17:661–671

Rossan RN, Young MD, Baerg DC (1975) Chemotherapy of *Plasmodium vivax* in *Saimiri* and *Aotus* models. Am J Trop Med Hyg 24:168–173

Rothe WE, Jacobus DP (1968) Laboratory evaluation of the phototoxic potency of quinolinemethanols. J Med Chem 11:366–368

Rothe WE, Jacobus DP, Walter WG (1969) Treatment of trophozoite-induced *Plasmodium knowlesi* infection in the rhesus monkey with trimethoprim and sulfalene. Am J Trop Med Hyg 18:491–494

Schmidt LH (1973) Infections with *Plasmodium falciparum* and *Plasmodium vivax* in the owl monkey – model systems for basic biological and chemotherapeutic studies. Trans R Soc Trop Med Hyg 67:446–474

Schmidt LH (1978a) *Plasmodium falciparum* and *Plasmodium vivax* infections in the owl monkey (*Aotus trivirgatus*). I. The courses of untreated infections. Am J Trop Med Hyg 27:671–702

Schmidt LH (1978b) *Plasmodium falciparum* and *Plasmodium vivax* infections in the owl monkey (*Aotus trivirgatus*). II. Responses to chloroquine, quinine, and pyrimethamine. Am J Trop Med Hyg 27:703–717

Schmidt LH (1978c) *Plasmodium falciparum* and *Plasmodium vivax* infections in the owl monkey (*Aotus trivirgatus*). III. Methods employed in the search for new blood schizontocidal drugs. Am J Trop Med Hyg 27:718–737

Schmidt LH, Rossan RN, Fisher KF (1963) The activity of a repository form of 4,6-diamino-1(*p*-chlorophenyl)-1,2-dihydro-2,2-dimethyl-*s*-triazine against infections with *Plasmodium cynomolgi*. Am J Trop Med Hyg 12:494–503

Schüpbach ME (1979) Mutagenicity evaluation of the two antimalarial agents chloroquine and mefloquine, using a bacterial fluctuation test. Mutat Res 68:41–49

Terzian LA (1947) A method for screening antimalarial compounds in the mosquito host. Science 106:449–450

Terzian LA, Stahler N, Weathersby AB (1949) The action of antimalarial drug in mosquitoes infected with *Plasmodium gallinaceum*. J Infect Dis 84:47–55

Thompson PE, Werbel LM (1972) Antimalarial agents: Chemistry and pharmacology. In: DeStevens G (ed) Medicinal Chemistry: A series of monographs, vol 12. Academic, New York

Thompson PE, Olszewski BJ, Elslager EF, Worth DF (1963) Laboratory studies on 4,6-diamino-1-(*p*-chlorophenyl)-1,2-dihydro-2,2-dimethyl-*s*-triazine pamoate (CI-501) as a repository antimalarial drug. Am J Trop Med Hyg 12:481–493

Thompson PE, Bayles A, Olszewski B, Waitz JA (1965) Qunine-resistant *Plasmodium berghei* in mice. Science 148:1240–1241

Thompson PE, Olszewski B, Bayles A, Waitz JA (1967) Relations among antimalarial drugs: Results of studies with cycloguanil-, sulfone-, or chloroquine-resistant *Plasmodium berghei* in mice. Am J Trop Med Hyg 16:133–145

Trager W, Jensen JB (1976) Human malaria parasites in continuous culture. Science 193:673–675

Wiselogle FY (1946) A survey of antimalarial drugs, 1941–1945. J. W. Edwards, Ann Arbor, MI

World Health Organization (1971) Report of conference on procedures for screening potential antimalarial compounds. WHO Document WHO/MAL 72:763

World Health Organization (1973) Chemotherapy of malaria and resistance to antimalarials. WHO Tech Rep Ser 529

Young MD, Baerg DC, Rossan RN (1975) Parasitological reviews. Experimental monkey hosts for human plasmodia. Exp Parasitol 38:136–152

CHAPTER 13

# Clinical Trials – Phases I and II

M. FERNEX

## A. Introduction

The need for developing new antimalarials has been expressed on various occasions by the World Health Organization (WHO). The "Special Programme for Research and Training in Tropical Diseases" (TDR), established in 1975 under the auspices of the UNDP, World Bank and WHO (1980), has stimulated new efforts in this field. The highest priority has been given to the development of new antimalarials.

When the TDR Programme was established in 1975, "malaria research was at its lowest ebb since World War II. The pharmaceutical industry had largely phased out the development of new antimalarial drugs, the only major effort in this area being that of the Walter Reed Army Institute of Research (WRAIR), USA and field research had virtually come to a standstill" (UNDP/WORLD BANK/WHO 1980).

WHO has already published a series of valuable documents and recommendations on the clinical assessment of antimalarials (WHO 1961, 1968, 1973, 1974). The WHO monograph published by COVELL et al. (1956) quotes 181 papers on clinical trials which contributed to establishing the basic clinical knowledge of the existing standard antimalarials, quinine, mepacrine, 4-aminoquinolines, proguanil, and antifol combinations. A recent publication of WHO (1980) on the clinical management of acute malaria describes the clinical patterns of malaria and summarises the requisite laboratory tests and treatment for all forms of the disease.

The TDR programme has gone some way towards improving the situation in the field of malaria chemotherapy and immunology. The aim of this chapter is to facilitate the work of new research groups intending to develop antimalarial drugs.

### I. Objectives of Trials in Individual Subjects

Therapeutic trials in humans may have two major objectives:

1. To test new compounds which have been proved by adequate, preclinical, pharmacological, and toxicological investigations to be potentially safe and effective antimalarials.

2. To assess more accurately the safety of a drug that is already introduced, when administered to a particular group of subjects, for instance, patients with low levels of erythrocyte glucose 6-phosphate dehydrogenase (G6PD). The efficacy of familiar drugs (for example, antibiotics) or combinations of drugs may be investigated in phase IV. Studies to determine clinically the susceptibility of *Plasmodium*

*falciparum* to standard antimalarials in a given area can also be considered as phase IV trials.

## II. Prerequisites for Administering a New Drug in Man

The prerequisites for first administering a new antimalarial in man are summarised elsewhere (see Chap. 12). In all cases official documents including the *Guidelines for Evaluation of Drugs for Use in Man* by WHO (1975 b), the *Clinical Guidelines* edited by the Food and Drug Administration (FDA 1977 a–c), as well as recommendations issued in the respective countries on this topic, must be consulted by investigators. When developing new antimalarial drugs, special consideration must be given to the following points

1. The target populations which need such drugs live in a particular tropical and subtropical ecological environment where malnutrition and associated infections are common. Certain genetic factors known to interfere with drug metabolism and/or with the disease (erythrocyte G6PD deficiency, haemoglobinopathies, rapid acetylator phenotypes, etc.) are highly prevalent in some areas.
2. Antimalarials are usually administered without medical supervision or may even be distributed prophylactically for a prolonged period in mass campaigns. New compounds must therefore be very safe. Such compounds must also be non-fetotoxic, non-mutagenic, and non-carcinogenic in experimental models since, in endemic areas, pregnant women, children, and infants represent the most vulnerable group for the disease.

## III. Definition of Phases for Clinical Trials

Some discrepancies exist regarding the definition of the phases of clinical trials, depending on the regulatory bodies of various countries.

In a basic report of WHO (1973) six phases were described, whereas the development of a new drug is usually divided into only four phases. However, the WHO document describes *steps* in the study of a new compound depending on the stage of development of the parasite at which the drug is thought to be active, and differentiates between tests performed in individual subjects or in the field.

In this chapter, the usual classification (phase I–IV) proposed by most of the national regulatory authorities will be used, although the steps to be carried out in each phase may differ slightly from country to country.

1. *Phase I* trials correspond to the initial administration of a new drug to man. At this stage, apparently healthy or oligosymptomatic volunteers will be selected to determine if this drug has a potentially beneficial effect (FDA 1977 a). For this purpose a qualified clinical pharmacologist will study:

The safety of the new compound.

Its bioavailability, mode of elimination and, if possible, its pharmacokinetics and metabolism (FDA 1977 a, b; GOLDBERG et al. 1975).

When appropriate, the pharmacological effect and evidence of tolerance and effectiveness and early dose-ranging studies will be included (FDA 1977 a, b).

For antimalarials it is essential to perform phase I trials also in endemic areas of Latin America, Asia, and Africa, in healthy or oligosymptomatic volunteers belonging to the target population and who are potentially carriers of malaria parasites.

2. *Phase II* consists of controlled clinical trials designed to demonstrate effectiveness and safety. These studies will make it possible to find the optimal dosage schedule for each potential indication, i.e. causal prophylaxis, blood schizontocidal activity, anti-relapse activity, and gametocytocidal and sporontocidal activity. These terms have been defined in previous chapters, as well as by BRUCE-CHWATT (1967), PETERS (1970), and KILLICK-KENDRICK and PETERS (1978).

3. *Phase III* includes expanded (usually comparative) trials in which effectiveness and safety are confirmed in larger groups of patients. More severe cases and patients with particular risk factors such as associated diseases, associated medication, genetic anomalies, and special age groups – children, infants, and women of child-bearing age – will be included. The main objective of this phase is to assess the safety of the drug when given in an optimal dosage to a larger group of patients under field conditions, and to compare its activity with standard treatments.

4. *Phase IV* applies to all aspects of drug investigation following the approval of a New Drug Application (BLACKWELL et al. 1975). The most important data to be collected at this stage are on tolerance, and a prospective or retrospective assessment of possible, rare, adverse reactions, or reactions occurring after prolonged use in different categories of patients. The efficacy must be constantly reassessed because of the potential development of resistance. These postmarketing clinical trials include:

a) Special studies to elucidate the incidence and mechanism of adverse reactions, or means of preventing them.
b) Large-scale, long-term, epidemiological studies to determine the effect of a drug on morbidity, mortality, fertility, and incidence of malformation of babies.
c) Comparative trials, as mentioned above, to assess the efficacy of a standard dosage regimen in a given epidemiological environment (e.g. where individual case reports or in vitro screening of parasites indicate an increased tolerance of the parasites to the antimalarial).
d) The benefit from concomitant medication administered in severe or complicated cases must also be assessed.

This chapter will be restricted to phase I and II clinical trials. Phase III, IV, and field trials are discussed in Chap. 14.

## IV. Classification of Antimalarials

Data provided by preclinical in vitro and in vivo experiments using various strains of rodent, avian, monkey or human malaria parasites – susceptible or resistant to standard antimalarials – indicate precisely in which situation or disease the new drug might be effective (PETERS 1970; KILLICK-KENDRICK and PETERS 1978). The susceptibility of each stage of development of the parasite to the new compound will be defined for various strains of *P. falciparum* and *P. vivax*. Less evidence will be available about its activity against *P. ovale* and *P. malariae*.

The following schedule (Fig. 1) indicates at which stage of the life cycle of a given species of parasite antimalarials are expected to act (BRUCE-CHWATT 1967; PETERS 1979).

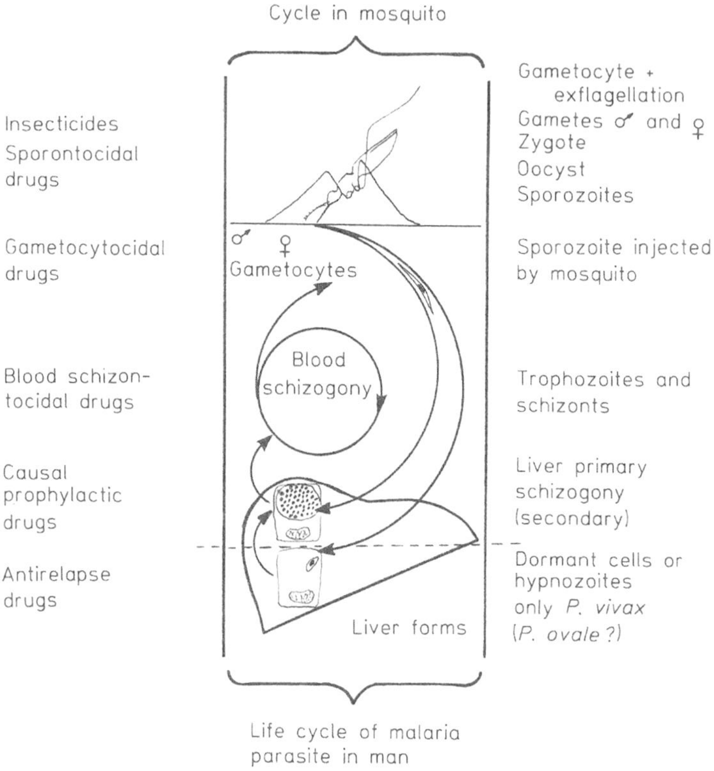


**Fig. 1.** Classification of antimalarials

1. *Causal prophylactic drugs* will eliminate the parasites before they reach the erythrocytes. Inoculated sporozoites may be destroyed even before being taken up, perhaps first by the macrophages, especially the Kupffer cells of the liver. Evidence for such activity against inoculated parasites is at present only available from experimental compounds. Medicaments such as 8-aminoquinolines, proguanil, pyrimethamine, antifol combinations, and antibiotics inhibit pre-erythrocytic schizogony in the liver, and are also considered to have potentially causal prophylactic activity in special circumstances. However, proguanil and pyrimethamine are the only drugs which are prescribed primarily for this purpose.

2. *Blood schizontocides* act on asexual intraerythrocytic forms and on young but not mature gametocytes of *P. falciparum,* whereas gametocytes of *P. vivax* and *P. malariae* are susceptible. Compounds such as quinine, mepacrine, chloroquine, antifol combinations and mefloquine belong to this group. These drugs may be used for *suppressive therapy* – i.e. the parasitaemia will be reduced below a level where symptoms become apparent – or for *radical treatment* in malaria due to *P. falciparum* or *P. malariae,* which implies the complete elimination of the parasites. In *P. vivax* only a clinical cure may be achieved.

3. *Antirelapse drugs* will destroy the dormant liver forms of *P. vivax,* the so-called hypnozoites, surviving in the liver cells (UNGUREANU et al. 1976; KROTOSKI

et al. 1980 (See also Chap. 1). They will achieve a radical cure in *P. vivax* infections after eradication of the erythrocytic forms. For the time being only 8-aminoquinoline derivatives such as primaquine are used as antirelapse drugs.

4. *Gametocytocides* will sterilise or destroy gametocytes (of *P. falciparum*) at certain stages of their development. If the gametocytes persist in the circulating blood but have lost their infectivity for the *Anopheles* vector, the drug is said to have a *sporontocidal activity*. The 8-aminoquinolines and pyrimethamine are the best sporontocidal compounds available for *P. falciparum*. This activity may be assessed in simple test systems (GERBERG 1971).

The risk of parasites developing resistance to the drug and the possibility of using a combination to prevent, or at least delay, such development must also be examined beforehand (PETERS 1970; MERKLI and RICHLE 1980; MERKLI et al. 1980).

## V. Resistance to Schizontocidal Drugs

The response of *P. falciparum* to schizontocidal drugs may be graded depending on the duration of the disappearance of asexual blood forms. If a standard dose of a drug provides permanent disappearance of parasites, the corresponding strain is considered to be susceptible (WHO 1973). Resistance to the antimalarial is graded RI, RII or RIII (see Chap. 17).

## VI. Ethical Considerations

Most nations have ratified the Declaration of Helsinki of 1975, adopted by the 18th World Medical Assembly in Helsinki, Finland, in 1964, and revised by the 29th World Medical Assembly in Tokyo, Japan, in 1975. The basic principles regarding the ethical aspects of any biomedical research involving human subjects have been clearly stated and must be considered as an essential minimum.

Some of the principles laid down in Helsinki may need to be quoted in detail in trial protocols:

2. The design and performance of each experimental procedure involving human subjects should be clearly formulated in an experimental protocol which should be transmitted to a specially appointed independent committee for consideration, comment, and guidance.

5. Every biomedical research project involving human subjects should be preceded by careful assessment of predictable risks in comparison with foreseeable benefits to the subject or to others. Concern for the interests of the subject must always prevail over the interests of science and society.

9. In any research on human beings, each potential subject must be adequately informed of the aims, methods, anticipated benefits, and potential hazards of the study and the discomfort it may entail. He or she should be informed that he or she is at liberty to abstain from participating in the study and that he or she is free to withdraw his or her consent to participating at any time. The doctor should then obtain the subject's freely-given informed consent, preferably in writing.

10. When obtaining informed consent for the research project the doctor should be particularly cautious if the subject is in a dependent relationship to him or her or may consent under duress. In that case the informed consent should be obtained by a doctor who is not engaged in the investigation and who is completely independent of this official relationship.

12. The research protocol should always contain a statement of the ethical considerations involved and should indicate that the principles enunciated in the present Declaration are complied with.

In phases I and II, informed consent of volunteers or patients must be obtained in every case. In tropical countries, this means that the information to be given to the patient must be written down or translated into a language and a form which is well understood by the patient. In phase III trials where children or severely ill patients might be included in trials, informed consent should be obtained from relatives in accordance with national legislation.

In the United States, especially during World War II and up to the end of the Vietnam War, and in some other countries, e.g. Australia, the United Kingdom and Brazil, healthy prison inmates or military personnel were allowed to volunteer for safety and phase II efficacy studies. Experimental infections in non-immune volunteers or in neurosyphilitic patients have furnished an important part of our knowledge about the human malaria parasites (BRUCE-CHWATT 1967). Experiments using the owl monkey (*Aotus trivirgatus*) as an animal model for *P. falciparum* and *P. vivax* provided numerous new possibilities for the study of human parasites and the effect of drugs on them (HICKMAN 1969). Human experimental infections may thus lose part of their justification, even though the actual risks encountered in such trials have proved to be very low when all necessary precautions are taken. A concomitant breakthrough has been the development of in vitro culture techniques which in some situations have made the study of drug action on *P. falciparum* a practical alternative to in vivo testing (see, e.g. DESJARDINS et al. 1979 and Chap. 6).

## B. Phase I

The objective of phase I is to assess human tolerance and to provide circumstantial evidence for the clinical usefulness of a new drug. The FDA guidelines indicate "Phase I studies should include determination of absorption, excretion, and plasma clearance of the drug, and, if feasible, metabolic pathways" (FDA 1977a).

Qualified clinical pharmacologists working in well-equipped centres will need to discuss the proposed trial plans once the Investigational Drug Brochure summarising the required preclinical data (phase 0) has been completed. While requirements differ considerably from country to country, the trend seems to be for this phase to be considered as a part of the screening of new compounds. In this sense, a letter from J. R. Long, January 1980, of the British Committee on Safety of Drugs (CSM) indicates: "The CSM were particularly concerned to facilitate the conduct of early clinical trials to enable companies to decide as quickly as possible whether further development of a drug is justified." Such encouragement appears to be essential in the field of parasitic diseases and malaria, where very promising leads are often abandoned, because of premature cost-benefit considerations (LASAGNA 1979).

### I. Initial Trials in Volunteers

#### 1. Objective

The aim of early trials is twofold, comprising on the one hand the assessment of safety and, on the other, a study of the pharmacokinetics, including absorption, distribution, rate, and mechanism of elimination of the new drug and of its main metabolites. Such information makes it possible to predict how human subjects will react to the compound (FDA 1977a, b). The potential activity and toxicity of a given dose or concentration obtained in human plasma may be calculated on the basis of corresponding concentrations measured in the animal species in which toxicity (and efficacy) trials were performed. Such a comparison of the pharmacokinetics increases the predictive value of animal toxicology (GEORGE 1974).

The selection of volunteers has become a significant problem (LASAGNA 1975). For antimalarials, healthy volunteers from industrial countries may be involved in early trials, but more representative subjects, i.e. oligosymptomatic patient volunteers living in the endemic area, must be included already in phase I trials (WHO 1975b).

## 2. Initial Dosage

The initial doses chosen will be based on toxicological findings in the most susceptible animal species. For instance, 5 mg/kg per day of mefloquine proved to be nontoxic when given for 28 days to dogs (the most susceptible species). The first dose administered to healthy male volunteers was therefore a single administration of about 1 mg/kg body wt., i.e. 50 mg given once (GOLDBERG et al. 1975).

If the first dose does not provoke any relevant unwanted effect, a second dose, chosen arbitrarily at a certain level above the first one, can be given after a "washout" period of 3 days to 1 week (GOLDBERG et al. 1975). Doses may be increased according to toxicological considerations. If a given organ toxicity has been noticed, adequate laboratory tests must be used to determine very early alterations in the corresponding parenchyma. If bioavailability is being studied, the wash-out period should be about six biological plasma half-lives ($t^1/_2$) of the drug. For mefloquine, with a half-life of about 20 days, this would represent 120 days, which is exceptionally long.

## 3. Pharmacokinetics

The aim of pharmacokinetic studies is to enable us to predict with greater accuracy the potential toxicity and efficacy of a new drug in the clinic. To this end, the pharmacokinetic and metabolic data found in man are compared with those obtained during toxicity and efficacy studies in various animal species. These findings also facilitate the selection of suitable doses and dosage intervals on a rational basis.

The results of pharmacokinetic trials may indicate the rate of absorption, the bioavailability, the distribution, and the type of metabolic transformation of a drug, as well as its mode and rate of elimination. It is further of importance to determine whether the plasma concentrations are dose dependent and whether repeated administration will modify the handling of the drug by the body. This requires studying different dose levels and multiple doses.

The penetration of the active substance into the erythrocyte, and especially into the target cell, the infected erythrocyte, is essential for schizontocidal compounds. The concentration of the active drug required to inhibit in vitro schizogony of *P. falciparum* can actually be determined during the preclinical development phase. A good correlation exists between the in vitro and the clinical activity of schizontocidal compounds (WHO 1973, 1977).

Classical antimalarials such as quinine, primaquine, and even chloroquine were introduced with no or very little knowledge of their kinetics. Only one early paper by BERLINER et al. (1948) reported on the plasma concentration of chloroquine achieved in volunteers during treatment of induced malaria. Rational pharmacokinetic arguments for the curative and prophylactic dosage recommendations for chloroquine were provided only recently by BROHULT et al. (1979), ARONSSON et al. (1981), and STAIGER et al. (1981). In contrast, a considerable number of studies have already been performed for the most recently developed antimalarials. A summary of these data follows as an example of the pharmacokinetic approach to antimalarial drug evaluation.

Mefloquine, a 4-quinoline methanol derivative selected by the Walter Reed Army Institute of Research (WRAIR) (see Part II, chap. 9), has been further developed since 1976 by WHO, in collaboration with WRAIR and Roche, through the Special Programme for Research and Training in Tropical Diseases (TDR).

Using $^{14}C$-labelled mefloquine, the absorption, distribution in different organs and elimination of the labelled material was determined in mice, rats, and owl monkeys (SMITH et al. 1973; MU et al. 1975; LISS and KENSLER 1976; ROZMAN et al. 1978). The structure of several metabolites in rats was elucidated by JAUCH et al. (1980). SCHWARTZ (1980) developed new methods of assessing the concentration of the parent (active) substance and of its main metabolite in different body fluids. Since this metabolite is about as toxic as mefloquine in mice and rats, it was essential to have some knowledge of its kinetics.

Following the single-dose kinetic study of mefloquine in man by DESJARDINS et al. (1979), SCHWARTZ et al. (1980, 1982) described the fate of unchanged mefloquine and of its main metabolites in animals and man.

The absolute bioavailability of the tablet used in clinical trials was determined in dogs and was found to amount to approximately 80% of the dose. No such precise assessment

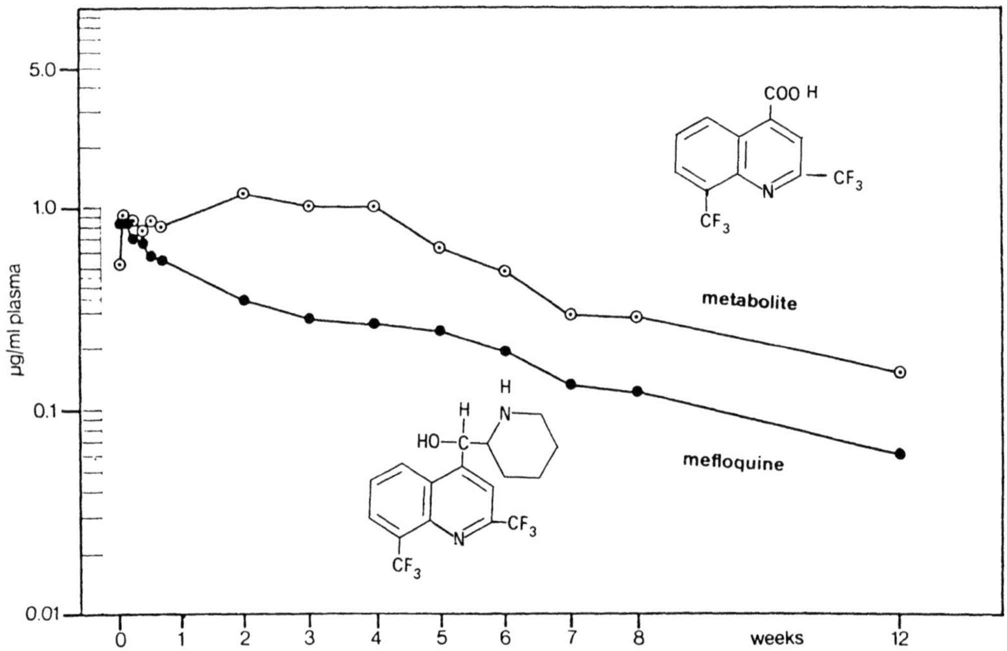


**Fig. 2.** Plasma levels of unchanged mefloquine and of its main metabolite following oral administration of 1 000 mg mefloquine base. After SCHWARTZ et al. (1980)

can be made in man because direct intravenous injection of mefloquine causes irritation of the vein.

SCHWARTZ et al. (1980, 1982) described the single-dose kinetics of mefloquine and of its metabolite in volunteers (from Europe and from Africa) following oral administration of four tablets, which corresponds to 1 g mefloquine base in the form of its hydrochloride (Fig. 2). The absorption was rapid, the apparent half-life of absorption being 0.36–2.0 h. Between 2 and 12 h after administration plasma concentrations of about 1.0 µg/ml of mefloquine could be measured. Thereafter, the plasma concentration time curve showed fluctuations, probably due to irregular biliary excretion and reabsorption. The decline of the plasma concentration was extremely gradual, the calculated terminal half-life of elimination ($t^1/_2$) ranging from 15 to 33 (mean ~21.4) days. In the plasma, although mefloquine is highly bound to protein (>99%), the concentration in or on human erythrocytes is nearly 170% of that in the plasma. It seems that about half of the mefloquine retained by the red blood cells is bound to the cell membrane (MU et al. 1975).

For simplification, SCHWARTZ et al. (1982) assumed that the dose administered was totally absorbed. The volume of distribution of mefloquine would then range between 27 and 50 litres/kg, indicating that the drug is widely distributed in tissue compartments.

The elimination of unchanged mefloquine in the urine is very slow, about 5% of the dose within the first 4 weeks. The drug is mainly eliminated by biotransformation and already 4 h after oral intake, measurable amounts of the main metabolite can be detected in the plasma. After a few days, the concentration of this metabolite exceeds that of mefloquine and the area under the plasma concentration time curve (AUC) is about 3.4 times greater than that of the active unchanged drug. However, the volume of distribution of the metabolite is small (in the dog about 30 times smaller than that of mefloquine), i.e. it does not diffuse into either tissue compartments or into the erythrocytes. One can therefore assume that the metabolite will not unfavourably influence the tolerance of mefloquine.

As expected from the results of one-dose kinetic studies, plasma levels gradually increase when repeated weekly doses of mefloquine are administered. In a tolerance trial in which volunteers received 250 mg mefloquine base (one tablet) at weekly intervals, mean mefloquine steady-state plasma level minima of 0.56–1.25 µg/ml were found. Mean plasma levels of the metabolite, measured at the same time, were 3.5–8.6 times greater than those of mefloquine. The half-life of elimination of the metabolite from the plasma is about equal to or slightly shorter than that of mefloquine. After 6 months of weekly administration (multiple-dose kinetics) the elimination half-life of mefloquine from plasma was assessed and was found to range from 17 to 35 (mean ~22.5) days. These values correspond to those found after administration of a single dose (SCHWARTZ et al. 1980, 1982), and indicate that no enzyme induction or inhibition is to be expected after prolonged therapy. Preliminary data suggest that the $t^1/_2$ of mefloquine is shorter in children than in adults.

## 4. Design of Phase I Trials

Tolerance trials should be randomised, prospective, double-blind comparisons of the test drug with either placebo or a standard drug such as chloroquine. In some cases, crossover studies versus placebo may be undertaken. The necessity to include placebo groups is due to the high incidence of subjective adverse reactions occurring after the intake of drugs, including placebo. Volunteers often complain of nausea, dizziness, restlessness, fatigue, headache, etc. after drug administration. The relevance of such subjective findings can only be assessed if the groups for comparison are sufficiently large and if differences found between subjects receiving placebo and those treated with active compounds show a significant difference, or at least a trend (CHAPUT DE SAINTONGE 1978).

The acceptability of the drug depends on the appearance, size, and taste of the tablets. The gastrointestinal tolerance as well as the bioavailability can be greatly influenced by the rate of dissolution of the compound from the pharmaceutic dosage form. When the drug has a bitter taste as, for example, chloroquine, lacquered or coated tablets should be used.

In early trials drugs are normally taken on an empty stomach with a glass of water. At a later stage the influence of food intake must be assessed.

Although occurring frequently with placebo, subjective adverse effects must be noted carefully. GEORGE (1974) has drawn up a checklist of findings which the volunteer has to tick off each day including the following points:

1. Loss of appetite
2. Increased appetite
3. Drowsiness
4. Dizziness
5. Nervousness
6. Weakness
7. Inability to sleep
8. Tiredness
9. Sleepiness
10. Light-headedness
11. Forgetfulness
12. Nightmares
13. Shakiness
14. Confusion
15. Jitteriness
16. Thirst
17. Headache
18. Stiffness
19. Pain
20. Change in physical activity or work
21. Numbness
22. Ringing in ears
23. Blurred vision
24. Skin rash
25. Hives
26. Itching
27. Unusual perspiration
28. Hot flushes
29. Dry mouth
30. Unpleasant taste
31. Easy bruising
32. Muscle cramps
33. Leg pains
34. Stuffy nose
35. Fast heartbeat
36. Irregular heartbeat
37. Nausea
38. Belching
39. Heartburn
40. Vomiting
41. Abdominal or stomach pain
42. Diarrhoea or frequent bowel movements
43. Constipation
44. Intestinal gas
45. Black stools
46. Dark urine
47. Painful urination
48. Getting up at night to urinate
49. Chest pain
50. Fever or chills
51. Change in sexual ability and/or desire
52. Others–specify.

Such questionnaires may also be used to check the acceptability and tolerance of suppressive therapy in non-hospitalised subjects.

Intramuscular or intravenous administration may be painful, even when local inflammation or necrosis is absent. Single injections may be subjectively well tolerated even though local necrosis, infiltration or thrombophlebitis may occur in animals after repeated injections. *The site of injection must therefore be carefully examined in every case.*

Volunteers must be kept under very close medical supervision. Clinical examination must be undertaken at least twice daily. This may require ECG, EEG, and other investigations, depending on the organs which seem most likely to be affected by the drug.

Laboratory tests performed daily will comprise a representative series of haematological and biochemical measurements. Complementary tests may be added if the drug is thought to be potentially toxic for a given tissue or system. For mefloquine, special studies were undertaken as a consequence of early clinical findings (dizziness) or toxicological observations (histological changes in the epididymis of a single species after very high dosage and prolonged administration), as well as routine clinical examinations and laboratory tests. These included neurological examination, cold pressure tests, caloric stimulation and orthokinetic nystagmus testing, audiograms and electroencephalograms, besides repeated monthly spermatograms during the long-term study in normal volunteers. These test results remained within the normal range both in the mefloquine-treated group and in subjects receiving placebo at weekly intervals in studies lasting 1 year or 26 weeks.

Physiological variations and a relatively broad range within the normal values for any given laboratory test must be taken into account. Furthermore, external factors such as violent physical activity, associated drugs, alcohol consumption and heavy smoking may affect the pharmacokinetics and the tolerance of the test medicament (Kahl 1978; Jusko 1981).

### 5. Recording and Processing of Data

Appropriate record forms should be used to facilitate the correct recording of all findings by the principal investigator. These questionnaires, designed so as to allow rapid data processing by a computer programme, must be prepared before the initiation of the study. Results must be assessed continuously to facilitate the close monitoring of the trial.

### 6. Selection of Volunteers

Selection of volunteers for phase I trials must be very strict. Apparently healthy male adults who are neither heavy smokers nor drug or alcohol addicts will be examined medically.

The very first group of volunteers is often composed of the staff of a pharmaceutical company, a research institute or a hospital. In some countries healthy adult prison inmates may still volunteer. Diet, activity and environment must be identical for all treatment groups. In order to be able to enter the trial, the prospective volunteer must show normal pre-treatment findings.

## II. Tolerance and Pharmacokinetics in the Target Population

### 1. Single-Dose Administration

Bioavailability, pharmacokinetics, and tolerance studies of a new drug must be repeated as soon as possible in apparently healthy or oligosymptomatic subjects belonging to the target population in areas where malaria is being transmitted, e.g. Latin America, Africa or Asia (WHO 1975b). The adult, healthy male volunteers are selected from among semi-immune, oligosymptomatic, healthy *P. falciparum* or *P. vivax* carriers. Such safety and bioavailability studies permit determination, at the same time, of the efficacy of a given single dose. Parasitological follow-up should be carried out to determine the dose required for radical cure, provided that the subjects are protected from reinfection in a mosquito-proof environment.

In trials with drugs possessing potential sporontocidal activity, repeated feeding of *Anopheles* mosquitoes on treated volunteers who present a high gametocytaemia, before and repeatedly after medication, would permit assessment of this property in the test compound. Indirect feeding of mosquitoes on infected blood withdrawn from the patients (e.g. through membranes) seems to give less accurate results.

### 2. Repeated Dosage

If a single dose of the new drug proves to be safe and effective, repeated administration may be undertaken. This requires complementary subacute or chronic toxicity data in two animal species. The dosage interval for repeated administration in a suppressive trial should correspond approximately to the biological half-life of the drug in man. The single doses administered would amount to about one-fourth of an effective, well-tolerated single dose. These trials should be designed whenever possible as randomised, double-blind, comparative trials versus a standard drug such as chloroquine. Good acceptability and tolerance are essential for drugs to be used prophylactically. These studies make it possible to demonstrate whether unexpectedly high accumulation or change in the t ½ occurs after repeated dosage. The steady-state pharmacokinetics of new antimalarials at different dose levels should be assessed. Six subjects should be included in each group. If results vary markedly between subjects, the number of volunteers would have to be increased.

# C. Phase II

## I. General Considerations

The aim of phase II studies will be to determine the optimal dosage required to achieve a given antimalarial response. The activity of the drug may vary depending on the geographical origin of the parasite strain.

All relevant information concerning chemistry, pharmacy, pharmacology, the completed toxicology, as well as the results of the phase I clinical trials should be summarised in the phase II Investigational Drug Brochure.

If the dosage formulation needs to be modified, the method of preparation, specification including stability data, and comparative bioavailability of the old and new formulations must be provided.

## II. Trials in Experimentally Infected Patients or Volunteers

### 1. Advantages

There are many advantages in undertaking dose-finding efficacy trials in experimentally infected subjects:

1. Such volunteers, living far from endemic areas, are non-immune, whereas naturally infected subjects usually have some degree of immunity which may influence the course of infection and enhance the antiparasitic effect of drugs.

2. As the risk of reinfection is nil in a subject living far from the endemic area, this will facilitate long-term (over 1 year) follow-up of patients with mosquito-induced *P. vivax* or *P. malariae*.

3. The parasite strains used for experimental infections have a predictable pattern of resistance to the standard antimalarials and to the test medicaments, whereas the resistance pattern of "wild," naturally acquired strains may exhibit different resistance patterns even when originating from a restricted transmission area.

4. Mixed infections which are frequently encountered in endemic areas are often difficult to detect and they represent a potential source of error. This difficulty does not occur with experimental infections.

5. Comparison of the protective activity of a compound against mosquito- and blood-induced infection can indicate whether a drug has a suppressive or a causal prophylactic activity as do, for instance proguanil or its metabolite (CONTACOS et al. 1964).

6. To test malaria vaccines, it will be necessary to study first the immunological changes in non-immunes. Vaccinated volunteers with positive antibody response may have to be challenged with repeated bites of infective mosquitos (CLYDE et al. 1973, 1975).

## 2. Trials in Neurosyphilitic Patients

Malaria therapy using various strains of *P. vivax* or *P. falciparum* was used from 1917 until the early 1970s and considered to have therapeutic value in the treatment of neurosyphilis, optic atrophy, and thromboangiitis obliterans (BRUCE-CHWATT 1967; GRIN et al. 1973; LUPASCU 1974). This technique gave an excellent opportunity for the close study of the effect of antimalarials on mosquito- and blood-induced infections. Today malaria therapy is rarely used, and trials of new drugs in such patients would be considered unethical.

## 3. Trials in Experimentally Infected Volunteers

Drug trials in hundreds of healthy volunteers deliberately infected with selected strains of *P. falciparum* or *P. vivax* were undertaken between World War II and the end of the Vietnam War, mainly in the United Kingdom, the United States, Australia, and other countries (WISELOGLE 1946; BALLIF-NEGULICI and CONSTANTINESCO 1963; BLACK et al. 1966; CANFIELD and ROZMAN 1974; ALVING and COGGESHALL 1974; UNGUREANU et al. 1976). These studies furnished "a steady flow of invaluable information on the course of malaria in the non-immune subjects and on the action of drugs against the various stages of the parasite. This information could not have been obtained in any other way" (WHO 1961).

Mosquito-induced falciparum infection is followed by a 5- to 7-day tissue phase, during which the blood is not infective. Thereafter the erythrocytic phase provokes clinical episodes. The size of the inoculum can be calculated by dissecting the salivary glands of the insects used for the experimental infection.

The tissue phase in mosquito-induced *P. vivax* infection is more prolonged. Depending on the strain, irregular fever starts between days 13 and 15 and the classical tertian type of temperature curve becomes manifest only after the 3rd week. Spontaneous relief may be expected within $1^1/_2$–2 months.

Causal prophylactic activity against *P. falciparum* still requires the involvement of volunteers deliberately infected with selected strains (POWELL and BREWER 1967).

The eradication of blood forms will not prevent relapses within a year in 60% of the cases. These are due to persisting "dormant" liver stages (hypnozoites). The incubation period is more prolonged in strains originating from temperate countries than those originating from tropical countries; the interval between relapses may vary between a few weeks and 1 year.

The response to therapy depends on the drug plasma concentration reached, the parasite species and the strains chosen, the mode of infection, the inoculum size (for instance 0.5 or 4 million blood parasites) and the number of days parasitaemia is permitted before therapy is commenced (2 or 4 days). Repeated inoculation after treatment may show the influence of certain immunity factors.

The research in the United States during World War II included clinical trials with quinine, 9-aminoacridine derivatives, 4- and 8-aminoquinolines, sulphonamides, diaminopyrimidines, and several other compounds tested in experimentally infected volunteers (WISELOGLE 1946). Other major studies were conducted in volunteers in Australia (FAIRLEY 1946).

From more than 230000 chemical compounds screened for antimalarial activity by the US Army Antimalarial Drug Development Programme between 1964 and 1974 about 30 were selected for clinical study in human volunteers (CANFIELD and ROZMAN 1974). Several promising new compounds reached phase II clinical trials; phase III was completed for mefloquine in 1983.

The dose-range finding trials in experimentally infected volunteers with compounds selected by the Walter Reed Army Institute of Research were conducted by highly qualified groups of investigators such as CONTACOS et al. (1964), CLYDE et al. (1971, 1976), ARNOLD et al. (1973), RIECKMANN et al. (1974), and TRENHOLME et al. (1975).

## III. Trials in Naturally Infected Subjects

### 1. Problems of Selection and Evaluation

How to cope with the difficulties arising from the selection of naturally infected subjects in early therapeutic trials requires special consideration.

1. Since the immune status of the patients will often be unknown, the presence of severe infections will constitute a criterion for exclusion in order to reduce the risks. Whenever possible, serological tests such as the indirect haemagglutination or immunofluorescence test should be performed prior to therapy. In the future, the radioimmunoassay or enzyme-linked immunosorbent assay (ELISA) techniques may be employed. Positive tests do not indicate the degree of protective immunity that exists in the subjects (CHIN et al. 1973; MEUWISSEN et al. 1974; AMBROISE-THOMAS 1974; WHO 1975a; MANNWEILER et al. 1976). False-positive, indirect immunofluorescence tests are encountered in only 2% of the cases (WILSON et al. 1975).

Non-immunes require higher doses than semi-immunes for the clinical cure of malaria. However, if the follow-up period of the semi-immune patients is sufficiently long, the differences measured in clinical response may be less marked where radical cure is concerned. For instance, the mefloquine dose required for the radical cure of falciparum malaria in non-immune patient volunteers and in semi-immune, naturally infected subjects, is of the same order of magnitude, i.e. a single dose of 750–1 250 mg mefloquine base for adult patients.

For greater clinical safety during early phase II therapeutic trials in falciparum malaria, the new compound can be given together with the short-term administration of quinine (MILLER et al. 1974; HALL et al. 1975a, b, 1977).

With regard to the immune status, some groups of patients living in rural endemic areas may be considered as semi-immune, while others living in towns where malaria is not transmitted may be considered as non-immunes. Trials in these two groups of patients in tropical countries may be carried out independently.

2. Mosquito-proof centres close to transmission areas may be selected for such therapeutic trials. The optimal acceptable follow-up period seems to be 63 days at this stage for *P. falciparum* infections. It should be longer for *P. vivax* if radical cure is being assessed.

3. Recent technological advances make it possible to characterise the *P. falciparum* strains isolated from patients. In vitro sensitivity tests to various antimalarials should be performed prior to therapy and especially in case of recrudescences (RIECKMANN 1971; RIECKMANN et al. 1968, 1978; WERNSDORFER 1980; WHO 1979). In cases of failure, cryopreservation and transport of the strain to specialised laboratories for further in vitro or in vivo tests in monkeys should be considered. [This procedure made possible the discovery of *P. knowlesi* in one patient by CHIN et al. (1965)].

4. The parasitologists must be experienced; parasitaemia must be assessed quantitatively and qualitatively. If possible, two separate technologists should check the blood slides independently. Should discrepancies be found, unstained preparations collected for this purpose must be re-examined and, if necessary, sent to a reference centre. The laboratory diagnosis of malaria from thin blood films and thick films has been well described by DRAPER (1971), WHO (1980) and in textbooks of parasitology.

Mixed infections can be sources of error and are difficult to eliminate. Young ring forms of *P. vivax* emerging some weeks after treatment of a *P. falciparum* infection may erroneously be described as a recrudescence of the primary infection. In naturally infected subjects from Latin America or Southeast Asia, mixed infections with *P. vivax* and *P. falciparum* are common, whereas in Africa *P. malariae* may frequently be associated with *P. falciparum*.

When treating naturally transmitted *P. vivax* infections, *P. falciparum* may also emerge when the most susceptible species, *P. vivax*, has been eliminated from the blood. This was the case, for instance, when low doses of mefloquine (250–500 mg base adult dose) were given for the clinical cure of vivax malaria in patients in whom *P. falciparum* had not been detected prior to therapy.

5. The assessment of the activity of a new drug against erythrocytic forms of naturally transmitted *P. vivax* infections necessitates the administration of an antirelapse compound known to have very few schizontocidal properties, such as primaquine, after elimination of the blood forms. In blood-induced *P. vivax* infections, relapses do not occur and the response to blood schizontocidal drugs can be better assessed.

6. Non-compliance with therapy is a further source of error in therapeutic trials. In severely ill patients vomiting or incomplete absorption of the active substance may occur. Malabsorption may be a consequence of the malarial infection itself or of an underlying disease (HERZOG et al. 1983). Abnormal handling of the drug in a subject such as a rapid acetylator phenotype or a patient with malabsorption syndrome must also be considered, especially when the isolated parasite has proved to be sensitive to the drug in vitro and in vivo.

One way of discovering such anomalies or non-compliance to the drug would be to collect urine or one or more samples of plasma in all treated patients at the beginning of the beta phase of elimination of the antimalarial, and to hold these samples, correctly labelled with the time interval between sampling and intake of the drug, frozen at −20 °C. CANFIELD et al. (1973), for example, demonstrated a correlation between poor absorption and drug failure in patients treated with new phenanthrene methanol derivatives.

7. A further difficulty in studying patients in curative trials may be the presence in the organism of antimalarials taken for prophylaxis before entering the trial. Here again, urine tests for chloroquine (e.g. HASKINS 1958), sulphonamides (RIEDER 1976) or pyrimethamine (AHMAD and ROGERS 1981) can be performed.

8. Besides genetic factors such as the rapid acetylator phenotype (GILLES and CLYDE 1974), other factors may influence the efficacy of antifols. The increased oral intake of *p*-aminobenzoic acid (PABA), for example, may suppress the antimalarial activity of dapsone in man (DEGOWIN et al. 1966). Reduced oral intake of PABA may eradicate the malaria parasites from the blood of children, e.g. on a predominantly milk diet. Drug interference or severe underlying diseases may also influence the response of patients to drugs (RAWLINS 1974).

## 2. Trial Plans

In phase II trials, the greatest attention must be paid to the trial protocol, so as to avoid risks in a potentially dangerous infection. Signs of clinical severity will be one reason for exclusion. The optimal dosage of a new compound in phase II trials is at first unknown; therefore two or more different dosage regimens are compared at this stage.

A protocol or trial plan must contain the following items:

### a) Title

The title will indicate briefly the aim of the study, the indication, the design of the trial, the drugs used and the phase.

### b) Location

The site where the trial is being undertaken must include the names of the principal investigator and of his deputy as well as the facilities to be used for the parasitological and laboratory work.

### c) Rationale

The rationale of the study will summarise the background knowledge already described in greater detail in the Investigational Drug Brochure. New publications should be quoted, and all recent information, especially on tolerance, must be given.

### d) Objectives

The objectives of the study must be precisely stated, for example, "The aim of this randomised, double-blind, comparative trial is to determine the efficacy and tolerance of a single administration of either 500 mg or 1 000 mg of mefloquine base compared with those of a standard treatment (quinine + sulfadoxine + pyrimethamine) in symptomatic, uncomplicated, falciparum malaria in semi-immune patients, living in an area where chloroquine resistant P. falciparum malaria is highly prevalent."

The main goals may include for instance, a comparison of:

1. The rapidity of clearance of asexual parasitaemia
2. The radical cure rate (eradication of asexual forms of *P. falciparum*), within a 63-day follow-up period, the patients not being exposed to reinfection
3. The speed of the clinical response in symptomatic patients, using clinical parameters listed in the enclosed record form
4. The safety and acceptability of the drugs (clinical adverse reactions and changes in the laboratory tests)

### e) Patient Selection

The criteria for patient selection must be adequate to provide results which are comparable in homogeneous groups. In malaria the age range should be narrow; adults 18–45 years, adolescents and subgroups of schoolchildren must be assessed separately. Except for children (under 12 years of age), male and female patients should also be grouped separately. The selection should take into consideration the following factors:

The immune status should be similar in all patients (epidemiological considerations or serological tests)

The severity of the disease should be of the same order, i.e. same single parasite species in the blood, similar parasite counts (e.g. asexual forms of *P. falciparum* ranging between 4 000 and 50 000/$mm^3$)

Patients with severe malaria or severe underlying diseases should be excluded.

Patients should be included in the trial, i.e. receive a trial number, only if they fulfill the above-mentioned conditions and when they have given their written or oral consent in the presence of the chief investigator or his deputy, who has provided them with all the necessary information on the drug to be utilised and the tests planned in the trial. The number of patients to be included in each group must be indicated.

### f) Exclusions

Exclusion criteria: age groups not required for the study, signs indicating a more severe prognosis such as temperature above 40 °C, fever lasting for more than 7 days, signs of meningism or encephalitis, cardiovascular involvement such as systolic blood pressure below 100 mmHg, blood dyscrasias including platelet counts below 60 000/$mm^3$, haemoglobin values below 9 g%, haemorrhagic diathesis, jaundice, severe dehydration, severe renal involvement or any severe underlying diseases or accompanying infection requiring specific treatment.

### g) Trial Design

Patients fulfilling the above conditions should be numbered according to their order of entry into the trial. The allocation to therapy must be based on the use of random tables. In double-blind (or double-dummy) trials, the antimalarials should be provided in numbered boxes containing tablets (or ampoules) of identical appearance.

The principal investigator should receive sealed, numbered, key envelopes. These must be sent back for checking together with the completed, corresponding record form. There is practically no reason to open the key in double-blind studies where the drug is administered only once, except in cases of severe adverse reaction.

### h) Treatment

The drug must be administered in the same way to all subjects. Even in double-blind trials, the dose may be adjusted depending on body weight. Precise information must be given on how and when to administer the drug, e.g. together with a given amount of water, before or after a meal. The intake of the medicament must be supervised by the principal investigator or his deputy.

### i) Parameters to be Measured

These include demographic data, clinical and parasitological findings, and diagnosis. The clinical and laboratory parameters to be assessed and the time when the tests or clinical investigation are to be performed are tabulated in the corresponding record form and/or on an attached schedule.

The parasite count must be repeated at regular 6-h intervals during the first 2 days, every 12 h up to day 6 and at weekly intervals up to the end of the trial (day 63). Early morphological changes occurring in the parasites should be noted (e.g. PICQ et al. 1972; EBISAWA et al. 1974). For subjective findings semiquantitative parameters or rating scales described in the record form should be used. Rating scales may also be employed to group objective findings such as parasite counts.

The recorded clinical data should correspond to the findings at the investigator's visit in the morning while the patient is still at rest.

Laboratory tests should usually be performed once a day, the specimen being collected before breakfast, while the patient is still at rest.

### j) Adverse Reactions

All adverse reactions encountered during the study must be reported on the case record forms. The side effects are graded on a three-point scale (mild/moderate/severe) and reported in detail, including date of onset and date of disappearance. In cases of severe adverse reactions, the monitor must be informed immediately by telephone or cable. Should unexplained abnormalities occur in laboratory tests, corroborative tests must be carried out until values have returned to normal and/or an adequate explanation is found.

In cases of severe adverse reactions, samples of 4 ml plasma should be taken and kept in a correctly labelled glass container at −20 °C. Under "Remarks," the investigator should state his opinion on the relationship between the adverse experience and the test drug. The likelihood of a relationship would be considered as remote when the adverse reaction does not follow within a reasonable space of time after administration of the drug, or if the symptoms correspond to the underlying disease. The adverse effect may be considered as drug related if it follows a reasonable temporal sequence from administration of the medicament, and if it differs from the usual symptoms of the infection. An adverse reaction may be considered as due to the drug if it cannot be explained by the clinical state of the patient, or if it follows a known pattern of response to the corresponding drug.

### k) Removing Patients from Study

Every effort must be made by the investigator to maintain the subjects in the study until the end of the follow-up period. All treated patients must be assessed, even if the follow-up is incomplete. The reasons for removing patients from the study must be clearly stated on the record forms. They may be one of the following:

1. Treatment failure:
   Occurrence of complications
   Absence of clinical improvement within 48 h
   No parasite cure within 7 days; in this case, the strain must be tested in vitro again for susceptibility to various antimalarials and, if possible, it should be sent to reference laboratories
2. Adverse reactions can be a cause of withdrawal from the trial if special treatment is required
3. Severe intercurrent illness
4. Administrative reasons:
   If the patient proves to be completely unreliable
   If the patient must leave, e.g. for family reasons

### l) Case Record Forms (Questionnaires)

These should be provided by the monitor and should enable the investigator to record all relevant information and findings including:

Demographic data, subject identification and code number
Past history, especially the duration and severity of the present episode
Clinical examination, before treatment and daily following treatment for 1 week, and body temperature and pulse rate twice daily for 1 week
Parasitological results four times daily during the first day, twice daily during the second half of the week and once a week during the 2-month observation period
Laboratory data, before and repeatedly after treatment (day 3, 6, 27)
Adverse reactions with the grade of severity, date of onset and date of disappearance
Double-checked abnormal laboratory values and date of normalisation

Completed questionnaires should be sent in batches of ten to the monitor after having been signed by the chief investigator. A copy of the patient consent forms and the corresponding sealed key envelopes should also be attached.

### m) Data Analysis

The monitor will have to check the files and laboratory work at regular intervals. He must describe the type of data processing and statistical analysis to be used, and provide the investigator with interim reports which may lead to modifications of the trial plan.

n) Publication of the Results

After completion of the study and on the basis of the results of the final evaluation and statistical analysis of the findings, the investigator and callaborators may envisage publication of the results.

The manuscript must be checked and discussed with the monitor of the trial.

The results, and especially findings concerning adverse reactions, must be communicated to the health authorities and to other investigators even if they are not to be published.

o) Ethical Considerations

After having been agreed upon and signed by the chief investigator and the monitor of the trial, the protocol must be subjected to review by the ethical committee of the relevant institution. The minimum requirements include all basic principles of the Declaration of Helsinki as revised in 1975 in Tokyo. The original wording of these principles could be attached or quoted.

Written or verbal consent is required from all patients who are willing to participate in the study after having been given adequate explanation of the trial and the potential adverse effects of the medicaments being tested.

p) Trial Plan

A copy of the trial plan must be signed and dated by the chief investigator indicating his willingness and capacity to treat within a limited period of time a given number of correctly selected patients. The monitor may accept amendments proposed by the investigator, but must also sign the revised, finalised version.

## References


Ahmad RA, Rogers HJ (1981) Salivary elimination of pyrimethamine. Br J Clin Pharmacol 11:101–102

Alving AS, Coggeshall LT (1974) Clinical testing of antimalarial drugs at Stateville Penitentiary, Malaria report 30. National Institute of Health, Washington

Ambroise-Thomas P (1974) La réaction d'immunofluorescence dans l'étude séro-immunologique du paludisme. Bull WHO 50:267–276

Arnold JD, Martin DC, Carson PE, Rieckmann KH, Willerson D Jr, Clyde DF, Miller RM (1973) A phenanthrene methanol (WR 33063) for treatment of acute malaria. Antimicrob Agents Chemother 3:207–213

Aronsson L, Bengtsson E, Björkan A, Pehrson PO, Rombo L, Wahlgren M (1981) Chloroquine-resistant falciparum malaria in Madagascar and Kenya. Ann Trop Med Parasitol 75:367–373

Ballif-Negulici E, Constantinesco P (1963) Therapeutic effects of a single dose of pyrimethamine in malaria inoculation with local or imported strains of *P. vivax* and *P. falciparum*. Arch Roum Pathol Exp Microbiol 22:997–1002

Berliner RW, Earle P Jr, Taggart JV et al. (1948) Studies on the chemotherapy of the human malarias VI. The physiological disposition, antimalarial activity, and toxicity of several derivatives of 4-aminoquinoline. J Clin Invest 27:98–107

Black RH, Dew BB, Hennessy WB, McMillan B, Torpy DC (1966) Studies on depot antimalarials: I. The effect of a single injection of the depot antimalarial CI-501 (Camolar) on relapsing vivax malaria acquired in New Guinea. Med J Aust 2:588–592

Blackwell B, Stolley PD, Buncher R, Klimt CR, Temple R, Venn D, Wardell WM (1975) Panel 4: Phase IV investigations. Clin Pharmacol Ther 18:653–656

Brohult J, Rombo L, Sirleaf V, Bengtsson E (1979) The concentration of chloroquine in serum during short- and long-term malaria prophylaxis with standard and "double" dosage in non-immunes: clinical implications. Ann Trop Med Parasitol 73:401–405
Bruce-Chwatt LJ (1967) Clinical trials of antimalarial drugs. Trans R Soc Trop Med Hyg 61:412–426
Canfield CJ, Hall AP, MacDonald BS, Neumann DA, Shaw JA (1973) Treatment of falciparum malaria from Vietnam with a phenanthrene methanol (WR 33063) and a quinoline methanol (WR 30090). Antimicrob Agents Chemother 3:224–227
Canfield CR, Rozman RS (1974) Clinical testing of new antimalarial compounds. Bull WHO 50:203–212
Chaput de Saintonge DM (1978) Klinische Prüfungen – leichter gesagt als getan. Internist (Berlin) 19:349–356
Chin W, Contacos PG, Coatney GR, Kimball HR (1965) A naturally acquired quotidian-type malaria in man transferable to monkeys. Science 149:865
Chin W, Rattanartihikul M (1973) The evaluation of the presumptive and radical treatments against falciparum malaria in Thailand. Southeast Asian J Trop Med Public Health 4:400–406
Clyde DF, Miller RM, DuPont HL, Hornick RB (1971) Antimalarial effects of tetracyclines in man. J Trop Med Hyg 74:238–242
Clyde DF, McCarthy VC, Miller RM, Hornick RB (1973) Specificity of protection of man immunized against sporozoite-induced falciparum malaria. Am J Med Sci 266:398–403
Clyde DF, McCarthy VC, Miller RM, Woodward WE (1975) Immunization of man against falciparum and vivax malaria by use of attenuated sporozoites. Am J Trop Med Hyg 4:397–401
Contacos PG, Coatney GR, Lunn JS, Kilpatrick JW (1964) The antimalarial activity of CI-501 (Camolar) against falciparum malaria. Am J Trop Med Hyg 13:386–390
Covell G, Coatney GR, Field JW, Singh I (1956) La chimiothérapie du paludisme. Monograph Series WHO 27:1–132
Degowin RL, Eppes RB, Carson PE, Powell RD (1966) The effects of diaphenyl-sulfone (DDS) against chloroquine-resistant *Plasmodium falciparum*. Bull WHO 34:671–681
Desjardins RE, Pamplin CL, Von Bredow J, Barry KG, Canfield CJ (1979) Kinetics of a new antimalarial, mefloquine. Clin Pharmacol Ther 26:372–379
Draper CC (1971) Laboratory diagnosis. Br Med J 2:93–95
Ebisawa I, Komoriya T, Kimura M, Muto T (1974) Morphological and clinical effects of pyrimethamine-sulfonamide combinations (sulformethoxine-pyrimethamine or sulfamonomethoxine-pyrimethamine) on *P. vivax* and its infection. Jpn J Exp Med 44:151–163
Food and Drug Administration (1977 a) General considerations for the clinical evaluation of drugs. US Department of Health, Education and Welfare, Washington, DC
Food and Drug Administration (1977 b) Guidelines for the clinical evaluation of anti-infective drugs (systemic adults and children) US Department of Health, Education and Welfare, Washington, DC
Food and Drug Administration (1977 c) General considerations for the clinical evaluation of drugs in infants and children. US Department of Health, Education and Welfare, Washington, DC
George CF (1974) The investigation of new drugs in man. Br J Hosp Med 780–787
Gerberg EJ (1971) Evaluation of antimalarial compounds in mosquito test systems. Trans R Soc Trop Med Hyg 65:358–363
Gilles HM, Clyde DF (1974) Acetylator phenotype in sulphonamide-resistant falciparum malaria. Ann Trop Med Parasitol 68:367–368
Goldberg LI, Besselaar GH, Arnold JD, Lemberger L, Mitchell JR, Whitset TL (1975) Panel 1: Phase I investigations. Clin Pharmacol Ther 18:643–646
Grin EI, Pirnat L, Dimitrijevic E, Simic L (1973) Thromboangiitis and results obtained by pyretotherapy using malaria. Excerpta Medica, Public Health Social Medicine and Hygiene 21:1–53
Hall AP, Doberstyn EB, Nanakorn A, Sonkom A (1975 a) Falciparum malaria semi-resistant to clindamycin. Br Med J 2:12–14

Hall AP, Doberstyn EB, Mettaprakong V, Sonkom P (1975b) Falciparum malaria cured by quinine followed by sulfadoxine-pyrimethamine. Br Med J 2:15–17
Haskins WT (1958) A simple qualitative test for chloroquine in urine. Am J Trop Med 7:199–222
Hickman RL (1969) The use of subhuman primates for experimental studies of human malaria. Milit Med 134:741–756
Jauch R, Griesser E, Oesterhelt G (1980) Metabolismus von Ro 21-5998 (Mefloquin) bei der Ratte. Arzneimittelforsch 30:60–67
Jusko WJ (1981) Smoking and drug response. Trends Pharm Int 2:10–13
Kahl GF (1978) Interaktionen von Arzneimitteln: Ein Problem bei der Therapie. Internist (Berlin) 19:366–374
Killick-Kendrick R, Peters W (1978) Rodent malaria. Academic, London, p 406
Krotoski WA, Garnham PCC, Bray RS, Krotoski DM, Killick-Kendrick R, Draper CC, Targett GAT, Guy WM (1980) The hypnozoite of *Plasmodium cynomolgi:* true latent stage in malarial relapse? 29 th Annual meeting. Am Soc Trop Med Hyg, Atlanta
Lasagna L (1975) Clinical trials of drugs from the viewpoint of the academic investigator (a satire). Clin Pharmacol Ther 18:629–633
Lasagna L (1979) The diseases and drug needs of the Third World. J Chronic Dis 32:413–414
Liss RL, Kensler CJ (1976) Advances in modern toxicology. In: Mehlman MA, Shapiro RE, Blumenthal H (eds) New concepts in safety evaluation. Hemisphere, Washington, DC, p 273
Lupascu G (1974) Applications actuelles de la malaria thérapie. Bull WHO 50:165–168
Mannweiler E, Mohr W, Felde I zum, Hinrichs A, Haas J (1976) Zur Serodiagnostik der Malaria. MMW 118:1139–1144
Merkli B, Richle R (1980) Studies on the resistance to single and combined antimalarials in the *Plasmodium berghei* mouse model. Acta Trop (Basel) 37:228–231
Merkli B, Richle R, Peters W (1980) The inhibitory effect of a drug combination on the development of mefloquine resistance in *Plasmodium berghei.* Ann Trop Med Parasitol 74:1–9
Meuwissen JHET, Leeuwenberg ADEM, Voller A, Matola Y (1974) Specificity of the indirect haemagglutination test with *Plasmodium falciparum* test cells. Bull WHO 50:513–519
Miller LH, Glew RH, Wyler DJ, Howard WA, Collins WE, Contacos PG, Neva FA (1974) Evaluation of clindamycin in combination with quinine against multidrug-resistant strains of *Plasmodium falciparum.* Am J Trop Med Hyg 23:565–569
Mu JY, Iraili ZH, Dayton PG (1975) Studies of the disposition and metabolism of mefloquine HCl (WR 142490), a quinoline-methanol antimalarial, in the rat. Drug Metab Dispos 3:198–210
Peters W (1970) Chemotherapy and drug resistance in malaria. Academic, New York
Peters W (1979) 4- and 8-Aminoquinoline, Chinin und Chinin-ähnliche Verbindungen. Hahnenklee Symposium Roche Grenzach, BRD
Picq JJ, Charmot G, Ricosse JH (1972) A comparative study between a single dose of pyrimethamine-sulfamethopyrazine compound and a single dose of chloroquine for the treatment of acute attack of *P. falciparum* malaria in "semi-immune" subjects living in an endemic area (Bobo-Dioulasso, Upper Volta). Méd Trop 32:527–546
Powell RD, Brewer GJ (1967) Effects of pyrimethamine, chlorguanide, and primaquine against exoerythrocytic forms of a strain of chloroquine-resistant *Plasmodium falciparum* from Thailand. Am J Trop Med Hyg 16:693–698
Rawlins MD (1974) Variability of response to drugs in man. Br J Hosp Med 803–811
Rieckmann KH (1971) Determination of the drug sensitivity of *Plasmodium falciparum.* JAMA 217:573–578
Rieckmann KH, McNamara JV, Frischer H, Stockert TA, Carson PE, Powell RD (1968) Effects of chloroquine, quinine, and cycloguanil upon the maturation of asexual erythrocytic forms of two strains of *Plasmodium falciparum* in vitro. Am J Trop Med Hyg 17:661–671

Rieckmann KH, Trenholme GM, Williams RL, Carson PE, Frischer H, Desjardins RE (1974) Prophylactic activity of mefloquine hydrochloride (WR 142490) in drug-resistant malaria. Bull WHO 51:375–377
Rieder J (1976) The simultaneous quantitative determination of total, "active," acetylated and conjugated sulfonamide in biological fluids. Chemotherapy 22:84–87
Rozman RS, Molek NA, Koby R (1978) The absorption, distribution, and excretion in mice of the antimalarial mefloquine, erythro-2,8-bis(trifluoromethyl)-α-(2-piperidyl)-4-quinoline-methanol hydrochloride. Drug Metab Dispos 6:654–658
Schwartz DE (1980) Quantitative determination of the antimalarial drug mefloquine and of its main metabolite in plasma by direct densitometric measurement on TLC plates. In: Frigerio, McCamish (eds) Recent developments in chromatography and electrophoresis, vol 10. Elsevier, Amsterdam, pp 69–74
Schwartz DE, Weber W, Richard-Lenoble D, Gentillini M (1980) Kinetic studies of mefloquine and one of its metabolites, Ro 21-5104, in the dog and in man. Acta Trop (Basel) 37:238–242
Schwartz DE, Eckert G, Hartmann D, Weber B, Richard-Lenoble D, Ekue JMK, Gentilini M (1982) Single-dose kinetics of mefloquine in man. Plasma levels of the unchanged drug and of one of its metabolites. Chemotherapy 28:70–84
Smith CC, Weigel WW, Wolfe GF (1973) Excretion and tissue localization patterns of experimental antimalarial agents. Fed Proc 32:701
Staiger MA, Nguyen-Dinh P, Churchill C (1981) Sensitive high-performance liquid chromatographic analysis for chloroquine in body fluids. Application to studies of drug resistance in *Plasmodium falciparum*. J Chromatogr 225:139–149
Trenholme GM, Williams RL, Desjardins RE, Frischer H, Carson PE, Rieckmann KH, Canfield CJ (1975) Mefloquine (WR 142490) in the treatment of human malaria. Science 190:792–794
Ungureanu E, Killick-Kendrick R, Garnham PCC, Branzei P, Romanescu C, Shute PG (1976) Prepatent periods of a tropical strain of *Plasmodium vivax* after inoculations of tenfold dilutions of sporozoites. Trans R Soc Trop Med Hyg 70:482–483
Wernsdorfer WH (1980) Field evaluation of drug resistance in malaria. In vitro micro-test. Acta Trop (Basel) 37:222–227
WHO (1961) Chemotherapy of malaria. WHO Tech Rep Ser 226
WHO (1968) WHO expert committee on malaria. 14th Report. Tech Rep Ser 382
WHO (1973) Chemotherapy of malaria and resistance to antimalarials. WHO Tech Rep Ser 529
WHO (1974) Symposium on Malaria Research. Bull WHO 50:1–372
WHO (1975a) Developments in malaria immunology. WHO Tech Rep Ser 579
WHO (1975b) Guidelines for evaluation of drugs for use in man. WHO Tech Rep Ser 563
WHO (1977) USAID/WHO Workshops on the biology and in vitro cultivation of malaria parasites. Bull WHO 55, n. 2–3:121–429
WHO (1979) Instruction for the use of the WHO Test Kit for the assessment of the response of *Plasmodium falciparum* to chloroquine. WHO Document MAP/79.1
WHO (1980) The clinical management of acute malaria. WHO Reg Publ SE Asia Ser 9
Wilson M, Fife EH Jr, Methews HM, Sulzer AJ (1975) Comparison of the complement fixation, indirect immunofluorescence, and indirect hemagglutination tests for malaria. Am J Trop Med Hyg 24:755–759
Wiselogle FY (1946) A survey of antimalarial drugs 1941–1945. Edwards, Ann Arbor

CHAPTER 14

# Clinical Trials – Phases III and IV and Field Trials

M. FERNEX

## A. Phase III

### I. Objective and Design of the Studies

Well-tolerated and effective dosages of a new antimalarial in a number of precise indications will have been defined during phase II. Phase III clinical trials are required to confirm that the drug is effective and safe when it is administered to all patients, including children, infants, women during pregnancy, and severely ill patients who may be semi-immunes or non-immunes, as well as patients with associated diseases requiring concomitant medication (drug interaction studies).

These studies can only be initiated when the finalised dosage forms and the statutory toxicological data, including chronic toxicity and reproductive studies, are available. Complementary information on pharmacokinetics in special conditions – younger age, subjects with impaired renal or liver function, the bioavailability of the drug in malnourished subjects – needs to be investigated early in phase III.

Although the design of phase III trials will not differ basically from that of phase II, it may be simplified. The follow-up period may be reduced to 28 days and the list of laboratory tests may be considerably shortened.

Since at each stage of the studies, comparative groups should be included, the trials will usually be designed as randomised, prospective, comparative studies. It is essential that the two treatment groups be as equal as possible with regard to severity of the disease or concomitant medications prescribed.

Specific antimalarial drug trials in phase III will *not* involve the assessment of the value of concomitant, symptomatic therapy. If associated drugs do have to be administered in severe cases, the choice of medicaments and dosages should be identical in the two treatment groups.

When considering the objective nature of the measurable findings in an antimalarial trial, e.g. the asexual parasite count and body temperature, it might be suggested that a double-blind study would be superfluous. However, one must also consider that the clinical and subjective improvement of the patient has to be assessed in severe cases. For instance, after three infusions of quinine at 8-h intervals, the improvement is often marked. Patients receiving only tablets but no infusions may subjectively be assessed less optimistically by the investigator. Using a double-blind design, this source of error will be avoided. Furthermore, the evaluation of subjective adverse reactions or minor adverse reactions may be easier to compare. Transient erythema, for example, will not be judged in the same way if one patient has taken, for example, sulphonamides or chloroquine. In the first case, the investigator might interrupt the treatment, and in the other he might continue and perhaps consider the skin reaction to be a consequence of the disease, rather than an adverse reaction to the drug. Double-blind trial design will prevent such discrepancies.

The need to use commercial brand drugs such as quinine or Fansidar, in combinations or for the control group, necessitates the use of a rather complicated double-dummy test system; each drug has to have its placebo counterpart. For example, group 1 receives four tablets of mefloquine containing 250 mg base and six vials for infusion containing quinine-placebo plus three tablets of Fansidar-placebo; group 2 receives six vials containing quinine corresponding to 650 mg dihydrochloride for 8-h infusions and three tablets of commercially available Fansidar (each tablet containing 500 mg sulfadoxine and 25 mg pyrimethamine) plus four tablets of mefloquine placebo.

## II. Selection of Patients and Risk Factors

### 1. Infants and Children

During studies in children, risks should be avoided as far as possible. The optimal existing treatment schedule will be taken as standard for the control group (JELIFFE 1966). Infants may be included in the trials only if favourable results have already been obtained in adults and children. The FDA (1977c) summarises the special problems of paediatric drug therapy and indicates that the investigator and the review board must ensure that any risks involved are minimal, and that the research is scientifically sound and significant. It must be stressed that children have the greatest need for better, safe and well-acceptable antimalarials as they represent the most vulnerable group with the highest morbidity and mortality. "The rights of the child to receive treatment with adequately tested drugs must not be abridged" (MIRKIN et al. 1975).

### 2. Genetic Blood Dyscrasias

During phase III, pilot tolerance studies may be conducted among subjects with genetic anomalies of the red blood cells (G6PD deficiency, thalassaemia, sickle cell anaemia, and other haemoglobinopathies), if competent haematologists are available to undertake the required controls. Subjects suffering from such anomalies may be less susceptible to malarial infection (REY et al. 1967) and, therefore, these genetic factors must be checked in patients who are included in comparative trials.

### 3. Pregnancy

The deleterious role of malaria on the outcome of pregnancy has been well established, and pregnant patients have a significant decrease in their resistance to malaria parasites (KORTMANN 1973; MACGREGOR and AVERY 1974). Unfortunately, in some areas of Southeast Asia and Brazil, *P. falciparum* now responds neither to 4-aminoquinoline derivatives nor to antifol combinations. Even prolonged treatment with quinine may not eliminate the asexual forms and there is an increase of RII resistance to the standard quinine treatment, especially in foci surrounding

Kampuchea (FERNEX 1981). It is therefore ethically acceptable, and indeed even compulsory and scientifically justified, to administer new life-saving drugs which may protect the fetus or the baby, as well as the mother, in controlled studies during any stage of pregnancy in such areas. It would, in fact, even be difficult to include any control group if, in a restricted area, only quinine + tetracycline combination therapy remained effective, since these two compounds are contraindicated during pregnancy. Accurate follow-up of the pregnancy and of the baby is, of course, essential in such cases (FLYNT and HAY 1979).

#### 4. Non-Immunes

In non-immunes the prognosis of falciparum malaria may be serious. The prognosis depends on the level of the parasitaemia, the duration of the symptoms and the degree of involvement of the central nervous or cardiovascular system, and of the kidney or liver parenchyma (WHO 1980).

### III. Special Tests Required

#### 1. Absorption

In severe falciparum malaria failure may be due to poor absorption of the drug due to the disease itself or due to an underlying condition (KARNEY and TONG 1972; CANFIELD et al. 1973). The pharmacokinetics of antimalarials might also be altered by hyperthermia (TRENHOLME et al. 1975) and, as a consequence, the toxicity of the drug may be enhanced. Therefore the pharmacokinetics of antimalarials should also be studied in severely ill patients.

Plasma samples should be taken to determine the concentration of the drug in case of treatment failure, or when severe adverse reactions occur. Even when the drug is taken in the presence of the chief investigator, it may be useful to measure the concentration of compound in the urine, both prior to therapy (as already mentioned, to determine if antimalarials were taken previously), and after treatment to ensure that the drug has actually been taken. Qualitative methods have been described for determining the presence of chloroquine or of sulphonamides in the urine (e.g. HASKINS 1958; RIEDER 1976). Recently, AHMAD and ROGERS (1981) have described a rather precise method for the evaluation of pyrimethamine in the saliva which reflects quite accurately the plasma concentration.

#### 2. Drug Susceptibility Tests

The sensitivity of the parasites to standard drugs should be assessed if possible. In vitro methods have been standardised and WHO can provide investigators with simplified test kits (RIECKMANN 1971; RIECKMANN et al. 1978; WHO 1979; WERNSDORFER 1980).

#### 3. Immunity

The immune status of the patients should be assessed in such studies. The immunofluorescence test usually gives high titres earlier than the indirect haemagglutination test. In non-immune subjects or those taking chemoprophylaxis, these tests can indicate whether the malaria episode really is the first attack.

Examples of comparative phase III drug trials in chloroquine-resistant falciparum malaria have been published, for instance, by BARTELLONI et al. (1967); HARINASUTA et al. (1967); PICQ et al. (1972); CHIN et al. (1973a); HALL et al. (1975, 1977); HALL (1974, 1976).

Trials with well-established drugs but tested in a new indication, e.g. antibiotics in chloroquine-resistant falciparum malaria are also regarded as phase III trials (COLWELL et al. 1972a, b; WALKER et al. 1969; MILLER et al. 1974).

No fundamental differences exist between phase III and IV clinical studies except as regards the stage of registration of the compound.

## B. Phase IV

Drug trials undertaken after registration of a drug, especially when it achieves widespread clinical use, may be defined as phase IV trials (BLACKWELL et al. 1975).

### I. Safety Studies

Complementary evaluation of safety and research into rare adverse reactions represent important goals for such studies which should be undertaken in all ethnic groups in which the compound is to be employed. EBISAWA and MUTO (1972), for instance, compared the tolerance of antimalarials in Laotian and in Japanese subjects.

The adverse reactions that may occur with quinine, for example, are still being investigated to determine the mechanisms responsible for severe haemolysis. Prevention and treatment of such complications still need to be improved (BENNETT and DESFORGES 1967). CANFIELD et al. (1968) studied erythrokinetics following the treatment of falciparum malaria with pyrimethamine. This antifol did not show any significant adverse influence on recovery from anaemia in patients treated for malaria.

### II. Pharmacokinetics

Even studies that are considered essential already in the early phases of drug development may need to be undertaken many years after its introduction if such data are still missing. For example, BROOKS et al. (1969), COLWELL et al. (1972c) HALL (1972, 1974), and SEGAL et al. (1974) have studied the safety and bioavailability of quinine, a drug which was introduced more than a century earlier. The pharmacokinetics of 8-aminoquinolines, first developed in 1925, and especially those of the newer derivative primaquine were not investigated until the late 1970s under the auspices of the WHO TDR programme. The active and/or toxic metabolites remain to be discovered. The pharmacokinetics of pyrimethamine are also still being studied after 20 years. Better methods for the analysis of the unchanged compounds and their metabolites are only now being developed.

### III. Efficacy Studies

When drug resistance is suspected in a given area, controlled trials are required to compare the standard treatment schedule with various new drug regimens, in order to find an optimal dosage, or the best drug combination for the current treatment of malaria. This has been the aim of many recent phase IV studies involving volunteers experimentally infected with strains from various tropical areas (HARINASUTA et al. 1965; CHIN et al. 1973b; CLYDE et al. 1973; COLLINS et al. 1973; CONTACOS et al. 1973; DENNIS et al. 1974; CLYDE and MCCARTHY 1977).

## IV. Symptomatic Treatment of Malaria

The assessment of the value of symptomatic treatment, besides the specific treatment of falciparum malaria, will have to be studied in phase IV when the optimal schizontocidal treatment schedule has already been established.

Resorting to exchange transfusion (KURATHONG et al. 1979) in cases with extremely high parasitaemia may be considered justified in isolated cases with no comparative studies being required. The necessity to give blood transfusions or packed cells to patients with severe anaemia may be accepted as routine procedure, but the time of survival of transfused erythrocytes should be carefully studied in patients with increased haemolysis.

Acute renal failure is a common complication of severe malaria. Haemodialysis or peritoneal dialysis may be compared when such complications occur (CANFIELD et al. 1968). It has been suggested that corticosteroids and especially dexamethasone may improve the clinical situation in cerebral malaria due to the reduction of cerebral edema (WOODRUFF and DICKINSON 1968; EALES 1974). Due to the price and risk of such compounds it would be worthwhile to demonstrate whether they really are more effective than aspirin or even placebo. Hydergine has also been used for the symptomatic treatment of cerebral malaria (DIOP MAR and SOW 1973). Controlled studies would be justified to find the optimal drug to be associated in the treatment of cerebral malaria. Anticonvulsant drugs such as phenobarbitone or diazepam are being prescribed in malaria, especially for children. However, a careful follow-up of such patients with encephalitis or febrile convulsions should be undertaken (MORLEY 1971; NATIONAL INSTITUTE OF HEALTH CONSENSUS STATEMENT 1980).

Parenteral fluid and electrolyte replacement (without giving an excess), low molecular weight dextran and diuretics are sometimes also prescribed for such conditions (SMITSKAMP and WOLTHOIS 1971; MITCHELL 1974; VACHON et al. 1974). The disseminated intravascular coagulation syndrome associated with a decrease of the level of circulating platelets and of coagulation factors such as fibrinogen is a complication requiring heparin therapy (VACHON et al. 1974; ARMENGAUD et al. 1975).

For all these forms of symptomatic treatment precise data regarding drug interaction and their real value are still being collected, this being the objective of phase IV trials.

Other complications of malaria, such as the nephrotic syndrome associated with *P. malariae* infections, are treated specifically and with various immunosuppressant drugs (KIBUKAMUSOKE 1968; ADENIJI et al. 1970; WOLFENSBERGER 1972).

## V. Conclusion

Controlled clinical trials in phase IV must be based on strict, scientifically sound plans. Ethical considerations at this stage must be as respected as in any other clinical study. Concomitant symptomatic therapy should be investigated only when the specific treatment regimen has been well established.

## C. Field Trials

### I. Introduction and Objectives

Field trials are required for the evaluation of blood schizontocidal- and sometimes also of sporontocidal compounds in naturally infected, most often partially immune groups, living in endemic areas (WHO 1973). Since it is becoming increasingly difficult to infect volunteers with *P. vivax* and *P. falciparum* deliberately, and it is considered essential to test the tolerance of an antimalarial in populations living in areas where malaria is transmitted, the importance of field trials is increasing.

Field trials must be considered independently of the four above-mentioned clinical trial phases. Pilot field trials may be begun during phase II, and extended field trials usually take place during phases III or IV. Field trials are planned studies not confined to modern clinics with continuous close medical surveillance. Suppressive treatment of groups of subjects in field conditions or curative treatment in less sophisticated centres, such as malaria clinics in conditions resembling those found in other rural hospitals, provides an opportunity for careful study of a drug in a larger number of subjects.

The objectives of pilot field trials were summarised in the report of the first Technical Meeting on Chemotherapy of Malaria (WHO 1961) and are to establish:

1. Optimum dosage and regimen
2. Further evidence of side effects
3. Evidence of possible resistance and cross-resistance
4. Acceptability of the drug to the population

Extended field trials represent an attempt to observe the consequences of mass drug administration in a given population (BRUCE-CHWATT 1967). Their objectives are the following:

1. To confirm the antiparasitic property of the drug and to compare its activity with that of a well-established standard antimalarial
2. To assess the acceptability and tolerance in a larger group of population, special attention being paid to discovering possible rare or delayed adverse reactions
3. To determine whether some strains of plasmodia are resistant to the drug (in such cases in vitro sensitivity testing would be indicated)
4. To evaluate the effect of mass drug administration on the degree of transmission in the area. This is possible when all groups of the population (including infants and pregnant women) can be treated. This will rarely be the case before the end of phase III or the registration of the drug (i.e. in phase IV). Such extended field trials may provide basic operational data for planning large-scale chemotherapeutic measures (BRUCE-CHWATT 1967).

### II. Design and Selection of Participants

Fewer than 200 selected subjects participate in pilot field trials, whereas in extended field trials often more than 1 000 subjects are involved. At the end of phase

III, the selection criteria for the participants will become less stringent. Phase IV studies may be conducted in all types of subjects, including infants and pregnant women, unless contraindicated in any particular group. BRUCE-CHWATT (1951), CLYDE (1961), and MCGREGOR et al. (1966) were pioneers in conducting such trials.

As field trials will always be prospective, randomised comparative trials versus a standard antimalarial, the groups to be compared will have to be very similar from the parasitological, epidemiological, and immunological points of view. Therefore, in holoendemic areas, children from 5 to 15 years represent a homogeneous group with high parasite density and mild symptomatology, splenomegaly, and anaemia. Malaria attacks occur mainly during the rainy season when the transmission rate is the highest. For these children suppressive treatment is beneficial. Therefore, local authorities, parents, teachers and children themselves will support the idea of cooperating in such a trial. BRUCE-CHWATT (1967) insists upon the importance of having "the full understanding and cooperation of the community. The success of such a trial depends on the goodwill of the whole population and must be carried out with every consideration for local customs and modes."

The inclusion of non-immune subjects is essential to determine the dosage schedule to be used in travellers entering the endemic area. However, there are only few papers dealing with such trials. Army personnel transferred from a non-malarious area into an endemic area represent a relatively homogeneous group of non-immunes which is easy to supervise.

EBISAWA et al. (1971) treated large numbers of non-immune Japanese workers in Laos using different treatment schedules for malaria prophylaxis. This was an excellent opportunity to assess the efficacy of a new drug (sulfadoxine + pyrimethamine) in an area where *P. falciparum* had proved to be highly resistant to chloroquine. It is interesting to note that protection of non-immunes and semi-immune subjects requires approximately the same dosage (EBISAWA et al. 1971; PEARLMAN et al. 1977, 1980).

## III. Extended Field Trials

Under the auspices of the Walter Reed Army Institute of Research, field trials of a very high standard were conducted in Thailand in a valley close to the Kampuchean border during the 1970 s.

Excellent logistic support, with participation of physicians, epidemiologists, well-trained nurses, and technicians with transport facilities, and well-equipped field laboratories, was available and must be considered as a prerequisite. One or 2 years before drug administration longitudinal malaria studies in the corresponding area were completed (SEGAL et al. 1974).

The population which participated in these trials lived in four villages. The eligible villagers were children over 10 years of age and adults, excluding women of child-bearing age (15–44 years). After having been informed in detail about the planned study and the drugs to be tested – including the use of a placebo in one group – the subjects had the opportunity to sign a consent form. They were then placed in the study pool (600–1 000 subjects) and divided at random into different treatment groups of about 200 subjects each.

Only a limited number of parameters should be measured in field trials, the most important being the asexual parasite and gametocyte count. The parasite clearance time requires 12-h or daily counts for 7 days in curative treatment. Blood slides must be examined at weekly intervals up to the 4th week; more prolonged examinations up to the 8th week of therapy would be required when long-acting drugs, such as mefloquine, are being used, in order to assess the radical cure rate, in cases where there is no risk of reinfection.

The viability of gametocytes can be checked to determine whether the drug has sporontocidal properties. Locally bred mosquitos can be used for this purpose.

In suppressive treatment, parasitaemia will be examined at 1- or 2-week intervals. After completion of drug administration, the follow-up of parasitaemia will indicate the duration of protection after different treatment schedules as well as the actual risk of reinfection.

Some laboratory tests may be performed if accurate techniques are available, e.g. microhaematocrits, red and white blood cell counts and urinalysis. The size of the spleen and the body weight may also be recorded. Analysis of urine samples can be carried out to check whether the drug has actually been taken. As it is essential to know whether any adverse reaction or any intercurrent disease occurred during prolonged suppressive treatment, medical examinations are required at regular intervals.

The drug trials were designed as prospective, randomised double-blind comparative studies. Demographic and parasitological findings were analysed statistically before and at the end of the study to verify comparability of the groups (same age and sex distribution, same incidence of risk factors, same initial parasitaemia, etc.).

The suppressive treatment lasted for 26 weeks, each study subject being visited weekly at his home on a prearranged day. The drug was always taken under the supervision of a technician. Besides weekly parasitological tests, haematological and immunological parameters were checked to assess safety. All participants were again examined 1, 3, and 15 weeks after the end of the suppressive treatment.

The blood slides were examined independently by three technicians. When discrepancy between the findings occurred, the slides were sent to and examined by the principal investigator for examination.

The results of 6 months of chemosuppression were analysed separately for *P. falciparum* and *P. vivax*. The protection provided by the different drug regimens was statistically compared. The new drug mefloquine given at weekly or 2-weekly intervals was the most active drug in preventing vivax parasitaemia and falciparum parasitaemia. Figure 1 summarises the results of the last trial by PEARLMAN et al. (1980).

Sulfadoxine-pyrimethamine (500 mg + 25 mg respectively) once weekly was the most effective commercially available drug in preventing falciparum malaria in this area where chloroquine-resistant malaria is highly prevalent. Mefloquine was significantly more active than this standard drug in preventing falciparum and vivax parasitaemia.

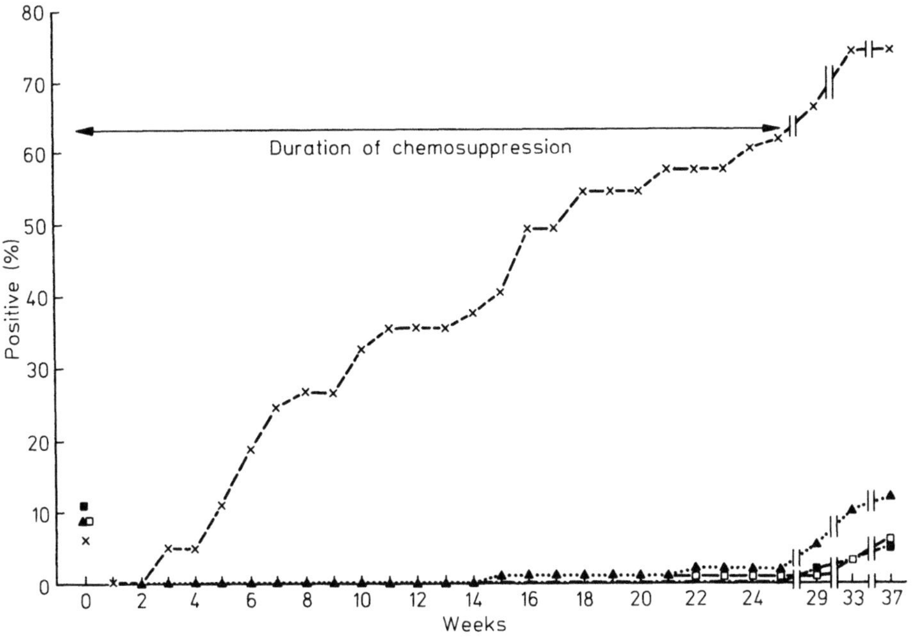


**Fig. 1.** Cumulative proportion of subjects with *P. falciparum* parasitaemias in four treatment groups. ▲® sulfadoxine (500 mg), pyrimethamine (25 mg) weekly; □, mefloquine (180 mg) weekly; ■, mefloquine (360 mg) biweekly; x, placebo. After PEARLMAN et al. (1980)

Papers on several trials performed by this group are worth studying before planning future field trials (SEGAL et al. 1973, 1974, 1975; PEARLMAN et al. 1975, 1977, 1980).

## IV. Conclusion

Once a new compound has completed the first three phases of clinical trials and enters phase IV it becomes necessary to design and conduct trials in communities within endemic areas, rather than in individuals. The detailed planning of clinical trials on a larger scale, often called "field trials," is beyond the scope of this book, but should be considered within the context of phase IV. There is some diversity of opinion as to whether field trials can be commenced prior to the registration of a new drug in a given country, or whether such trials must await this phase of a drug's development. Practical considerations, such as the availability of alternative compounds, for example, must obviously be taken into account. In certain countries where multiple drug-resistant falciparum malaria is prevalent, considerable pressure may be exerted on those responsible for the trials of a new compound (e.g. mefloquine) to release it prematurely for use in a greater number of people at risk or actually infected. While there may well be a case for initiating *carefully controlled* field trials under such circumstances, it would be mistaken policy to permit the compound to be widely disseminated until the information sought in phases I–III is as complete as possible.

## References

Adeniyi A, Hendrickse RG, Houba V (1970) Selectivity of proteinuria and response to prednisolone or immunosuppressive drugs in children with malarial nephrosis. Trop Dis Bull 67:27

Ahmad RA, Rogers HJ (1981) Salivary elimination of pyrimethamine. Br J Clin Pharmacol 11:101–102

Armengaud M, Auvergnat JC, Bonen B, Baraoat G, Cujus G (1975) Paludisme pernicieux et coagulopathie de consommation. Médecine d'Afrique Noire 22:363–367

Bartelloni PJ, Sheehy TW, Tigertt WD (1967) Combined therapy for chloroquine-resistant *Plasmodium falciparum* infection. Concurrent use of long-acting sulphormethoxine and pyrimethamine. JAMA 199:173–177

Bennett JM, Desforges JF (1967) Quinine-induced haemolysis: mechanism of action. Br J Haematol 13:706–712

Blackwell B, Stolley PD, Buncher R, Klimt CR, Temple R, Venn D, Wardell WM (1975) Panel 4: Phase IV investigations. Clin Pharmacol Ther 18:653–656

Brooks MH, Malloy JP, Bartelloni PJ, Sheehy TW, Barry KG (1969) Quinine pyrimethamine and sulphorthodimethoxine: Clinical response, plasma levels, and urinary excretion during initial attack of naturally acquired falciparum malaria. Clin Pharmacol Ther 10:85–91

Bruce-Chwatt LJ (1951) Evaluation of synthetic anti-malarial drugs in children from a hyperendemic area in West Africa. Trans R Soc Trop Med Hyg 44:563–592

Bruce-Chwatt LJ (1967) Clinical trials of antimalarial drugs. Trans R Soc Trop Med Hyg 61:412–426

Canfield CJ, Miller LH, Bartelloni PJ, Eichler P, Barry KG (1968) Acute renal failure in *Plasmodium falciparum* malaria. Treatment by peritoneal dialysis. Arch Intern Med 122:199–203

Canfield CJ, Hall AP, MacDonald BS, Neumann DA, Shaw JA (1973) Treatment of falciparum malaria from Vietnam with a phenanthrene methanol (WR 33063) and a quinoline methanol (WR 30090). Antimicrob Agents Chemother 3:224–227

Canfield CR, Rozman RS (1974) Clinical testing of new antimalarial compounds. Bull WHO 50:203–212

Chin W, Bear DM, Colwell CJ, Kosakal S (1973a) A comparative evaluation of sulfalene-trimethoprim and sulphormethoxine-pyrimethamine against falciparum malaria in Thailand. Am J Trop Med Hyg 22:308–312

Chin W, Rattarnarithikul M (1973b) The evaluation of the presumptive and radical treatments against falciparum malaria in Thailand. Asian J Trop Med Public Health 4:400–406

Clyde DF (1961) Chloroquine treatment for malaria in semi-immune patients. Am J Trop Med Hyg 10:1

Clyde DF, McCarthy VC (1977) Radical cure of Chesson-strain vivax malaria in man by 7, not 14, days of treatment with primaquine. Am J Trop Med Hyg 26:562–563

Clyde DF, McCarthy VC, Miller RM, Hornick RB (1973) Specificity of protection of man immunized against sporozoite-induced falciparum malaria. Am J Med Sci 266:398–403

Collins WE, Contacos PG, Chin W (1973) Experimental infection in man with *Plasmodium malariae*. Am J Trop Med Hyg 22:685–692

Colwell EJ, Hickman RL, Intraprasert R, Tirabutana C (1972a) Minocycline and tetracycline treatment of acute falciparum malaria in Thailand. Am J Trop Med Hyg 21:144–149

Colwell EJ, Hickman RL, Kosakal S (1972b) Tetracycline treatment of chloroquine-resistant falciparum malaria in Thailand. JAMA 220:684–686

Colwell EJ, Neoypatimanondh S, Saduddee N (1972c) Investigations of the quinine sensitivity of *Plasmodium falciparum* in central Thailand. Southeast Asian J Trop Med Public Health 3:496–500

Contacos PG, Coatney GR, Collins WE, Briesch PE, Jeter MH (1973) Five-day primaquine therapy – an evaluation of radical curative activity against vivax malaria infection. Am J Trop Med Hyg 22:693–695

Dennis DT, Doberstyn EB, Sissay A, Tesfai GK (1974) Chloroquine tolerance of Ethiopian strains of *P. falciparum*. Trans R Soc Trop Med Hyg 68:241–245
Diop Mar I, Sow A (1973) Treatment of cerebral malaria with Fansidar and Hydergin. Bulletin de la Société Médicale d'Afrique Noire de Langue Française 18:357–366
Eales L (1974) Acute falciparum malaria. Complications and treatment. S Afr Med J 48:1386–1389
Ebisawa I, Muto T (1972) Malaria in Laos. III. Primaquine sensitivity of the Laotians and the Japanese. Jpn J Exp Med 42:415–417
Ebisawa I, Muto T, Mitsui G (1971) Treatment and suppression of malaria with combined folic inhibitors (pyrimethamine with sulformethoxine or sulfamonomethoxine) in Laos. Symposium on Chemotherapy, Bangkok, 26.–30.10.1971
Fernex M (1981) The need to develop new antimalarials. Praxis (Bern) 70:1025–1032
Flynt JW, Hay S (1979) International clearinghouse for birth defects monitoring systems. Contr Epidem Biostatist 1:44–52
Food and Drug Administration (1977) General considerations for the clinical evaluation of drugs in infants and children. US Department of Health, Education and Welfare, Washington, DC
Hall AP (1972) Quinine infusion of recrudescences of falciparum malaria in Vietnam: a controlled study. Am J Trop Med Hyg 21:851–856
Hall AP (1974) Quinine fever in falciparum malaria. Southeast Asian J Trop Med Public Health 5:413–416
Hall AP (1976) The treatment of malaria. Br Med J 1:323–328
Hall AP, Doberstyn EB, Nanakorn A, Sonkom A (1975) Falciparum malaria semi-resistant to clindamycin. Br Med J 2:12–14
Hall AP, Doberstyn EB, Karnchanachetanee C, Samransamruajkit S, Laixuthal B, Pearlman EJ, Lampe RM, Miller CF, Phintuyothin P (1977) Sequential treatment with quinine and mefloquine or quinine and pyrimethamine-sulfadoxine for falciparum malaria. Br Med J 1:1626–1628
Harinasuta T, Suntharasamai P, Viravan C (1965) Chloroquine-resistant falciparum malaria in Thailand. Lancet II:657–660
Harinasuta T, Viravan C, Reid HA (1967) Sulphormethoxine in chloroquine-resistant falciparum malaria in Thailand. Lancet I:1117–1119
Jelliffe DB (1966) The therapy of cerebral malaria in children. J Pediatr 69:483–484
Karney WW, Tong MJ (1972) Malabsorption in *Plasmodium falciparum* malaria. Am J Trop Med Hyg 21:1–5
Kibukamusoke JW (1968) Malaria prophylaxis and immuno-suppressant therapy in management of nephrotic syndrome associated with quartan malaria. Arch Dis Child 43:598–600
Kortmann HFCM (1973) Malaria and pregnancy. Trop Dis Bull 70:607–609
Kurathong S, Srichaikul T, Isarangkura P, Phanichphant S (1979) Exchange transfusion in cerebral malaria complicated by disseminated intravascular coagulation. Southeast Asian J Trop Med Public Health 10:389–392
MacGregor JD, Avery JG (1974) Malaria transmission and fetal growth. Br Med J 3:433–439
McGregor IA, William K, Walker GH, Rahman AK (1966) Cycloguanil pamoate in the treatment and suppression of malaria in the Gambia, West Africa. Br Med J 1:695–701
Miller LH, Glew RH, Wyler DJ, Howard WA, Collins WE, Contacos PG, Neva FA (1974) Evaluation of clindamycin in combination with quinine against multidrug-resistant strains of *Plasmodium falciparum*. Am J Trop Med Hyg 23:565–569
Mirkin BL, Done AK, Christensen CN, Cohen SN, Howie VM, Lockhart JD (1975) Panel on pediatric trials. Clin Pharmacol Ther 18:657–658
Mitchell AD (1974) Recent experiences with severe and cerebral malaria. S Afr Med J 48:1353–1354
Morley D (1971) Malaria in childhood. Trop Doct 1:159–161
National Institutes of Health Consensus Statement (1980) Febrile seizures: long-term management of children with fever-associated seizures. Br Med J 281:277–279

Pearlman EJ, Thiemanun W, Castaneda BF (1975) Chemosuppressive field trials in Thailand. II. The suppression of *Plasmodium falciparum* and *Plasmodium vivax* parasitemias by a diformyldapsone-pyrimethamine combination. Am J Trop Med Hyg 24:901–909

Pearlman EJ, Lampe RM, Thiemanun W, Kennedy RS (1977) Chemosuppressive field trials in Thailand. III. The suppression of *Plasmodium falciparum* and *Plasmodium vivax* parasitemias by a sulfadoxine-pyrimethamine combination. Am J Trop Med Hyg 26:1108–1115

Pearlman EJ, Doberstyn EG, Sudsok S, Thiemanun W, Kennedy R, Canfield CJ (1980) Chemosuppressive field trials with mefloquine in Thailand. Am J Trop Med Hyg 29:1131–1137

Picq JJ, Charmot G, Ricosse JH (1972) A comparative study between a single dose of pyrimethamine-sulfametopyrazine compound and a single dose of chloroquine for the treatment of acute attack of *P. falciparum* malaria in "semi-immune" subjects living in an endemic area (Bobo-Dioulasso, Upper Volta). Méd Trop (mars) 32:527–546

Rey M, Oudart JL, Diop Mar I, Nouhouayi A, Camerlynck P (1967) Erythrocytopathies héréditaires et paludisme. Médecine d'Afrique Noire 14:253–255

Rieckmann KH (1971) Determination of the drug sensitivity of *Plasmodium falciparum*. JAMA 217:573–578

Rieckmann KH, Campbell GH, Sax CJ, Mrema JE (1978) Drug sensitivity of *Plasmodium falciparum*. An in vitro microtechnique. Lancet I:22–23

Rieder J (1976) The simultaneous quantitative determination of total, "active," acetylated, and conjugated sulfonamide in biological fluids. Chemotherapy 22:84–87

Segal HE, Pearlman EJ, Thiemanun W, Castaneda BF, Ames CW (1973) The suppression of *Plasmodium falciparum* and *Plasmodium vivax* parasitemias by a dapsone-pyrimethamine combination. J Trop Med Hyg 76:285–290

Segal HE, Hall AP, Jewell JS, Pearlman EJ, Na-Nakorn A, Mettaprakong V (1974) Gastrointestinal function, quinine absorption, and parasite response in falciparum malaria. Southeast Asian J Trop Med Public Health 5:499–503

Segal HE, Gresso WE, Thiemanun W (1975) Longitudinal malaria studies in rural northeast Thailand. Chloroquine treatment of falciparum malaria infections. Trop Geogr Med 27:160–164

Smitskamp H, Wolthuis FH (1971) New concepts in treatment of malignant tertian malaria with cerebral involvement. Br Med J 1:714–716

Trenholme GM, Williams RL, Desjardins RE, Frischer H, Carson PE, Rieckmann KH, Canfield CJ (1975) Mefloquine (WR 142490) in the treatment of human malaria. Science 190:792–794

UNDP (1980) World Bank, WHO (July 1st, 1979–June 30th, 1980) Special programme for research and training in tropical diseases. Fourth Annual Report, Geneva, p 346

Vachon F, Arbon C, Gilbert C (1974) Diagnostic et traitement du paludisme cérébral en zone non endémique. Bull WHO 50:169–175

Walker AJ, Lopez-Antuñano FJ (1969) Studies on the response to drugs of blood-induced falciparum malaria: South American parasite strains. Trans R Soc Trop Med Hyg 62:654

Wernsdorfer WH (1980) Field evaluation of drug resistance in malaria. In vitro micro-test. Acta Trop (Basel) 37:222–227

WHO (1961) Chemotherapy of malaria. WHO Tech Rep Ser 226

WHO (1973) Chemotherapy of malaria and resistance to antimalarials. WHO Tech Rep Ser 529

WHO (1979) Instruction for the use of the WHO Test Kit for the assessment of the response of *Plasmodium falciparum* to chloroquine. WHO Document MAP/79.1

WHO (1980) The clinical management of acute malaria. WHO Reg Publ SE Asia Ser 9

Wolfenberger HR (1972) Suppressive and curative trials in *Plasmodium malariae* infection with Fansidar. East Afr Med J 49:338–345

Woodruff AW, Dickinson CJ (1968) Use of dexamethasone in cerebral malaria. Br Med J 3:31–32

CHAPTER 15

# Pharmacogenetic Factors in Antimalarial Drug Testing

H. M. GILLES

The pharmacogenetic factors that are of importance in antimalarial drug testing (which in the final analysis must be conducted in the endemic areas) are (a) red-cell genetic factors, (b) acetylator phenotype and, possibly, (c) blood groups.

## A. Red-Cell Genetic Factors

Factors of special relevance in malaria chemotherapy are widespread in many parts of the tropics, with high gene frequencies in some countries. The ones considered in this section as relevant to antimalarial drug testing are the haemoglobinopathies, the thalassaemias, and the enzyme deficiencies.

Even if on pharmacological grounds there may be no reason to believe that these genetic factors are likely to influence either the pharmacokinetics of the antimalarial concerned or its toxic effects, it is prudent in phase I and phase II clinical trials to test the drug in these special groups, especially in areas of the tropics where gene frequencies are high, such as haemoglobin AS in Africa or haemoglobin AE in Thailand. In such areas phase I and II clinical trials should always include the following categories as separate study groups: (a) normal homozygotes (AA); (b) abnormal homozygotes (SS); (c) double heterozygotes (SC); and (d) heterozygotes (AS), even if the latter are rarely associated with clinical manifestations.

### I. The Haemoglobinopathies

The haemoglobinopathies are inherited as autosomal codominant traits, and heterozygous carriers have both the normal and the abnormal haemoglobin in each red cell. More than 300 structural variants have been described, but for the clinical pharmacologist concerned with antimalarial drug trials in the tropics those of greatest importance with high gene frequencies in some areas are: (a) haemoglobin S, (b) haemoglobin C, (c) haemoglobin D, (d) haemoglobin E, and (e) the thalassaemias (Fig. 1). In the Carribean and the Americas some of these genetic traits are found in persons of African, Mediterranean or Asian ancestry.

#### 1. Haemoglobin S

a) Sickle Cell Trait

Persons heterozygous for haemoglobin S (HbS) are said to have sickle cell trait (AS). Sickle cell trait is found among all Africans, Greeks, Italians, Saudis, Israeli, Arabs, and the Veddoids of Southern India. The highest prevalence, around 30%, is found in some areas of tropical Africa. Although in the majority of cases the trait

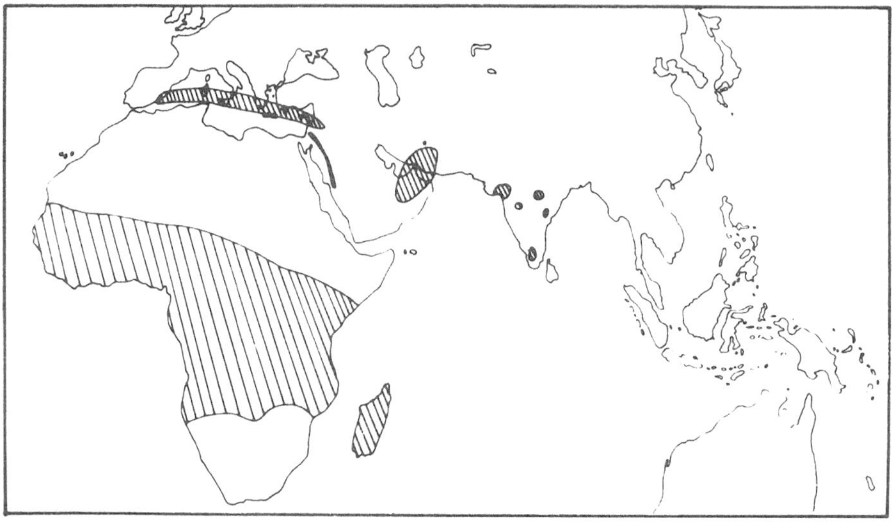

**Fig. 1.** Distribution of haemoglobin S. Courtesy of Medicine Digest and Dr. A. FLEMING

is rarely associated with clinical disease, it would be prudent in phase I and II clinical trials to assess them initially as a distinct group.

b) Sickle Cell Disease

Sickle cell disease is a serious condition characterised by a severe haemolytic anaemia, episodes of pain and fever, and manifestations of specific organ damage. Since patients with sickle cell disease in malarious areas should be kept on regular chemoprophylaxis, it is important that the pharmacokinetics of any new antimalarial should be studied in this special group of patients, especially in areas where they can make up as much as 1% of the total population. This concept becomes additionally pertinent in relation to the known involvement of hepatic and renal function in such patients.

The kidneys are known to play an important role in the control of drug therapy, particularly with regard to excretion and metabolism. By virtue of their blood supply and unique concentrating powers they are exposed to high levels of drugs and are therefore potentially vulnerable to damage. Furthermore, in states of diminished renal function they are unable to excrete certain drugs and their metabolites at an adequate rate and keep blood concentrations below the limits of toxicity. Careful attention must therefore be paid to dosage regimens, particularly with drugs that are in clinical trial. In SS disease renal haemodynamics are altered in a variety of ways (KOJO ADDAE 1975) and the kidney is often considered a repository of sickle cell pathology.

c) Double Heterozygous Conditions

As might be expected of a gene with the high frequency of HbS, it is not infrequently encountered in association with another abnormality of either the alpha or beta polypeptide chains of haemoglobin. The most common associations are: (a) haemoglobin SC disease, (b) sickle cell thalassaemia, (c) sickle cell/HbD disease, and (d) haemoglobin S/hereditary persistence of fetal haemoglobin (HPFH).

d) Haemoglobin SC Disease

This condition is particularly common in West Africa and occurs in other areas where HbS and C overlap, e.g. the West Indies. Indeed, in older adults, patients with HbSC are more often encountered than SS homozygotes because SC is a milder disease associated with a longer life span.

e) Sickle Cell B Thalassaemia

This double heterozygous condition is the second most common genetic variant of sickling.

f) Sickle Cell/HbD Disease

This rare disease is due to the presence of HbS and HbD-Punjab and has many of the features of sickle cell anaemia.

g) Haemoglobin S/HPFH

Hereditary persistence of fetal haemoglobin is an anomaly in which HbF is present in the red cells throughout life without anaemia. In association with HbS, it results in a benign disorder because it is known that HbF inhibits the sickling of HbS. Its incidence is about 0.1% in West Africa, Mediterranean areas, Jamaica, and East Africa.

## 2. Haemoglobin C

Haemoglobin C is found in its highest incidence in Northern Ghana (18%) and falls in incidence to the south, where it is not found east or south of the River Niger. It is rare in Liberia and Sierra Leone. The incidence in Southern Ghana is about 12% and in Western Nigeria 6%. It is absent from East Africa (see Fig. 2).

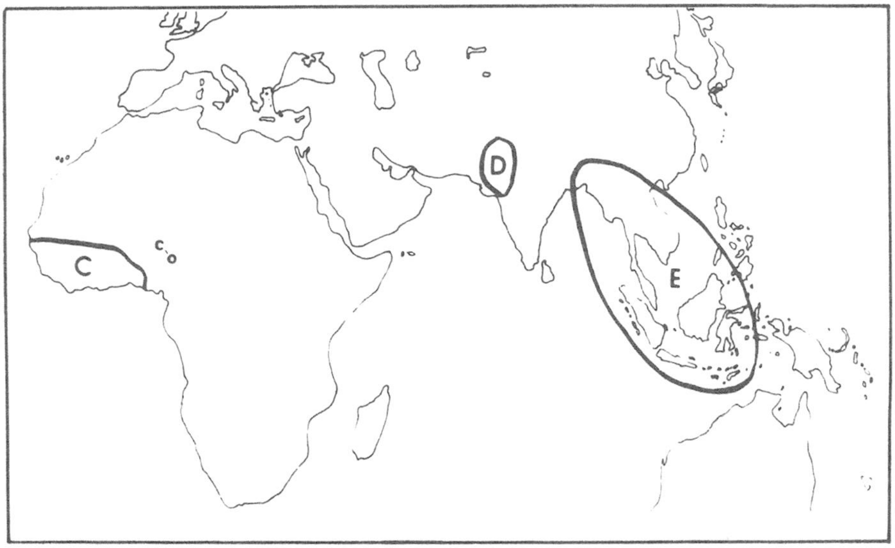


**Fig. 2.** Distribution of haemoglobin C, D, and E. Courtesy of Medicine Digest and Dr. A. FLEMING

a) Haemoglobin C Trait

In the heterozygote (AC), haemoglobin C forms about 30%–40% of the haemoglobin and the condition is harmless. Target cells may be present in the peripheral blood film and the osmotic fragility may be increased.

b) Haemoglobin C Disease

In the homozygote (CC), patients may suffer from a mild haemolytic anaemia with splenomegaly. They are frequently unaware of the condition, which is often detected accidentally in surveys. Target cells are numerous in the peripheral blood.

### 3. Haemoglobin D

The most commonly encountered of the D haemoglobins in HbD-Punjab. It is found in 3% of Sikhs in the Punjab and in lower incidence in Bombay, in the Mediterranean area, in Turks, Persians, Nigerians, Congolese, and Indonesians. The heterozygotes (AD) are completely symptomless. The homozygotes (DD) show a mild haemolytic anaemia, splenomegaly, and target cells in the peripheral blood.

### 4. Haemoglobin E

The abnormality is in the $\beta$ chain. Haemoglobin E is found in high incidence in Burma, Thailand, and Eastern Malaysia, where frequencies of 19%–35% have been reported. In India the highest incidence recorded was 3.9% in Bengalis. Foci have been reported in the Veddas of Ceylon, Turkey, Egypt, and Vietnam. The heterozygote (AE) is symptomless while the homozygote (EE) exhibits a mild haemolytic anaemia with target cells in the peripheral blood. Persons heterozygous for HbE and beta ($\beta$) thalassaemia have a more severe anaemia and the spleen is usually enlarged.

## II. Thalassaemias

There are two major varieties of thalassaemia: $\beta$ thalassaemia, where the deficit of synthesis is in the $\beta$ chains of haemoglobin, and $\alpha$ thalassaemia, in which there is retarded production of $\alpha$ chains of globin (WEATHERALL and CLEGG 1972).

### 1. Heterozygous $\beta$ Thalassaemia

Heterozygous thalassaemia has a worldwide distribution, with high incidence areas (10%–20%) in the Mediterranean region, and the Middle and Far East. It occurs sporadically in nearly every ethnic group. It has a relatively low incidence in tropical Africa, excluding Liberia where the incidence may be as high as 10%. $\beta$ Thalassaemia minor shows great variability in its clinical manifestations. At one end of the scale there may be no symptoms and the blood picture merely shows minor morphological changes of the red cells with diminished saline fragility. At the other end, the symptomatology and clinical signs may be so severe as to resemble the homozygous state. An intermediate form with mild anaemia, moderate

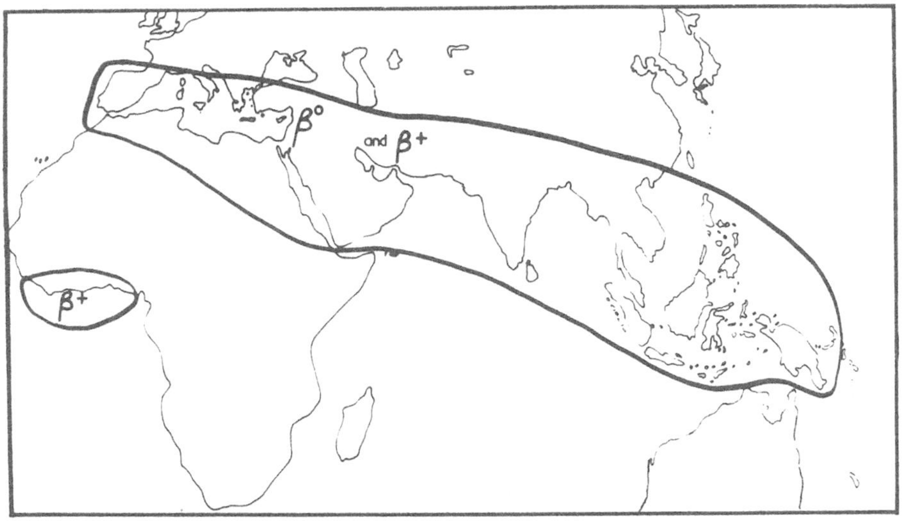


**Fig. 3.** Distribution of β thalassaemia. Courtesy of Medicine Digest and Dr. A. Fleming

splenomegaly, gallstones, bone pains, leg ulcers, and chronic jaundice – thalassaemia minor – also occurs.

### 2. Homozygous β Thalassaemia

This is a severe disease characterised by profound anaemia and marked hepatosplenomegaly. A typical facies develops with frontal bossing, prominent malar bones, protruding upper jaw, and the typical "hair on end" appearance on skull X-ray. Intercurrent infection is extremely common, as is hepatic insufficiency.

Double Heterozygous Conditions

Apart from *sickle cell-β thalassaemia,* which has already been referred to, the most important association of β thalassaemia with another β-chain structural variant is *haemoglobin E-β thalassaemia,* which is a common as well as a severe disease in Thailand.

### 3. Heterozygous α Thalassaemia

Alpha thalassaemia I trait is a benign condition found in persons of oriental or Mediterranean ancestry. These asymptomatic carriers of the gene are detected on routine haematological examination or during family studies of patients with homozygous disease.

### 4. Homozygous α Thalassaemia

There are two important clinical forms of homozygous disease: (a) a severe form which is incompatible with life and results in hydrops foetalis and (b) a milder form which presents in adult life as haemoglobin H disease.

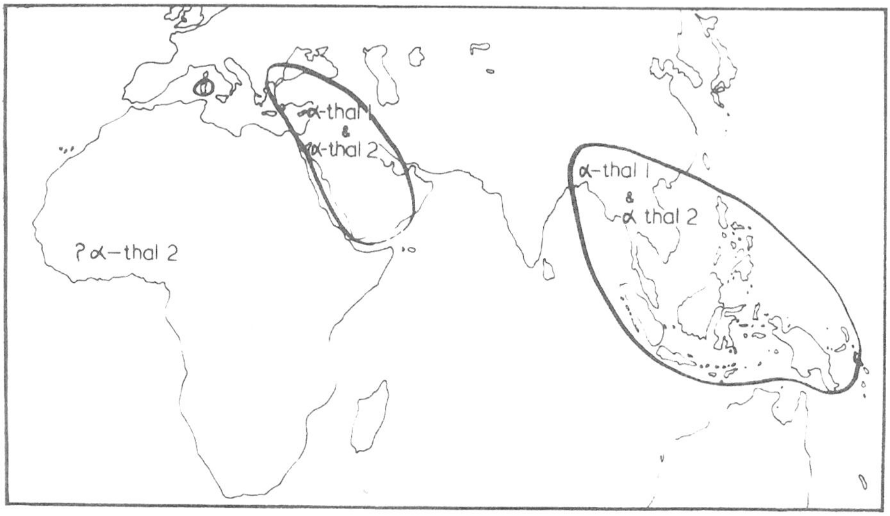


**Fig. 4.** Distribution of α thalassaemia. Courtesy of Medicine Digest and Dr. A. FLEMING

Haemoglobin H Disease

This homozygous condition is common in Chinese, Greeks, Italians, Indians, Indonesians, Burmese, and Thais. Clinically the manifestations are very variable. They include lassitude due to the long-standing anaemia, recurrent attacks of jaundice and fever, generalised joint pains and splenomegaly. The chronic haemolytic anaemia may become worse if sulphonamides are administered.

## III. Enzyme Deficiencies

Several enzyme deficiencies involved in the anaerobic pathway of glycolysis (the Embden-Meyerhof pathway) are genetically determined, e.g. pyruvate kinase (PK) deficiency and hexokinase deficiency. The most widespread and important in the context of this section is glucose-6-phosphate dehydrogenase (G6PD) deficiency.

Another enzyme to be considered here is methaemoglobin reductase, which is responsible for the reduction of methaemoglobin in human erythrocytes and which is also genetically determined (JAFFE 1966).

### 1. Glucose-6-Phosphate Dehydrogenase Deficiency

Glucose-6-phosphate dehydrogenase deficiency is a common inherited defect found all over the world, affecting over 100 million people. The three geographical areas where the deficiency is most common are Africa, the Mediterranean area, and Southeast Asia. In China, G6PD deficiency is common among Hakkanese and people of the Kwantung region (LEE et al. 1963; CHAN et al. 1964) affecting about 5% of the male population. At least 100 different forms of G6PD have been demonstrated. The most common variant in the southern Chinese is G6PD Canton, while G6PD Mahidol is the most common variant among Thais, Laotians, and Cambodians. The two clinically most important deficiencies are the "Negro" type $A^-$ ($Gd^{A-}$) and the "Mediterranean" type $B^-$ ($Gd^{B-}$).

**Table 1.** Some potentially haemolytic substances in G6PD-deficient subjects

| | |
|---|---|
| 1. Antimalarials | 5. Nitrofurans |
| Primaquine | Nitrofurantoin (Furadantin) |
| Pamaquine | Furazolidone (Furoxone) |
| Quinocide | Nitrofurazone (Furacin) |
| Pentaquine | 6. Other drugs |
| Mepacrine | Dimercaprol (BAL) |
| Chloroquine | Methylene blue |
| 2. Sulphonamides | Naphthalene (moth balls) |
| 3. Sulphones | Ascorbic acid |
| | Phenylhydrazine |
| 4. Antipyretics and analgesics | Probenecid (Benemid) |
| Acetylsalicylic acid | Vitamin K |
| Acetanilide | Trinitrotoluene |
| Acetophenetidin (Phenacetin) | Neosalvarsan |
| Phenazone | Quinidine (C)[a] |
| Aminophenazone | Chloramphenicol |
| | Niridazole |
| | Co-trimoxazole |
| | 7. Peas, beans, other vegetables |

[a] (C), Haemolysis so far only observed in Caucasians

The deficiency is inherited as a sex-linked trait, and the gene coding for G6PD has been proved to be located on the X-chromosome. The defect is therefore fully expressed in male hemizygotes and female homozygotes, while in female heterozygotes the expression is variable according to the varying proportions of normal and G6PD-deficient cells. In the negro type of deficiency haemolysis is less severe than in the Mediterranean type and limited in duration, since only relatively old cells are vulnerable.

Many drugs have been found to produce haemolysis in G6PD-deficient persons (Table 1). Reports on chloroquine-induced haemolysis have been extremely rare (Choudhry et al. 1977; D. J. Warrell 1980, personal communication), bearing in mind the widespread use of this drug in many areas where the incidence of G6PD deficiency is high. It is clearly very important, however, in clinical trials of antimalarial drugs, especially with chemical structures similar to those listed in Table 1, that a meticulous search is undertaken to assess their potential haemolytic effects in G6PD-deficient individuals.

## 2. NADH-Methaemoglobin Reductase Deficiency

Methaemoglobinaemia occurs when a significant amount of the oxygen-carrying ferrous haemoglobin is oxidised to the non-oxygen carrying ferric state and accumulates in the erythrocytes. The reduction of methaemoglobin in red cells depends on the activity of a reduced nicotinamide adenine dinucleotide (NADH)-dependent methaemoglobin reductase system. *Hereditary methaemoglobinaemia* due to the presence of the abnormal haemoglobin M is very rare.

Family and biochemical studies have demonstrated that NADH-methaemoglobin reductase is inherited as an autosomal codominant. Methaemoglobinaemia has been shown to occur in individuals heterozygous for NADH-methaemoglobin reductase deficiency while receiving drugs such as primaquine, chloroquine or diaminodiphenylsulphone (DDS) for chemoprophylaxis (COHEN et al. 1968; SIETSMA et al. 1968, 1971). Combinations of drugs seem to increase methaemoglobin production even in normal individuals (GREAVES et al. 1980).

If cyanosis occurs during the course of antimalarial clinical trials the possibility of this enzymatic defect should be borne in mind, over and above the possibility of the more complex reactions responsible for the methaemoglobin-forming properties of the aromatic amino and nitro compounds such as acetanilide, phenacetin, primaquine, and sulphonamides.

## B. Acetylator Phenotype

The enzyme *N*-acetyltransferase influences the metabolism of a wide variety of drugs. "Slow inactivators" are homozygous for a recessive gene that leads to lack of the hepatic enzyme acetyltransferase. "Rapid inactivators" are normal homozygotes or heterozygotes. The gene for slow inactivation shows marked differences in geographical distribution (Table 2). SUNAHARA (1961) has observed that there was a "cline" in frequency (q) of the allele ($A^s$) controlling slow acetylator along the Pacific Asian littoral in that the frequency steadily rose from a very low level in the far north to a fairly high level in Thailand. Apart from the Pacific area, a clear pattern is not discernible in data from Europe, Africa, Asia or the Americas.

**Table 2.** Global frequency (q) of allele controlling slow acetylation ($A^s$)

| Ethnic group | Location collected | q | (SE) |
|---|---|---|---|
| Japanese | Japan | 0.34 | 0.01 |
| Koreans | Korea | 0.33 | 0.06 |
| Chinese | Singapore | 0.46 | 0.02 |
| Thais | Thailand | 0.54 | 0.04 |
| Philippinos | Cebu | 0.82 | 0.04 |
| Burmese | Rangoon | 0.61 | 0.04 |
| Indians | Madras | 0.80 | 0.04 |
| Libyans | Benghazi | 0.81 | 0.05 |
| Egyptians | Cairo | 0.91 | 0.03 |
| Sudanese (non-Arab) | Khartoum | 0.81 | 0.03 |
| Kenyans | East Africa | 0.74 | 0.05 |
| Ugandans | | 0.74[a] | 0.02 |
| Tanzanians | | | |
| Zambians | | | |
| Northern Nigerians | Zaria | 0.70 | 0.03 |
| Southern Nigerians | Nsukka | 0.64 | 0.04 |
| Italians | Rome | 0.74 | 0.03 |
| British whites | Liverpool | 0.81 | 0.03 |
| Swedes | Stockholm | 0.82 | 0.02 |
| Eskimos | Hudson and Jones Bay | 0.22 | 0.03 |
| American Indians | Denver | 0.47 | 0.05 |
| Shuara Indians | Ecuador | 0.47 | 0.05 |

[a] Random selection from 953 patients in 35 tuberculosis treatment centres in East Africa

The enzyme acetylates, for example, isoniazid, sulphamethazine, sulphadimidine, sulfisoxazole, hydralazine, dapsone, procainamide, and phenelzine (EVANS et al. 1960; EVANS 1969; GELBER et al. 1971; ELLARD et al. 1972; PETERS et al. 1972). Even when the acetylator status of a person does not affect the outcome of treatment, as in the case of isoniazid, slow acetylators are more likely to develop cumulative toxicity leading to peripheral neuritis. On the other hand, there is always the danger that rapid inactivators may not be able to maintain adequate blood levels unless they are given their drugs on a carefully regulated schedule (JEANES et al. 1972).

Quite clearly, therefore, acetylator status is a consideration to be borne in mind when testing antimalarial drugs with chemical formulae similar to those drugs mentioned above, both from the point of view of adverse reactions as well as efficacy or drug failure (CHIN et al. 1966; GILLES and CLYDE 1974).

## C. Blood Groups

There is no evidence to date that blood groups influence the metabolism of drugs, but the finding by MILLER et al. (1975) that the Duffy antigen Fy is associated with the receptor for *P. vivax* has sharpened the focus on parasite – red cell membrane interactions and, by inference, on the effects of other, possibly genetically controlled, blood group antigen "receptors" within the general context of "targeted" antimalarial chemotherapy.

## D. Conclusion

In this chapter are covered some of the more important and geographically widespread genetic factors, with particular reference to the endemic areas where clinical trials of antimalarial drugs must eventually be tested.

It is essential to re-emphasise the importance and, indeed, the obligation for investigators to include these particular potential risk groups in all their studies, and certainly before a final evaluation of the antimalarial in question is made. Without doubt the effect of the above pharmacogenetic factors must be carefully evaluated before phase III trials are undertaken. The finding that, in phase I and II clinical trials, these genetic factors do *not* influence the pharmacokinetics of the antimalarial drug concerned would simplify and expedite phase III trials in the community, as well as satisfy an important ethical criterion.

## References

Chan TK, Todd D, Wong CG (1964) Erythrocyte glucose-6-phosphate dehydrogenase deficiency in Chinese. Br Med J 2:102

Chin W, Contacos PG, Coatney GR, King HK (1966) The evaluation of sulfonamides, alone or in combination with pyrimethamine, in the treatment of multi-resistant falciparum malaria. Am J Trop Med Hyg 15:823–829

Choudhry VP, Nishi M, Sood SK, Ghai OP (1977) Chloroquine induced haemolysis and acute renal failure in subjects with G-6-PD deficiency. Trop Geogr Med 30:331–335

Cohen R, Sachs JR, Wicker DJ, Conrad ME (1968) Methaemoglobinaemia provoked by malaria chemoprophylaxis in Vietnam. N Engl J Med 279:1127–1131

Ellard GA, Gammon PT, Helmy HS, Rees RJW (1972) Dapsone acetylation and the treatment of leprosy. Nature 239:159–160

Evans DAP (1969) An improved and simplified method of detecting the acetylator phenotype. J Med Genet 6:405–407
Evans DAP, Manley KA, McKusick VA (1960) Genetic control of isoniazid metabolism in man. Br Med J 2:485–491
Gelber R, Peters JH, Ross Gordon G, Glazko AJ, Levy MD (1971) The polymorphic acetylation of dapsone in man. Clin Pharmacol Ther 12:225–237
Gilles HM, Clyde DF (1974) Acetylator phenotype in sulphonamide resistant falciparum malaria. Ann Trop Med Parasitol 68:367
Greaves J, Evans DAP, Fletcher KA (1980) Urinary primaquine excretion and red cell methaemoglobin levels in man following a primaquine: chloroquine regimen. Br J Clin Pharmacol 10:293–295
Jaffe ER (1966) Hereditary methemoglobinemias associated with abnormalities in the metabolism. Am J Med 41:786–798
Jeanes CWL, Schaefer O, Eidus L (1972) Inactivation of isoniazid by Canadian Eskimos and Indians. Can Med Assoc J 106:331–335
Kojo Addae S (1975) The kidney in sickle cell disease. Ghana Universities Press, Accra
Lee TC, Shin LY, Huang PC, Lin CC, Blackwell BN, Blackwell RQ, Hsia DYY (1963) Glucose-6-phosphate dehydrogenase deficiency in Taiwan. Am J Hum Genet 15:126
Miller LH, Mason SJ, Dvorak JA, McGinniss MH, Rothman IK (1975) Erythrocyte receptors for *Plasmodium knowlesi* malaria: Duffy blood group determinants. Science 189:561
Peters JH, Ross Gordon G, Ghoul DC, Tolentino JG, Walsh GP, Levy L (1972) The disposition of the antileprotic drug dapsone (DDS) in Philippine subjects. Am J Trop Med Hyg 21:450–457
Sietsma A, Naughton MA, Harley JD (1968) "Blue soldiers." Med J Aust 55:911
Sietsma A, Naughton MA, Harley JD (1971) Methaemoglobin levels in soldiers receiving antimalarial drugs. Med J Aust 58:473–475
Sunahara S (1961) Genetic geographical and clinical studies on isoniazid metabolism. In: Proceedings of the XVI international tuberculosis conference, Toronto, Canada. Excerpta Medica, Amsterdam (Excerpta Medica International Congress Series No. 44, pp 513–540)
Weatherall DJ, Clegg JB (1972) The thalassaemia syndromes, 2 edn. Blackwell, Oxford

# Antimalarial Drug Resistance

CHAPTER 16

# History and Current Status of Drug Resistance

W. PETERS

## A. Introduction

Biologists and physicians define drug resistance in different terms (PETERS 1970 a), the former being more concerned with the parasite and the latter with the host. In this book the definition of WHO (1965) has been adopted. This states that, in malaria, resistance to drugs is the ability of the parasites to survive and/or multiply despite the administration and absorption of a drug given in doses equal to or higher than those usually recommended but within the limits of tolerance of the host. This definition points out that, while it may apply to any species or stage of malaria parasites, it is most commonly used with reference to the action of blood schizontocides, especially the 4-aminoquinolines when used in the treatment of infections with *Plasmodium falciparum*. This itself is a reflection of the serious impact made by the recognition of chloroquine resistance in *P. falciparum* in 1959 and 1960 since, in spite of the well-known problem of resistance to proguanil and pyrimethamine that had appeared in various parts of the world from 1949 onwards, no real attempt had been made to define the problem before 1963 (WHO 1963) and it was only in 1967 that a WHO Scientific Group established criteria by which the level of clinical response could be measured.

The graphical representation set out in the earlier report (WHO 1967) was modified to the form shown in Fig. 1 (WHO 1973), this representing the response to a standard oral dose of 1.5 g chloroquine base administered over a 3-day period. In recent years two in vitro procedures for the determination of the response of *P. falciparum* in field conditions have been described. Details of the macro test (RIECKMANN et al. 1968 a) and the micro test (RIECKMANN et al. 1978) are given elsewhere in this book (see Chap. 18). While the first of these has been employed extensively to evaluate the response of *P. falciparum* to chloroquine in a number of countries, the latter is still in the development stage under the auspices of WHO for use not only with chloroquine but also with mefloquine, sulphonamides, and pyrimethamine (WERNSDORFER 1980; KOUZNETSOV et al. 1980).

## B. History of Experimental Research on Antimalarial Drug Resistance

The literature on this topic up to 1970 was covered in an exhaustive review by PETERS (1970 a) and updated by PETERS (1974) and ROZMAN and CANFIELD (1979). A further but brief review has just appeared (PETERS 1980). In this chapter, there-

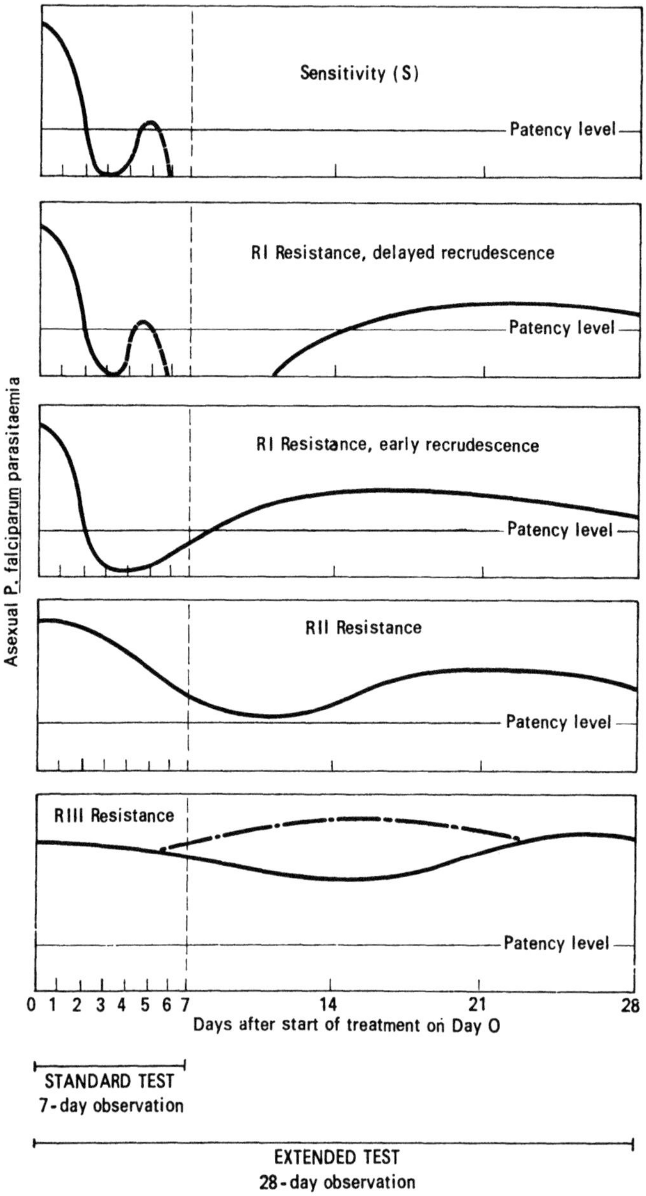


**Fig. 1.** Response to WHO field test for sensitivity of *P. falciparum* to chloroquine in vivo in man. Reproduced by permission from WHO (1973)

fore, no attempt is made to go over the same ground in full detail but the outstanding work and recent reports will be considered in the light of the current and future perspectives of antimalarial chemotherapy. Structures of antimalarial compounds are shown in Figs. 2 and 3. Since the advent of potent, often highly specific chemotherapeutic agents (among which, it must be pointed out, quinine was one of the

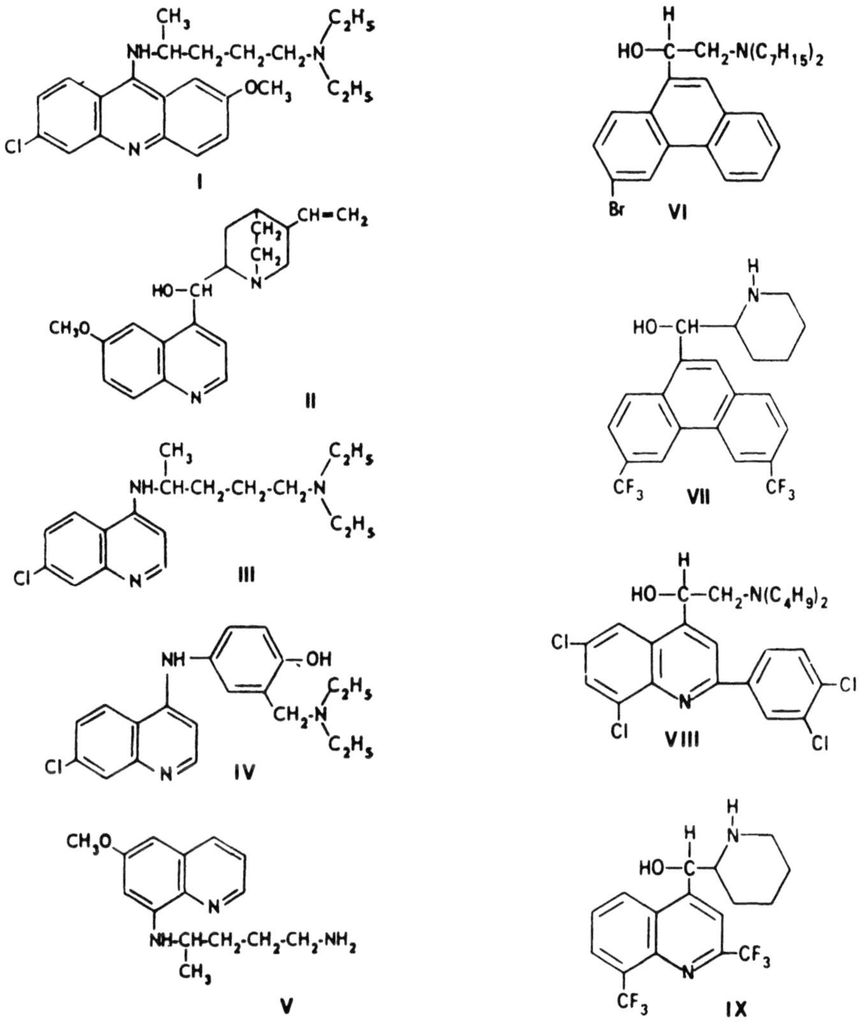


**Fig. 2.** Structures of antimalarial compounds. *I*, mepacrine (atebrine); *II*, quinine; *III*, chloroquine; *IV*, amodiaquine; *V*, primaquine; *VI*, WR 33063; *VII*, WR 122455; *VIII*, WR 30090; *IX*, mefloquine (WR 142490)

first), particularly the sulphonamides and then the antibiotics, the history of chemotherapy has been one long saga of disaster, the target organisms "leapfrogging," as it were, over each new therapeutic hurdle placed in their path by the ingenuity of the chemotherapists. While the seemingly limitless genetic lability of the organisms can be blamed for the multitude of drug-resistant mutants that have appeared in both prokaryotes and eukaryotes, much of the problem in drug resistance must be attributed to the misuse of the drugs themselves by man, a theme that is taken up again by the writer in the final chapter of this book. The experimental techniques for the study of drug resistance are considered in Chap. 18.

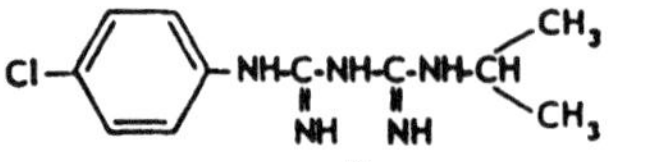

X

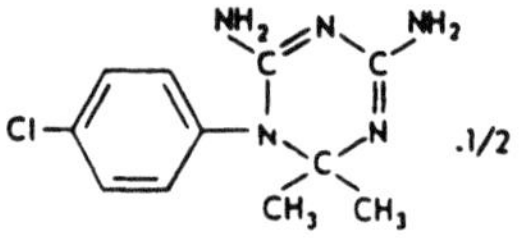

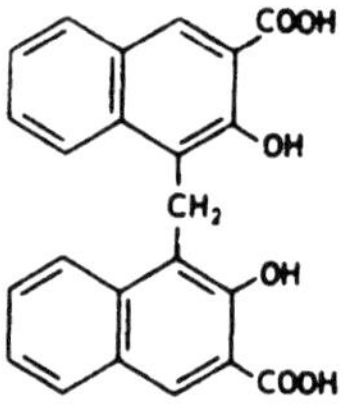

XI

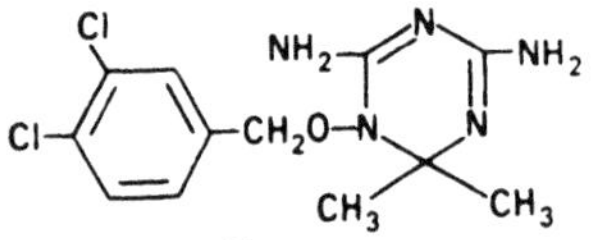

XII

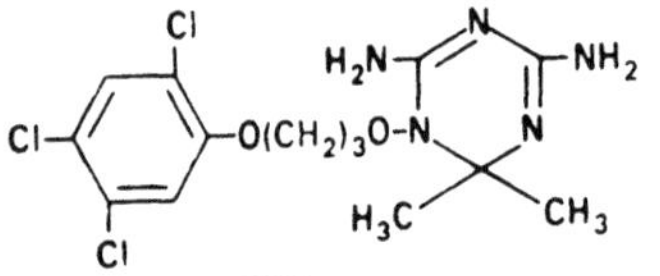

XIII

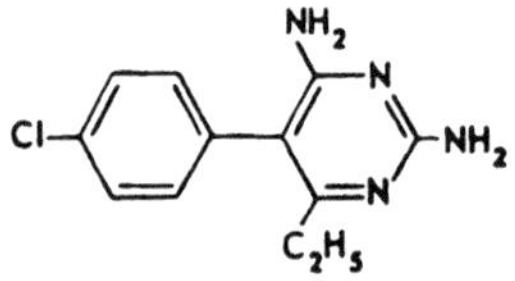

XIV

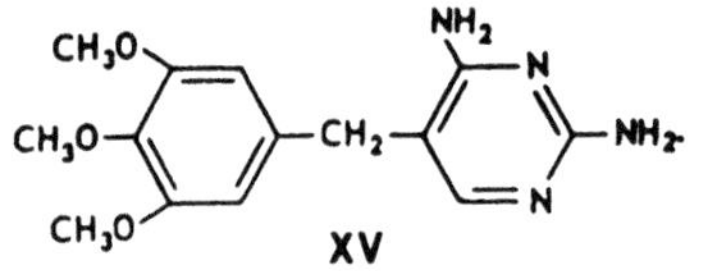

XV

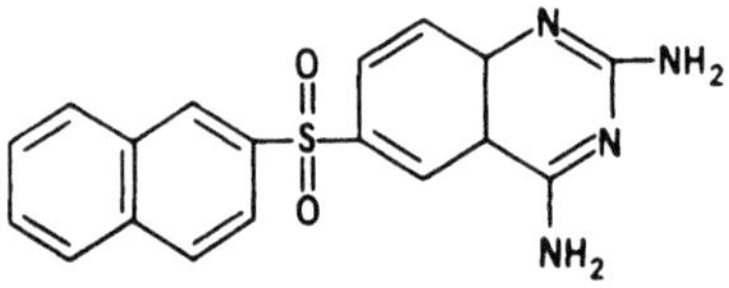

XVI

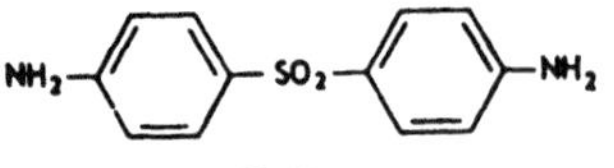

XVII

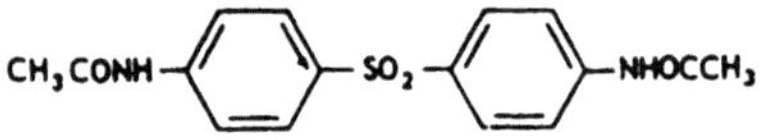

XVIII

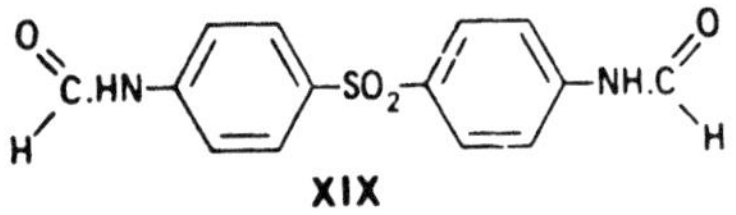

XIX

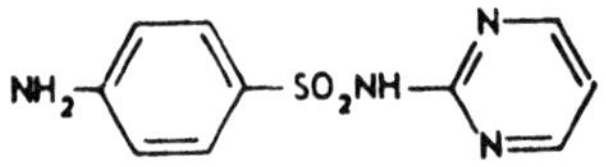

XX

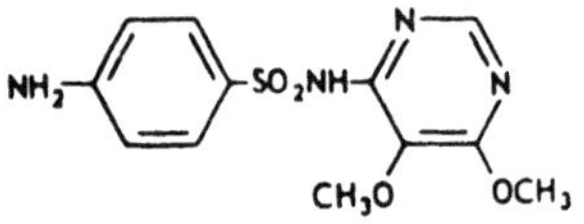

XXI

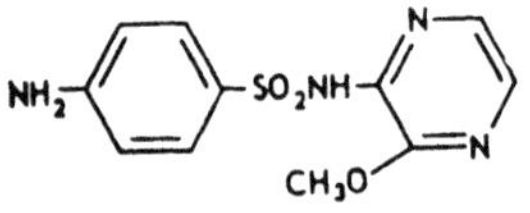

XXII

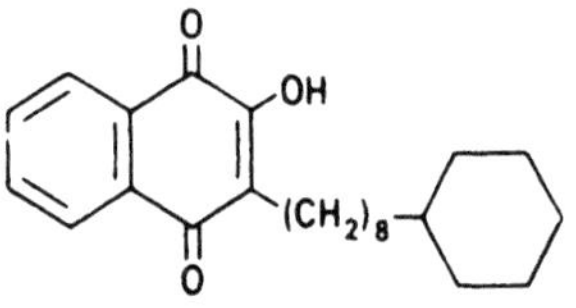

XXIII

**Fig. 3.** Structures of antimalarial compounds, *X*, proguanil; *XI*, cycloguanil embonate; *XII*, clociguanil; *XIII*, WR 99210; *XIV*, pyrimethamine; *XV*, trimethoprim; *XVI*, WR 158122; *XVII*, dapsone; *XVIII*, acedapsone; *XIX*, diformyl dapsone (DFD); *XX*, sulphadiazine; *XXI*, sulfadoxine; *XXII*, sulfalene; *XXIII*, menoctone

**Table 1.** Dates of introduction of antimalarials and the first recognition of resistance to them. Modified from PETERS (1970a) in which full details of references are given

| Compound | Year first used in therapy | Year resistance first strongly suspected or confirmed | | | | Remarks |
|---|---|---|---|---|---|---|
| | | Laboratory studies | Therapy in man | | | |
| | | | *P. falciparum* | *P. vivax* | *P. malariae* | |
| Quinine | c. 1630 | *P. relictum* 1921 | Brazil 1910 [a]<br>Malaya 1967 | Macedonia 1918 [a] | | Possibly only strain differences [a] |
| Methylene blue | 1891 | *P. berghei* 1953 | | | | Little used in clinic after 1910 |
| Pamaquine | 1926 | *P. knowlesi* 1934 | | | | Withdrawn after about 1946 |
| Mepacrine | 1935 | *P. berghei* 1965 | New Guinea 1946 | | | Little used after about 1950 |
| Chloroquine | 1945 | *P. gallinaceum* 1956 | Venezuela 1960 [a]<br>Colombia 1961 [b] | | | |
| Proguanil | 1948 | *P. gallinaceum* 1947 | Liverpool 1949 | Liverpool 1949 | Java 1950 | |
| Primaquine | 1951 | *P. knowlesi* 1956 | Colombia 1963 | New Guinea 1958 [c] | | Strain difference [c] |
| Pyrimethamine | 1952 | *P. gallinaceum* 1951 | Gambia 1952 | United States 1953 | Kenya and Tanzania 1954 | |
| Cycloguanil embonate | 1963 | *P. berghei* 1964 | S. Rhodesia 1964 | | | Hydrochloride in mouse |
| Sulphadiazine | 1964 | *P. gallinaceum* 1948 | | | | Only used with pyrimethamine |
| Sulphadoxine | 1964 | *P. berghei* 1968 | Cambodia 1968 | | | Only used with pyrimethamine |
| Dapsone | 1965 | *P. cynomolgi* 1962 | Cambodia 1968 | | | Only used with pyrimethamine |
| Mefloquine | ? | *P. berghei* [c] 1977 | ? Thailand 1980 [d] | | | |

[a] Only suspected [b] First confirmation [c] PETERS et al. (1977) [d] Unpublished data

The history of experimental antimalarial resistance and its relation to the problem of drug resistance in human malaria are summarised in Table 1. It is quite apparent that resistance can be produced to virtually every drug with which malaria parasites can be challenged, and some are inherently unresponsive e.g. *P. yoelii* to chloroquine (WARHURST and KILLICK-KENDRICK 1967). To the drugs shown in Table 1 should be added the following compounds that failed to achieve clinical acceptance or, in some cases, did not even reach clinical trial.

## I. Dihydrofolate Reductase Inhibitors

SCHMIDT (1973) reported that WR 158122 (Fig. 3, XVI), a quinazoline with remarkable inhibitory effect on the dihydrofolate reductase of *P. berghei*, rapidly lost its effectiveness when used alone in *Aotus* monkeys infected with *P. falciparum* and *P. vivax* but was extremely effective in combination with sulphadiazine (SCHMIDT 1979). The future of this compound is still being weighed in the balance. It is clear that it, like other antifols, should not be deployed alone, and experiments are currently in hand to determine whether it could form one of the components of a potentiating combination with a sulphonamide or sulphone for use as a repository preparation in a biodegradable polymer (WISE et al. 1979).

Clociguanil (Fig. 3, XII), a close analogue of cycloguanil, which is the active metabolite of proguanil, received a preliminary clinical trial against *P. falciparum* in The Gambia (LAING 1974) but was not further followed up because it appeared to offer no advantage over proguanil or pyrimethamine. It was also studied by RIECKMANN (1971) in volunteers infected with a multiple-resistant strain of *P. falciparum* in whom it failed to protect against sporozoite challenge. The rodent malaria parasite *P. berghei* readily develops resistance to clociguanil when it is used alone (KNIGHT and WILLIAMSON 1980). These workers used two techniques, the application of gradually increasing drug-selection pressure and the use of single high doses with transfer of "relapsed" parasites in successive passages, and compared the ease with which resistance developed to clociguanil and cycloguanil in a parallel experiment. With the relapse technique resistance developed rapidly to cycloguanil but not to clociguanil. However, resistance to clociguanil was achieved with the application of gradually increasing drug-selection pressure and the use of the relapse procedure from passage 22 onwards. The clociguanil-resistant line proved to be somewhat less virulent than the parent N strain but the resistance was stable in the absence of drug-selection pressure. The resistant parasites showed a curious pattern of response to other antifols, being fully cross-resistant to cycloguanil but normally sensitive to sulphadimethoxine and hypersensitive to pyrimethamine. This finding parallels an earlier observation (PETERS et al. 1975) that clociguanil is fully active against a pyrimethamine-resistant line.

A further triazine in the clociguanil series (BR 26231 or WR 99210) (Fig. 3, XIII) (KNIGHT et al. 1982) has proved of particular interest because it retains a high level of activity against lines of *P. berghei* (PETERS et al. 1975) and *P. falciparum* (RIECKMANN 1973, cited by WHO 1973) that are highly resistant to proguanil and pyrimethamine. KNIGHT and WILLIAMSON (1982) have demonstrated that *P. berghei* develops resistance to this compound used alone in mice far more slowly than to cycloguanil or to clociguanil, both of which share the property shown by most antifols of rapidly losing their efficacy because of resistance. Indeed, the remarkable lack of cross-resistance of WR 99210 with other antifols, together with the slowness with which *P. berghei*-resistant mutants emerge and a tendency for it to inhibit pigment clumping in the CIPC test (see p. 303) (PETERS et al. 1975), would suggest that this triazine may have another mode of action against *P. berghei* in addition to the inhibitory action on parasite dihydrofolate reductase. GENTHER and SMITH (1977), for example, found that WR 99210 inhibits the growth of *Escherichia coli* at a far lower concentration than pyrimethamine, while this organism is hardly affected at all by cycloguanil. Clociguanil, too, inhibits the growth of *E. coli*.

## II. Naphthoquinones and Related Compounds

Little difficulty was experienced by the writer in developing a line of *P. berghei* resistant to the naphthoquinone compound, menoctone (WR 49808, Fig. 3, XXIII) (unpublished observation), and HOWELLS et al. (1970) suggested that the asexual intraerythrocytic parasites may survive the damaging effects of this compound on parasite mitochondria by increasing the biogenesis of these organelles. In studies on a quinolone ester (ICI 56780) RILEY and PETERS (1970) observed a very rapid development of resistance by *P. berghei*, which could be interpreted as a single-step resistance in the face of a high drug dose-selection pressure. Resistance to this compound was stable in further drug-free passages. In contrast to menoctone, which displayed synergism with cycloguanil (PETERS 1970b), ICI 56780 gave some indication of synergism with chlorcycloguanil and also with sulphonamides. Neither menoctone nor ICI 56780 were synergistic with primaquine.

## III. Primaquine

Since the experiments of ARNOLD et al. (1961), in which a strain of *P. vivax* was made highly resistant to primaquine in a succession of human volunteers, no further studies of this nature have been reported. In that work the strain lost not only the sensitivity of the asexual blood stages but also of the gametocytes. Fortunately the gametocytocidal action of primaquine appears to have been retained in highly chloroquine-resistant lines of *P. falciparum* (RIECKMANN et al. 1968b). In mice MERKLI and PETERS (1976) showed that primaquine resistance was more readily induced by the application of slowly increasing drug-selection pressure than by the application of large, single doses in the relapse technique.

## IV. Aminoalcohols Related to Quinine

THOMPSON (1972) reported that a phenanthrenemethanol, WR 33063 (Fig. 2, VI), and a quinolinemethanol, WR 30090 (Fig. 2, VIII), were less active against a highly chloroquine-resistant line of *P. berghei*, but he did not actually attempt to produce lines resistant to these two aminoalcohols. PETERS and PORTER (1976) found that they could rapidly produce a line of *P. berghei* resistant to a related phenanthrenemethanol, WR 122455 (Fig. 2, VII), and in 1977 PETERS et al. reported similar observations with the quinolinemethanol mefloquine (WR 142490, Fig. 2, IX). In both these cases resistance emerged more rapidly if the starting point was a line of *P. berghei* that was already resistant to chloroquine. Mefloquine is currently in extensive clinical trial against chloroquine-resistant *P. falciparum*. If experimental data on *P. berghei* bear any relevance to the situation in *P. falciparum* (as most workers believe they do), the implications for the future of mefloquine, if deployed alone for the prevention or treatment of human malaria, are self-evident.

## C. History of Drug Resistance in Man

From the summary in Table 1 it will be apparent that drug resistance has always presented problems for the prevention and treatment of malaria in man. It must be remembered, however, that the distinction between the therapeutic response to the first generally used antimalarial, quinine, against *P. falciparum* and *P. vivax* only became clear during the early part of this century, and particularly when malariotherapy came into favour as a treatment for neurosyphilis. At that point it soon became apparent that there was a marked difference between the two species, depending upon whether infection had been induced by mosquito bite or by the inoculation of intraerythrocytic parasites, although the true significance of this did not become apparent until the discovery of the existence of a secondary exoerythrocytic cycle of *P. vivax*, the nature of which is still being actively investigated (KROTOSKI et al. 1980, and Chap. 1 of this book). The difference between *P. falciparum* and *P. vivax* is still apparent in relation to chemotherapy in that only the first of these two species has been shown so far to have the ability to become resistant to 4-aminoquinolines or aminoalcohols. No such resistance has ever been found in *P. vivax, P. ovale* or *P. malariae*. We refer here, of course, to resistance of the asexual intraerythrocytic stages since none of these compounds has any activity against the exoerythrocytic stages, primary or (in *P. vivax* and *P. ovale*) secondary.

### I. Quinine and 4-Aminoalcohols

The earliest suggestions that some strains of *P. falciparum* could be relatively insensitive to quinine came from German malariologists who were responsible for treating falciparum malaria in patients who had become infected in Brazil. PETERS (1970a), reviewing this history, showed how suspicions of "quinine fastness," first aired by COUTO (1908) and NOCHT and WERNER (1910), were lost in a confusion of reports from other parts of the world where no evidence for this could be demonstrated, and by confusion between the action of quinine against *P. vivax* as opposed to *P. falciparum*. Only in recent years have reports been given of clearly defined loss of sensitivity of *P. falciparum* to quinine in individuals who were infected with strains of this parasite from Southeast Asia that were already highly resistant to chloroquine. The observation that the response to therapeutic quinine diminished progressively in successive passages in human volunteers infected with the Vietnam Camp strain (MCNAMARA et al. 1967) was particularly relevant. This work culminated in a report indicating that the response of the late passages of this line of the Camp strain to quinine in vitro was significantly poorer than that of the original material. Parasite maturation which was completely inhibited in parent material by a quinine concentration of 12–14 nmol required some 20–50 nmol in the late-passage parasites. Subsequently other reports of relative quinine resistance have emerged including detailed case histories of Thai patients by JAROONVESAMA et al. (1974), who also reviewed earlier experiences in that region. Two of the patients gave what could be called an RIII response to quinine but all three were radically cured with a single dose of 1 g sulphadoxine with 50 mg pyrimethamine. A further Thai case was reported by MIGASENA et al. (1980). In 1978 GLEW et al. reported the deliberate selection of RIII resistance to quinine by the passage under drug-selection pressure of *P. falciparum* in *Aotus* monkeys. They drew particular attention to the potential risk of resistance to quinine or its analogues (such as mefloquine) arising when these drugs are used to treat patients infected with strains of *P. falciparum* that are already resistant to chloroquine, a problem to which THOMPSON (1972) also alluded on the basis of his experience in rodent malaria. On the African continent *P. falciparum* has enjoyed the reputation of being highly responsive to quinine and, until recently, to chloroquine. The possible reasons why this should be so could include factors related to the inherent response to the parasites, to the kinetics and metabolism of the drugs in the host, or to the nature of the immune responses of the African to infection. The latter is, of course, vitally important since it is likely that no drug is totally effective against any pathogen without the active participation of host immune responses (WHITESIDE 1962; PETERS 1969). It was, therefore, particularly salutary to read a report from NGUYEN-DINH and TRAGER (1978) indicating that chloroquine resistance had been selected in a West African isolate of *P. falciparum* maintained in vitro, in view of the close links between resistance to chloroquine and quinine. In other words, resistance to chloroquine *can* develop in at least one African strain of this parasite given appropriate conditions, and the same may well be shown to be true for quinine.

At the time of writing the use of mefloquine has been restricted to the treatment of falciparum malaria in areas where chloroquine resistance is a major problem, and its prophylactic use has been limited to a few carefully controlled field studies in endemic populations (e.g. that of PEARLMAN et al. 1980). Because of the need to evaluate this compound before releasing it for general use, and of the potential risk that its unrestricted marketing may lead to its misuse and devaluation through drug resistance, a careful watch has been maintained on its distribution by all concerned. Nevertheless, reports, unconfirmed at the time of writing, are beginning to appear suggesting that the response of acute falciparum malaria in refugees near the Thai-Kampuchean border, where chloroquine resistance is maximum, is less impressive than that reported in other parts of areas of Southeast Asia and Latin America.

## II. Mepacrine and 4-Aminoquinolines

Mepacrine, which has long since been abandoned for the prevention or treatment of malaria, is referred to here because (a) its mode of action and pattern of drug response are virtually identical to those of the 4-aminoquinolines and (b) it was the first of this group to which drug resistance was found in *P. falciparum* (see Table 1). The first observations of chloroquine resistance were made in 1959 in Latin America and in Thailand. A report by MABERTI (1960) from Venezuela was quickly followed by that of MOORE and LANIER (1961) from Colombia. Chloroquine resistance was suspected in Thailand as long ago as 1957 but the first proven cases were those reported by HARINASUTA et al. (1962). Since that time numerous reports have appeared indicating that chloroquine resistance is restricted to *P. falciparum* but that resistant strains of this parasite are widely distributed throughout the endemic areas of South and Central America, Southeast Asia, and the southwest Pacific (Fig. 4). Until 1979 no clearly substantiated cases of chloroquine resistance were reported from the African continent and the few reports that did suggest that chloroquine resistance was present were unconvincing. However, there remained an uneasy feeling that not all patients responded to the standard oral dose of chloroquine (1.5 g base in 3 days) as would be anticipated, especially non-immune expatriate or short-term visitors to Africa. Inadequate attention was paid by many clinicians to the simple fact that non-immune patients may well need more than the "standard" dose of chloroquine, a fact recently stressed in the new WHO monograph on malaria chemotherapy (BRUCE-CHWATT et al. 1981).

Unfortunately the question mark that lay over Africa at the time when earlier versions of Fig. 4 were drawn up must now be replaced by definite locations for the detection of chloroquine resistance in non-immune expatriates. The first reliable information was that disseminated by the Center for Disease Control, Atlanta (MORBIDITY MORTALITY WEEKLY REPORT 1978), which referred to three visitors to East Africa (two from the United States and one Dane) who developed *P. falciparum* infections that yielded an RI response to chloroquine.

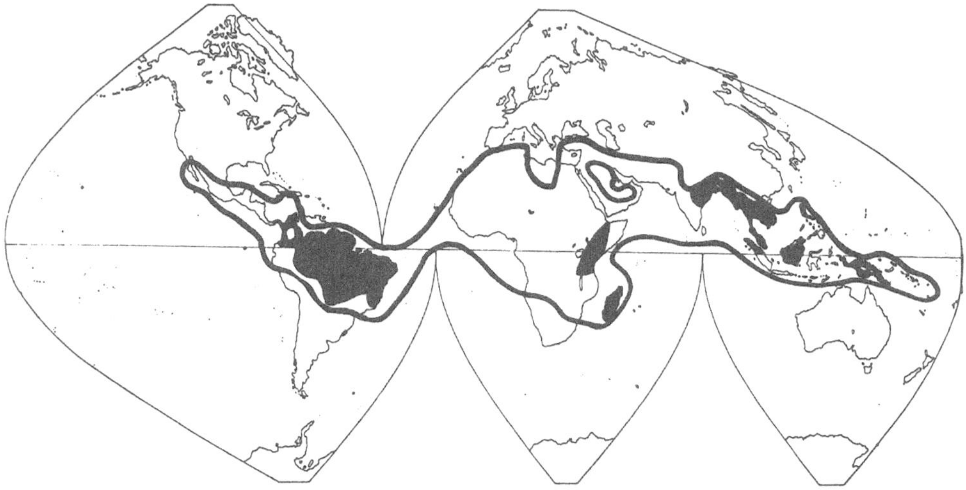

**Fig. 4.** Distribution of chloroquine resistance in *P. falciparum*. Malaria occurs within most of the areas contained within the *heavy line*, except the deserts of the Middle East (as indicated) and the Sahara. Areas of chloroquine resistance are indicated by *solid black shading*. (Note a small area in East Africa)

A hypothesis on how the innate resistance of Africans to *P. falciparum* may have accounted for the relative delay before chloroquine resistance became established in Africa was proposed in 1969 by PETERS and is illustrated in Fig. 5.

According to this hypothesis resistance to compounds which display a relatively flat dose-activity relationship (compound B in Fig. 5) can develop rapidly since numerous parasites evade the action of the drug and are present in sufficient numbers to survive the immune attack of the host. On the contrary, drugs such as A have a steep dose-activity curve, which implies that only a few survive the drug action and, therefore, the infection has less chance of persisting, since immune mechanisms will mop up the few survivors. If in the African context we translate B as, for example, pyrimethamine and A as chloroquine, we find ourselves in the actual situation that exists on that continent where pyrimethamine resistance has existed since 1952 and chloroquine resistance has only just appeared, both compounds having been in use for a similar period of time, i.e. nearly 30 years. Only now have the rapidly increasing numbers of foreign visitors to Africa, many taking inadequate prophylaxis, provided a sufficient pool of non-immune "sentinel guinea pigs" to detect the presence of a small number of chloroquine-resistant mutants in the falciparum population. Current surveys being carried out under the auspices of WHO with the micro in vitro sensitivity test (see Chap. 18) indicate that RI resistance to chloroquine may well be relatively common among the indigenous population, but that this does not show up in standard in vivo testing of these semi-immune people (KOUZNETSOV et al. 1980; WERNSDORFER and KOUZNETSOV 1980).

Details of two of the three earliest proven cases of chloroquine-resistant falciparum malaria acquired in East Africa (referred to above) were given by KEAN (1979) and FOGH et al. (1979). In addition the first of these authors described a fourth case, also from the United States. A further study of the third of the original cases, a man infected in the Selous area of southern Tanzania, was made by CAMPBELL et al. (1979), who both passaged parasites from this patient into *Aotus* monkeys and carried out a modified in vitro chloroquine sensitivity test on the strain maintained in culture. The response to chloroquine in the *Aotus* monkeys indicated a low level of resistance (corresponding to the RI response found in the patient). In vitro the parasites were highly resistant but the significance of these observations using this particular technique is uncertain. EICHENLAUB and POHLE (1980) reported that an African from the Comoros Islands, long resident in West Germany, acquired falciparum malaria when on holiday in his homeland. On return to Berlin his infection became patent and his response to chloroquine therapy indicated that RI resistance was present. This case is particularly interesting as it illustrates the danger that exists when people from highly endemic areas lose their immunity in the presence of a spreading, low-grade chloroquine resistance. A further indication of chloroquine resistance from Kenya and Tanzania are two case reports of Danish patients in whom serum chloroquine determinations showed that drug concentrations above 40 μg/litre were likely to have failed to control parasitaemia (PETTERSSON et al., 1981). RI resistance has also been proven in two Swedish women who were infected in Madagascar (ARONSSON et al. 1981).

Elsewhere in Africa the situation is less clear. There are indications that in Ethiopia *P. falciparum* is slightly less sensitive on the whole to chloroquine than in other parts of Africa (DENNIS et al. 1974; ARMSTRONG et al. 1976), and this has

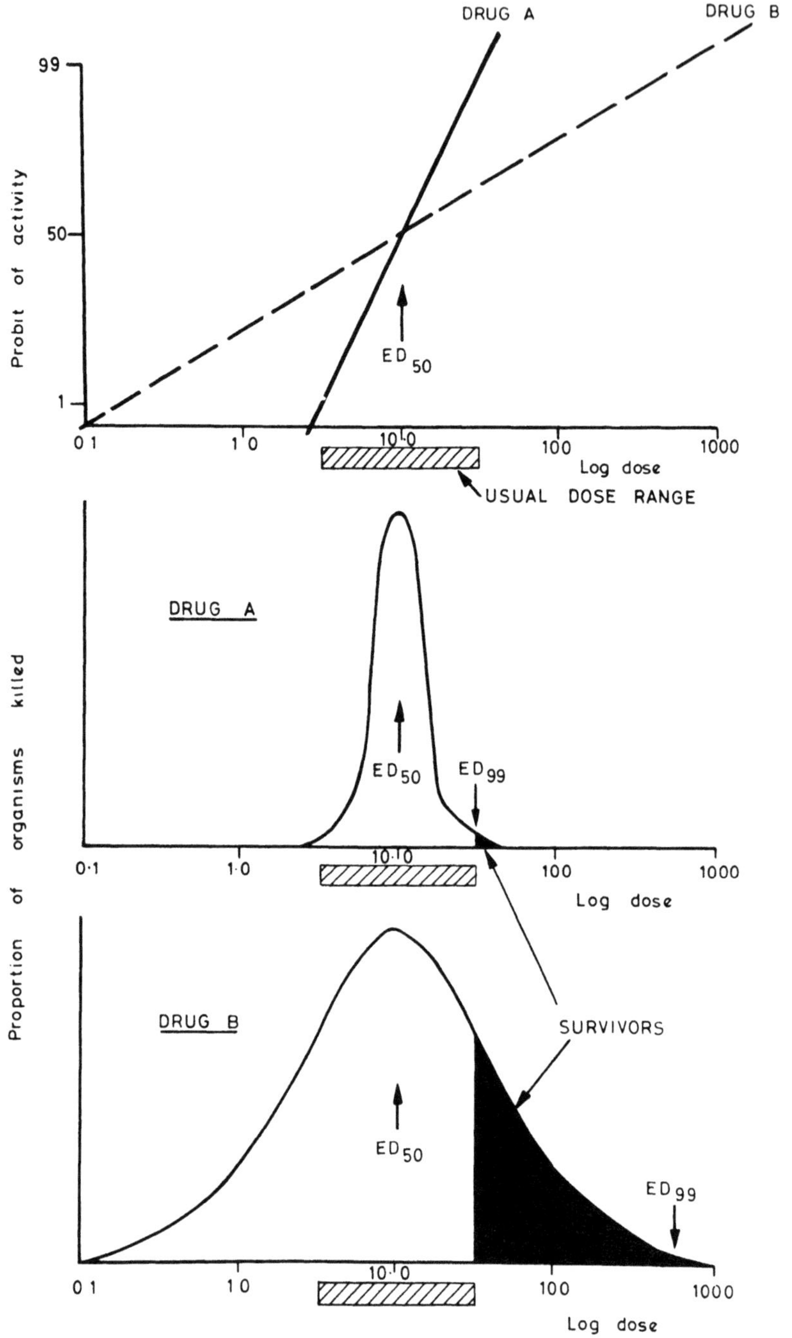


**Fig. 5.** A diagrammatic representation of drug response to two compounds, one (*A*) with a steep dose-activity regression line (e.g. chloroquine), and the other with a shallow dose-activity regression line (e.g. proguanil). Many more parasites can survive a smaller dose increase of drug *B* than of drug *A*. In the latter case host immunity may destroy the few survivors but the chances of this happening with drug *B* are less. Reproduced by permission from PETERS (1969)

been confirmed by the in vitro macro test (PALMER et al. 1976). In the Sudan OMER (1978) and KOUZNETSOV et al. (1979) found a similar suggestion of a slight decrease in response to chloroquine in vivo, and the latter workers pointed out that in the Sennar area the mean parasite-clearance time was unusually prolonged. While their in vitro micro test data were considered inconclusive because of the lack of comparative data from the same test in other areas, it did appear that a low level of chloroquine resistance was present in the blood of some patients. Whether this represents, as in Ethiopia, an inherent difference in drug susceptibility of the local falciparum strains or an acquired resistance in the face of drug-selection pressure will only be determined in the light of future experience.

The situation in West Africa is also uncertain at the present time but, at least in Nigeria *P. falciparum* appears still to be chloroquine sensitive (ADEROUNMU et al. 1981). No absolutely convincing case report of chloroquine resistance has been published to date although several suggestive reports have appeared (e.g. EBISAWA et al. 1979; EKE 1979). Nevertheless, for the time being chloroquine remains the drug of choice for the therapy of acute falciparum malaria in Africa (BRUCE-CHWATT and PETERS 1979). Failure to take the drugs is a far more likely cause of "drug failure" than true drug resistance (BROHULT et al. 1979).

## III. Dihydrofolate Reductase Inhibitors

The two antifols that have been most widely used for malaria prophylaxis are proguanil and pyrimethamine. Chlorproguanil is a halogenated analogue of proguanil that has a significantly longer half-life and that was recommended for single weekly (as opposed to daily) prophylactic dosage. Pyrimethamine has also a long half-life and is generally recommended also as a weekly prophylactic. Since these compounds are plasmodistatic and not plasmodicidal, and hence control established blood infections only slowly, their use alone is restricted to prophylaxis. The members of this group share additional activities, namely a sporontocidal action against the mosquito stages of all species and a causal prophylactic action against the pre-erythrocytic stages of *P. falciparum*.

Resistance to proguanil was first produced in a human volunteer infected with *P. vivax* by LOURIE and SEATON (1949), and subsequently in this species and in *P. falciparum* (ADAMS and SEATON 1949) by these and other workers. In 1949 the first field reports of proguanil resistance in *P. falciparum* arrived from Malaya (FIELD and EDESON 1949) and India (CHAUDHURI and CHAUDHURI 1949). In 1952 GUNTHER et al. found proguanil resistance in *P. vivax* in New Guinea, and other strains were later reported from India and Malaya. *P. malariae* was first found resistant to proguanil in Indonesia in 1952 (VAN GOOR and LODENS 1950). However, numerous workers even before that had remarked that *P. malariae* responded significantly more slowly than other infections to *treatment* with proguanil. (This is not surprising in the light of the mode of action of the antifols, which is to block the parasites during early schizogony, an event that occurs only once in 72 h in *P. malariae*.) A similar comment was made by SCHNEIDER et al. (1948), who found that in Tunisia and Morocco proguanil was most effective against *P. falciparum*, less against *P. vivax* and least against *P. malariae*. The first significant report of the failure of proguanil prophylaxis in an African (Lagos) strain of *P. falciparum* was that of COVELL et al. (1949) in neurosyphilitics. The prophylactic daily dose of proguanil, 100 mg, was established from the work of FAIRLEY (1946). In the Lagos area this dose, which initially was highly successful, later appeared to be less so, and NICOL (1953) recommended that 200 mg daily would be better than 100 mg. Since that time there have been numerous reports of the failure of daily proguanil prophylaxis (100 mg) to prevent the development of *P. falciparum*, but very few well-documented case histories. The real incidence of proguanil prophylactic resistance appears to be in doubt, but many British authorities retain a firm belief in the continuing efficacy of this compound as a prophylactic against falciparum malaria.

There are, however, several pieces of evidence that indicate another view. In Vietnam BLACK (1973) showed clearly that proguanil alone was *not* adequate to prevent infection with multiple drug-resistant *P. falciparum*, but that a combination of proguanil with dapsone was far more effective (see Part II, Chap. 6). [Recently RAY et al. (1979) have demonstrated a potentiating effect between proguanil and dapsone on chloroquine-resistant *P. berghei*.] In a number of clinical trials with the repository formulation of cycloguanil (which is the active metabolite of proguanil) (under the code name CI 501) in Africa, in Pakistan and in New Guinea proguanil failed to control infection in patients in whom *P. falciparum* breakthroughs occurred (see review in PETERS 1970a). Moreover, chlorproguanil failed to control falciparum infection in school children in a prophylactic trial in Nigeria (DODGE 1967). There must now be little doubt that resistance to proguanil used as a prophylactic against *P. falciparum* and *P. vivax* is very widespread geographically, although resistance may be focal in any given country. Doubling the daily dose to 200 mg is believed by some to overcome the problem but, as stated above, good documentary data are lacking. One major problem is that most strains of *P. falciparum* that display resistance to chloroquine exhibit also resistance both to proguanil and to pyrimethamine. A reason for this was proposed by PETERS et al. (1973), who drew attention to the possible common mechanisms of survival by parasites that have the ability to resist the action of both chloroquine and an antifol, e.g. pyrimethamine. In both cases the host cell appears to be stimulated to produce more of the basic metabolites that are required by the parasites and of which they otherwise be deprived through the intervention of the drug.

Pyrimethamine resistance has followed a similar history to that against proguanil. Strains of *P. vivax, P. malariae,* and then *P. falciparum* in human volunteers were made resistant to pyrimethamine by COATNEY et al. (1952); YOUNG (1957), and BURGESS and YOUNG (1959). "Natural" resistance of *P. vivax* and *P. malariae* was first found in Kenya in 1952 and 1953 by AVERY JONES (1954, 1958) and in Malaysia in 1952 (WILSON 1952), and of *P. falciparum* in West Africa in 1952 by MCGREGOR and SMITH. Since then numerous reports have appeared from every country and today pyrimethamine resistance appears to be a major problem everywhere. As noted above, multiple drug resistance with chloroquine is the rule, with the consequence that pyrimethamine used alone is of very little value wherever chloroquine resistant *P. falciparum* is present. Of the two commonly used prophylactic antifols, a number of authorities believe that proguanil has retained most value. However, there is an increasing tendency today to recommend antifol-sulphonamide combinations rather than antifols alone, a point that is discussed at length in Part II, Chap. 16).

## IV. Primaquine and Other 8-Aminoquinolines

The only 8-aminoquinoline in common use today is primaquine, but it is likely that new compounds in this class will be developed for clinical trial in the near future (see Part II, Chap. 10). Primaquine is indicated for two purposes. The first of these is as a radical curative agent in *P. vivax* infections. Whether the drug destroys hypnozoites in hepatocytes, or some other relapsing but dormant stage of the parasite, is currently under investigation. What does appear to be proven is that the radical curative dose is a function of the total drug dosage. The normally recommended dosage of 15 mg base daily for 14 successive days which produces a radical cure in the great majority of infections in most areas other than the southwest Pacific (BLACK 1958) can be replaced in certain individuals who tolerate the drug by double the dosage given in half the time (CLYDE and McCARTHY 1977). However, primaquine is poorly tolerated by many people, and particularly by those with G6PD deficiency who may develop a severe haemolytic anaemia, or with congenital NADH methaemoglobin reductase deficiency who may become methaemoglobinaemic. In the light of the remarkably brief half-life of primaquine in man (FLETCHER, cited in BRUCE-CHWATT et al. 1981) it is difficult to understand how this dose-time relationship operates unless possibly the drug or a metabolite accumulate in the parasites themselves or their host cells up to an effective plateau level, a point yet to be investigated.

There are several reports indicating that the sensitivity of *P. vivax* exoerythrocytic stages to primaquine varies significantly from area to area. The relative insensitivity of the so-called Chesson strain, originally isolated in a patient infected in New Guinea, was first recorded by ALVING et al. (1959). More recently it has been suggested that some strains of *P. vivax* in Thailand are less responsive to primaquine than anticipated (CHAROENLARP and HARINASUTA 1973) and that the response is not dissimilar from that of the Chesson strain (HARINASUTA et al. 1976). Eighty per cent of infections relapse after 5 and 30% after 14 day's treatment with primaquine. In India, where there was a massive resurgence of malaria transmission from 1965 onwards, several reports indicated that the old 5-day regimen of primaquine that had proved highly effective as a radical curative regimen in the early days of the Indian National Malaria Eradication Programme was no longer producing more than about 90% cures, and CONTACOS et al. (1973) noted that a West Pakistan strain of *P. vivax* in volunteers relapsed in all five volunteers who received only a 5-day course. It must be remembered that, in the Indian epidemic, many of the population had had time to lose their hard-gained immunity to *P. vivax* in the years between the pre-eradication days and 1965 onwards. Hence they were responding to therapy just as would non-immune volunteers. Under these circumstances it is remarkable that at least 90% were apparently cured on only a 5-day course of primaquine, an observation documented recently by Indian workers [e.g. ROY et al. (1977) reported a mere 1.3% relapse rate in Tamil Nadu at the end of a 1-year follow-up of 8 329 patients].

Several reports indicate that 8-aminoquinolines are less effective as blood schizontocides against chloroquine-resistant strains of *P. falciparum* than against chloroquine-sensitive ones (a somewhat academic exercise, since the 8-aminoquinolines available so far are too toxic to be used as blood schizontocides). MOORE and LANIER (1961) reported that primaquine was ineffective against their Colombian strain. POWELL (1965) observed that WIN 5037 had no effect on asexual parasitaemia of a Thai strain, while POWELL et al. (1964) found that another 8-aminoquinoline, BW 377C54, was ineffective against other Southeast Asian strains. A number of reports and several years of bitter experience bear witness to the failure of the prophylactic use of a mixture of 300 mg chloroquine base with 45 mg primaquine base administered once weekly (the famous CP tablet) to protect US troops during the Vietnam war. The report of EPPES et al. (1967) clearly demonstrated the failure of this regimen to protect volunteers against sporozoite challenge with two Vietnamese strains. However, RIECKMANN et al. (1968 b) showed convincingly that a single 45-mg dose of primaquine would render gametocytes of these strains non-infective to anophelines for several days, thus offering a means of minimising the transmission of infective chloroquine-resistant gametocytes in the continuing presence of the vectors.

## D. Future Problems and Prospects

While this topic will be dealt with at some length in the final chapters of this book, it is appropriate to consider several points in the present context.

### I. Biological Factors in the Dissemination of Chloroquine Resistance

Drug resistance as a general rule carries with it certain biological disadvantages, for example slower division time, so that the removal of drug pressure permits drug-sensitive organisms in a mixture of drug-sensitive and drug-resistant organisms to overgrow and replace the resistant ones. Thus, for example, CLYDE and SHUTE (1959) found that pyrimethamine resistance in *P. falciparum* had almost disappeared some 26 months following withdrawal of chemoprophylaxis after it had been shown to be present in a high proportion of school children who had received pyrimethamine prophylaxis up to that point. Early experimental data in *P. berghei* indicated that the high level of chloroquine resistance produced by slowly increasing drug-selection pressure was initially very unstable (PETERS 1965), but subsequent studies in inherently resistant organisms such as *P. yoelii* 17X (WARHURST and KILLICK-KENDRICK 1967) and the NS lines of *P. berghei* (PETERS et al. 1978) showed that, in these, chloroquine resistance is a stable, cyclically transmissible character. All the evidence indicates that chloroquine resistance in *P. falciparum* too is stable both in Nature and in vitro (NGUYEN-DINH and TRAGER 1978).

Chloroquine-resistant *P. berghei* and *P. yoelii* respond paradoxically to chloroquine in that infections from chloroquine-treated mice are transmitted through anophelines more readily than gametocytes of the same lines from untreated animals. This observation was first reported by RAMKARAN and PETERS (1969). More significantly, similar findings were obtained by WILKINSON et al. (1976) in chloroquine-resistant *P. falciparum* transmitted through *A. balabacensis* in Thailand. Viewed from the point of view of the population dynamics of *P. falciparum* in a country were chloroquine is still in use, the implication is that the continuing use of this and related blood schizontocides may actually favour a geographical spread of chloroquine resistance. A second biologically favourable factor has been demonstrated by ROSARIO et al. (1978), who showed that, in mice infected with a mixture of chloroquine-sensitive and chloroquine-resistant *P. chabaudi,* the resistant parasites overgrew the sensitive ones. It remains to be seen whether the same applies to *P. falciparum.*

### II. The Geographical Extension of Chloroquine Resistance in *P. falciparum*

Whatever the reasons may be, there is no doubt that chloroquine-resistant strains of *P. falciparum* are extending their geographical boundaries wherever conditions permit the continuation of malaria transmission. In the Americas resistant strains have long since been identified in Panama (WHO 1967). The presence of resistant *P. falciparum* has been proven in isolated foci in East Africa, and there are increasing anxieties about the possibility of the establishment of such strains in West Africa (see above) although proof there is still lacking. However, the potential for West African *P. falciparum* to become resistant to chloroquine has been established. In Southeast Asia resistance has now been confirmed from several parts of the northeastern States of India as well as Bangladesh and as far south in India as Orissa State (GUHA et al. 1979). Resistant strains have spread over the Vietnamese border into adjacent parts of the People's Republic of China and Hainan Island. In the southwest Pacific, parts of Sabah, Kalimantan, and Sumatra, West Iran and Papua New Guinea are involved. In the older-established areas such as Thailand the proportion of chloroquine-resistant to chloroquine-sensitive strains of *P. falciparum* has greatly increased over the past decade. In Thailand, for example, it was estimated (COLWELL et al. 1972) that 26% of 57 falciparum infections were resistant to chloroquine at the RI level, 63% at the RII and 7% at the RIII level (reinfections could not be excluded in this series). At least 2.5–3.5 nmol chloroquine/ml blood were required to stop falciparum erythrocytic schizogony in 12 of 14 Thai patients with RI infections and 4 nmol in two with RII infections (SUCHARIT et al. 1977; SUCHARIT and EAMSOBHANA 1980). Most ominously, reports have now been confirmed indicating that resistance has also arisen to the combination of sulphadoxine with pyrimethamine (Fansidar), which until now has been one of the mainstays for prophylaxis and treatment in areas where chloroquine resistance is prevalent. Of 30 Thai children given Fansidar alone for acute falciparum malaria only 23 were cured, 5 showing an RI and 2 an RII response (CHONGSUPHAJAISIDDHI et al. 1979). DIXON et al. (1982) reported a poor therapeutic response to Fansidar in Thai marines, while BLACK et al. (1981) obtained an RIII response in a Vietnamese refugee who was possibly infected in West Malaysia. As mentioned earlier, there are hints also that some resistance to mefloquine is also being encountered among refugees on the Thai-Kampuchean border.

## E. Conclusion

While this is not the appropriate forum for a lengthy discussion on the future of malaria control, several basic principles must be stated. These are:

1. Malaria parasites have a remarkable ability to overcome any drug that is directed against them.
2. No new drugs are available today that are likely to last more then a few years before resistance to them emerges *if they are deployed alone*. Even combinations of two drugs are at risk.
3. The reliance solely on chemoprophylaxis or therapy for malaria control is doomed to failure. Nevertheless, a completely new generation of antimalarial drugs is urgently needed.
4. All possible measures of malaria control should be thrown into the fight against malaria. These include the use of vaccines for immunoprophylaxis and of insecticides against larval and adult vectors.
5. Research is urgently needed to find out how parasites become resistant to the various drugs and how to overcome or slow down this phenomenon.

A number of these points are taken up elsewhere in this book (e.g. Part II, Chaps. 6, 16).

## References

Adams ARD, Seaton DR (1949) Resistance to paludrine developed by a strain of *Plasmodium falciparum*. Trans R Soc Trop Med Hyg 42:314–315

Aderounmu AF, Salako LA, Walker O (1981) Chloroquine sensitivity of *Plasmodium falciparum* in Ibadan, Nigeria: II. correlation of in vitro and in vivo sensitivity. Trans R Soc Trop Med Hyg 75:637–640

Alving AS, Rucker K, Flanagan CL, Carson PE, Schrier SL, Kellermeyer RW, Tralov AR (1959) Observations on primaquine in the prophylaxis and cure of vivax malaria. Proc 6th int congr trop med malar, Lisbon 5–13 Sep 1958. Vol 7, pp 203–209. Anais Inst Med Trop 16:Suppl. II

Armstrong JC, Asfaha W, Palmer TT (1976) Chloroquine sensitivity of *Plasmodium falciparum* in Ethiopia, I. Results of an in vivo test. Am J Trop Med Hyg 25:2–9

Arnold J, Alving AS, Clayman CB (1961) Induced primaquine resistance in vivax malaria. Trans R Soc Trop Med Hyg 55:345–350

Aronsson B, Bengtsson E, Björkman A, Pehrson PI, Rombo L, Wahlgren M (1981) Chloroquine-resistant falciparum malaria in Madagascar and Kenya. Ann Trop Med Parasitol 75:367–373

Avery Jones S (1954) Resistance of *P. falciparum* and *P. malariae* to pyrimethamine (Daraprim) following mass treatment with this drug. A preliminary note. East Afr Med J 31:47–49

Avery Jones S (1958) Mass treatment with pyrimethamine: a study of resistance and cross resistance resulting from a field trial in the hyperendemic malarious area of Makueni, Kenya, Sept 1952–Sept 1953. Trans R Soc Trop Med Hyg 52:547–561

Black F, Bygbjerg I, Effersøe P, Gomme G, Jepsen S, Jensen GA (1981) RIII Fansidar resistant falciparum malaria acquired in Southeast Asia. Trans R Soc Trop Med Hyg 75:715–716

Black RH (1958) Results of the clinical use of primaquine for the eradication of relapsing vivax malaria of south-west Pacific origin. Australas Ann Med 7:259

Black RH (1973) Malaria in the Australian army in South vietnam: successful use of a proguanil-dapsone combination for chemoprophylaxis of chloroquine-resistant falciparum malaria. Med J Aust 1:1265–1270

Brohult J, Hedman P, Rombo L, Sirleaf V, Bengtsson E (1979) Habits of malaria chemoprophylaxis and an analysis of breakdowns in a West African mining town. Ann Trop Med Parasitol 73:327–331

Bruce-Chwatt LJ, Peters W (1979) Chloroquine-resistant *Plasmodium falciparum* in Africa. Br Med J II:1374–1375

Bruce-Chwatt LJ, Black RH, Canfield CJ, Clyde DF, Peters W, Wernsdorfer W (1981) Chemotherapy of malaria, 2 nd edn. WHO, Geneva

Burgess RW, Young MD (1959) The development of pyrimethamine resistance by *Plasmodium falciparum*. Bull WHO 20:37–46

Campbell CC, Collins WE, Chin W, Teutsch SM, Moss DM (1979) Chloroquine-resistant *Plasmodium falciparum* from East Africa. Lancet II:1151–1154

Charoenlarp P, Harinasuta T (1973) Relapses of vivax malaria after a conventional course of primaquine and chloroquine: report of two cases. Southeast Asian J Trop Med Public Health 4:135–137

Chaudhuri RN, Chaudhuri MN (1949) Falciparum infection refractory to Paludrine. Indian J Malariol 3:365–369

Chongsuphajaisiddhi T, Subchareon A, Puangpartk S, Harinasuta T (1979) Treatment of falciparum malaria in Thai children. Southeast Asian J Trop Med Public Health 10:132–137

Clyde DF, McCarthy VC (1977) Radical cure of Chesson strain vivax malaria in man by seven, not 14, days of treatment with primaquine. Am J Trop Med Hyg 26:562–563

Clyde DF, Shute GT (1959) Survival of pyrimethamine-resistant *Plasmodium falciparum*. Trans R Soc Trop Med Hyg 53:170–172

Coatney GR, Myatt AV, Hernandez T, Jeffrey GM, Cooper WC (1952) Studies on the compound 50–63. Trans R Soc Trop Med Hyg 46:496–508

Colwell EJ, Phintuyothin P, Sadudee N, Benjapong W, Neoypatimandondh S (1972) Evaluation of an in vitro technique for detecting chloroquine-resistant falciparum malaria in Thailand. Am J Trop Med Hyg 21:6–12

Contacos PG, Coatney GR, Collins WE, Briesch PE, Jeter MH (1973) Five-day primaquine therapy: an evaluation of radical curative activity against vivax malaria infection. Am J Trop Med Hyg 22:693–695

Couto M (1908) Les injections endo-veineuses du bleu de méthylène dans le paludisme. Bull Soc Pathol Exot 1:292–295

Covell G, Nicol WD, Shute PG, Maryon M (1949) Studies on a West African strain of *Plasmodium falciparum*, II. The efficacy of paludrine (Proguanil) as a therapeutic agent. Trans R Soc Trop Med Hyg 42:465–476

Dennis DT, Doberstyn EB, Sissay A, Tesfai GK (1974) Chloroquine tolerance of Ethiopian strains of *P. falciparum*. Trans R Soc Trop Med Hyg 68:241–245

Dixon KE, Williams RG, Ponsupat T, Pitaktong U, Phintuyothin P (1982) A comparative trial of mefloquine and Fansidar in the treatment of falciparum malaria: failure of Fansidar. Trans R Soc Trop Med Hyg 76:664–667

Dodge JS, (1967) Malaria chemoprophylaxis in four schools in Kaduna, Northern Nigeria. West Afr Med J 16:55–58

Ebisawa I, Muto T, Tanabe S (1979) Chemotherapy of falciparum malaria: regional differences in responsiveness to treatment. Jpn J Exp Med 49:405–412

Eichenlaub D, Pohle HD (1980) Ein Fall von Falciparum-Malaria mit Chloroquine-Resistenz (RI) von den ostafrikanischen Komoren-Inseln. Infection 8:90–91

Eke RE (1979) Possible chloroquine-resistant *Plasmodium falciparum* in Nigeria. Am J Trop Med Hyg 28:1074–1075

Eppes RB, McNamara JV, DeGowin RL, Carson PE, Powell RD (1967) Chloroquine-resistant *Plasmodium falciparum*: protective and hemolytic effects of 4,4′-diaminodiphenylsulfone (DDS) administered daily together with weekly chloroquine and primaquine. Milit Med 132:163–175

Fairley NH (1946) Researches on Paludrine (M 4888) in malaria: an experimental investigation undertaken by the LHQ Medical Research Unit (AIF), Cairns, Australia. Trans R Soc Trop Med Hyg 40:105–151

Field JW, Edeson JFB (1949) Paludrine-resistant falciparum malaria. Trans R Soc Trop Med Hyg 43:233–236

Fogh S, Jepsen S, Effersøe P (1979) Chloroquine-resistant *Plasmodium falciparum* malaria in Kenya. Trans R Soc Trop Med Hyg 73:228–229

Genther CS, Smith CC (1977) Antifolate studies: activities of 40 potential antimalarial compounds against sensitive and chlorguanide triazine-resistant strains of folate-requiring bacteria and *Escherichia coli*. J Med Chem 20:237–243

Glew RH, Collins WE, Miller LH (1978) Selection of increased quinine resistance in *Plasmodium falciparum* in *Aotus* monkeys. Am J Trop Med Hyg 27:9–13

Guha AK, Roy JR, Das S, Roy RG, Pattanayak S (1979) Results of chloroquine sensitivity tests in *Plasmodium falciparum* in Orissa State. Indian J Mes Res [Suppl] 70:40–47

Gunther CEM, Fraser NM, Wright WG (1952) Proguanil and malaria among non-tolerant New Guinea natives. Trans R Soc Trop Med Hyg 46:185–190

Harinasuta T, Migasen S, Boonag D (1962) Chloroquine resistance in *Plasmodium falciparum* in Thailand. UNESCO 1st regional symposium on scientific knowledge of tropical parasites. 5–9 Nov. 1962, University of Singapore, Singapore, pp 148–153

Harinasuta T, Gilles HM, Sandosham AA (1976) Malaria in Southeast Asia. Southeast Asian J Trop Med Public Health 7:641–678

Howells RE, Peters W, Fullard J (1970) The chemotherapy of rodent malaria, XIII. Fine structural changes observed in the erythrocytic stages of *Plasmodium berghei berghei* following exposure to primaquine and menoctone. Ann Trop Med Parasitol 64:203–207

Jaroonvesama N, Harinasuta T, Muangmanee L (1974) Recrudescence, poor response or resistance to quinine of falciparum malaria in Thailand. Southeast Asian J Trop Med Public Health 5:504–509

Kean BH (1979) Chloroquine-resistant falciparum malaria from Africa. JAMA 241:395

Knight DJ, Williamson P (1980) The antimalarial activity of *N*-benzyl oxydihydrotriazines, II. The development of resistance to clociguanil (BRL 50216) and cycloguanil by *P. berghei*. Ann Trop Med Parasitol 74:407–413

Knight DJ, Williamson P (1982) The antimalarial activity of *N*-benzyl oxydihydrotriazines, IV. The development of resistance to BRL 6231 [4,6-diamino-1,2-2,2-dimethyl-1-(2,4,5,trichloropropyloxy)-1,3,5,-triazine hydrochloride] by *P. berghei*. Ibid 76:9–14

Knight DJ, Mamalis P, Peters W (1982) The antimalarial activity of *N*-benzyl oxydihydrotriazines, III. The activity of 4,6-diamino-1,2-dihydro-2,2-dimethyl-1-(2,4,5-trichloropropyloxy)- 1,3,5,-triazine-hydrobromide (BRL 51084) and hydrochloride (BRL 6231). Ann Trop Med Parasitol 76:1–7

Kouznetsov RL, Rooney W, Wernsdorfer W, El Gaddal AA, Payne D, Abdalla RE (1979) Assessment of the sensitivity of *Plasmodium falciparum* to antimalarial drugs at Sennar, Sudan: use of the in vitro microtechnique and the in vivo method. WHO/MAL/79.910. WHO Cyclostyled Report, Geneva

Kouznetsov RL, Rooney W, Wernsdorfer WH, El Gaddal AA, Payne D, Abdalla RE (1980) Use of the in vitro microtechnique for the assessment of drug sensitivity of *Plasmodium falciparum* in Sennar, Sudan. Bull WHO 58:785–789

Krotoski WA, Krotoski DM, Garnham PCC, Bray RS, Killick-Kendrick R, Draper CC, Targett GAT, Guy MW (1980) Relapses in primate malaria: discovery of two populations of exoerythrocytic stages: preliminary note. Br Med J I:153–154

Laing ABG (1974) Studies on the chemotherapy of malaria, III. Treatment of falciparum malaria in the Gambia, with BRL 50216 [4,6-diamino-(3,4-dichlorobenzyloxy)-1,2,dihydro-2,2-dimethyl -1,3,5,-triazine hydrochloride] alone and in combination with sulphonamides. Trans R Soc Trop Med Hyg 68:133–138

Lourie EM, Seaton DR (1949) Resistance to paludrine developed by a strain of *Plasmodium vivax*. Trans R Soc Trop Med Hyg 42:315

Maberti S (1960) Desarrollo de resistencia a la pirimetamina: presentacion de 15 cases estudiados en Trujilo, Venezuela. Arch Venez Med Trop Parasitol Med 3:239–259

McGregor IA, Smith DA (1952) Daraprim in treatment of malaria: a study of its effects in falciparum and quartan infections in West Africa. Br Med J I:730–734

McNamara JV, Rieckmann KH, Frischer H, Stockert TA, Carson PE, Powell RD (1967) Acquired decrease in sensitivity to quinine observed during studies with a strain of chloroquine-resistant *Plasmodium falciparum*. Ann Trop Med Parasitol 61:386–395

Merkli B, Peters W (1976) A comparison of two different methods for the selection of primaquine resistance in *Plasmodium berghei berghei*. Ann Trop Med Parasitol 70:473–474

Migasena S, Bunnag D, Harinasuta T (1980) A case of *P. falciparum* malaria in Thailand apparently resistant to quinine. Ann Trop Med Parasitol 74:243–244

Moore DV, Lanier JE (1961) Observations on two *Plasmodium falciparum* infections with an abnormal response to chloroquine. Am J Trop Med Hyg 10:5–9

Morbidity Mortality Weekly Report (1978) Chloroquine-resistant malaria acquired in Kenya and Tanzania. Denmark, Georgia, New York, No 47, 27:463–464

Nicol BM (1953) Use and effectiveness of antimalarial drugs: experience of non-native resident populations of Nigeria, West Africa. Br Med J II:177–180

Nguyen-Dinh P, Trager W (1978) Chloroquine resistance produced in vitro in an African strain of human malaria. Science 200:1397–1398

Nocht B, Werner H (1910) Beobachtungen über relative Chininresistenz bei Malaria aus Brasilien. Dtsch Med Wochenschr 36:1557–1560

Omer AHS (1978) Response of *Plasmodium falciparum* in Sudan to oral chloroquine. Am J Trop Med Hyg 27:853–857

Palmer TT, Townley LB, Yigzaw M, Armstrong JC (1976) Chloroquine sensitivity of *Plasmodium falciparum* in Ethiopia, II. Results of an in vitro test. Am J Trop Med Hyg 25:10–13

Pearlman EJ, Doberstyn EB, Sudsok S, Thiemanum W, Kennedy R, Canfield CJ (1980) Chemosuppressive field trials in Thailand IV. The suppression of *Plasmodium falciparum* and *Plasmodium vivax* parasitemias by mefloquine (WR 142490, a 4-quinolinemethanol). Am J Trop Med Hyg 29:1131–1137

Peters W (1965) Drug resistance in *Plasmodium berghei,* Vincke and Lips, 1948, I. Chloroquine resistance. Exp Parasitol 17:80–89

Peters W (1969) Drug resistance in malaria: a perspective. Trans R Soc Trop Med Hyg 63:25–45

Peters W (1970 a) Chemotherapy and drug resistance in malaria. Academic, London

Peters W (1970 b) A new type of antimalarial drug potentiation. Trans R Soc Trop Med Hyg 64:462–464

Peters W (1974) Recent advances in antimalarial chemotherapy and drug resistance. Adv Parasitol 12:69–114

Peters W (1980) Chemotherapy of malaria. In: Kreier JP (ed) Malaria, vol 1. Academic, New York, pp 145–283

Peters W, Porter M (1976) The chemotherapy of rodent malaria, XXVI. The potential value of WR 122455 (a 9-phenanthrenemethanol) against drug-resistant malaria parasites. Ann Trop Med Parasitol 70:271–281

Peters W, Portus JH, Robinson BL (1973) The chemotherapy of rodent malaria, XVII. Dynamics of drug resistance, Part 3: influence of drug combinations on the development of resistance to chloroquine in *P. berghei.* Ann Trop Med Parasitol 67:143–154

Peters W, Portus J, Robinson BL (1975) The chemotherapy of rodent malaria, XXII. The value of drug-resistant strains of *P. berghei* in screening for blood schizontocidal activity. Ann Trop Med Parasitol 69:155–171

Peters W, Portus JH, Robinson BL (1977) The chemotherapy of rodent malaria, XXVIII. The development of resistance to mefloquine (WR 142490). Ann Trop Med Parasitol 71:419–427

Peters W, Chance ML, Lissner R, Momen H, Warhurst DC (1978) The chemotherapy of rodent malaria, XXX. The enigmas of the "NS Lines" of *P. berghei.* Ann Trop Med Parasitol 72:23–36

Petterson T, Kyrönseppä H, Pitkänen T (1981) Chloroquine-resistant falciparum malaria from East Africa. Trans R Soc Trop Med Hyg 75:112–113

Powell RD (1965) The effect of 6-methoxy-8-(5′-propylaminoamylamino)-quinoline phosphate against the asexual erythrocytic forms of a strain of chloroquine-resistant *Plasmodium falciparum* from Thailand. Bull WHO 32:591–593

Powell RD, Brewer GJ, Alving AS, Millar JW (1964) Studies on a strain of chloroquine-resistant *Plasmodium falciparum* from Thailand. Bull WHO 30:29–44

Ramkaran AE, Peters W (1969) Infectivity of chloroquine-resistant *Plasmodium berghei* to *Anopheles stephensi* enhanced by chloroquine. Nature 223:635–636

Ray AP, Parkinson AD, Black RH (1979) Experimental studies on the effect of proguanil and dapsone against chloroquine-resistant *Plasmodium berghei* (ANKA) in white mice. Ann Trop Med Hyg 73:19–22
Rieckmann KH (1971) Drug potentiation against pre-erythrocytic stages of *Plasmodium falciparum*. Trans R Soc Trop Med Hyg 65:533–535
Rieckmann KH (1973) Data in Table 5. In: WHO (1973)
Rieckmann KH, McNamara JV, Frischer H, Stockert TA, Carson PE, Powell RD (1968a) Effects of chloroquine, quinine, and cycloguanil upon maturation of asexual erythrocytic forms of two strains of *Plasmodium falciparum* in vitro. Am J Trop Med Hyg 17:661–671
Rieckmann KH, McNamara JV, Frischer H, Stockert TA, Carson PE, Powell RD (1968b) Gametocytocidal and sporontocidal effects of primaquine and sulfadiazine with pyrimethamine in a chloroquine-resistant strain of *P. falciparum*. Bull WHO 38:625–632
Rieckmann KH, Campbell GH, Sax LJ, Mrema JE (1978) Drug sensitivity of *Plasmodium falciparum*: an in vitro technique. Lancet I:22–23
Rosario VE, Walliker D, Hall R, Beale GH (1978) Persistence of drug-resistant malaria parasites. Lancet I:185–187
Roy RG, Chakrapani KP, Dhinagaran D, Sitaraman NL, Ghosh RB (1977) Efficacy of 5-day radical treatment of *P. vivax* infection in Tamil Nadu. Indian J Med Res 65:652–656
Rozman RS, Canfield CJ (1979) New experimental antimalarial drugs. Adv Pharmacol Chemother 16:1–43
Ryley JF, Peters W (1970) The antimalarial activity of some quinoline esters. Ann Trop Med Parasitol 64:209–222
Schmidt LH (1973) Infections with *Plasmodium falciparum* and *Plasmodium vivax* in the owl monkey: model systems for basic biological and chemotherapeutic studies. Trans R Soc Trop Med Hyg 67:446–474
Schmidt LH (1979) Studies on the 2,4-diamino-6-substituted quinazolines, III. The capacity of sulfadiazine to enhance the activities of WR 158122 and WR 159412 against infections with various drug-susceptible and drug-resistant strains of *Plasmodium falciparum* and *Plasmodium vivax* in owl monkeys. Am J Trop Med Hyg 28:808–818
Schneider J, Decourt P, Méchali D (1948) Nouveaux médicaments du paludisme-étude comparée de leur activité dans le traitement curatif et en prophylaxie. Proc 4th int congr trop med malar, 10–18 May 1948, (Washington) I, pp 756–775. Available from: Department of State, Washington, DC
Sucharit P, Eamsobhana P (1980) In vitro response of *Plasmodium falciparum* in Thailand to antimalarial drugs. Ann Trop Med Hyg 74:11–15
Sucharit P, Harinasuta T, Chongsuphajaisiddhi T, Tongprasoeth N, Kasemsuth R (1977) In vivo and in vitro studies of chloroquine-resistant malaria in Thailand. Ann Trop Med Parasitol 71:401–405
Thompson PE (1972) Studies on a quinolinemethanol (WR 30090) and on a phenanthrene-methanol (WR 33063) against drug-resistant *Plasmodium berghei* in mice. Proc Helminthol Soc Wash [Suppl] 39:297–308
Van Goor WT, Lodens JG (1950) Clinical malarial prophylaxis with proguanil. Doc Neerl Indones Morbis Trop 2:62–81
Warhurst DC, Killick-Kendrick R (1967) Spontaneous resistance to chloroquine in a strain of rodent malaria (*Plasmodium berghei yoelii*). Nature 213:1048–1049
Wernsdorfer WH (1980) Field evaluation of drug resistance in malaria. In vitro micro-test. Acta Trop 37:222–227
Wernsdorfer WH, Kouznetsov RL (1980) Drug-resistant malaria – occurrence, control, and surveillance. Bull WHO 58:341–352
Whiteside EF (1962) Interactions between drugs, trypanosomes, and cattle in the field. In: Goodwin LG, Nimmo-Smith RH (eds) Drugs, parasites, and hosts. Churchill, London, pp 116–141
WHO (1963) Terminology of malaria and of malaria eradication. Report of a Drafting Committee. WHO, Geneva
WHO (1965) Resistance of malaria parasites to drugs. Report of a WHO Scientific Group. WHO Tech Rep Ser No. 296

WHO (1967) Chemotherapy of malaria. WHO Rep Ser No. 375
WHO (1973) Chemotherapy of malaria and resistance to antimalarials. WHO Rep Ser No. 529
Wilkinson RN, Noeypatimanondh S, Gould DJ (1976) Infectivity of falciparum patients for anopheline mosquitoes before and after chloroquine treatment. Trans R Soc Trop Med Hyg 70:306–307
Wilson T (1952) Discussion. In: Symposium on Daraprim. Trans R Soc Trop Med Hyg 46:499–500
Wise DL, Gresser JD, McCormick GJ (1979) Sustained release of a dual antimalarial system. J Pharm Pharmacol 31:210–204
Young MD (1957) Resistance of *Plasmodium malariae* to pyrimethamine (Daraprim). Am J Trop Med Hyg 6:621–624

CHAPTER 17

# Evaluation of Drug Resistance in Man

K. H. RIECKMANN

## A. Introduction

Drug resistance in malaria can be defined as the "ability of a parasite strain to survive and/or multiply despite the administration and absorption of a drug given in doses equal to or higher than those usually recommended but within the limits of tolerance of the subject" (WHO 1967). Although this definition could logically be applied to include all plasmodial stages, it has generally been restricted to describe the drug susceptibility of asexual blood forms, presumably because this stage in the life cycle of the parasite produces the acute clinical symptoms observed during the course of a malaria infection. Resistance of asexual blood forms to drugs has been reported in all species of human plasmodia. However, because of the appearance of chloroquine-resistant infections of falciparum malaria about 2 decades ago, attention has been focused on developing procedures for assessing the response of *Plasmodium falciparum* to chloroquine and other antimalarial drugs.

## B. Evaluation of Drug Resistance In Vivo

### I. Resistance to Chloroquine

The efficacy of a drug against falciparum infections has been determined traditionally by observing whether the level of parasites in the blood stream changes after drug administration and, if clearance occurs, by noting whether there is a subsequent recrudescence of parasitaemia. Soon after the emergence of chloroquine-resistant strains of *P. falciparum*, it became obvious that resistance to chloroquine varied from a level at which the drug had no apparent effect on the course of the infection to one at which the infection responded to treatment but was associated with a recrudescence of parasites 3–4 weeks after treatment. In an effort to standardise the spectrum of response observed in chloroquine-resistant strains of *P. falciparum*, an arbitrary system to grade the level of chloroquine resistance was proposed in 1967 (WHO 1967) and slightly modified in 1973 (WHO 1973).

#### 1. Procedure for Grading Level of Resistance

The WHO Field Test (WHO 1973) consists of the administration of 25 mg chloroquine base/kg body wt. over a period of 3 days and a follow-up observation period of 7 days ("standard test") or 28 days ("extended test") to determine the response of parasites to treatment. As the "standard test" will not detect the presence of low levels of chloroquine resistance, its use should be restricted to circumstances where reinfection is likely within 2 or 3 weeks after drug administration or where it is impossible to carry out follow-up examinations over a period of 4 weeks after treatment with chloroquine. The "alternative test," consisting of the administration of a single dose of 10 mg chloroquine/kg body wt., is sometimes used where treatment cannot be given for 3 days or where a single dose of chloroquine has been accepted as the standard form of treatment.

The procedure involves the following steps:

1. Thick and thin blood films are collected from a patient suspected of having falciparum malaria and examined for the presence of asexual forms of *P. falciparum*.
2. Patients who have taken antimalarial drugs recently, who are severely ill or vomiting, or who have excessively high levels of parasitaemia, mixed species infection or only gametocytes of *P. falciparum*, are excluded from the test.
3. Urine specimens are collected from suitable patients who are willing to participate in the test and examined for the presence of chloroquine and, if possible, for other antimalarials. Patients who are shown to have drugs in their urine are excluded from the test.
4. A record should be kept of the duration of symptoms during the current episode of malaria, the number of previous fever episodes during the past 6 months and the probable location where the infection was acquired. Such information may be helpful in assessing the possible role of immunity in influencing the outcome of the test and in identifying the location of chloroquine-resistant strains of *P. falciparum*.
5. Uncoated chloroquine tablets, conforming to International Pharmacopoeia standards, are administered once on each of three successive days starting on day 0.10 mg chloroquine base on day 0, 10 mg chloroquine base on day 1, and 5 mg chloroquine base on day 2. Individuals who vomit after drug administration should not be used for the test. This risk can be minimised by swallowing the tablets after a light meal.
6. Individuals should be seen daily for 7 days after drug administration. The clinical condition of the patient always takes precedence over the conduct of the test and, if necessary, the clinical attack of malaria should be aborted by the use of alternative drugs such as quinine. Thick and thin blood films should be made each day to determine the concentration of asexual parasites of *P. falciparum*. Thick films are considered negative when careful examination of 100 fields (about 0.1 μl) shows no evidence of asexual parasites. Absorption of chloroquine should be confirmed by examining urine specimens for the presence of the drug 1–3 days after the beginning of treatment.
7. In the "extended test," individuals whose asexual parasitaemia cleared by the end of 7 days are followed up for an additional 21 days. Blood films are examined at least once a week to monitor any recurrence of asexual parasites during this period.

## 2. Interpretation of Tests (see Chap. 16, Fig. 1, p. 424)

1. Absence of asexual parasites by day 6 and 7 after the start of treatment indicates that the infection is either sensitive or resistant at the RI level to the drug. A sensitive (S) response can only be distinguished from an RI level of resistance (delayed recrudescence) by the 28-day observation period of the "extended test," providing there is no opportunity for the individual to be bitten by infected mosquitoes dur-

ing the first 3 weeks of the test. Absence of asexual parasites during these 28 days means that parasites are sensitive to the drug whereas, if parasitaemia reappears during this period of time, reinfection having been excluded, the parasites are resistant at the RI level.

2. Disappearance of asexual parasites for at least two consecutive days after treatment, but reappearance by day 7, is also classified as an RI level of resistance (early recrudescence).

3. Reduction of asexual parasitaemia to 25% or less (but without clearance) of the original pretest level during the first 48 h of treatment indicates that parasites are resistant at the RII level.

4. Reduction of asexual parasites by less than 75%, or an increase in parasitaemia, during the first 48 h of treatment indicates an RIII level of resistance. In these cases, the test should be suspended and the patients given alternative antimalarial therapy appropriate to their clinical condition.

## II. Resistance to Other Antimalarials

The grading system used for chloroquine can also be applied to other antimalarial drugs, if they act as rapidly as chloroquine and other 4-aminoquinolines against asexual erythrocytic blood stages of *P. falciparum.*

This grading can, obviously, not be used to determine the early response to treatment with slower-acting blood schizontocides, such as the tetracyclines or sulphones. Furthermore, assessment of the response of parasites to such drugs, not given in combination with rapidly acting schizontocides, should only be determined in partially immune individuals. Non-immune or acutely ill persons might develop dangerously high levels of parasitaemia before an infection could be brought under effective control (RIECKMANN et al. 1972).

In assessing the efficacy of blood schizontocides with a long duration of activity, patients included in the "extended test" should be followed-up beyond 28 days after drug administration. Drugs belonging to this category include Fansidar (combination of sulfadoxine and pyrimethamine) and mefloquine. The former is widely used for the treatment of chloroquine-resistant infections and the latter is a new drug receiving considerable attention as a promising antimalarial agent (see Part II, Chap. 9). Recrudescences of parasitaemia have been observed between 28 and 42 days after the administration of pyrimethamine and long-acting sulphonamides (personal observations). Late recrudescences can also be anticipated if parasites become resistant to mefloquine, owing to the prolonged suppressive activity of this drug (RIECKMANN et al. 1974).

## III. Disadvantages of In Vivo Evaluation of Drug Resistance

### 1. Variability in Response to Drugs

The response of falciparum infections to drug treatment varies from one individual to another. Some variability in response can be observed when non-immune individuals, infected with the same strain of chloroquine-resistant *P. falciparum*, are treated with antimalarial drugs (POWELL et al. 1964; WALKER and LOPEZ ANTUÑANO 1968). The response to treatment varies more widely, however, when previous exposure to falciparum malaria is taken into account because the immunity acquired by the host tends to supplement the antimalarial activity of the drug (see also Chap. 11). Thus partially immune persons may be cured of infections with strains of *P. falciparum* which show an RI level of resistance in non-immunes. The response of fever and parasitaemia to treatment is often more rapid and complete in individuals living in endemic areas than in those living in non-endemic areas (WHO 1967). For example, in a study involving patients with drug-resistant falciparum malaria in Brazil, it was noted that clearance of parasitaemia and lack of subsequent recrudescences occurred more frequently when chloroquine was administered during the later stages of an infection than when it was given during the earlier stages (WALKER and LOPEZ ANTUÑANO 1968). In another study in Brazil, individuals who had experienced symptoms suggestive of malaria for a short period of time were, in general, less responsive to treatment (RII response) than those who had experienced them for a longer time (RI or S response). The virtual absence of gametocytes in individuals with an RII response suggested that they had acquired their infections recently and that they had, consequently, developed a lower level of immunity to their infections than their counterparts with an RI or S response (RIECKMANN and LOPEZ ANTUÑANO 1971). In a study in Colombia, chloroquine resistance was detected only in children, presumably because adults living in this endemic area had had more time to acquire a level of immunity which was sufficiently marked to cure them of their infection after treatment with chloroquine (COMER et al. 1968). In many areas of high endemicity in Africa where strains are still susceptible to chloroquine, a single dose of chloroquine (10 mg/kg) has been accepted as the standard form of treatment because the elevated level of immunity in the population does not necessitate administration of the usual dose (25 mg/kg) of the drug.

### 2. Prolonged Follow-up of Patients After Drug Administration

Follow-up of patients for 1–4 weeks after drug administration often poses a problem because patients do not want to submit to further examination after they feel better. Asymptomatic individuals also frequently change their mind regarding continued participation in a study, particularly in the "extended test," because they do not want to be interrupted from pursuing their normal activities. Consequently, the proportion of individuals available for complete follow-up can be disappointingly low if inadequate precautions have been taken in selecting participants for the study.

### 3. Uncertainty Concerning the Retention and Absorption of Drug

Necessary observations to monitor that the drug is swallowed and retained after drug administration are sometimes not carried out. Individual variation in the absorption or metabolism of a drug raises further uncertainty concerning the reliability and reproducibility of test results to determine the drug susceptibility of parasites of *P. falciparum*.

Examination of urine specimens for the presence of the drug will confirm that the entire medication was not vomited after being administered to the patient. As the tests are usually qualitative, the results will not indicate any deficiencies in the absorption or metabolism of a drug. Quantitative serum or erythrocyte levels of the drug are also not necessarily useful in comparing the drug susceptibility of parasites between different individuals (RIECKMANN and LOPEZ ANTUÑANO 1971).

#### 4. Difficulty in Distinguishing Between Sensitive and Resistant Strains in Endemic Areas

Low levels of emerging drug resistance cannot be confirmed in areas with continuous malaria transmission. Recurrence of parasitaemia within a few weeks after drug administration provides only presumptive evidence of a drug-resistant infection in areas where reinfection cannot be ruled out. This means that a drug-sensitive (S) infection can only be differentiated from a drug-resistant (RI) infection by isolating an individual in a mosquito-free environment for a few weeks or carrying out follow-up observations in a non-endemic area known to be free of malaria transmission. These requirements limit the circumstances under which testing for drug susceptibility can be carried out and, therefore, represent an important disadvantage in determining the presence of drug-resistant strains of *P. falciparum*.

## C. Evaluation of Drug Resistance In Vitro

### I. Macrotechnique Using Venous Blood Specimens

The problem associated with the in vivo determination of the drug susceptibility of parasites of *P. falciparum* led to the development of a simple in vitro test which could be performed using a single specimen of venous blood (RIECKMANN et al. 1968). The test measured the extent to which maturation of ring forms to schizonts was inhibited after incubation of parasitised blood at various drug concentrations for a period of 24 h. In this short-term culture system, a marked difference in the maturation of sensitive and resistant parasites was observed in the presence of drug plasma levels comparable to those observed after administration of the drug in vivo. Evaluation of this technique under laboratory and field conditions proved that it was a quick and reliable method for estimating the presence, prevalence or degree of chloroquine resistance found in various areas of the world (RIECKMANN and LOPEZ ANTUÑANO 1971; PETERS and SEATON 1971; COLWELL et al. 1972; RIECKMANN 1972; VALERA and SHUTE 1975; PALMER et al. 1976; EBISAWA et al. 1976; SUCHARIT et al. 1977). The test has been adopted as a standard in vitro method for determining the susceptibility of parasites of *P. falciparum* to chloroquine, and test kits to carry out this procedure are available from the World Health Organization (WHO 1979).

#### 1. Procedure

The procedure involves the following steps:

1. Preliminary examination of patients suspected of having falciparum malaria should follow steps 1–3 outlined under Sect. B.I.1. In addition, patients with predominantly *young* ring forms, or parasite counts exceeding 80000/mm$^3$, should be excluded from the test.

2. About 10 ml blood are collected from the patient, transferred immediately to a sterile 25- or 50-ml Erlenmeyer flask containing glass beads and defibrinated by rotation of the flask for 5 min.
3. One-millilitre aliquots of blood are placed into sterile, screw-capped, flat-bottomed glass vials (1.5 cm internal diameter) that contain glucose (5 mg) and either no drug (control) or various amounts of drug.
4. Blood in the vials is swirled gently to mix the contents well, the caps are unscrewed about half a turn and the vials are then placed in an incubator or water bath at 38°–40 °C for a period of about 24 h.
5. After incubation, vials are shaken to resuspend erythrocytes in plasma, then thick films are prepared and stained for 20 min with 5% Giemsa stain (pH 7.0).
6. Inhibition of the maturation of ring forms to normal-appearing schizonts by the drug is determined by comparing the degree of maturation in control samples with that in samples containing various concentrations of the drug. The percentage of ring forms that mature to normal-appearing schizonts containing more than two nuclei is determined by microscopic examination and provides a useful end point for quantitative assessment of maturation. It is customary to examine at least 200 asexual parasites per sample and to express results by dividing the number of schizonts per 100 parasites in a sample containing drug by the corresponding value observed in the control samples. For example, 20% of parasites were able to mature to schizonts, relative to the control, if the drug sample contained 12 schizonts/100 parasites and the control sample contained 60 schizonts/100 parasites.

## 2. Resistance to Chloroquine

The in vitro susceptibility of different strains of *P. falciparum* to chloroquine has been studied more thoroughly and extensively than that to other antimalarial drugs. The results of some of these investigations are shown in Fig. 1. As comparative in vitro-in vivo testing was carried out in a few studies, it is now possible to relate the parasite susceptibility in vitro to the response of non-immune individuals treated with chloroquine. Complete inhibition of schizont formation at a concentration of 1.0 nmol chloroquine/ml blood indicates infection with chloroquine-sensitive parasites, whereas chloroquine-resistant parasites show maturation to schizonts at this concentration of the drug. Maturation to schizonts is often observed up to 1.5 or 2.0 nmol chloroquine/ml blood with an RI level of resistance, up to 2.5 or 3.0 nmol with an RII level of resistance and from 4.0 to 8.0 nmol with an RIII level of resistance.

In recording the maturation of ring forms to schizonts at different concentrations of chloroquine, it has been customary to plot regression lines for comparing the chloroquine susceptibility of *P. falciparum* from different malarious areas. Detailed microscopic examination of parasite maturation at each concentration of chloroquine and the recording of results involves much time and effort. Satisfactory evaluation of the relative drug susceptibilities of parasites should be possible just by scanning the blood films and noting the concentrations of drug at which inhibition of schizonts is complete ($ED_{100}$) and almost complete ($ED_{95}$). Such a procedure would simplify the performance, evaluation and statistical analysis of a large number of in vitro tests.

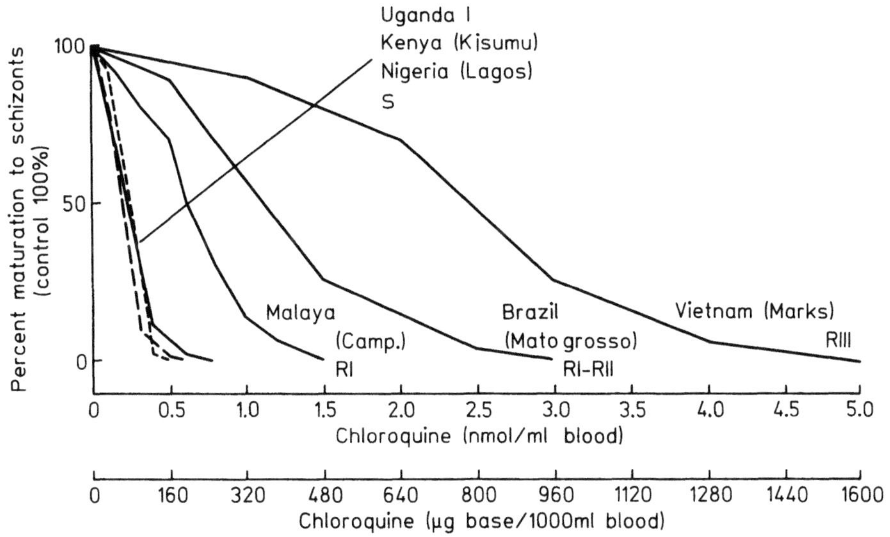


**Fig. 1.** Susceptibility of some isolates of *P. falciparum* to chloroquine in vitro. (Reproduced by permission from WHO 1973)

In areas where both *P. falciparum* and *P. malariae* are prevalent, findings obtained with the in vitro test must be interpreted with caution (RIECKMANN 1972). "Unidentified" young ring forms of *P. malariae* (easily confused with more mature *P. falciparum* rings) may mature to schizonts at chloroquine concentrations which invariably prevent schizogony of chloroquine-sensitive parasites of *P. falciparum*. In mixed infections, with only a few *P. malariae* parasites, the mistaken diagnosis of chloroquine resistance can only be avoided by a careful search for typical *P. malariae* parasites in pre- and postculture thick and thin blood films.

## 3. Resistance to Other Antimalarial Drugs

### a) Amodiaquine

The effects of amodiaquine upon the morphological appearance of parasites of *P. falciparum* is identical to that of chloroquine. The most striking effect of both these 4-aminoquinolines is an inhibition of maturation at successively earlier stages of development as ring forms are exposed to increasing concentrations of these drugs. Mole for mole, the activity of amodiaquine in vitro is greater than that of chloroquine against a strain of *P. falciparum* with a high level of resistance to chloroquine. This was subsequently also shown to be the case in vivo (RIECKMANN 1971).

### b) Quinine

The effects of quinine upon the morphological appearance of parasites are similar to those observed with the 4-aminoquinolines (RIECKMANN et al. 1968). In chloroquine-sensitive strains, the amount of quinine required to inhibit the maturation of schizonts is about ten times greater than the amount of chloroquine needed to produce a similar effect. A tenfold difference in plasma levels is also observed in patients treated with either quinine or chloroquine.

c) Mefloquine

The new antimalarial drug, mefloquine (WR 142490), exerts a similar in vitro effect upon the morphology of parasites as observed with chloroquine in this test. However, it is considerably more effective than chloroquine, both in vitro and in vivo, against strains of *P. falciparum* with a high level of resistance to chloroquine (RIECKMANN et al. 1974).

d) Dihydrofolate Reductase Inhibitors

The effects of dihydrofolate reductase (DHFR) inhibitors, such as cycloguanil and pyrimethamine, upon the maturation of parasites are different from the afore mentioned drugs (RIECKMANN et al. 1968). In contrast to the effect of these drugs, even large amounts of the DHFR inhibitors do not prevent maturation of ring forms to trophozoites. The most conspicuous effect of DHFR inhibitors is the formation of abnormal-appearing parasites (RIECKMANN et al. 1968). This had been noted previously after patients were treated with proguanil, presumably because parasites weres exposed to the dihydrotriazine metabolite of the drug (BLACK 1946; MACKERRAS and ERCOLE 1948). After exposure to DHFR inhibitors, the chromatin of parasites, instead of dividing normally to form schizonts, is split into indistinct fragments of varying size and shape. The difference in susceptibility to DHFR inhibitors between drug-sensitive and drug-resistant strains is usually much greater than that observed with other antimalarial drugs.

e) Drugs Which Show no Activity In Vitro

Maturation of parasites is not affected by the addition of drugs which exert antimalarial activity only after metabolic transformation by the host. Thus proguanil shows no activity in vitro, but its dihydrotriazine metabolite, cycloguanil, shows a marked DHFR inhibitor effect upon maturing parasites. This feature of the in vitro test could be used to appraise the relative antimalarial activity of a parent compound with that of its metabolites.

Determination of the susceptibility of parasites to some slow-acting drugs, such as the sulphonamides, sulphones, and tetracyclines, is also not possible in this short-term in vitro system, which cannot support parasite maturation in excess of 30 h. If a slow-acting drug does not exert its activity through its metabolite(s), it should be possible to determine the drug's antimalarial activity by the in vitro microtechnique (see below). As this technique can support parasite growth through one or more complete life cycles, the effects of a slow-acting drug can be studied over a longer period of time.

## II. Microtechnique Using Capillary Blood Specimens

The recent introduction of a microtechnique for assessing the drug susceptibility of *P. falciparum* (RIECKMANN et al. 1978) has made it easier to carry out susceptibility testing in young children. The decreased volume of blood required for this technique means that specimens can now be collected by fingerprick rather than by venepuncture. In contrast to the macrotechnique, parasites are able to mature to schizonts when counts exceed 80 000/µl and, as parasites do not degenerate when incubated for longer than 30 h, the period of incubation can be extended to enable young rings to develop into schizonts (RIECKMANN 1980). The period of incubation can be prolonged up to 48 h, without changing medium, to study the effect of the drug on parasite reinvasion of erythrocytes (YISUNSRI and RIECKMANN 1980).

### 1. **Procedure** (see Fig. 2)

The procedure involves the following steps:
1. Preliminary examination of patients suspected of having falciparum malaria should follow steps 1–4 outlined under Sect. B.I.1.
2. From the tip of a finger 50–100 µl of blood is collected and transferred immediately into presterilised plastic vials containing 0.5–1.0 ml recently prepared sterile culture medium. The medium consists of powdered RPMI 1640 (10.4 mg/ml), sodium bicarbonate (2 mg/ml), HEPES buffer (6 mg/ml) and gentamicin sulphate (4 µg/ml).
3. The blood-medium (1:10) mixture should then be transferred in 50-µl quantities to flat-bottomed wells (diameter, 6.5 mm) of a plastic microculture plate containing various concentrations of the drug.
4. If necessary, the blood-medium mixture can be transported to the laboratory in the vials, keeping the vials fairly close to body temperature (e.g. in shirt pocket) during transportation, and transferring the blood-medium mixture to the culture plates within 6 h of collection of the blood specimens.
5. The plate, covered with a lid, is then agitated gently and placed in a jar containing a pure paraffin candle and a damp sponge. After lighting the candle, the greased lid of the jar is screwed on tightly and the culture plate incubated at 37 °C for 24–48 h. The duration of incubation will vary depending on the maturity of rings at the start of culture and the maturity of parasites desired at the end of culture.
6. After incubation, about 30 µl supernatant culture medium is removed from each well and thick films are prepared from the sediment.
7. Giemsa-stained thick films are examined for parasite maturation. As a higher proportion of ring forms mature to schizonts than is observed in the macrotechnique, it is usually sufficient to count only 100 asexual parasites to obtain an accurate estimate of the extent of maturation. Results may be expressed as described previously in this section. However, as noted above, performance and analysis of a large number of tests could be simplified by simply determining the lowest concentration of the drug in which the formation of normal schizonts is inhibited by more than 95% and 100% of that observed in the control wells.

### 2. Advantages and Applications of Test

#### a) Comparison to Macrotechnique

Following the initial laboratory studies with two strains of *P. falciparum* (RIECKMANN et al. 1978), a number of studies have shown the value of this technique in

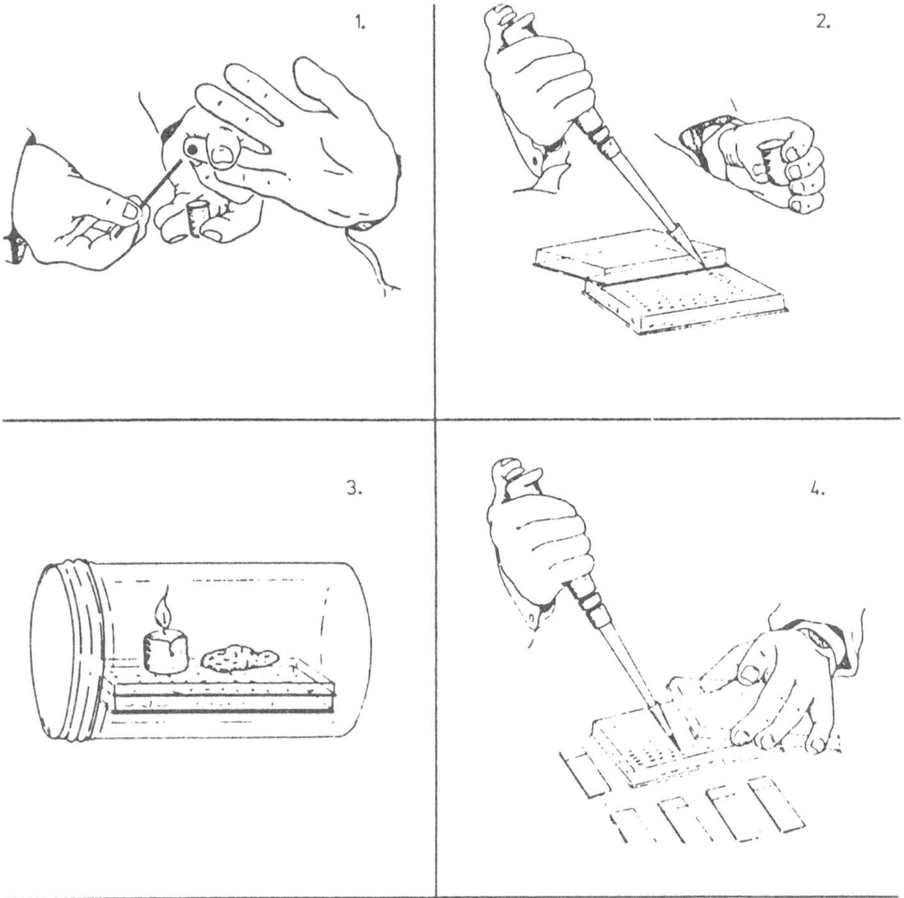


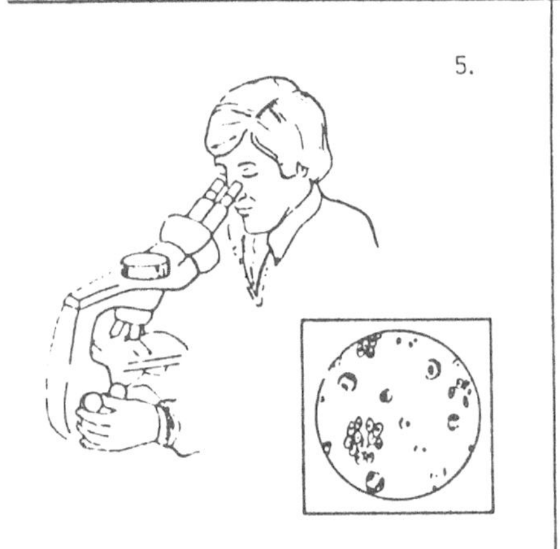


*Procedure for processing slides* 6.

1. Count the number of normal schizonts per 100 asexual parasites.
2. Determine the lowest concentration of drug in which the formation of normal schizonts is inhibited by more than 95% of that observed in the control wells.
3. Record results as follows, for example:

| Patient No. | Drug concentration (nmol/ml blood) 0.5 | 1.0 | 1.5 | 2.0 | 4.0 |
|---|---|---|---|---|---|
| 1 | * | | | | |
| 2 | | | * | | |
| 3 | | | | | * |

* Represents >95% normal schizont inhibition

**Fig. 2.** Procedural steps for determining the drug susceptibility of *P. falciparum* by the in vitro microtechnique (see text for details) assessing the susceptibility of *P. falciparum* to chloroquine and other drugs under both field and laboratory conditions (RIECKMANN 1980; LOPEZ ANTUÑANO and WERNSDORFER 1980; KOUZNETSOV et al. 1980; YISUNSRI and RIECKMANN 1980). At equivalent blood concentrations of chloroquine, inhibition of growth in the microtechnique is similar to that observed in the macrotechnique (RIECKMANN 1980; WERNSDORFER and KOUZNETSOV 1980). Blood specimens containing more than 80000 or 100000 parasites/μl blood require higher concentrations of chloroquine to achieve similar inhibition of growth (RIECKMANN 1980; KOUZNETSOV et al. 1980). As growth at such high parasite densities is not attainable in the macrotechnique, this difference in drug effect need only be considered in relation to the microtechnique.

b) Advantages

The main advantages of the microtechnique are that parasitised specimens of blood can be obtained by fingerprick and that they can be used irrespective of the stage of development or density of the parasites. Because of these advantages and the successful performance of the test under field conditions, the microtechnique should replace the macrotechnique as the standard procedure for assessing the presence, prevalence, and degree of drug resistance in various parts of the world. An inexpensive field incubator, developed specifically for use with the microtechnique and operated by a battery, will make it feasible to apply the technique in remote areas (EASTHAM and RIECKMANN 1981). The drug susceptibility of parasites in patients with acute falciparum malaria can be determined more readily by the microtechnique because young ring forms, the predominant stage during acute febrile episodes, are able to mature to schizonts during 30–42 h of incubation. As the results of the sensitivity test are available within 2 days of the start of the treatment, the initial chemotherapeutic regimen can be modified if the in vitro results show that alternative drugs might be more effective in achieving a radical cure of the infection.

c) Availability of Test Kits

Comparison and evaluation of results obtained from one area of the world with another will only be possible if test kits are prepared at a Central Reference Laboratory. Meticulous standardisation is particularly important in this test because microculture plates must contain precise and minute (picogram or nanogram) quantities of drug (in dried form) at the bottom of the wells and any variability could have a profound effect on the interpretation of the test. Further studies are needed to determine the shelf-life of these compounds after their addition to the culture plates. To safeguard against any possible technical errors, each new batch of kits should be tested against *P. falciparum* isolates of known drug susceptibility before dispatch from the laboratory. Standard kits are now available from WHO.

d) Baseline Susceptibility to Chloroquine and Other Drugs

Evaluation of the drug susceptibility of *P. falciparum* should not be confined to those locations where drug resistance is a problem. The test should also be carried out in areas where falciparum infections are still susceptible to treatment with chloroquine. Such determinations would provide baseline values against which subsequent changes in chloroquine susceptibility of parasites could be measured. The susceptibility of local strains of *P. falciparum* to new drugs, e.g. mefloquine, should be determined in areas where these drugs might be used in the future to provide more effective control of malaria infections (LOPEZ ANTUÑANO and WERNSDORFER 1980). The minute quantities of drug required for the microtechnique are particularly advantageous when only a limited amount of a new drug is available for obtaining baseline values of parasite susceptibility.

e) Susceptibility to Sulphonamide-Pyrimethamine Combinations

As there is increasing evidence that a single dose of sulfadoxine and pyrimethamine is becoming less effective as the alternative antimalarial medication in chloroquine-resistant areas, it seems important to determine the parasite susceptibility to the sulphonamides and pyrimethamine. Although sulphonamides do not show a well-defined activity during short-term in vitro culture, they potentiate the antimalarial activity of pyrimethamine during incubation (YISUNSRI and RIECKMANN 1980). Further studies are needed to ascertain whether the microtechnique can eventually be used to define the susceptibility of parasites to sulphonamide-pyrimethamine combinations. As some individuals are not cured by such drug combinations (CHIN et al. 1966) due to a host erythrocyte factor, rather than to parasite resistance (TRENHOLME et al. 1975), an in vitro test should be helpful in clarifying whether parasite or host resistance is responsible for an inadequate response to treatment.

f) Susceptibility to Slow-Acting Antimalarial Drugs

The activity of slow-acting antimalarials can be determined in this in vitro system because parasites can be exposed to the drug over a number of developmental life cycles. The only disadvantages are that it is necessary to replace medium and drugs on one or more occasions and to extend observations over a longer period of time.

## D. Monitoring of Drug Resistance

The World Health Organization has developed a global programme to monitor the susceptibility of *P. falciparum* to chloroquine and other drugs (WERNSDORFER and KOUZNETSOV 1980). These activities are carried out by the malaria services and research institutes of individual countries and through Regional Advisory Committees on Medical Research and WHO regional offices. Global research efforts are coordinated by WHO Scientific Working Groups on Applied Field Research and on Chemotherapy of Malaria and the results of drug susceptibility tests are published once a year in the *WHO Weekly Epidemiological Record.*

"The global programme has the following objectives in relation to falciparum malaria:
- Assessment of the current geographical distribution, prevalence and degree of resistance to 4-aminoquinolines
- Monitoring of sensitivity levels and the spread, relative prevalence, and degree of resistance to 4-aminoquinolines, with the aim of facilitating the implementation of operational countermeasures

– Assessment of sensitivity to currently used drugs other than 4-aminoquinolines and to candidate antimalarial compounds in order to determine their clinical and operational usefulness and baseline data
– Methodological research on the determination of drug sensitivity
– Studies on the epidemiology of drug-resistant malaria
– Elaboration of guidelines on the clinical management of malaria resistant to 4-aminoquinolines
– Development of operational measures for limiting the spread and eliminating of drug-resistant malaria" (WERNSDORFER and KOUZNETSOV 1980).

## References

Black RH (1946) The effect of antimalarial drugs on *Plasmodium falciparum* (New Guinea strains) developing in vitro. Trans R Soc Trop Med Hyg 40:163–170

Chin W, Contacos PG, Coatney GR, King HK (1966) The evaluation of sulfonamides, alone or in combination with pyrimethamine, in the treatment of multi-resistant falciparum malaria. Am J Trop Med Hyg 15:823–820

Colwell EJ, Phintuyothin P, Sadudee N, Benjapong W, Neoypatimanondh S (1972) Evaluation of an in vitro technique for detecting chloroquine resistant falciparum malaria in Thailand. Am J Trop Med Hyg 21:6–12

Comer RD, Young MD, Porter JA Jr, Gauld JR, Merritt W (1968) Chloroquine resistance in *Plasmodium falciparum* on the Pacific coast of Colombia. Am J Trop Med Hyg 17:795–799

Eastham GM, Rieckmann KH (1981) Field incubator for measuring drug susceptibility of *Plasmodium falciparum*. J Trop Med Hyg 84:27–28

Ebisawa I, Fukuyama T, Kawamura Y (1976) Additional foci of chloroquine-resistant falciparum malaria in East Kalimantan and West Irian, Indonesia. Trop Geogr Med 28:349–354

Kouznetsov RL, Rooney W, Wernsdorfer WH, El Gaddal AA, Payne D, Abdallas RE (1980) Use of the in vitro microtechnique for the assessment of drug sensitivity of *Plasmodium falciparum* in Sennar, Sudan. Bull WHO 58:785–789

Lopez Antuñano FJ, Wernsdorfer WH (1980) In vitro response of chloroquine-resistant *Plasmodium falciparum* to mefloquine. Bull WHO 57:663–665

Mackerras MJ, Ercole QN (1948) Observations on the action of paludrine on malarial parasites. Trans R Soc Trop Med Hyg 41:365–376

Palmer TT, Townley LB, Yigzaw M, Armstrong JC (1976) Chloroquine sensitivity of *Plasmodium falciparum* in Ethiopia. II. Results of an in vitro test. Am J Trop Med Hyg 25:10–13

Peters W, Seaton DR (1971) Sensitivity of *Plasmodium falciparum* to chloroquine in Africa. Ann Trop Med Parasitol 65:267–269

Powell RD, Brewer GJ, Alving AS, Millar JW (1964) Studies on a strain of chloroquine-resistant *Plasmodium falciparum* from Thailand. Bull WHO 30:29–44

Rieckmann KH (1971) Determination of the drug sensitivity of *Plasmodium falciparum*. JAMA 217:573–578

Rieckmann KH (1972) In vitro assessment of the sensitivity of *Plasmodium falciparum* to chloroquine at Kisumu, Kenya and Lagos, Nigeria. WHO/MAL 72:792 (Cyclostyled report) WHO, Geneva

Rieckmann KH (1980) Susceptibility of cultured parasites of *Plasmodium falciparum* to antimalarial drugs. In: Rowe DS, Hirumi H (eds) The in vitro cultivation of the pathogens of tropical diseases. Tropical diseases research series, No. 3. Schwabe, Basel, pp 35–50

Rieckmann KH, Lopez Antuñano FJ (1971) Chloroquine resistance of *Plasmodium falciparum* in Brazil detected by a simple in vitro method. Bull WHO 45:157–167

Rieckmann KH, McNamara JV, Frischer H, Stockert TA, Carson PE, Powell RD (1968) Effects of chloroquine, quinine, and cycloguanil upon the maturation of asexual erythrocytic forms of two strains of *Plasmodium falciparum* in vitro. Am J Trop Med Hyg 17:661–671

Rieckmann KH, Willerson WD Jr, Carson PE, Frischer H (1972) Effects of tetracycline against drug-resistant falciparum malaria. Proc Helminthol Soc Wash 39:339–347

Rieckmann KH, Trenholme GM, Williams RL, Carson PE, Frischer H, Desjardins RE (1974) Prophylactic activity of mefloquine hydrochloride (WR 142490) in drug-resistant malaria. Bull WHO 51:431–434

Rieckmann KH, Sax LJ, Campbell GH, Mrema JE (1978) Drug sensitivity of *Plasmodium falciparum*. An in vitro microtechnique. Lancet I:22–23

Sucharit P, Harinasuta T, Chongsuphajaisiddhi T, Tongprasroeth N, Kasemsuth R (1977) In vivo and in vitro studies of chloroquine-resistant malaria in Thailand. Ann Trop Med Parasitol 71:401–405

Trenholme GM, Williams RL, Frischer H, Carson PE, Rieckmann KH (1975) Host failure in treatment of malaria with sulfalene and pyrimethamine. Ann Intern Med 82:219–223

Valera CV, Shute GT (1975) Preliminary studies on the response of *Plasmodium falciparum* to chloroquine in the Philippines using the in vitro technique. WHO/MAL 75:852 (Cyclostyled report) WHO, Geneva

Walker AJ, Lopez Antuñano FJ (1968) Response to drugs of South American strains of *Plasmodium falciparum*. Trans R Soc Trop Med Hyg 62:654–667

Wernsdorfer WH, Kouznetsov RL (1980) Drug-resistant malaria – occurrence, control, and surveillance. Bull WHO 58:341–352

WHO (1967) Chemotherapy of malaria. Report of a WHO scientific group. WHO Tech Rep Ser 375:42

WHO (1973) Chemotherapy of malaria and resistance to antimalarials. Report of a WHO scientific working group. WHO Tech Rep Ser 529:30

WHO (1979) Instructions for use of the WHO test kit for assessment of the response of *Plasmodium falciparum* to chloroquine. WHO/MAP 79:1 (Cyclostyled report) WHO Geneva

Yisunsri L, Rieckmann KH (1980) In vitro microtechnique for determining the drug susceptibility of cultured parasites of *Plasmodium falciparum*. Trans R Soc Trop Med Hyg 74:809–810

CHAPTER 18

# Experimental Production of Drug Resistance

W. Peters

## A. Introduction

A decade ago I made the following statement: "reviewing the literature now with the wisdom bestowed by hindsight one is impressed by the relative ease with which resistance can be induced to almost any antimalarial drug. The method employed may facilitate the process but is, in most cases, not over-important" (Peters 1970). This statement is still valid. A number of additional techniques for the experimental production of drug resistance have since been published and these are incorporated in Table 1.

**Table 1.** Classification of techniques for inducing drug resistance. Modified from Peters (1970)

- 1 In vitro (Nguyen-Dinh and Trager 1978)
- 2 Semi in vitro (not yet reported. Could be used with or without the aid of a mutagenic agent)
- 3 Tissue culture (not yet reported in *Plasmodium* but used successfully to produce pyrimethamine resistance in *Toxoplasma gondii* by Cook 1958)
- 4 In vivo
  - 4.1 Serial passage
    - 4.1.1 Single treatment (or course of treatment) per passage
      - (i) Constant dose
        - a) Intermittent exposure (in alternate passages)
        - b) Constant exposure (e.g. drug-diet method)
      - (ii) Low dosage–increased progressively (favours 'adaptation')
      - (iii) High dosage
        - a) Rapid passage } (favours selection of mutants)
        - b) Passage in relapse } (favours selection of mutants)
    - 4.1.2 Multiple treatment (or course) in each passage
      - (i) High infection rate
        - a) Low dosage increased progressively at each relapse
        - b) High doses, passage in relapse (favours selection of mutants)
      - (ii) Low infection rate (latent infections)
        - a) Low dosage, increased progressively } unfavourable to production of resistance
        - b) Constant dose } unfavourable to production of resistance
  - 4.2 Single treatment
  - 4.3 Hybridisation
    - 4.3.1 In vertebrate host (Yoeli et al. 1969)
    - 4.3.2 In invertebrate host (Greenberg and Trembley 1954; Greenberg 1956; Beale et al. 1978)
- 5 Indirect methods
  - 5.1 Withhold essential metabolites (Ramakrishnan et al. 1956)
  - 5.2 Produce resistance to other compounds working on same metabolic pathways or by similar mechanisms of action

## B. Modes of Drug Resistance Development

The development of drug resistance by microorganisms depends on a variety of factors, which are summarised in Table 2.

The only clearly defined ways in which malaria parasites have been shown to become resistant to drugs are: (a) the selection under drug pressure of pre-existing mutants, e.g. BISHOP (1958), who, selecting for metachloridine resistance in *Plasmodium gallinaceum*, came to the conclusion that mutants were present in her original line at a frequency possibly less than 1 in $10^9$; (b) simple Mendelian inheritance, as shown for several antimalarials by the group headed by BEALE in Edinburgh (see review of BEALE et al. 1978); and (c) phenotypic adaptation, as is apparent in the highly chloroquine-resistant RC-type lines of *P. berghei* (PETERS 1965).

**Table 2.** Classification of possible modes of drug resistance. From PETERS (1970), after BRYSON and SZYBALSKI (1955)

A. Resistance primarily dependent upon change of genotype
- (i) Mutation
  - Spontaneous (the expression of the mutant may be delayed by 'phenomic lag', i.e. several generations may elapse between the genetic event and its phenotypic expression
  - Induced (usually by non-specific mutagenic agents rather than the drug itself but the latter is possible if subinhibitory drug concentrations are used)
- (ii) Genetic exchange (chromosomal or extrachromosomal)
  - By gametes (sexual recombination)
  - By 'unpackaged' DNA
    - Transduction } (see discussion above)
    - Transformation } (see discussion above)

B. Resistance dependent upon non-genetic change of phenotype (i.e. inducible organisms)
- (i) Induction of a new physiological function
  - Production of inducer-inactivating enzymes
    - Single enzyme
    - Chain of enzymes
- (ii) Elimination of a cytoplasmic particle
- (iii) Accumulation of a drug-inactivating factor
- (iv) Selection of an alternative physiological function, e.g. selective change in the relative emphasis upon two or more pre-existent enzymatic pathways, leading to the formation of an essential metabolite
- (v) 'Reorganisation of the cytoplasm' (a general term quoted from BEALE to cover a variety of phenotypic adaptations leading to resistance, e.g. altered membrane structure and permeability).

C. Resistance involving no adaptive change

D. Borderline cases

E. Resistance dependent upon composite changes (the most likely process in most cases of drug resistance).

## C. Techniques

### I. In Vitro Procedure

The seminal papers of TRAGER and JENSEN (1976) and HAYNES et al. (1976), describing methods for the continuous cultivation of the blood stages of *P. falciparum* in vitro have opened the way to the use of cultures for the selection or induction of drug resistance in malaria parasites.

NGUYEN-DINH and TRAGER (1978) have reported the development of a chloroquine-resistant line of *P. falciparum* from an isolate originating in The Gambia in West Africa using the following technique:

*P. falciparum* (FCR-3) was isolated from a patient infected in The Gambia in 1976 and maintained in vitro by the technique of TRAGER and JENSEN (1976). In a simple Petri-dish test system (TRAGER et al. 1978) or a "multiwells" procedure (see below) a constant response to chloroquine was observed over an 8-month period, i.e. 48 h exposure to 0.1 μg base/ml completely inhibited growth. Parasites were passaged serially in 35-mm Petri dishes with daily medium change and subculture to fresh blood cells every 4th day. Starting with a concentration of 0.01 μg/ml, the chloroquine-base content of the medium was progressively increased in successive passages as rapidly as the parasite growth permitted. After 15 asexual cycles in 1 month the parasites supported a concentration of 0.1 μg/ml. Further progress was made up to 0.16 μg/ml at the time of the report on this work but no success had met efforts to step up the level to 0.2 μg/ml over the last 6 months of the experiment.

The sensitivity of the line to chloroquine was tested either in Petri dishes or in 16-mm wells. In the first method, parasites were grown without drug for 2 days, then in different concentrations of chloroquine for a further 2 days. Counts were made on days 0, 2, and 4. In the second "multiwells" method, parasites were grown

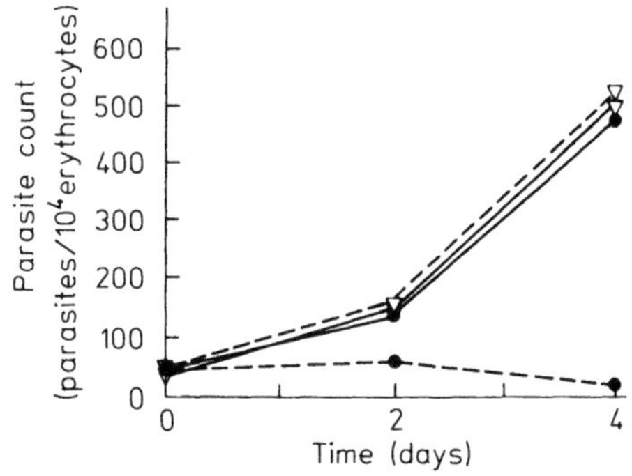


**Fig. 1.** Effect of chloroquine on an African strain of *P. falciparum* maintained with or without chloroquine in vitro. Growth in vitro of the original FCR-3 strain in normal medium (*full circle line*) is compared with the same strain in 0.1 μg chloroquine/ml (*full circle broken line*), the resistant R-FCR-3 line in normal medium (*triangle line*) and this line in 0.1 μg chloroquine/ml (*triangle broken line*). Each *point* represents the average of triplicate dishes. (Reproduced by permission of the American Association for the Advancement of Science from NGUYEN-DINH and TRAGER (1978)

1 day in medium in a 50-mm Petri dish, then distributed into 16-mm wells containing control or chloroquine-supplemented medium. Parasite counts were made on day 0, then on days 1 and 3. Concentrations of 0.01, 0.03, 0.06, 0.1, and 0.3 μg chloroquine base/ml were used. In Fig. 1 are shown the data obtained when the response of the parent and derived line to 0.1 μg/ml were compared at the end of 1 month. After being passaged for 4 months in drug-free medium no decrease in drug resistance was deteced. The maximum resistance level obtained after 5 months of drug exposure was considered to be equivalent to the level encountered in Nature in the highly resistant Vietnam (FVO) line, which is RIII in vivo.

This work is particularly important, not only because it is the first example of an in vitro method for producing antimalarial drug resistance but because it also demonstrates that at least one African strain of *P. falciparum* has the genetic capability of becoming chloroquine resistant, a point that has been much debated up to now. Of perhaps even greater significance is the development by BROCKELMAN et al. (1981) of a line of *P. falciparum* of Thai origin highly resistant to mefloquine using a similar technique to that described above.

## II. Semi In Vitro Techniques

None has yet been reported. However, the way is now open through the in vitro system referred to above, which is adaptable to species other than *P. falciparum*. It is clear that the use of *P. falciparum* itself is limited since the only animals into which parasites exposed, for example, to mutagenic agents in vitro, can be passaged are New World monkeys (*Aotus trivirgatus* or *Saimiri sciureus*) which are scarce and expensive. *P. berghei* has also been cultured in vitro although no publications on this work have appeared to date. Since this parasite readily infects most laboratory rodents it would easily lend itself to a semi in vitro application of chemical or physical mutagenic agents for the rapid induction of drug resistance.

## III. Tissue Culture

Although techniques have long been available for the growth of exoerythrocytic stages of avian malaria in tissue culture, there are no reports to date of the exploitation of this model for the development of drug resistance. COOK (1958) has used a tissue-culture system to develop pyrimethamine resistance in *Toxoplasma gondii*.

The system described by STROME et al. (1979) for the growth of the exoerythrocytic schizonts of *P. berghei* in tissue culture (see Chap. 6) is probably not yet suitable for adaptation as a model for the development of drug resistance since, as SINDEN and SMITH (1980) have pointed out, the schizonts fail to reach maturity and produce cryptozoites which could be used to infect new rodent hosts. Further improvements of the technique may, however, provide a suitable model for such experiments in the foreseeable future. HOLLINGDALE et al. (1981), for example, have succeeded in growing exoerythrocyte schizonts of *P. berghei* to maturity in a human lung cell line in tissue culture.

# IV. In Vivo Techniques

## 1. Serial Passage

Procedures involving serial passage under drug pressure are the most widely used for the production of drug-resistant lines of *Plasmodium*. The techniques fall into two broad groups: (a) those involving exposure to progressively increasing drug doses in successive passages and (b) relapse techniques in which parasites are exposed to a single high dose at each passage.

### a) Progressive Increase of Drug Dosage

This widely used technique involves the regular passage of parasites in an appropriate host to which the drug is administered daily. Usually a higher and lower dose are given to different groups of animals, the doses remaining constant in each passage but being advanced progressively in consecutive passages to the maximum that will permit the survival of enough parasites to initiate a further passage. The example of Fig. 2 will help to illustrate the procedure, which was described by PETERS (1968, 1980).

Mice were given an intraperitoneal inoculum of approximately $10^7$ donor erythrocytes infected with *P. berghei*, the day of inoculation being called D O. Four

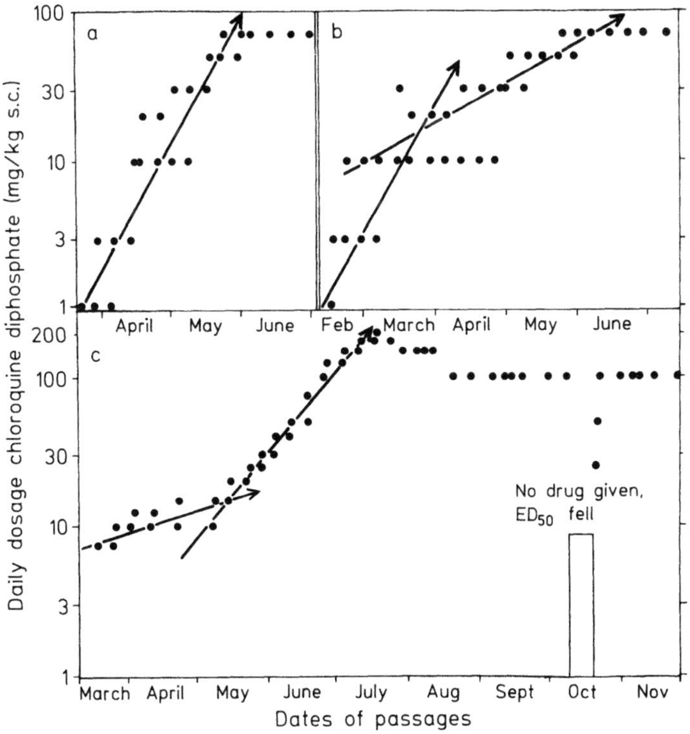


**Fig. 2.** The acquisition of resistance by three lines of *P. berghei* to chloroquine as reflected by the increasing dosage applied to infected mice in succeeding passages. *a*, NK65 line 41A; *b*, NK65 line 41; *c*, K173 N strain (giving rise to the RC strain). Reproduced with permission from PETERS (1968)

consecutive daily doses of drug were administered on D O, D+1, D+2, and D+3, starting with the dose that experience has shown would permit the survival of about a 1% parasitaemia level on D+6. Three groups of five animals were used at each passage, one group receiving no drug (as an insurance for the survival of the line), one receiving the dose given in the previous passage and the third receiving a somewhat higher dosage (the exact level being judged on experience). The highest dose was increased if possible at each passage, which was made once a week from parasites surviving the maximum dose. Occasionally it may be found necessary to reduce the dose or hold it constant for several passages. The development of resistance may be monitored at intervals for stability (by passaging only in untreated mice) and for the level of resistance (by the "4-day test" of PETERS 1980). In the examples shown here resistance to chloroquine developed up to the maximum dose tolerated by the hosts (60 mg/kg salt × 4) in 8, 13, and 13 passages respectively in the A, B, and C lines.

The highly resistant parasites produced by this technique display an unusual morphology. The asexual intraerythrocytic trophozoites and schizonts appear to

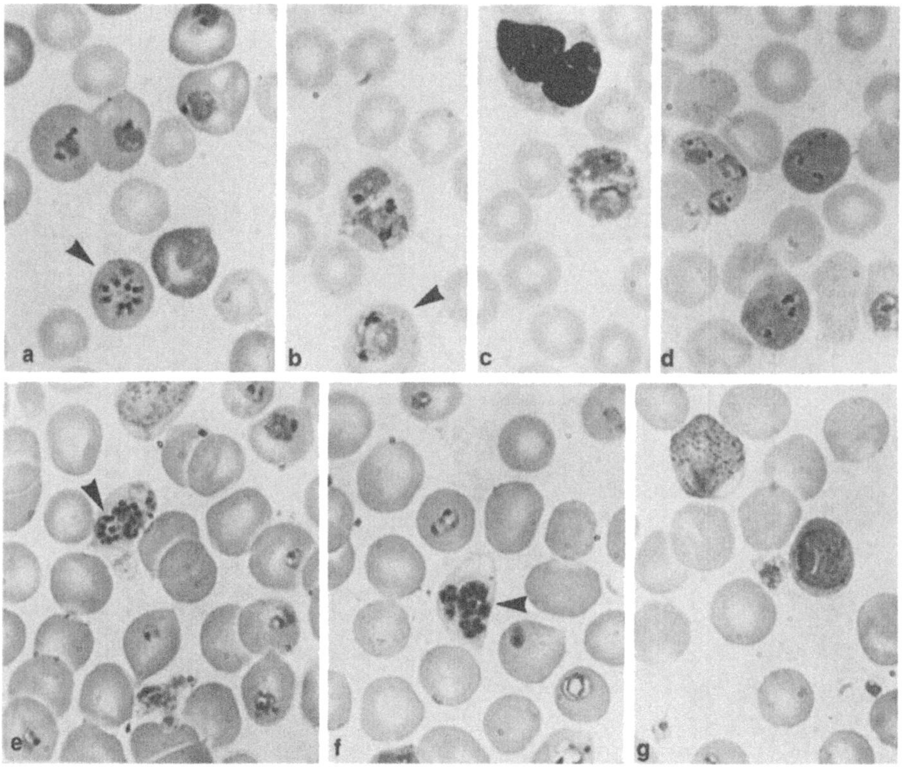


**Fig. 3 a–g.** Morphology of intraerythrocytic parasites of the highly chloroquine-resistant RC line of *P. berghei* compared with the drug-sensitive parent K173 (N) strain. **a–d** RC line; **e–g** parent strain. Note the lack of pigment indicated by *arrows* in **a** and **b**, compared with conspicuous haemozoin grains in schizonts indicated by arrows in **e, f** and in the gametocytes seen in **g**. Giemsa stain, × 1140 lack the malaria pigment haemozoin, and their cytoplasm has a "foamy" appearance well seen in Fig. 3.

b) Relapse Technique

A simple bioassay procedure was described (WARHURST and FOLWELL 1968) to determine the potency of inocula of rodent malaria parasites. This procedure, which is based on an estimate of the time required for parasitaemia to reach a 2% level, has been adapted for the simultaneous production and monitoring of drug resistance. In principle the technique is carried out as follows. The host is infected on D O with approximately $10^7$ infected donor erythrocytes and, on the same day, receives a single, large dose of the drug. Daily blood films are made and parasitaemia levels determined during the log phase of multiplication (i.e. until about 5% of red cells are infected). From a graph of the daily parasite levels the time required to reach a 2% level is interpolated. A figure is also obtained from parasites in a parallel group of sham-treated animals. In subtracting the "2% time" of the latter from the figure for treated groups the difference represents the delay caused by the drug, and this is termed the "2% delay time." This is then plotted for each successive passage as illustrated in Figs. 4 and 5.

Resistance is shown by a progressive decrease in the "2% delay time." These figures show the different rates at which resistance to the phenanthrenemethanol WR 122455 develops, depending upon whether one commences with the chloroquine-sensitive *P. berghei* N strain or a chloroquine-resistant NS derivative, the latter becoming resistant much more readily (PETERS and PORTER 1976).

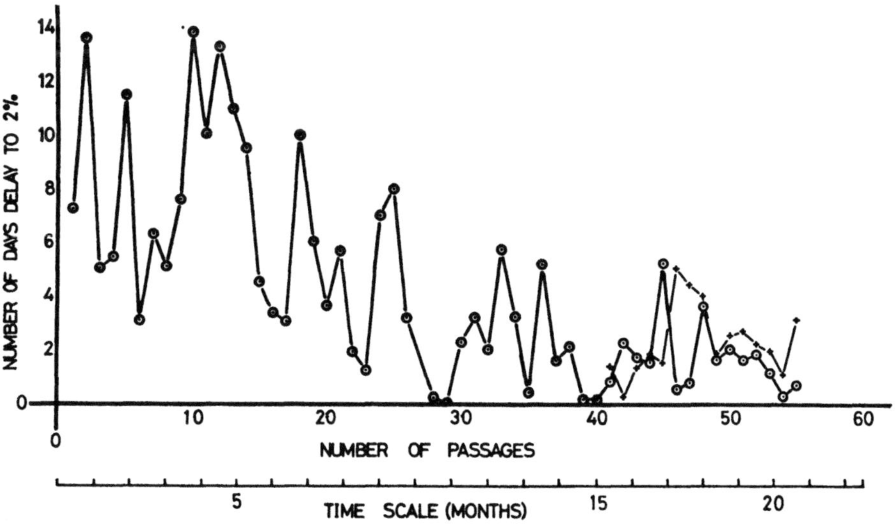


**Fig. 4.** Use of the relapse technique to produce resistance in the *P. berghei* N strain (a strain sensitive to chloroquine) against WR 122455. The acquisition of resistance is indicated by a progressive fall in the time required to reach a 2% level of parasitaemia following a single dose of 60 mg/kg on the day of infection. Drug-treated passages (*circle*); untreated passages (*cross*). Reproduced with permission from PETERS and PORTER (1976)

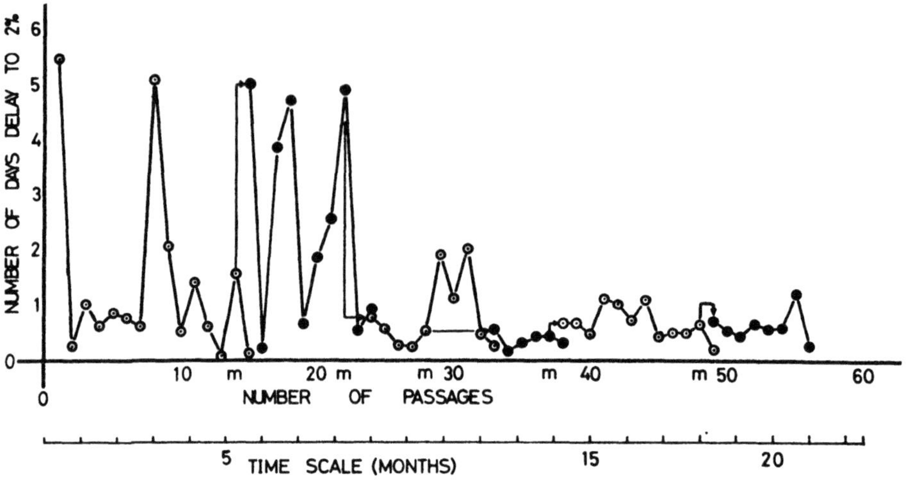


**Fig. 5.** Resistance to WR 122455 in the slightly chloroquine-resistant NS line of *P. berghei*. Mosquito passages were made at intervals and are indicated by an *m*. *Arrows* indicate from which passage the main line was continued. Following the feeding of mosquitos the line was continued by blood passage until further infective sporozoites became available, and these were then used to continue the main line. Compare the rapid development of resistance in this line with the rate in Fig. 3. Reproduced with permission from PETERS and PORTER (1976)

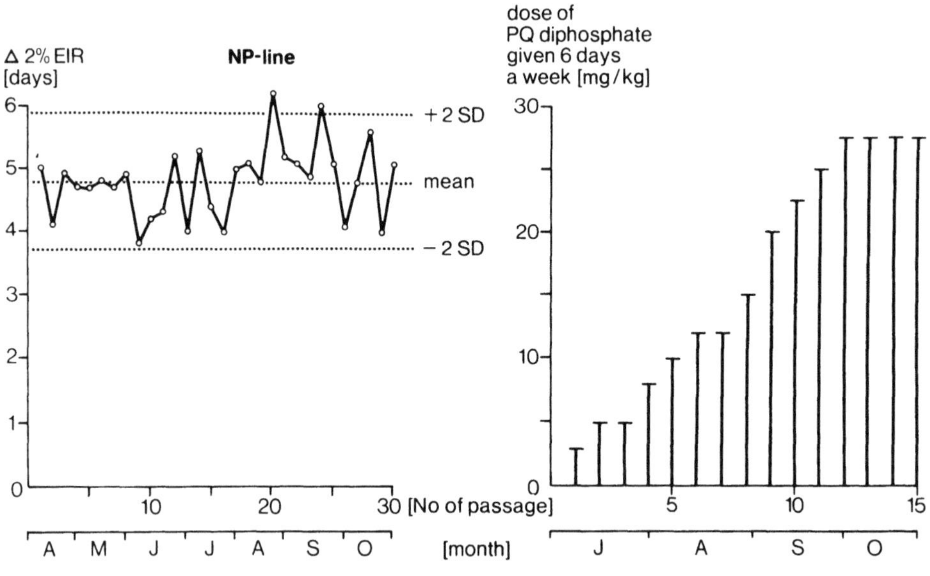


**Fig. 6.** The serial and relapse techniques compared in experiments to produce primaquine resistance in *P. berghei* N strain. No change in response to the drug was observed over 30 serial passages using the relapse technique (*left*), whereas significant resistance developed when the serial technique was used (*right*). Reproduced with permission from MERKLI and PETERS (1976)

Quite different results may be attained with the two different approaches, and this is exemplified by data of MERKLI and PETERS (1976), illustrated in Fig. 6, showing that primaquine resistance could readily be produced in *P. berghei* by method (a) but not by method (b).

Whether the use of progressively increased drug dosage or the high-dosage relapse technique in vivo selects resistant parasites obviously depends on the changes in the parasites that enable them to survive in the presence of the drug. Experience with chloroquine in *P. berghei,* for example, suggests that the use of slowly increasing drug dosage enables the parasites initially to undergo various physiological adaptive processes, one of these being a limitation to growth within immature red cells (reticulocytes) and an inability to mature in older erythrocytes. Initially these RC-type parasites displayed a very unstable resistance which disappeared rapidly once the drug-selection pressure was removed. With continuing selection pressure, however, the resistance became stabilised at a high level, indicating probably that a subsequent change, perhaps in the form of a mutation, had occurred. Sequential changes during the development of drug resistance are a familiar phenomenon in bacteria, so that it is not surprising to find the same phenomenon in eukaryotic *Plasmodium,* which after all possess a far more complex genetic repertoire than prokaryotes and are hence far more genetically labile.

Our experience with chloroquine resistance in rodent malaria led us to the conclusion that the application of method (b) in old laboratory strains of *P. berghei* selected out chloroquine-resistant organisms which, initially named by us the "NS lines of *P. berghei,*" in fact represented rare trophozoites of a *P. yoelii* subspecies which had formed a cryptic mixture in these long blood-passaged, laboratory lines (PETERS et al. 1978). Our attention was first drawn to this possibility when we submitted the parent and resistant lines to biochemical characterisation of their enzymes and discovered that they belonged to quite different isoenzyme groups. In order to test the hypothesis we attempted to develop NS-type parasites from uncloned and cloned parent material of an old line of *P. berghei* N strain that had been maintained by blood passage and cryopreserved in a laboratory that did not hold a stock of the parasite which our NS lines most closely resemble, namely *P. yoelii nigeriensis.* In Fig. 7 the actual "2% times" rather than the "2% delay times" are plotted for uncloned and cloned material subjected to two dose levels of chloroquine, 20 and 40 mg/kg, or no drug (controls) in successive passages.

Whereas resistance developed rapidly at both drug levels in the parasites of the uncloned material, no change in drug response could be observed in the cloned line, thus giving some support for our hypothesis (PETERS et al. 1978).

Parasites of the *P. berghei* NS type, unlike the parent *P. berghei* N strain, produce gametocytes and are cyclically transmissible. The level of chloroquine resistance is less than that of the RC-type parasites and highly stable (PETERS et al. 1970). In many ways they resemble the chloroquine-resistant strains of *P. falciparum* found in Nature. ROSARIO (1976) has provided evidence indicating that low-level chloroquine resistance in another rodent parasite, *P. chabaudi,* is a genotypic character that follows a normal Mendelian pattern of inheritance, resistant parasites apparently being dominant both in rodent and cyclical passage (BEALE et al. 1978). It is interesting to note, incidentally, that both ROSARIO (1976), working with *P. chabaudi,* and POWERS et al. (1969), working with *P. vinckei,* were only able to

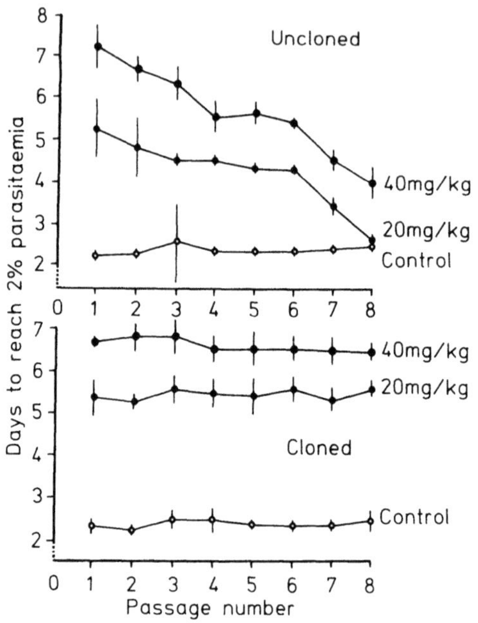


**Fig. 7.** Time taken to reach a 2% parasitaemia in uncloned *P. berghei* MH line, compared with the response in parallel experiments with a cloned line of this parasite. No resistance developed to chloroquine in the latter over the same period of exposure using the relapse technique. Reproduced with permission from PETERS et al. (1978)

achieve chloroquine resistance by starting with lines of these parasites that were already resistant to pyrimethamine.

## 2. Single Treatment

There are a number of instances of drug resistance being produced by a single exposure of infected hosts to a large dose of drug. One example is that of BURGESS and YOUNG (1959), who obtained a pyrimethamine-resistant infection of *P. falciparum* in man following a single 25-mg dose. DIGGENS et al. (1970) selected a pyrimethamine-resistant line from *P. berghei* NK 65 by a single exposure of infected hamsters and mice to a large drug dose. Resistant parasites were found to have a mutant dihydrofolate reductase.

## 3. Hybridisation

Hybridisation of malaria parasites does not appear to occur in the vertebrate host, and the claim by YOELI et al. (1969) that they had observed this phenomenon (for which they coined the term "synpholia") must now be considered invalid.

Considerable use has been made of hybridisation during the sexual phase of plasmodial development in the invertebrate host for the study of the genetics of antimalarial drug resistance. A review of this topic by BEALE et al. (1978), who have contributed the most to this field, should be read by those interested. Drug-resistance markers combined with isoenzyme markers have provided an invaluable tool for the exploration of patterns of inheritance of resistance to sulphonamides, pyrimethamine, and chloroquine in rodent-malaria parasites and to such features as parasite virulence, which, in *P. yoelii,* is a genetically determined character (WALLIKER et al. 1976).

## V. Indirect Methods

### 1. Withholding of Essential Metabolites

A classical example of this technique is the production of a line of *P. berghei* resistant to sulphonamides through the simple measure of retaining mice in successive passages on a milk diet which contained a minimal quantity of *p*-aminobenzoic acid (RAMAKRISHNAN et al. 1956). This line proved highly resistant to sulphadiazine, which, of course, normally functions by blocking the incorporation of *p*-aminobenzoic acid by *Plasmodium.*

### 2. Associated Resistance

Resistance to sulphonamides may carry with it resistance to dihydrofolate reductase inhibitors, although the reverse is not usually true. Thus, for example, BISHOP and MCCONNACHIE (1950) observed that a sulphonamide-resistant line of *P. gallinaceum* was resistant also to proguanil, with which the parasites had never been in contact. No general rules, however, can be laid down for cross-resistance between compounds acting on the folate pathways, and several inconsistencies have been described (see PETERS 1970).

# D. Conclusion

The experimental production of drug-resistant lines of *Plasmodium* serves a number of distinct purposes. Firstly it provides a tool for the investigation of the nature and genetics of resistance to a given compound (BEALE et al. 1978); secondly it provides an insight, through patterns of cross-resistance, of the mode of action of a drug (ROLLO 1968); thirdly the evaluation of the activity of a new compound in a battery of drug-resistant parasite lines and the study of the ease with which parasites can become resistant to it provide a means of forecasting the future usefulness of that compound if it is eventually released to the public (PETERS et al. 1975; PETERS and PORTER 1976).

Now that suitable techniques are available both for the cultivation of erythrocytic stages of *Plasmodium* and for the evaluation of their sensitivities to antimalarial drugs (see Chaps. 6, 17), increasing attention should be paid to the study of drug resistance and the selection of resistant parasite lines in vitro, since this opens many possibilities that would otherwise not be available in vivo. It may, for example, be possible to employ far higher drug concentrations and hence produce parasites with a correspondingly higher level of drug resistance than could be achieved in vivo because of the limited tolerance of the host to the compound being studied. The use of physical or chemical mutagens will also be possible. Moreover, in the absence of host immunity, even minimal numbers of surviving parasites will have a chance to grow. Cloning of cultures will also contribute to the genetic analysis of drug resistance, and the use of cultures will considerably facilitate biochemical studies on mechanisms of drug action and drug resistance.

## References

Beale GH, Carter R, Walliker D (1978) Genetics. In: Killick-Kendrick R, Peters W (eds) Rodent malaria. Academic, London

Bishop A (1958) An analysis of the development of resistance to metachloridine in clones of *Plasmodium gallinaceum*. Parasitology 48:210–234

Bishop A, McConnachie EW (1950) Cross resistance between sulphanilamide and Paludrine (proguanil) in a strain of *Plasmodium gallinaceum* resistant to sulphanilamide. Parasitology 40:175–178

Brockleman CR, Monkolkeha S, Tanariya P (1981) Decrease in susceptibility of *Plasmodium falciparum* to mefloquine in continuous culture. Bull WHO 59:249–252

Bryson V, Szybalski W (1955) Microbial drug resistance. Adv Genet 7:1–46

Burgess RW, Young MD (1959) The development of pyrimethamine resistance by *Plasmodium falciparum*. Bull WHO 20:37–46

Cook MK (1958) The development of a pyrimethamine-resistant line of *Toxoplasma* under in vitro conditions. Am J Trop Med Hyg 7:400–402

Diggens SM, Gutteridge WE, Trigg PI (1970) Altered dihydrofolate reductase associated with a pyrimethamine-resistant *Plasmodium berghei* produced in a single step. Nature 228:579–580

Greenberg J (1956) Mixed lethal strains of *Plasmodium gallinaceum:* drug-sensitive, transferable (SP) × drug-resistant, non-transferable (BI). Exp Parasitol 5:359–370

Greenberg J, Trembley HL (1954) The apparent transfer of pyrimethamine resistance from the BI strain of *Plasmodium gallinaceum* to the M strain. J Parasitol 40:667–672

Haynes JD, Diggs CL, Hines CL, Desjardins RE (1976) Culture of human malaria parasites, *Plasmodium falciparum*. Nature 263:767–769

Hollingdale MR, Leef JL, McCullough M, Beaudoin RL (1981) In vitro cultivation of the exoerythrocytic stage of *Plasmodium berghei* from sporozoites. Science 213:1021–1022

Merkli B, Peters W (1976) A comparison of two different methods for the selection of primaquine resistance in *Plasmodium berghei berghei*. Ann Trop Med Parasitol 70:473–474

Nguyen-Dinh P, Trager W (1978) Chloroquine resistance produced in vitro in an African strain of human malaria. Science 200:1397–1398

Peters W (1965) Morphological and physiological variations in chloroquine-resistant *Plasmodium berghei*, Vincke and Lips, 1948. Ann Soc Belg Med Trop 45:365–378

Peters W (1968) The chemotherapy of rodent malaria, V: dynamics of drug resistance, Part I: methods for studying the acquisition and loss of resistance to chloroquine by *Plasmodium berghei*. Ann Trop Med Parasitol 62:277–287

Peters W (1970) Chemotherapy and drug resistance in malaria. Academic, London

Peters W (1980) Chemotherapy of malaria. In: Kreier JP (ed) Malaria, vol 1. Academic, New York, pp 145–283

Peters W, Porter M (1976) The chemotherapy of rodent malaria, XXVI: the potential value of WR 122455 (a 9-phenanthrenemethanol) against drug-resistant malaria parasites. Ann Trop Med Parasitol 70:271–281

Peters W, Portus JH, Robinson BL (1975) The chemotherapy of rodent malaria, XXII: the value of drug-resistant strains of *P. berghei* in screening for blood schizontocidal activity. Ann Trop Med Parasitol 69:155–171

Peters W, Bafort J, Ramkaran AE, Portus JH, Robinson BL (1970) The chemotherapy of rodent malaria, XI: cyclically transmitted, chloroquine-resistant variants of the Keyberg 173 strain of *Plasmodium berghei*. Ann Trop Med Parasitol 64:41–51

Peters W, Chance ML, Lissner R, Momen M, Warhurst DC (1978) The chemotherapy of rodent malaria, XXX: the enigmas of the "NS line" of *P. berghei*. Ann Trop Med Parasitol 72:23–36

Powers KG, Jacobs RL, Good WC, Koontz LC (1969) *Plasmodium vinckei:* production of chloroquine-resistant strain. Exp Parasitol 26:193–202

Ramakrishnan SP, Satya P, Sen Gupta GP (1956) Studies on *Plasmodium berghei,* Vincke and Lips, 1948, XXIII: isolation of and observations on a "milk-resistant" strain. Indian J Malariol 10:175–182

Rollo IM (1968) The mode of action of antimalarials. In: Da Silva JR, Ferreira MJ (eds) Proceedings of the 3 rd international pharmacological meeting, São Paulo, 1966. Pergamon, Oxford, pp 45–50

Rosario VE (1976) Genetics of chloroquine resistance in malaria parasites. Nature 261:585–586

Sinden RE, Smith J (1980) Culture of the liver stages (exoerythrocytic schizonts) of rodent malaria parasites from sporozoites in vitro. Trans R Soc Trop Med Hyg 74:134–136

Strome CPA, De Santis PL, Beaudoin RL (1979) The cultivation of the exoerythrocytic stages of *Plasmodium berghei* from sporozoites. In Vitro 15:531–536

Trager W, Jensen JB (1976) Human malaria parasites in continuous culture. Science 193:673–675

Trager W, Robert-Gero M, Lederer E (1978) Antimalarial activity of *S*-isobutyl adenosine against *Plasmodium falciparum* in culture. FEBS Lett 85:264–266

Walliker D, Sanderson A, Yoeli M, Hargreaves BJ (1976) A genetic investigation of virulence in a rodent malaria parasite. Parasitology 72:183–194

Warhurst DC, Folwell RO (1968) Measurement of the growth rate of the erythrocytic stages of *Plasmodium berghei* and comparison of the potency of inocula after various treatments. Ann Trop Med Parasitol 62:349–360

Yoeli M, Upmanis RS, Most H (1969) Drug resistance transfer among rodent plasmodia, I: acquisition of resistance to pyrimethamine by a drug-sensitive strain of *P. berghei* in the course of its concomitant development with a pyrimethamine-resistant *P. vinckei* strain. Parasitology 59:429–447

# Subject Index

# Handbook of Experimental Pharmacology

Continuation of "Handbuch der experimentellen Pharmakologie"



Springer-Verlag
Berlin
Heidelberg
GmbH

Volume 22: Part 1
**Die Gestagene I**

Part 2
**Die Gestagene II**

Volume 23
**Neurohypophysial Hormones and Similar Polypeptides**

Volume 24
**Diuretica**

Volume 25
**Bradykinin, Kallidin and Kallikrein**

Volume 26
**Vergleichende Pharmakologie von Überträgersubstanzen in tiersystematischer Darstellung**

Volume 27
**Anticoagulantien**

Volume 28: Part 1
**Concepts in Biochemical Pharmacology I**

Part 3
**Concepts in Biochemical Pharmacology III**

Volume 29
**Oral wirksame Antidiabetika**

Volume 30
**Modern Inhalation Anesthetics**

Volume 32: Part 2
**Insulin II**

Volume 34
**Secretin, Cholecystokinin Pancreozymin and Gastrin**

Volume 35: Part 1
**Androgene I**

Part 2
**Androgens II and Antiandrogens/Androgene II und Antiandrogene**

Volume 36
**Uranium - Plutonium - Transplutonic Elements**

Volume 37
**Angiotensin**

Volume 38: Part 1
**Antineoplastic and Immunosuppressive Agents I**

Part 2
**Antineoplastic and Immunosuppressive Agents II**

Volume 39
**Antihypertensive Agents**

Volume 40
**Organic Nitrates**

Volume 41
**Hypolipidemic Agents**

Volume 42
**Neuromuscular Junction**

Volume 43
**Anabolic-Androgenic Steroids**

Volume 44
**Heme and Hemoproteins**

Volume 45: Part 1
**Drug Addiction I**

Part 2
**Drug Addiction II**

Volume 46
**Fibrinolytics and Antifibronolytics**

# Handbook of Experimental Pharmacology

Continuation of
"Handbuch der experimentellen
Pharmakologie"



Springer-Verlag
Berlin
Heidelberg
GmbH

Volume 47
**Kinetics of Drug Action**

Volume 48
**Arthropod Venoms**

Volume 50: Part 1
**Inflammation**

Part 2
**Anti-Inflammatory Drugs**

Volume 51
**Uric Acids**

Volume 52
**Snake Venoms**

Volume 53
**Pharmacology of Ganglionic Transmission**

Volume 54: Part 1
**Adrenergic Activators and Inhibitors I**

Part 2
**Adrenergic Activators and Inhibitors II**

Volume 55
**Psychotropic Agents**

Part 1
**Antipsychotics and Antidepressants I**

Part 2
**Anxiolytics, Gerontopsychopharmacological Agents and Psychomotor Stimulants**

Part 3
**Alcohol and Psychotomimetics, Psychotropic Effects of Central Acting Drugs**

Volume 56
**Cardiac Glycosides**

Part 1
**Experimental Pharmacology**

Part 2
**Pharmacokinetics and Clinical Pharmacology**

Volume 57
**Tissue Growth Factors**

Volume 58
**Cyclic Nucleotides**

Part 1: **Biochemistry**

Part 2: **Physiology and Pharmacology**

Volume 59:
**Mediators and Drugs in Gastrointestinal Motility**

Part 1: **Morphological Basis and Neurophysiological Control**

Part 2: **Endogenous and Exogenous Agents**

Volume 60
**Pyretics and Antipyretics**

Volume 61
**Chemotherapy of Viral Infections**

Volume 62
**Aminoglycoside Antibiotics**

Volume 64
**Inhibition of Folate Metabolism in Chemotherapy**

Volume 65
**Teratogenesis and Reproductive Toxicology**

Volume 66
Part 1: **Glucagon I**
Part 2: **Glucagon II**

Volume 67
Part 1
**Antibiotics Containing the Beta-Lactam Structure I**

Part 2
**Antibiotics Containing the Beta-Lactam Structure II**

GPSR Compliance

*The European Union's (EU) General Product Safety Regulation (GPSR) is a set of rules that requires consumer products to be safe and our obligations to ensure this.*

*If you have any concerns about our products, you can contact us on ProductSafety@springernature.com*

In case Publisher is established outside the EU, the EU authorized representative is:

Springer Nature Customer Service Center GmbH
Europaplatz 3
69115 Heidelberg, Germany

Batch number: 10838062

Printed by Printforce, the Netherlands